We are grateful first and foremost to the families that have entrusted us with the care of their children. We acknowledge with grateful humility their trust in our ability, though occasionally limited, to heal.

The constant patience, support, understanding and love of my family, especially my wife Susan, and our children, Robin, Katie and Scott, through all of my academic pediatric life, no matter how trying at times, is what makes it all worth it.

ANTHONY J. ALARIO, MD

For Dr. Diana Lidofsky – your guidance and support are so much more appreciated than words can relate. I want to thank you for always being there with kindness, generosity, and patience. As with many things in my life, this book is an example of the difference you have made.

For Mom and Mitch, my parents, who have supported me always. I have so much to thank you for. And for my Aunt Natasha, whose creativity and personality are always there. I've learned so much from you and just wanted to thank you. I also want to thank my Aunt Ruth for her artistry in life.

For Andrea, whose friendship, support, guidance, and love are always appreciated, this book would not have been finished without your help. For Sonia, a sister I never had, a colleague I value, a friend I cherish, for your brilliant mind; you have helped me through so many of life's challenges, including this book. For Michelle and Kambis, two of the best people I know, your friendship has meant the world to me — Darius and Jackson are very lucky to have you both. For both Joes, whose friendship I appreciate, whose technically analytic and creative minds I admire, and whose work ethic is a model I take with me always, especially while completing this book. For Ellen, who I miss. For Jenny, who has made a huge difference in a short time. And of course, for Albert and Jackson (and Sax), the dogs in my life, the joy in my life.

JONATHAN D. BIRNKRANT, MD

Contributors

Dianne N. Abuelo, MD
Associate Professor, Department of Pediatrics, The Warren Alpert
  Medical School of Brown University
Director, Genetic Counseling Center, Rhode Island Hospital
Providence, Rhode Island
Dysmorphology and Common Syndromes

Anthony J. Alario, MD
Professor of Pediatrics, The Warren Alpert Medical School of
  Brown University
Director, Academic General Pediatrics, Hasbro Children's Hospital
Providence, Rhode Island
*Approach to the Pediatric Patient, Routine Health Maintenance and Preventive
Medicine, Differential Diagnoses, Renal Disorders, Fluids and Electrolytes,
Acid-Base Disturbances, Rheumatic Disorders, Pulmonary and Allergic
Diseases, Infectious Diseases*

Christine Barron, MD
Assistant Professor of Pediatrics, The Warren Alpert Medical School of
  Brown University
Clinical Director, Child Protection Program, Hasbro Children's Hospital
Providence, Rhode Island
Child Maltreatment

Jeffrey M. Becker, MD
Staff Urologist, Lourdes Medical Center of Burlington County,
  Willingboro, New Jersey
Staff Urologist, Virtua Hospital of Burlington County, Mount Holly,
  New Jersey
Staff Urologist, Mid Atlantic Stone Center, Marlton, New Jersey
Urologic Conditions

Sulaiman Bharwani, MD, FAAP, FRCP(C), FACG
Associate Professor of Pediatrics, University of Western Ontario
Section Chief, Pediatric Gastroenterology, Children's Hospital of Western
  Ontario, and Associate Professor of Pathology, London Health
  Sciences Centre
Pediatric Gastrointestinal Consultant, St. Joseph's Hospital
London, Ontario, Canada
Gastrointestinal Disorders

Jo-Ann Blaymore Bier, MD
Assistant Professor of Pediatrics, Harvard Medical School
Attending Developmental Pediatrician, Complex Care Services,
    Department of Medicine, Children's Hospital Boston
Boston, Massachusetts
Developmental Disabilities

Jonathan D. Birnkrant, MD
Attending Physician, Pediatrics, Child and Adolescent Psychiatry,
    Adult Psychiatry, New Hampshire
Differential Diagnoses, Behavioral and Psychiatric Disorders of Childhood

Bradley J. Bloom, MD
Translational Medicine Lead, Inflammation Therapeutic Area, Pfizer
    Global Research and Development, New London, Connecticut
Rheumatic Disorders

Anthony A. Caldamone, MD, MMS, FAAP, FACS
Professor of Surgery (Urology) and Pediatrics, The Warren Alpert
    Medical School of Brown University
Director of Pediatric Urology, Hasbro Children's Hospital
Providence, Rhode Island
Urologic Conditions

Andrea R. Carlsen, MD
Private Practice, Child and Adolescent Psychiatry
    Cold Spring Harbor, New York
Voluntary Staff, Department of Psychiatry, North Shore-Long Island
    Jewish Health System, Great Neck, New York
Behavioral and Psychiatric Disorders of Childhood

William J. Cashore, MD
Professor of Pediatrics, The Warren Alpert Medical School of
    Brown University
Associate Chief, Department of Pediatrics, Women & Infants Hospital
Attending Pediatrician, Hasbro Children's Hospital
Providence, Rhode Island
The Newborn Infant

Thomas H. Chun, MD
Assistant Professor, Division of Pediatric Emergency Medicine,
    The Warren Alpert Medical School of Brown University
Attending Physician, Emergency Department, Hasbro Children's Hospital
Providence, Rhode Island
General Approach to Trauma

Steven T. Cobery, MD, MC, USN
Chief Resident and Clinical Instructor, Department of Neurosurgery,
    The Warren Alpert Medical School of Brown University, and
    Rhode Island Hospital
Providence, Rhode Island
Surgical Conditions in Infants and Children

Monika Upadhye Curlin, MD
Staff Dermatologist, Kaiser Permanente
Fontana, California
Pediatric Dermatology

Idris Dahod, MD
Clinical Associate, Department of Pediatrics, University of Massachusetts
Pediatric Gastroenterologist, Department of Pediatrics, St. Vincent Hospital
Worcester, Massachusetts
Gastrointestinal Disorders

Manuel F. DaSilva, MD
Clinical Assistant Professor, Department of Orthopedic Surgery,
    The Warren Alpert Medical School of Brown University
Orthopedic Surgeon, Rhode Island Hospital and the Miriam Hospital
Providence, Rhode Island
Orthopedic Conditions

Christopher DiGiovanni, MD
Associate Professor and Chief, Division of Foot and Ankle Surgery,
    Department of Orthopedic Surgery, The Warren Alpert Medical School
    of Brown University and Rhode Island Hospital,
Providence, Rhode Island
Orthopedic Conditions

Craig P. Eberson, MD
Assistant Professor, Department of Pediatric Orthopaedics, The Warren
    Alpert Medical School of Brown University
Director, Pediatric Spine Service, Department of Pediatric Orthopaedics,
    Hasbro Children's Hospital
Providence, Rhode Island
Orthopedic Conditions

Michael G. Ehrlich, MD
Vincent Zecchino Professor and Chairman, Department of Orthopedics,
    The Warren Alpert Medical School of Brown University
Surgeon-in-Chief, Department of Orthopedics, Rhode Island Hospital
Providence, Rhode Island
Orthopedic Conditions

M. Khurram Faizan, MD
Assistant Clinical Professor of Pediatrics, Division of Pediatric Nephrology,
    The Warren Alpert Medical School of Brown University
Director, Division of Pediatric Nephrology, Hasbro Children's Hospital
Providence, Rhode Island
Renal Disorders

Lloyd R. Feit, MD
Associate Professor of Pediatrics, The Warren Alpert Medical School of
   Brown University
Attending Cardiologist, Department of Pediatrics, Hasbro Children's
   Hospital
Providence, Rhode Island
Cardiovascular Disorders

Fred F. Ferri, MD, FACP
Clinical Professor, The Warren Alpert Medical School of Brown
   University, Providence, Rhode Island
Acid-Base Disturbances

Patricia Flanagan, MD
Associate Professor of Pediatrics, Division of Adolescent Medicine,
   The Warren Alpert Medical School of Brown University
Director, Teens with Tots Program, Department of Pediatrics, and
   Medical Director, Outpatient Services, Hasbro Children's Hospital
Providence, Rhode Island
Adolescent Medicine

Edwin N. Forman, MD
Alan G. Hassenfeld Professor of Pediatrics, The Warren Alpert Medical
   School of Brown University
Associate, Pediatric Hematology/Oncology, Hasbro Children's Hospital
Consultant in Neonatology, Women & Infants Hospital
Providence, Rhode Island
Hematologic/Oncologic Disorders

Aris C. Garro, MD, MPH
Assistant Professor, Division of Pediatric Emergency Medicine,
   The Warren Alpert Medical School of Brown University
Attending Physician, Emergency Department, Hasbro Children's Hospital
Providence, Rhode Island
General Approach to Trauma

Natalia Golova, MD
Clinical Assistant Professor of Pediatrics, The Warren Alpert Medical
   School of Brown University
Fellow of the AAP, Assistant Professor of Pediatrics, Division of
   Academic General Pediatrics, Hasbro Children's Hospital
Providence, Rhode Island
*Approach to the Pediatric Patient, Routine Health Maintenance and
   Preventive Medicine, Renal Disorders, Behavioral and Psychiatric Disorders
   of Childhood*

Philip A. Gruppuso, MD
Professor of Pediatrics, The Warren Alpert Medical School of
    Brown University
Staff Physician, Department of Pediatrics, Rhode Island Hospital
Providence, Rhode Island
Endocrinologic Disorders

Zeev Harel, MD
Associate Professor of Pediatrics, The Warren Alpert Medical School of
    Brown University
Attending Physician and Director of Research and Training, Division of
    Adolescent Medicine, Hasbro Children's Hospital
Providence, Rhode Island
Adolescent Medicine

Horacio B. Hojman, MD
Clinical Assistant Professor, Department of Psychiatry and Human
    Behavior, The Warren Alpert Medical School of Brown University
Staff Psychiatrist, Department of Child and Family Psychiatry, Rhode
    Island Hospital
Providence, Rhode Island
Behavioral and Psychiatric Disorders of Childhood

Hannah M. Huddleston, MD
Resident, Department of Surgery, The Warren Alpert Medical School of
    Brown University, Providence, Rhode Island
Surgical Conditions in Infants and Children

Christopher Paul Keuker, MD
Assistant Professor of Pediatrics, Division of Pediatric Hematology/
    Oncology, University of Massachusetts Medical School
Attending Physician, UMass Memorial Medical Center
Worcester, Massachusetts
Hematologic/Oncologic Disorders

Robert B. Klein, MD
Professor and Vice Chair, Department of Pediatrics, The Warren Alpert
    Medical School of Brown University
Director, Asthma and Allergy Center, Department of Pediatrics,
and Associate Pediatrician-in-Chief, Hasbro Children's Hospital
Providence, Rhode Island
Pulmonary and Allergic Diseases

Chandan N. Lakhiani, MD, FAAP
Clinical Assistant Professor of Pediatrics, The Warren Alpert Medical
    School of Brown University
Faculty, Division of Academic General Pediatrics, Hasbro Children's
    Hospital
Providence, Rhode Island
Gastrointestinal Disorders

Barry M. Lester, PhD
Professor of Psychiatry and Human Behavior, and Professor of Pediatrics,
   The Warren Alpert Medical School of Brown University
Director, Brown Center for the Study of Children at Risk,
   Women & Infants Hospital of Rhode Island
Providence, Rhode Island
Behavioral and Psychiatric Disorders of Childhood

William J. Lewander, MD
Professor of Emergency Medicine and Pediatrics, The Warren Alpert
   Medical School of Brown University
Director of Pediatric Emergency Medicine, Hasbro Children's Hospital
Toxicologic Emergencies

Gregory R. Lockhart, MD
Associate Professor (Clinical) of Emergency Medicine and Pediatrics,
   The Warren Alpert Medical School of Brown University
Attending Physician, Emergency Department, Hasbro Children's Hospital
Providence, Rhode Island
Toxicologic Emergencies

Maya Liza C. Lopez, MD
Clinical Instructor of Pediatrics, University of Arkansas Medical Sciences
Faculty, Department of Developmental and Behavioral Pediatrics,
   Arkansas Children's Hospital
Little Rock, Arkansas
Developmental Disabilities

Emily C. Lutterloh, MD
Attending Physician, Pediatric Infectious Diseases, Rhode Island Hospital
Providence, Rhode Island
Infectious Diseases

Shelly D. Martin, MD
Assistant Professor of Pediatrics, Uniformed Services University of the
   Health Sciences, Bethesda, Maryland
Staff Physician, Department of Pediatrics, National Naval Medical Center,
   Bethesda, Maryland
Staff Physician, Department of Pediatrics, Walter Reed Army Medical
   Center, Washington, District of Columbia
Child Maltreatment

Kelly L. Matson, PharmD
Clinical Assistant Professor, Department of Pharmacy Practice,
   University of Rhode Island, Kingston, Rhode Island
Pediatric Clinical Pharmacist, Hasbro Children's Hospital,
   Providence, Rhode Island
Infectious Diseases

Rebecca R. McEachern, MD
Assistant Professor of Pediatrics, The Warren Alpert Medical School of
    Brown University
Attending Physician, Division of Pediatric Endocrinology and
    Metabolism, Hasbro Children's Hospital
Providence, Rhode Island
Endocrinologic Disorders

Cynthia H. Meyers-Seifer, MD
Clinical Associate Professor of Pediatrics, University of Medicine and
    Dentistry of New Jersey, Robert Wood Johnson Medical School,
    New Brunswick, New Jersey
Co-Director, Pediatric Endocrinology, Jersey Shore University
    Medical Center, Neptune, New Jersey
Endocrinologic Disorders

Shelley D. Miyamoto, MD
Instructor of Pediatrics, University of Colorado at Denver and
    Health Sciences Center
Director, Heart Failure and Cardiomyopathy Program,
    The Children's Hospital
Denver, Colorado
Cardiovascular Disorders

Jennie J. Muglia, MD
Associate Professor (Clinical) of Dermatology, The Warren Alpert Medical
    School of Brown University
Director, Pediatric Dermatology Clinic, Hasbro Children's Hospital
Providence, Rhode Island
Pediatric Dermatology

Stephen K. Obaro, MD, FRCPCH, PhD
Associate Professor of Pediatrics, Department of Pediatrics and Human
    Development, College of Human Medicine, Michigan State University,
    East Lansing, Michigan
Infectious Diseases

Judith A. Owens, MD, MPH
Associate Professor of Pediatrics, The Warren Alpert Medical School of
    Brown University
Attending Physician, Department of Pediatrics, Hasbro Children's Hospital
Providence, Rhode Island
Behavioral and Psychiatric Disorders of Childhood

Sonia Partap, MD
Instructor, Department of Neurology, Stanford University,
    Lucille Packard Children's Hospital, Stanford, California
Formerly: Child Neurology Resident, University of Washington School of
    Medicine, and Children's Hospital and Regional Medical Center,
    Seattle, Washington
Neurologic Disorders

David Pugatch, MD
Associate Professor of Pediatrics, The Warren Alpert Medical School of
    Brown University
Attending Physician, Department of Pediatric Infectious Diseases,
    Hasbro Children's Hospital
Providence, Rhode Island
Infectious Diseases

Randal C. Richardson, MD, MMS
Chief Resident, Division of Pediatric Neurology, University of Washington
    School of Medicine, and Children's Hospital and Regional Medical
    Center, Seattle, Washington
Neurologic Disorders

Suzanne Riggs, MD
Professor of Pediatrics, The Warren Alpert Medical School of
    Brown University
Director, Division of Adolescent Medicine, Rhode Island Hospital
Providence, Rhode Island
Adolescent Medicine

Randy Rockney, MD
Associate Professor of Pediatrics and Family Medicine, The Warren
    Alpert Medical School of Brown University
Director, Undergraduate Medical Education in Pediatrics, Hasbro
    Children's Hospital
Providence, Rhode Island
Behavioral and Psychiatric Disorders of Childhood

Albert M. Ross IV, MD
Clinical Assistant Professor of Pediatrics, The Warren Alpert Medical
    School of Brown University
Director of Pediatric Endoscopy, Department of Pediatric Gastroenterology,
    Hasbro Children's Hospital
Providence, Rhode Island
Gastrointestinal Disorders

Michael S. Schechter, MD, MPH
Associate Professor of Pediatrics, Emery University School of Medicine
Atlanta, Georgia
Pulmonary and Allergic Diseases

Thomas F. Tracy, Jr., MD
Vice Chairman, Professor of Surgery and Pediatrics, The Warren Alpert
    Medical School of Brown University
Pediatric Surgeon-in-Chief, Division of Pediatric Surgery, Hasbro
    Children's Hospital
Providence, Rhode Island
Surgical Conditions in Infants and Children

Robert O. Wright, MD, MPH
Assistant Professor of Pediatrics and Environmental Health, Staff
Toxicologist, Rhode Island/Massachusetts Poison Control System,
    Harvard Medical School
Department of Pediatrics, Division of Emergency Medicine, Children's
    Hospital Boston
Boston, Massachusetts
Toxicologic Emergencies

Ali Yalcindag, MD
Assistant Professor of Pediatrics, The Warren Alpert Medical School of
    Brown University
Attending Physician, Department of Pediatric Rheumatology, Hasbro
    Children's Hospital
Providence, Rhode Island
Rheumatic Disorders

Priya Swamy Zeikus, MD
Assistant Professor, Department of Dermatology, University of Texas—
    Southwestern, Dallas, Texas
Private practice in dermatology, Sherman, Texas
Pediatric Dermatology

Preface

The first edition to this manual in 1997 emphasized the benefits of a "peripheral brain" because of rapidly evolving medical knowledge. What was true in 1997 is especially true with this second edition. We have tried to update this edition with new knowledge in pathophysiology as well as updating both the detailed and practical aspects of caring for children.

The second edition continues to provide the important and basic foundations, emphasizing a structured approach to pediatric primary care, routine health maintenance, and screening. The practical aspects of the clinical evaluation (history/examination), diagnosis, and treatment for a variety of the most commonly encountered pediatric conditions have been revised and enhanced. Whenever possible, the most recent, state-of-the-art, evidence-based information available is provided to the reader.

There is a new and expanded section on differential diagnoses; color photographic representation of common rashes in the chapter on pediatric dermatology; updates in the management of complex disorders such as cystic fibrosis and seizure disorders; latest guidelines on prescription of contraceptive drugs; as well as an update on behavioral and psychiatric disorders in childhood, with particular reference to attention deficit hyperactivity disorder, depression and bipolar disorders, and pediatric psychopharmacology. The prudent reader, however, understands that for any pediatric condition there is no substitute for genuine caring, thoughtful clinical judgment, and careful patient follow-up.

The authors hope that students of pediatrics at all levels, from medical, nursing, and paramedical schools, through pediatric and family medicine residents, to the wizened and veteran clinician, will continue to find this manual, particularly this edition, a helpful guide in the practical care of the pediatric patient. We continue to seek feedback from readers, and it is gratefully accepted to promote our own growth and development.

Anthony J. Alario, MD
Jonathan D. Birnkrant, MD

Acknowledgments

We would like to acknowledge all of our academic colleagues who have contributed to this manual, our mentors in various stages of our intellectual and human development. In particular, we would like to thank the residents of the Program in Pediatrics at Rhode Island Hospital/Hasbro Children's Hospital for their advice and guidance. We are also deeply indebted to our student editor, Dr. Stewart Mackie, currently an intern in Pediatrics, as well as Dr. Stephen Flynn, currently a second year resident at Children's Hospital in Philadelphia and a former Brown University medical student, both of whom were especially helpful in directing us toward what was important for the medical student reader. We would also like to thank our editors at Elsevier Publications, Jim Merritt, Andrea Vosburgh, and Joan Nikelsky for their perseverance, openness, detailed observations, and helpful direction. Finally, Judith daSilva, the administrative assistant in the Division of Academic General Pediatrics at Hasbro Children's Hospital, has been a driving force not only in manuscript preparation but also in the organization, design, and quality control of this manual. Without her efficiency and organizational abilities, this manual would still be on the drawing table. All of the people mentioned above had significant roles to play in the presentation and production of the manual you now hold in your hands, and for all their hard work, we are extremely grateful.

Contents

20. Neurologic Disorders, 612
Sonia Partap and Randal C. Richardson

21. Developmental Disabilities, 641
Maya Liza C. Lopez and Jo-Ann Blaymore Bier

22. Behavioral and Psychiatric Disorders of Childhood, 660
Andrea R. Carlsen, Jonathan D. Birnkrant, Judith A. Owens, Randy Rockney, Natalia Golova, Horacio B. Hojman, and Barry M. Lester

23. Surgical Conditions in Infants and Children, 732

Hannah M. Huddleston, Thomas F. Tracy, Jr., and Steven T. Cobery

24. Toxicologic Emergencies, 749

Robert O. Wright, Gregory R. Lockhart, and William J. Lewander

Approach to the Pediatric Patient: Gathering Data and Communicating Information

1

Natalia Golova and Anthony J. Alario

1.1 The Pediatric History

BASIC PRINCIPLES AND HELPFUL HINTS

1. Careful history taking can delineate the nature of most pediatric problems and assist in developing differential diagnoses and plans of management.
2. Identify yourself to make the child and caregivers comfortable and reassured; use language they can understand; take a moment to interact with the child in a friendly, nonthreatening way.
3. Be flexible—you may need to ask a question in several different ways.
4. With an acute problem or a hospitalized patient, begin at the beginning of the problem, then go back in time.
5. If appropriate, ask the child to provide information. Adolescents should be interviewed alone, their confidentiality respected.

COMPONENTS OF THE PEDIATRIC HISTORY

Depending on the age of the child and the nature of the visit, several of the following components of the history may be altered, combined, or eliminated (Box 1-1). (The routine well-child visit is detailed in Chapter 2.)

1. Chief complaint/reason for visit: a brief account of the present illness or the reason for the visit
2. History of present illness
   a. When was patient entirely well before this condition?
   b. When, where, and how did illness begin? Specify symptoms/signs.
   c. What is the duration of present symptoms? Determine order, onset, and date of new or changing symptoms.
   d. What factors or medications aggravate/alleviate symptoms?
3. Review of systems: See Chapter 3 for positive findings in review of systems
   a. General: Overall health, unusual weight loss or gain, personality or behavioral changes, fatigue, other (e.g., diabetes may be suspected with history of excessive thirst, weight loss, and bedwetting)
   b. Skin: Color changes, rashes, bruising, lumps/bumps, nail/hair changes
   c. Eyes: Visual problems, increase or decrease in tearing (e.g., recurrent pink eye may suggest uveitis)

1

Box 1-1   Basic Components of the Pediatric History

- Chief complaint/reason for visit
- History of present illness
- Review of systems
- Past and ancillary history
  - Pregnancy, labor delivery
  - Post natal/infancy history
  - Significant past illness
  - Hospitalizations
  - Operations
  - Accident/poisoning/injuries
- Current status
  - Immunizations
  - Allergies/allergic reactions
  - Medications
  - Nutrition
  - Elimination
  - Developmental/personal history
  - Social history
  - Habits
- Family history

---

   d. Ears, nose, throat: Frequency of colds, pharyngitis, otitis, hearing loss, tinnitus, nasal discharge, mouth breathing (e.g., snoring and/or periodic breathing may suggest obstructive sleep apnea)

   e. Lungs: Cough, dyspnea/shortness of breath, wheezing, heavy breathing, chest tightness, breathlessness (e.g., nocturnal cough may suggest asthma)

   f. Cardiovascular: Chest pain, previous murmur, syncope, tachycardia

   g. Gastrointestinal: Difficulty swallowing, nausea/vomiting, diarrhea, recurrent abdominal pain, spitting up/reflux, constipation, blood/mucus in stools

   h. Genitourinary: Dysuria, frequency, hematuria, polyuria, vaginal discharge, prior sexually transmitted diseases (STDs) or pregnancy/fathering a child

   i. Musculoskeletal: Weakness, joint swelling, morning stiffness, abnormality of gait, scoliosis, back pain (e.g., excessive bone pain in one area may suggest malignancy)

   j. Neurologic: Headache, double vision, previous seizures, ataxia, tics, dizziness

   k. Endocrine: Difficulty with growth, polyphagia, excessive thirst/fluid intake, goiter, age of onset of puberty/menarche, quality of menses (duration, amount of flow, number of pads/tampons used)

4. Past and ancillary history

   a. Pregnancy, labor, delivery

     (1) Health of mother, prenatal care, significant complications or infections (prenatal laboratory tests such as rapid plasma reagin,

hepatitis B, rubella, herpes, human immunodeficiency virus [HIV]), medication
   (2) Type of delivery (vaginal vs. cesarean section)
   (3) Birth weight, health of infant, Apgar scores, complications (e.g., infection, jaundice), length of hospital stay
 b. Postnatal/infancy
   (1) Immediate period: Congenital problems (neurologic, musculo-skeletal, cardiac)
   (2) Infancy: Nutrition (type of feedings), developmental problems, chronic medical conditions
 c. Illnesses: Significant childhood illnesses/infections
 d. Hospitalizations
 e. Operations: Type, age, complications
 f. Accidents/poisonings/injuries: Age, nature, severity, complications
5. Current status (some of the following are age dependent)
 a. Immunizations: Specify dates and special tests (e.g., tuberculosis, lead, sickle screen)
 b. Allergies: To medication or food and note type of reaction (e.g., hives)
 c. Medications: All current medications and herbal remedies as well as past medications related to the problem
 d. Nutrition
   (1) Infant: Type of feedings (bottle vs. breast), amount taken each feed (volume vs. time for breast-feed), age of introduction of solids, appetite and any changes in appetite or feeding habits, vitamin supplementation
   (2) Older child: Overall diet, personal eating habits (especially binge, purge, anorexic behavior), unusual family dietary habits (e.g., vegetarian, vegan)
 e. Elimination
   (1) Toilet training: Age of onset
   (2) Daily habits: Difficulties (there will always be some!)
   (3) Incontinence: Bladder or bowel—day versus night
 f. Developmental/personal history
   (1) Landmarks: Age of attainment of developmental milestones (see Chapter 2)—any delay/acceleration, growth or failure to grow
   (2) Psychosocial: Adjustment to new environments, comfort in social situations, relationships with siblings, peers, and adults
   (3) School: School readiness (e.g., toilet trained, attained age-appropriate developmental milestones), grade and performance, behavior problems
 g. Social history
   (1) Family framework: Adults/children living in home, relationship to child/each other
   (2) Household framework: Living conditions, sleeping arrangements, support systems
   (3) Environment: Type of neighborhood, violence, safety
   (4) Child care arrangements: Stay at home parent versus day care and type (relative, neighbor vs. day care center)
   (5) Insurance status: Health coverage
   (6) Child's physician/source of health care: Frequency of visits. Was he/she notified of this visit/hospitalization?

h. Habits
   (1) Sleeping: Number of hours, frequent night wakenings, snoring, bedtime routine
   (2) Recreation: Play, exercise, competitiveness
   (3) Behavioral: Thumb sucking, temper tantrums, tics, breath-holding, masturbation, anxiety, methods of discipline, amount of television watching and quality of programs
   (4) Adolescent habits: Substance use (tobacco, alcohol, illicit drugs), risk taking, sexual activity, STD/HIV knowledge, gang involvement, peer activities, future goals/education
   (5) Dental hygiene: Brushing, flossing, fluoride, frequency of dentist visits
   (6) Safety inventory: Automobile child restraints, smoke detectors, bicycle helmets, weapons secured with locks/in safe, poison control, avoidance of strangers
   (7) Family habits: Smoking, alcohol use, recreational interests
6. Family history: Age and health status of immediate family members and for two generations, with special attention to childhood illnesses. Major conditions such as diabetes, seizures, asthma, atopy, renal or gastrointestinal disease, anemia, mental illness, cardiovascular disease (especially in adults ≤55 years of age). Any hereditary or congenital familial conditions should be recorded.

1.2 Physical Examination

BASIC PRINCIPLES AND HELPFUL HINTS

1. Approach the child with respect and gentleness; gain the child's confidence through play.
2. Warm and wash hands (and instruments) and make friends.
3. Try to be at eye level with the child during the examination (e.g., examine the child in the caretaker's lap as you sit across from him/her).
4. Examine the child undressed but respect his/her modesty.
5. Perform the least-tolerated, most anxiety-producing procedures last, such as the ear and throat examination (if a tongue depressor must be used, moistening it with warm water will decrease gagging), genital examination in adolescents, rectal examination in anyone.
6. Become familiar with normal physical development; age-related ranges of normal and abnormal findings.
7. Proceed in a slow, deliberate manner. Be ready to hear the heart or lung sounds of a crying child the moment a breath is taken. Palpate the abdomen when there is transient relaxation after leaving your hands on the belly for several seconds (or with infant, giving a pacifier/gloved finger to suck will relax the abdominal muscles).

COMPONENTS OF THE PHYSICAL EXAMINATION

1. Observation
   a. Significant clinical information may be gained when first encountering the patient by observing the following:
      (1) The child's facial expressions (pain), eye contact, and response to play or social overtures (e.g., lack of response may mean serious bacterial illness)

      (2) Rate, depth, and rhythm of respirations (e.g., rapid, shallow respirations may mean pneumonia or acidosis vs. deep indrawing of chest wall, and the prolonged expiration seen in asthma)

      (3) Body posture and movements (e.g., guarding of a joint or extremity may mean arthritis, trauma, or infection)

      (4) Interaction with caretakers and examiner (e.g., a child who is overly cautious or solicitous during the genital examination may have been abused)

  b. Three key features to observe in a child: "Position, cry, eyes"

    (1) Position of child

      (a) Head deviation to one side: Congenital torticollis or acute torticollis (cervical adenitis), myositis, central nervous system (CNS) tumors, dislocated cervical vertebrae (trauma, arthritis, osteomyelitis, atlanto-occipital dislocation), ocular disease

      (b) Leaning forward in sitting position: Respiratory distress, asthma, upper airway obstruction, foreign body, epiglottitis, pericarditis

      (c) Head and back arched (opisthotonos): CNS infection, tumor, or an adverse (dystonic) reaction to phenothiazines

      (d) Lying on left side with leg flexed at hip and knee: Appendicitis

      (e) Lying on back with leg externally rotated and hip abducted with knee flexes: Septic arthritis/osteomyelitis of hip

    (2) Cry

      (a) Weak: Serious illness

      (b) High-pitched: Increased intracranial pressure

      (c) Infrequent: Hypothyroidism, drug sedation

      (d) Excessive: Colic, anxiety

      (e) Moaning: Serious illness, meningitis

      (f) Grunting: Respiratory distress, cardiac disease, hyperthermia, severe dehydration

    (3) Eyes

      (a) Sunken: Dehydration

      (b) Glossy or distant stare: Serious illness, increased intracranial pressure

      (c) Apprehensive expression: Impending respiratory failure, maltreatment

  c. For an overall impression of the patient that will be communicated to colleagues, ask yourself the following questions: Is the child

    (1) Well or acutely ill/toxic? Chronically ill, wasted, or malnourished?

    (2) Alert, active, or lethargic/fatigued?

    (3) Cooperative or combative/confused?

    (4) Pink, cyanotic, or pale?

    (5) Well hydrated or dehydrated?

    (6) Are there any unusual body odors? For example: Acetone smell, think diabetic ketoacidosis; foul odor, think foreign body; musty/"mousy," think phenylketonuria.

2. Measurements

  a. Vital signs: Temperature, pulse, respiratory rate, blood pressure—compared with standardized norms (see Appendix I).

b. Height and weight in all children, and head circumference in children ≤2 years of age: Plot and calculate body mass index on appropriate growth charts (see Appendix II). Comparison of multiple measurements made over a period of time will yield the most useful information.

3. Skin: Color (cyanosis, jaundice, pallor, erythema), texture, eruptions, hydration, edema, bruises, scars, hemangiomas, café au lait spots, pigmentation, elasticity, subcutaneous nodules, hair distribution, desquamation, capillary refill

a. Jaundice—visually evident once serum bilirubin is >5 mg/dL (first on sclera). Progresses downward with higher levels.

b. Dermal melanoses (also called *Mongolian spots*) are large, flat, black or blue-black areas seen in young children. They are frequently present over the lower back and buttocks but may also occur on upper back and shoulders. They are of no pathologic significance and fade over 5 to 6 years. Occasionally, they are mistaken for signs of child abuse by the inexperienced eye.

c. Cyanosis will not be visually evident unless at least 5 g/dL of reduced hemoglobin is present. Cyanosis may not be a reliable indicator of hypoxia; for example, if anemic, the patient may be hypoxic before cyanosis develops. Conversely, in polycythemia, the patient may appear cyanotic and not be hypoxic.

d. Infants who eat a large amount of yellow/orange vegetables will develop carotenemia, a yellow-orange "glow" to their skin, usually most prominent over the palms and soles and around the nose.

e. Rashes on dark-skinned children are difficult to see (e.g., the "sandpaper" rash of scarlet fever needs to be felt).

4. Lymph nodes: Location, size, sensitivity, mobility, consistency

a. Palpable lymph nodes, especially of cervical and inguinal chains, are common in normal children.

b. Mobile, nontender "shotty" nodes are commonly found during or after infection.

c. Supraclavicular, scalene, axillary, or epitrochlear nodes may be pathologic (e.g., infection/malignancy) and should be further investigated.

5. Head: Size, shape, circumference, asymmetry, cephalhematoma, bossing, craniotabes, head control, molding, bruits, fontanelles (size, tension, number, abnormally late or early closure), sutures, dilated veins, facial asymmetry, hair distribution

a. The head is measured at its greatest circumference (forehead to just above ears).

b. Fontanelle tension is best determined with the child quiet and in the sitting position.

c. The anterior fontanelle should be closed by 18 months. It may have slight pulsations.

d. The posterior fontanelle closes by the first month (it remains open in hypothyroidism).

e. Craniotabes (a "ping-pong ball" give to the skull when pressure is applied with a finger) may be found in normal newborn infants (especially premature infants) and for the first 2 to 3 months of life; afterward such a response is abnormal (e.g., hypothyroidism).

6. Eyes: Pupillary size, shape, and reaction to light including accommodation; muscular control and conjugate gaze; nystagmus; Mongolian slant; Brushfield's spots; epicanthic folds; lacrimation; discharge; lids; exophthalmos; conjunctiva; color of iris; corneal opacities/cataracts; fundi; photophobia; visual acuity; visual fields (in older children)
   a. Unequal pupil size may be normal.
   b. Strabismus (eye deviation) may be present intermittently during the first 6 months of life but after that time should be considered abnormal.
   c. Lack of a red reflex may indicate cataracts or retinoblastoma.
   d. Sclera: Newborns may have a bluish tinge because of a thin sclera, or a blue sclera may signify osteogenesis imperfecta or Ehlers-Danlos syndrome; black children may normally have a "muddy" color.
   e. Pseudostrabismus: Secondary to epicanthal folds and position of each fissure, tested by the following:
      (1) Light shone into eyes—reflection of beam falls symmetrically on each pupil with pseudostrabismus (i.e., normal eyes).
      (2) Cover test for older, cooperative children (see Chapter 2).
   f. Evaluation of vision (see Chapter 2): Does the infant see? Infant's blinking in response to a strong light indicates light perception. An infant who cannot see displays a constant searching movement of the eyes. Spinning an infant will produce nystagmus, which stops in 15 to 30 seconds as the infant fixes gaze, suggesting an intact visual axis.
7. Nose: Shape, septal integrity, mucosa, patency, discharge, bleeding, pressure over sinuses, flaring of nostrils (may indicate respiratory distress from pneumonia or even sepsis or severe illness)
   a. A crease over the nasal bridge suggests chronic (allergic) rhinitis (allergic salute).
   b. Chronic unilateral discharge with foul odor indicates a foreign body.
   c. Recurrent, difficult-to-control nosebleeds suggest a hemoglobinopathy or blood dyscrasia. Most common reason for nose bleed is picking!
8. Mouth: Lips (thinness, downturning, fissures, color, cleft), teeth (number, position, caries, mottling, discoloration, notching, malocclusion or malalignment) timing of tooth eruptions (see Appendix IV), mucosa (color, appearance of Stensen's duct, enanthems), gums, palate (Epstein's pearls are small white cysts on palate and are a normal variant), tongue (geographic is usually normal), uvula
   a. If the tongue can be extended as far as the alveolar ridge, there should be no interference with nursing or speaking.
   b. Gum hemorrhage may be a sign of bacteremia in an infant or leukemia in older children.
   c. Mental retardation is sometimes associated with a high arched palate.
9. Throat: Tonsils (size, inflammation, exudate, crypts, inflammation of the anterior pillars), hypertrophic lymphoid tissue, postnasal drip, voice (hoarseness, stridor, grunting, type of cry, speech)
   a. To make examining the mouth and throat easier, have the child "pant like a puppy" with the tongue blade moistened with warm water to reduce gagging.

   b. Young children seldom complain of sore throat even in the presence of significant infection of the pharynx and tonsils.

   c. Always examine the throat of a child with abdominal pain, especially if pain is on the right side (streptococcal pharyngitis may cause abdominal pain similar to appendicitis because of lymphoid tenderness in right lower quadrant). Epigastric pain and headache are also commonly associated with streptococcal pharyngitis.

10. Ears: Pinnas (position, size), canals, tympanic membranes (landmarks, mobility, perforation, inflammation, discharge), mastoid tenderness and swelling, hearing assessment.

   a. Hearing tests are an important part of the physical examination of every infant and child (see Chapter 2).

   b. Pneumatic insufflation to test mobility of the tympanic membrane should always be part of the examination. Gentle pressure on bulb is sufficient.

   c. Low-set ears are present in a number of congenital syndromes, including several associated with mental retardation. The ears may be considered low set if they are below a line drawn from the lateral angle of the eye to the external occipital protuberance.

   d. Congenital anomalies of the urinary tract are frequently associated with abnormalities of the pinnas (e.g., ear tags).

   e. To examine the ears of an infant, it is usually necessary ro pull the auricle backward and upward or down and forward.

   f. Bilateral erythema of the eardrum is normal with crying and blanches with insufflation.

   g. Shortening of the light reflex, erythema of the pars flaccida, and change in the normal 90-degree angle made by the manubrium of the malleus and the light reflex can be seen early in otitis media (see Fig. 1-1 for landmarks).

11. Neck: Position (torticollis, opisthotonos, inability to support head, mobility), swelling, thyroid (size, contour, isthmus, nodules, tenderness), lymph nodes, veins, position of trachea, sternocleidomastoid (swelling, shortening), webbing, edema, auscultation, movement. In the older child, the size and shape of the thyroid gland may be more clearly defined if the gland is palpated from behind.

12. Thorax: Shape and symmetry; pulsations of veins; size, shape, and position of nipples and breasts; intercostal and substernal retractions, asymmetry of respirations.

13. Lungs: Character and quality of breathing—rate, depth, and rhythm of respirations, presence of dyspnea, chest expansion, prolongation of expiration (obstructive, e.g., asthma), cough, fremitus, flatness or dullness to percussion, resonance, breath and voice sounds, rales (crackles, fine or coarse), wheezing

   a. Breath sounds in infants and children normally are more intense and bronchial, and expiration is more prolonged than in adults.

   b. Most of a young child's respiratory movement is produced by abdominal movement; there is very little intercostal motion.

   c. If a sound that is heard by auscultating the lungs is also heard when placing the stethoscope over the patient's mouth, it is usually

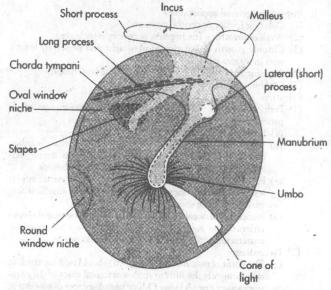

Figure 1-1   Anatomy of the tympanic membrane. (From Greene HL, Fincher RE, Johnson WP, et al [eds]: Clinical Medicine, 2nd ed. St. Louis, Mosby, 1995.)

considered to be an upper airway sound (i.e., its etiology is outside the lungs, at or above the vocal cords).

   d. Bilateral crackles heard in infants with upper respiratory symptoms during winter are most likely the result of small airways and alveoli opening up in a patient with bronchiolitis.

   e. Flaring of the alae nasi indicates air hunger, hypoxemia. Forced expiratory grunting is involuntary, but the effect is to maintain small airway opening (i.e., physiologic positive end-expiratory pressure). It is a sign of severe respiratory distress.

14. Heart/cardiovascular

   a. Vital signs (*be precise*—they are not called *vital* without good reason):

     (1) Respiratory rate (RR) and heart rate (HR) should be counted for a full minute with the child calm and at rest. Remember that fever will result in increased RR and HR; each degree Fahrenheit increases the HR 8 to 10 beats per minute.

     (2) Blood pressure (BP) must be taken with an appropriately sized cuff; width should be 125% to 150% of the diameter of the limb to be evaluated. BP values should be obtained in both arms and at least one leg—systolic BP more than 20 mm Hg higher in the arms than legs is suggestive of a coarctation of the aorta.

b. Inspection (general appearance)
   (1) Coloring (pallor or central cyanosis)
   (2) Work of breathing (tachypnea, accessory muscle use)
   (3) Chronic growth retardation (low weight and preserved length seen in infants with heart failure)
   (4) Asymmetry of the chest suggesting cardiac hypertrophy
   (5) Clubbing suggesting long-standing hypoxia
c. Palpation
   (1) Peripheral pulses: Essential portion of the examination of all patients, but especially infants
      (a) Evaluate rhythm for regularity.
      (b) Weak pulses throughout suggest reduced systemic cardiac output. Etiologies include severe aortic stenosis, decompensated heart failure, pericardial tamponade, and shock.
      (c) Full and bounding pulses throughout suggest aortic runoff lesions—patent ductus arteriosus, aortic insufficiency, Blalock-Taussig shunt.
      (d) Nonpalpable, weak, or delayed femoral pulses suggest coarctation of the aorta. If the right arm is also weak, consider coarctation with aberrant right subclavian artery.
   (2) Precordium
      (a) The point of maximal impulse (PMI) should be dime-sized, in approximately the fifth to sixth intercostal space of the anterior axillary line. A larger PMI or lateral, inferior displacement suggests left ventricular hypertrophy.
      (b) Parasternal heave (left sternal border) suggests right ventricular (RV) hypertrophy (RV pressure overload).
      (c) A hyperactive precordium is characteristic of myocardial volume overload (left-to-right shunt lesions, valvular insufficiency).
      (d) A thrill is appreciated in the presence of a grade IV/VI murmur.
      (e) A silent precordium (absent PMI) suggests severe cardiac pump dysfunction (as in myocarditis or other causes of heart failure).
d. Auscultation: Listen when the child is calm, in a quiet room, with careful attention to rate and rhythm, normal heart sounds, extra sounds (clicks, rubs, gallops), and murmurs. Each component should be evaluated in many locations (e.g., base, apex, axillae, back, suprasternal notch).
   (1) Heart sounds
      (a) S_1: Closure of the atrioventricular (AV) valves. It is best evaluated at the cardiac apex and may occasionally be normally split; a prominent split suggests Ebstein's anomaly or bundle branch block.
      (b) S_2: Closure of the semilunar valves. It is best evaluated at the cardiac base. Normally split, the aortic component precedes the pulmonary component, reflecting higher systemic vascular resistance. The S_2 split is augmented during the

inspiratory phase of respiratory cycle; increased negative intrathoracic pressure during inspiration results in increased systemic venous return and RV output, thus delaying closure of the pulmonary valve. A wide, fixed split S_2 (i.e., does not vary with respiratory cycle) suggests an atrial septal defect or other RV volume load. A narrow or single S_2 suggests increased pulmonary vascular resistance. A *loud, banging, or palpable S_2 is diagnostic of pulmonary hypertension.*

(2) Extra sounds

(a) S_3: Corresponds to the early, rapid phase of diastole. It may be normally heard, especially in school-age, active children. In pathologic states, it may represent high-volume flow across the AV valves.

(b) S_4: Heard later in the diastolic phase, particularly at the cardiac apex. It is almost always pathologic, suggesting diminished ventricular compliance and subsequent impedance to ventricular filling.

(c) Clicks: Clicks are associated with dilated great vessels or valve abnormalities. Pulmonic clicks are best heard at the mid-left sternal border, with aortic clicks being most prominent over the apex. A mid-systolic click, heard best at the apex, is characteristic of mitral valve prolapse. An associated mid-systolic blowing murmur suggests mitral regurgitation.

(3) Murmurs: Represent turbulent, high-volume, or disturbed (nonlaminar) blood flow (Fig. 1-2)

(a) Timing (phase of the cardiac cycle: Systolic, diastolic, or continuous)

(b) Grade (Table 1-1)

(c) Quality: Harsh, coarse, blowing, vibratory, high or low pitched

(d) Location: Identify where the murmur is loudest and points of maximal radiation (Fig. 1-3). Murmurs due to abnormal flow in the pulmonary trunk radiate to the back and axillae. Those associated with abnormal aortic flow radiate to the suprasternal notch and neck. Mitral valve flow disturbances are loudest at the apex and the left axilla.

(e) Relationship to S_1: Systolic *ejection* murmurs occur after the period of isovolumic contraction, a short silent period after S_1 in which there is no flow. These murmurs are due to flow across an abnormal semilunar valve (aortic valve stenosis, pulmonary valve stenosis), or increased flow across a normal semilunar valve (atrial septal defect, anemia, high-output heart failure). The *holosystolic* murmur occurs at the onset of S_1, often obscuring it. These murmurs are due to lesions such as a ventricular septal defect or mitral regurgitation, where turbulent flow occurs at the onset of systole. *Pansystolic* is the appropriate term for those murmurs whose duration is all or most of systole.

(f) Caveats about murmurs (Table 1-2)

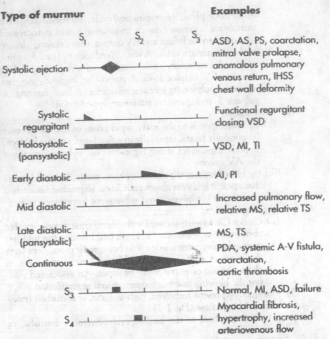

Figure 1-2 Types of murmurs and examples. AI, aortic valve insufficiency; AS, aortic valve stenosis; ASD, atrial septal defect; IHSS, idiopathic hypertrophic subaortic stenosis; MI, mitral valve insufficiency; MS, mitral valve stenosis; PDA, patent ductus arteriosus; PI, pulmonary valve insufficiency; PS, pulmonary valve stenosis; TI, tricuspid valve insufficiency; TS, tricuspid valve stenosis; VSD, ventricular septal defect. (From Barness L: Manual of Pediatric Physical Diagnoses, 6th ed. St. Louis, Mosby, 1991.)

Table 1-1	Grading of Cardiac Murmurs
Grade	**Description**
I	Faintest audible; can be heard only with special effort
II	Faint, but easily audible
III	Moderately loud
IV	Loud; associated with a thrill
V	Very loud; associated with a thrill
	May be heard with a stethoscope off chest
VI	Maximum loudness; associated with a thrill; heard without a stethoscope

From Ferri F: Practical Guide to the Care of the Medical Patient, 6th ed. St. Louis, Mosby, 2004.

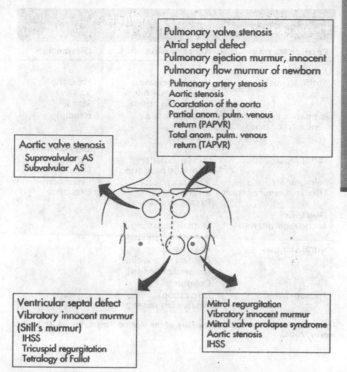

Aortic valve stenosis
  Supravalvular AS
  Subvalvular AS

Pulmonary valve stenosis
Atrial septal defect
Pulmonary ejection murmur, innocent
Pulmonary flow murmur of newborn
  Pulmonary artery stenosis
  Aortic stenosis
  Coarctation of the aorta
  Partial anom. pulm. venous
    return (PAPVR)
  Total anom. pulm. venous
    return (TAPVR)

Ventricular septal defect
Vibratory innocent murmur
(Still's murmur)
  IHSS
  Tricuspid regurgitation
  Tetralogy of Fallot

Mitral regurgitation
Vibratory innocent murmur
Mitral valve prolapse syndrome
Aortic stenosis
IHSS

Figure 1-3 Systolic murmurs audible at various locations. Less common conditions are shown in smaller type. AS, aortic valve stenosis; IHSS, idiopathic hypertrophic subaortic stenosis. (From Park MK: Pediatric Cardiology for Practitioners, 2nd ed. St. Louis, Mosby, 1988.)

    (i) Many children normally have a sinus dysrhythmia (i.e., the heart rate accelerates with inspiration). The child should be asked to take a deep breath to determine its effect on the rhythm.

    (ii) Extra systoles are not uncommon in childhood.

    (iii) The heart should be examined with the child in the following position: Sitting or standing erect, recumbent, supine, and left lateral decubitus. Innocent murmurs decrease in intensity when patient is examined while sitting or standing, compared with supine.

    (iv) A murmur that disappears when the child's head is turned side to side is likely to be a venous hum.

Table 1-2 Response of Selected Murmurs to Physiologic Intervention

Cardiac Murmur	Accentuation	Diminution
Systolic		
Aortic stenosis	Valsalva release	Handgrip
	Sudden squatting	Valsalva
	Passive leg raising	Standing
Idiopathic hypertrophic subaortic stenosis	Valsalva strain	Handgrip
	Standing	Squatting
		Leg elevation
Mitral regurgitation	Sudden squatting	Valsalva
	Isometric handgrip	Standing
Pulmonic stenosis	Valsalva release	Expiration
Tricuspid regurgitation	Inspiration	Expiration
	Passive leg raising	
Diastolic		
Aortic regurgitation	Sudden squatting	
	Isometric handgrip	
Mitral stenosis	Exercise	
	Left lateral position	
	Isometric handgrip	
	Coughing	
Tricuspid stenosis	Inspiration	Expiration
	Passive leg raising	

From Ferri F: Practical Guide to the Care of the Medical Patient, 6th ed. St. Louis, Mosby, 2004.

      (v) A murmur in an adolescent that increases in intensity when standing indicates possible hypertrophic cardiomyopathy and requires a cardiology evaluation.

  e. Other pertinent aspects of the cardiac examination
    (1) Extremities
      (a) Edema of lower extremities
      (b) Perfusion assessment by noting rapid or delayed capillary refill time
    (2) Jugular venous distention: Can be difficult to assess in the pediatric patient but can be important in a patient with heart failure
    (3) Abdomen
      (a) Hepatomegaly can be a sign of heart failure resulting in congested venous return to a stiff or volume-loaded ventricle.
      (b) Splenomegaly can be noted in patients with endocarditis.
15. Abdomen: Size and contour, visible peristalsis, respiratory movements, veins (distention, direction of flow), umbilicus, hernia, tenderness and rigidity, rebound tenderness, tympany, shifting dullness, palpable organs or masses (size, shape, position, mobility), fluid wave, reflexes, femoral pulsations, bowel sounds (Table 1-3)

Table 1-3 Evaluation of Acute Abdominal Pain

Test	Method	Interpretation	Significance
Rebound tenderness	Gentle, deep pressure over abdomen; quick release	Severe pain on release indicates positive test result	Localized or generalized peritonitis
Guarding (rigidity)	Careful, gentle pressure on abdominal wall	Patient resists palpation; may be voluntary or involuntary	May be positive in some normal patients; consider nervous state of patient; "boardlike" indicates perforated viscus
Hyperesthesia	Lightly stroke abdominal wall with point of a pin at slight angle	Stroke feels sharper in positive area	Positive along affected dermatome or in distribution of affected peripheral nerve
Iliopsoas sign	Place patient on side opposite pain; extend and hyperextend thigh	Causes pain or patient resists maneuver because of psoas spasm	Caused by direct or indirect psoas (retroperitoneal) irritation
Obturator sign (thigh rotation test)	Flex knee and thigh on affected side; rotate lower leg medially and thigh laterally	Lower quadrant pain indicates positive test result	Positive when focus in contact with obturator internus (e.g., perforated append x)
Alario's sign	Have patient hop on right leg	Pain in right lower quadrant indicates positive test	Possible localized peritoneal inflammation from appendicitis

Modified from Driscoll CE, Bope ET, Smith CW, Carter BL: Family Practice Desk Reference, 3rd ed. St. Louis, Mosby, 1996.

a. The abdomen may be examined with the child prone in the parent's lap, held over the shoulder, or seated on the examining table facing away from the doctor. These positions may be particularly helpful where tenderness, rigidity, or a mass must be palpated. In the infant, the examination may be aided by having the child suck on a pacifier or gloved finger.

b. Light palpation, especially for the spleen, often provides more information than deep palpation.

c. Umbilical hernias are common during the first 2 to 3 years. They usually disappear spontaneously by 5 years of age.

d. Percussive tenderness may indicate peritonitis.

e. Alario's sign (see Table 1-3) or a right heel strike of the extended straight leg in a supine patient that transmits pain to the right lower quadrant may suggest appendicitis.

f. Always examine the throat in a child with abdominal pain; streptococcal pharyngitis can produce enlargement and tenderness of Peyer's patches of the right abdomen, mimicking the pain of appendicitis.

16. Genitalia: All children should have their genitals examined.

a. Male genitalia (see also Chapter 6): Circumcision, meatal opening, hypospadias, phimosis (narrowing of the opening of the foreskin), adherent foreskin, size of testes, cryptorchidism, scrotum, hydrocele, hernia, pubertal changes. *Tanner stage* of sexual maturation (see Appendix X) should be noted.

(1) In a suspected case of cryptorchidism, examine the child in a warm bath to help testes descend. The older boy may be examined while sitting in a chair holding his own knees and with his heels on the seat so that increased intra-abdominal pressure may push the testes into the scrotum.

(2) Start the examination above the inguinal canal and work downward to prevent pushing the testes up into the canal or abdomen.

(3) In an adolescent, a scrotum that looks and feels like a bag of worms indicates varicoceles.

(4) In the first few days of life, breast enlargement and a small amount of lactation are common secondary to passive transfer of maternal hormones.

(5) Breast enlargement (symmetric or asymmetric) is not unusual in adolescent boys. They will need reassurance that this is normal.

b. Female breasts and genitalia (see also Chapter 6)

(1) Breasts: Stage of development, size, shape, symmetry, masses, discharge

(2) Vagina: Imperforate, discharge, adhesions, size of vaginal opening (in prepubertal children), hypertrophy of clitoris, pubertal changes. Perform pelvic examination as indicated. Tanner stage should be noted.

(a) Gentle pressure on the lower abdomen above the symphysis pubis during a midline rectal examination may elicit cervical motion tenderness consistent with pelvic inflammatory disease.

    (b) In the first few days of life, a small amount of vaginal bleed-
ing or milky discharge, as well as breast enlargement or lactation are common secondary to passive transfer of maternal
hormones.

17. Rectum and anus: Irritation, fissures, prolapse, imperforate anus, tags.
Note muscle tone, character of stool, masses, tenderness, sensation.
   a. The rectal examination should be performed with a lubricated little
   finger in infants (inserted with slow, gentle pressure).
   b. Paradoxical exaggerated relaxation of the rectal sphincter with
   gentle lateral traction on the buttocks or an absent anal wink suggests maltreatment.

18. Extremities
   a. General: Deformity, hemiatrophy, bowlegs (common in infancy),
   knock knee (common at 2 to 3 years of age), paralysis, edema, temperature, posture, gait, stance, asymmetry
   b. Joints: Range of motion, swelling, redness, pain, limitation, tenderness, rheumatic nodules, tibial torsion. Note: A "click" or "clunk"
   felt on rotation of hips may indicate congenital hip dislocation.
   c. Hands and feet: Extra digits, clubbing, simian lines, curvature of
   little finger, deformity or pitting of nails, splinter hemorrhages, flat
   feet (commonly appear flat during first 2 years of life), abnormalities of feet, width of thumbs and big toes, syndactyly, length of
   various segments, temperature
   d. Peripheral vessels: Presence, absence, or diminution of arterial
   pulses
   e. A "3-minute" screening orthopedic examination is described in
   Table 1-4.
   f. Normal femoral arterial pulsations during the newborn period do
   not definitely exclude coarctation.

19. Spine and back: Posture; curves (scoliosis); rigidity; webbed neck;
spina bifida; pilonidal dimple or cyst; tufts of hair; mobility; dermal
melanosis (Mongolian spots); tenderness over spine, pelvis, or kidneys
   a. Bruises/ecchymosis on the back suggest maltreatment.
   b. Point tenderness of a vertebral body requires evaluation for fracture
   or infections.

20. Neurologic examination
   a. Cerebral function/mental status: General behavior, level of consciousness, intelligence, emotional status, memory, orientation,
   hallucinations, cortical sensory interpretation, cortical motor integration, ability to understand and communicate, auditory-verbal
   and visual-verbal comprehension, visual recognition of objects,
   speech, ability to write, performance of skilled motor acts
   b. Cranial nerve testing (Table 1-5). Formal testing of cranial nerve
   function in young children is difficult, and usually observation will
   suffice.
   c. Motor system: Muscle size, consistency, and tone; muscle contours and
   outlines; muscle strength (graded on scale of 5; Table 1-6); myotonic contraction; slow relaxation; symmetry of posture; fasciculation;
   tremor; resistance to passive movement; involuntary movements.

Table 1-4 The 3-Minute Orthopedic Examination	
Have Patient:	**Observe For:**
Face examiner standing	Stature and position of acromioclavicular joints
Look at ceiling, floor, over both shoulders	Cervical spine mobility
Shrug shoulders (against your resistance)	Trapezius strength
Abduct shoulders 90 degrees (against your resistance)	Deltoid strength
Rotate arms	Shoulder mobility
Extend and flex elbows	Elbow mobility
Pronate and supinate wrists	Wrist mobility
Spread fingers, make fist	Hand or finger strength and mobility
Tighten quadriceps; relax quadriceps while you hold down patient	Patellar mobility and check for pain consistent with patellofemoral syndrome
"Duck walk" three or four steps (with buttocks on heels)	Hip, knee, and ankle mobility and muscle strength
Keep knees straight, touch toes	Scoliosis, hip motion, hamstring tightness
Raise up on toes, raise heels	Calf symmetry, leg strength
Heel–toe walk three or four steps	Coordination, maturation of central nervous system

Modified from American Academy of Pediatrics, Committee on Sports Medicine: Health Care for Young Athletes. Elk Grove, Ill, American Academy of Pediatrics, 1983.

Assess tone of trunk—examiner should suspend child from underarms and horizontally. To assess for dystrophy (proximal weakness), have child stand up from cross-legged position on floor (Gower's sign).

  d. Reflexes
    (1) Deep biceps, brachioradialis, triceps, patellar, and Achilles tendon reflexes; rapidity and strength of contraction and relaxation (Table 1-7)
    (2) Superficial-abdominal, cremasteric, plantar, anal wink
    (3) Developmental reflexes: Rooting (0 to 3 months), Moro (0 to 6 months), traction response (pulling the child by the hands to the sitting position; head lag, 0 to 1 month; increasing head flexion, 1 to 3 months; flexion at the elbow with head posture maintained, 3 to 5 months; grasp (0 to 6 months), and tonic neck reflexes (0 to 6 months), Babinski (downgoing by 6 to 12 months), Landau (flexion of the legs/trunk with head flexion while infant held in horizontal prone position; 10 to 24 months), parachute (arm extension toward floor in controlled fall; 9 months to adulthood)

Table 1-5 Testing of Cranial Nerves

Cranial Nerves	Action
I—Olfactory	Sense of smell
II—Optic	Vision (visual acuity, visual fields, color), assess optic nerve with funduscopy
III—Oculomotor IV—Trochlear VI—Abducens	Extraocular movements (EOMs), pupillary constriction (oculomotor), elevation of upper lids; tracking objects such as stuffed animals or lights helpful to assess EOMs. Helpful mnemonic is "LR6SO4"—lateral rectus VI, superior oblique IV, other muscles innervated by III
V—Trigeminal	Sensation of face, mastication Divided into V1, V2, V3
VII—Facial	Sensory of forehead, face, and jaw Facial expression, taste in anterior two thirds of tongue
VIII—Vestibulocochlear	Hearing and balance
IX—Glossopharyngeal X—Vagus	IX and X—Sensory and motor functions of pharynx and larynx (gag reflex, position of uvula, swallowing) IX—Taste of posterior one third tongue
XI—Accessory	Shoulder shrugging, rotary head movement
XII—Hypoglossal	Motor control of tongue

From Ferri F: Practical Guide to the Care of the Medical Patient, 6th ed. St. Louis, Mosby, 2004.

(4) Pathologic reflexes for upper motor neuron process
  (a) Spread of reflexes—for example, tapping right patella and eliciting contraction of left leg. Can be normal in infants.
  (b) Clonus—rapid rhythmic muscle contractions usually with provocation; most often seen in foot with ankle jerk and can be normal in the newborn period.

Table 1-6 Grading of Muscle Strength

0	Absent muscular contraction
1	Minimal contraction
2	Active movement with gravity eliminated
3	Active movement against gravity only
4	Active movement against gravity and some resistance
5	Normal muscle strength

From Ferri F: Practical Guide to the Care of the Medical Patient, 6th ed. St. Louis, Mosby, 2004.

Table 1-7	Grading of Deep Tendon Reflexes
0	Absent
+	Hypoactive
++	Normal
+++	Brisker than average
++++	Hyperactive, often indicative of disease

From Ferri F: Practical Guide to the Care of the Medical Patient, 6th ed. St. Louis, Mosby, 2004.

e. Sensation: Generally difficult to assess in child younger than 4 years of age. Assess by tickling or, if concerned about pathologic process, noxious stimuli such as applying nail bed pressure. Other avenues of testing include pinprick test (broken wooden cotton swab), light touch with cotton tip, vibration, temperature, and proprioception.

f. Cerebellar function: Finger to nose and then to examiner's finger; rapidly alternating pronation and supination of hands; ability to run heel down opposite shin; ability to stand with eyes closed (Romberg's test) also tests proprioception and vestibular input. Ataxia, nystagmus, abnormalities of muscle tone and speech all suggest cerebellar dysfunction.

g. Gait: If child ambulates, assess symmetry in arm swing and leg swing. Check regular gait, running, walking on toes and heels. Also important to assess tandem gait—walking one foot in front of other (walking a balance beam).

21. Developmental assessment: Should be performed on all children. It may be brief and to the point (i.e., a global evaluation—"Do you think your child is developing normally?"). How does he/she compare with his/her siblings or other children of the same age? Have the caretaker give examples. The developmental assessment may also be more detailed and formal (see Appendix VII—developmental reference material, including Denver Developmental Assessment, as well as Chapter 2, Section 2.6, Development).

1.3 Admission Orders

Use the mnemonic "ABC VANDALISM":

Admit: Ward and attending patient to be admitted to (e.g., floor, pediatric intensive care unit; and Dr. Jones service)

Because: Diagnosis (or reason if diagnosis unknown) for hospitalization (e.g., acute asthma exacerbation or progressive weakness)

Condition: Stable, fair, poor, critical.

Vitals: Specify frequency (e.g., Q4h, Q shift) and parameters when you want to be notified or a special intervention made (e.g., for temperature >100.4 call house officer and draw blood cultures). It is always good to specify types of vitals (temperature, HR, RR, BP, etc.).

Activity: Ad lib or restricted (bed rest). *Note:* Try not to limit a child's activity level if at all possible.

Nursing: Special orders (e.g., strict input and output recording, daily weights)

Diet: Regular for age or special (clears, soft, or restricted such as low salt, sugar, protein). Indicate if infant strictly breast-fed (i.e., NO bottle). Calculate caloric needs.

Allergies: Specify medications or foods as well as specific reaction (e.g., penicillin—rash; or peanut butter—stops breathing, anaphylaxis, and death).

Labs: Type and frequency (e.g., complete blood count with differential Q day and reticulocyte count Q3 days). Avoid unnecessary or extra blood draws if possible, try to group them Q AM, but indicate any stat labs.

Intravenous fluids: In addition to strict ins and outs, indicate any stat or maintenance fluids, types, and volume. (See Chapter 9 for types and rate of fluids.)

Special: Other diagnostic tests, including electrocardiogram (ECG), x-ray.

Medications: Indicate name, dose, frequency, and type.

Always remember to date and time your orders. Sign or print your name legibly, as well as your pager number.

SUGGESTIONS FOR PREVENTING/ REDUCING MEDICATION ERRORS

1. Always write dosages in milligrams, units, etc., and not in milliliters/ volumes, because most medications come in different concentrations.
2. Use generic names instead of brand names.
3. When calculating dosages, keep in mind convenient dosing for family.
4. When writing medications in micrograms, spell the entire word.
5. When writing medications in decimal figures, always write a zero before the first number and not just a dot (e.g., Digoxin 0.2 mg, not Digoxin .2 mg), and do not use trailing zero (e.g., Digoxin 0.2 mg, not 0.20 mg).
6. When obtaining medication dosages from parents, always check to make sure that the dose reported is appropriate for that child.

1.4 Progress Notes

Use the "SOAP" format:

S (subjective): How the patient feels that day. In nonverbal patients, you can rely on the parents' perception of the child's well-being or yours (e.g., "He looks more comfortable today").

O (objective): A description of the patient's vital signs, ins and outs, weight change, physical findings, laboratory data, and test results

A (assessment): Your analysis of data, thoughts about what is going on with the patient, pathophysiologic processes, differential diagnosis, and tentative diagnosis; analysis of pros and cons of your different diagnostic possibilities. Avoid long supermarket lists of diagnostic entities; focus your assessment on that particular patient.

P (plan): Both diagnostic and therapeutic. Your management plan should be consistent with your assessment of the patient's problems.

SUGGESTED READINGS

Barness L: Manual of Pediatric Physical Diagnosis, 6th ed. St. Louis, Mosby, 1991.

DeAngelis C: Pediatric Primary Care, 3rd ed. Boston, Little, Brown, 1984.
Gundy JH: The pediatric physical examination. In Hoekelman RA (ed): Primary
    Pediatric Care, 2nd ed. St. Louis, Mosby, 1992.
Schmitt B: Pediatric Telephone Advice. Boston, Little, Brown, 1980.
Ziai M: Pediatrics, 4th ed. Boston, Little, Brown, 1990.

Natalia Golova and Anthony J. Alario

Routine Health Maintenance and Preventive Medicine: A Guide to Well-Child Care

2

2.1 Parental (or Child's) Concerns and Issues

It is important to elicit concerns and issues from either the parent or child in their own words. Topics will range from traditional well-child care issues ("Why doesn't my 2-year-old eat?") to broader psychosocial concerns ("How can my son deal with the school bully?"). Most concerns can be addressed during the routine time allotted for a well-child encounter; however, more complex issues require further exploration, necessitating subsequent visits.

2.2 Growth: Gains in Stature and Weight

One of the most important tasks of routine health maintenance is the monitoring of a child's growth parameters. The purpose of this section is to provide basic principles of childhood growth related to stature and weight gain.

STATURE (HEIGHT)

1. Measurements: Serial, multiple, and correctly obtained measurements are necessary in all children to determine whether gain in height is appropriate. Infants should be measured supine using a standardized device; older children (>2 years) can be measured standing in socks with their heels and back against a wall, ideally using a standardized instrument. Standardized charts, based primarily on cross-sectionally derived measurements in white, middle-class children, are available (see Appendix II) and have traditionally been used to plot serial measurements and determine percentiles of growth.
2. Height velocity curve: Another type of plot, *the height velocity curve* (see Appendix II), may yield more information about growth status than the traditional growth curve (i.e., a low-percentile channel on a velocity reference curve might suggest a clinical condition that, if amenable to therapy, would then show "catch-up" growth after a successful intervention).
3. Growth in fetus, newborn, and infant (Box 2-1)
   a. Maternal (prenatal) factors have a major influence on postnatal growth in length for the first month of life. Note that birth length is a poor predictor of eventual adult height.

> **Box 2-1 Summary of Key Milestones in Stature (Height)**
>
> Average birth length is 50 cm (20 inches).
> By the end of the first year, birth length increases by 50%.
> Birth length doubles by 4 years.
> Birth length triples by 13 years.
> Average annual growth is 5 cm (2 inches) or more per year (2 years of age to puberty).

  b. Large newborns do not grow at a rate that would be suggested by their size (i.e., they may not be destined to be large). Their growth slows during the first 6 months of life, termed "catch-down" growth.
  c. Small-for-gestational-age infants: Growth can be predicted from head circumference at birth.
      (1) If head size is normal, catch-up growth will occur.
      (2) If head size is small (usually due to early and significant prenatal insult), little catch-up growth will occur.
  d. Premature infants do not have catch-up growth; they grow at the same rate as a fetus (with less deceleration as full term infants) and reach their destined growth track by 2 years of age. Growth parameters are corrected for the weeks of prematurity up to 2 years of age.
4. Growth in toddlers and prepubertal child
  a. Height gain occurs at a rate of 5 to 6 cm/year. This is the expected gain in height that should occur for most normal children.
  b. The genetically programmed growth curve that a child will follow (e.g., 18%, 75%) is reached by approximately 18 months to 2 years.
  c. Height and weight velocity are not synchronized.
      (1) Childhood height velocity exceeds weight velocity; therefore, toddlers lose the "fat-healthy" appearance they had in the previous 6 to 12 months. As they grow faster, they put on weight.
      (2) Before puberty, weight velocity exceeds height velocity; therefore, the prepubertal child looks chubby.
      (3) During the adolescent growth spurt, height velocity equals or surpasses weight velocity; therefore, the teen loses his or her "baby fat."
  e. Short stature (see Chapter 7) and growth failure
      (1) Short stature: By definition, 5% of children will be plotted at or below the 5th percentile (2 SD) for age. This means that 5% of the population is short stature. If these children grow at a normal rate, they should not be considered to have growth failure.
      (2) Growth failure: Classically defined as a failure to gain the expected 5 to 6 cm/year in height.
      (3) The three most common clinical associations with short stature as an outcome (see Chapter 7) include:
          (a) True growth failure: This is generally associated with congenital or chronic disease entities that lead to primary growth

failure or an acquired arrest of growth. These include prenatal insult, skeletal dysplasia, nutritional insult, chronic illness (e.g., arthritis, inflammatory bowel disease), congenital abnormality (i.e., Turner's, Down syndromes), hormonal deficiency (i.e., hypothyroidism, Cushing's syndrome), or a deprivational environment.

(b) Familial short stature
  (i) Growth occurs at or below 5th percentile by age 2 to 3 years.
  (ii) Growth occurs along child's own "normal" curve and growth rate.
  (iii) Bone age equals chronologic age (not height age—long bone growth is consistent with age).
  (iv) Puberty occurs at normal time.
  (v) Ultimate height is consistent with family stature but shorter than that of peers.

(c) Constitutional delay. These are the so-called "late bloomers."
  (i) Growth deceleration leads these children to grow along the 5th percentile early (9 months to 3 years).
  (ii) The prepubertal growth rate is normal.
  (iii) Bone age equals height age (not chronologic age—long bone growth is delayed).
  (iv) Pubertal development is also delayed.
  (v) A longer growth period and delayed epiphyseal fusion lead to normal adult height.
  (vi) A family history of delayed puberty is often identified.

f. Head growth: By 2 years of age, most (95%) of head (i.e., brain) growth is completed, but head circumference may increase until 60 years of age.

5. Adolescent growth (see also Appendix II)
  a. There is considerable variability in the peak and termination of the adolescent growth spurt, as much as 3 years from one normal child to another.
  b. Adolescent growth is related to the rate of sexual maturation.
  c. Girls tend to be 2 years ahead of boys; their growth spurt begins at 11 years of age and peaks at 12 years (i.e., girls are taller at 11 to 13 years of age). A girl's growth spurt precedes the onset of menarche. After menarche, a girl still grows, but at a much decelerated rate (approximately 1 to 3 inches). Estrogen secretion induces closure of long bone epiphyses.
  d. Boys' growth rate is more variable and marked; their growth spurt begins at 13 years of age, peaks at 14 years (rate = 10 cm/year in boys, 8 cm/year in girls).
  e. The growth spurt lasts 2 to 2.5 years in both sexes.
  f. A major gain in height results from growth of the trunk.
  g. Three variables are important to predict final adult height:
    (1) Height of parents: The following equation, using parental stature (mid-parental stature), is one of the many calculations that can

be used to provide an estimate of a child's *eventual* height (in centimeters; 1 SD = 5 cm):

$$\frac{(\text{maternal height} + \text{paternal height} + 13)}{2} = \text{boy's height}$$

$$\frac{(\text{maternal height} + \text{paternal height} - 13)}{2} = \text{girl's height}$$

(2) Bone age (at varying ages)
(3) Age of maternal menarche (for girls)

WEIGHT

1. Measurements: Sequential, accurate measurements are most helpful in differentiating normal from abnormal.
2. Weight gain: Fetus, newborn, infant, and school-age child (Box 2-2)
   a. Fetal weight velocity peaks at 32 to 34 weeks' gestation (unlike fetal gain in height, which peaks at 16 to 20 weeks).
   b. Increase in somatic growth and fat tissue occurs in the third trimester.
   c. Birth weight is influenced more by maternal health status (e.g., diabetes, preeclampsia, hypertension) and habits (e.g., smoking) than by maternal nutritional status.
   d. Infants lose up to 10% of their birth weight in the first week of life, and should at least regain birth weight by 2 weeks of age.
   e. Infants who are small for gestational age (weight ≤10th percentile for gestational age) fail to catch up.
   f. Maximum weight velocity (unlike height) is achieved after birth. A healthy newborn should gain approximately 30 g (1 oz) per day.
   g. A child of average birth weight will double birth weight by 4 to 5 months and triple it by 12 months.
3. Weight gain in the adolescent
   a. Adolescent growth spurt: Weight gain (see Appendix II):
      (1) Correlates with gain in height, but occurs over a longer period of time.

Box 2-2 Summary of Key Milestones in Weight Gain

1. Birth weight is regained by the 10th to 14th day.
2. During the first 3 months, the average gain is about 1 kg/month (about 0.5 to 1 oz/day).
3. Birth weight doubles at about 5 months, triples at 12 months, and quadruples at 24 months.
4. By the sixth month, the average gain per month is 0.5 kg.
5. During the second year, the average gain per month is 0.25 kg.
6. After 2 years of age, the average annual increment is 2.3 kg (5 lb) until the adolescent growth spurt.

(2) Occurs earlier in girls (10 to 12 years) than in boys (12 to 14 years).
(3) In girls, onset of growth spurt usually occurs 1 year before menarche.

b. A body mass index (BMI) helps quantify the weight-to-height relationship (Fig. 2-1): BMI = weight (kg)/[height (m)]^2. The BMI should be calculated at every well-child visit and plotted. It is a good indicator of obesity or risk of overweight.

c. Obesity is also defined as a weight more than 20% above the average for height, age, and sex. Morbid obesity is defined as a weight of more than 50% above the average for height, age, and sex.

SKELETAL GROWTH OF LEGS AND FEET AND RELATIONSHIP TO POSTURE

1. The fat and wide newborn foot aids in stability (fat pads obliterate the longitudinal arch until 3 to 4 years of age, so flat feet are a normal variation in toddlers).

2. With walking (10 to 14 months), the feet are turned out, pronated, and flattened for better balance; the heels may be everted, and a knock-kneed (genu valgum) or bowlegged (genu varum) appearance may be seen (Fig. 2-2A).

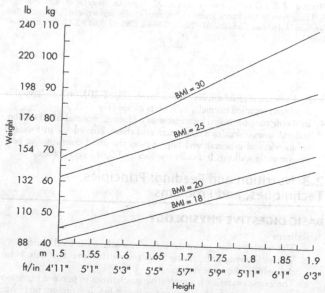

Figure 2-1 Relationship of weight to height using body mass index (BMI). (Adapted from Sinclair D: Human Growth after Birth, 5th ed. Oxford, Oxford University Press, 1989.)

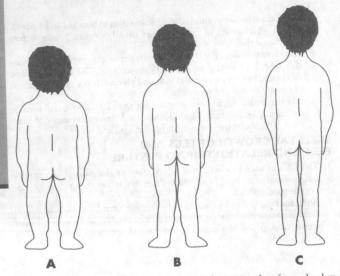

Figure 2-2 Development of stance. A, Eighteen months of age: bowlegs. B, Three years of age: knock knees. C, Six years of age: legs straight. (Adapted from Sinclair D: Human Growth after Birth, 5th ed. Oxford, Oxford University Press, 1989.)

3. By 3 years, the child displays knock knees (Fig. 2-2B), only to have this condition rectified normally by 6 years of age (Fig. 2-2C).
4. In-toeing may be caused by metatarsus adductus, internal tibial torsion, femoral anteversion, or a combination of these. Physiologic in-toeing is symmetric and bilateral, and improves as the child continues to bear weight while walking. It usually resolves by 2.5 to 3 years of age.

2.3 Nutrition and Feeding: Principles, Techniques, and Problems

BASIC DIGESTIVE PHYSIOLOGY

1. Reflexes
   a. The rooting reflex guides the infant's mouth to the food source.
   b. The swallowing reflex along with peristalsis move the milk bolus through the digestive system.
   c. The extrusion reflex is a protective mechanism to prevent ingestion of inappropriate food sources or foreign bodies. It is present up to 2 to 3 months of age and allows the infant to thrust the tongue forward, pushing material out from the anterior part of the mouth.

2. The development of the lower esophageal sphincter is incomplete at birth; thus, some form of reflux (spitting up) is not uncommon until about 3 to 4 months of age.
3. Although at birth salivary and pancreatic amylase are low, they rise to adult levels by 6 months of age, so *carbohydrates* are readily digestible.
4. Proteolytic enzymes for *protein* digestion and absorption are sufficiently functional at birth; the mucosal barrier to large, antigenic protein molecules is intact by 4 months of age.
5. Fats are readily absorbed by most term infants.
6. Because of immature kidney function in the first 4 months of life, especially with respect to handling osmolar loads, high-protein or high-electrolyte foods such as whole cow's milk are contraindicated in young infants.

BREAST-FEEDING AND BREAST MILK

In the first year of life, the infant requires between 105 and 117 kcal/kg/day to grow properly. Breast milk is the strongly recommended sole source of nutrition in the first 4 to 6 months of life. Breast milk provides approximately 7% of calories from protein, 55% from fat, and 38% from lactose.

1. The specific nutritional and immunochemical benefits of breast milk are:
   a. Colostrum (the initial milk produced in the first 7 to 10 days after delivery): High in fat, protein, calories, and immunoglobulins; stimulates passage of meconium
   b. Protein
      (1) Protein composition changes to meet nutritional and digestive requirements:
         (a) Premature or transitional human milk is 80% whey, 20% casein.
         (b) Mature human milk is 60% whey, 40% casein.
      (2) Cholesterol-stable amount regardless of intake—important in central nervous system growth and later cholesterol metabolism
      (3) High in omega-3 fatty acids (for brain growth and retinal maturation)
      (4) Rich in lipase (for rapid absorption of fats)
   c. Vitamins
      (1) Rich in A, C, and E
      (2) Lower than cow's milk in D and K
      (3) Variable levels of B vitamins; depends on intake
      (4) Vitamin deficiencies overcome by increased maternal intake (e.g., B_{12} supplements in strict vegetarian), sunlight exposure, and supplementation. Breast-fed infants may need to be supplemented with vitamins D and K, and fluoride (Note: Vitamin K is administered to all newborns at birth. No fluoride is needed until after 6 months of age, then add 0.25 mg/day.)
   d. Iron also is sufficiently bioavailable in breast milk, so iron supplementation is usually not required for the first 6 months of life. After 6 months, the breast-fed infant should be receiving foods high in bioavailable iron or iron supplements.
   e. Other factors making human milk more beneficial than cow's milk
      (1) Lower sodium content; less osmolar load

(2) Trace elements more bioavailable

(3) Macrophages present

(4) Development of beneficial intestinal microflora enhanced

(5) Thought to decrease the risk of development of diabetes, Crohn's disease, and celiac disease

(6) Thought to be protective against certain allergic conditions: eczema, asthma, allergic rhinitis

(7) Less constipating; a breast-fed infant's stools are loose, yellow, and seedy

(8) More vigorous sucking necessary, which is beneficial for infant dental and mandibular development

(9) Less cost and a readily available, convenient source

(10) Psychological benefits for both mother and infant (bonding)

  f. Supplementation: Extensively breast-fed infants may require supplementation with vitamins D and iron such as Tri-Vi-Sol with Iron (1 mL PO each day).

2. Practical aspects and techniques

  a. Encourage "feeding on demand" for first few weeks, usually every 1.5 to 2.5 hours with 8 to 10 feeds per day.

  b. Infant should have at least six wet diapers a day and may stool after every feeding (especially in breast-fed infants), but should stool at least once a day.

  c. Alternate breasts to start each feeding because infant suckles better on first breast.

  d. Gradually increase duration of feeding from 5 minutes each breast on days 1 and 2 to 10 to 15 minutes each breast.

  e. Try to avoid bottle supplementation in the first 3 to 6 weeks until ample maternal milk supply is attained. Water supplementation is not necessary (breast milk is 80% H_2O) and may actually be dangerous because of inability of immature kidneys to handle changes in osmolarity.

  f. Expect the infant to lose 7% to 10% of birth weight in the first week; the adequacy of feeding thereafter can be assessed by the infant's satisfaction with feeds, as well as the infant's voiding and stooling patterns and a weight gain of at least 0.5 to 1 oz/day (15 to 30 g/day).

3. Complications

  a. Engorgement

    (1) Usually occurs 2 to 3 days postpartum and is caused by an increase in blood flow and the start of milk production; usually decreases after 24 to 48 hours

    (2) Treatment

      (a) Nurse frequently every 1 to 3 hours for 10 to 20 minutes each side.

      (b) Express milk before nursing if areola is firm; apply warm compresses.

      (c) Massage breasts while nursing.

      (d) Use cold packs after nursing.

      (e) Wear a support bra.

      (f) Take acetaminophen as needed for pain relief.

        (g) Do not pump. Pumping will only increase milk production and cause further engorgement.

        (h) Manual expression under warm water may alleviate some of the discomfort.

b. Sore nipples

  (1) In most cases this is due to incorrect latching-on.

  (2) Position infant perpendicular to nipple, sit upright, and hold breast with a "C" hold.

  (3) Express or pump before nursing to soften areola; position infant carefully. Tickle bottom lip with nipple until infant opens mouth wide, then pull infant in close and quickly. If latched on wrong, break suction and reposition.

  (4) Nipple dermatitis: Irritated, red, swollen nipples with or without cracking and usually burning, usually caused by reaction to creams, most commonly those with vitamin E or lanolin. Stop the use of creams; apply cool compresses after nursing: if severe, use anti-inflammatory creams after nursing.

  (5) Thrush nipples: Red, swollen, tender nipples; may be cracked, itchy, flaking, or burning. Usually occurs after weeks or months of nursing and spreads from infant to mother. Apply anticandidal (e.g., nystatin) cream to breasts and give liquid suspension to infant after every other feeding. Let nipples air dry or blow dry. Change nursing pads frequently.

c. Plugged ducts and lumps

  (1) Presents as a tender lump on the breast. Occurs usually in early weeks, after a missed feeding or wearing bras that are too tight.

  (2) Treatment

    (a) Do not wear a bra too tightly.

    (b) Nurse frequently.

    (c) Infant should nurse on the affected breast first in order to empty it completely.

    (d) Increase fluid intake.

    (e) Apply moist heat and massage above sore area.

    (f) Position infant with chin close to involved area.

    (g) Watch for signs of infection.

d. Mastitis

  (1) Occurs in 30% of all nursing women, usually in first 3 months

  (2) Symptoms

    (a) Flulike fever, chills, aches, headache, nausea/vomiting

    (b) Usually in only one breast

    (c) Red streak or wedge is noted on the affected breast and is tender to palpation.

  (3) Causes: Cracked nipples, plugged milk duct, tight bras, or skipped feedings

  (4) Treatment

    (a) Wear loose or no bra.

    (b) Nurse frequently, beginning on affected side; decreasing or stopping nursing may lead to a breast abscess.

    (c) Increase fluid intake.

    (d) Apply moist heat.

(e) Take acetaminophen.

(f) If no improvement in 24 hours, begin antibiotics. *Staphylococcus* and *Streptococcus* are the most common pathogens. Dicloxacillin is the drug of choice.

4. Contraindications to breast-feeding
   a. Significant maternal mental illness; some psychotropic medication
   b. Uncontrollable seizure disorder in infant or mother
   c. Infantile inborn errors of metabolism (galactosemia, phenylketonuria, urea cycle defects)
   d. Maternal septicemia
   e. Maternal infections: Tuberculosis, malaria, hepatitis, human immunodeficiency virus (HIV)
   f. Maternal malnutrition

5. Medications and breast-feeding
   a. Most drugs and medications may be found in breast milk, usually in low concentrations.
   b. Always check that a drug is safe and will not potentially harm the infant if given to a nursing mother. U.S. Food and Drug Administration categories A and B are generally acceptable for nursing mothers.

FORMULA FEEDING

1. As with breast-fed infants, initial feedings with formula should be "on demand." Infants will adjust their intake (number and volume of feedings) depending on their growth requirements.
2. The midnight and early morning feeds are usually given up during the second or third month of life.
3. Most commercially available formulas are developed (and are continually evolving) to be more like human milk than cow's milk. (See Appendix VI for comparison of human with commercially prepared milk.)
4. For infants with special requirements, a number of specific formulas have been developed. Two basic categories include soy-based and protein-hydrolysate–based formulas. (These are more "elemental" formulas).
5. In addition, special formulas and caloric supplementations have been developed for premature infants or infants who need increased calories (see Appendix VI).

SUPPLEMENTS

1. Iron (Fe): Infants should receive 1 mg/kg/day of elemental Fe (maximum 15 mg/day) during the first year of life to prevent iron-deficiency anemia. Iron is supplemented in most commercial formulas (8 to 12 mg Fe/L).
2. Vitamins: Vitamin K is the only needed vitamin at birth; all others are stored in sufficient quantity. Commercially available formulas contain adequate vitamin content, so no supplementation is usually needed in healthy infants.

EARLY MILK INTOLERANCE DISORDERS

1. Cow's milk protein allergy
   a. Pathophysiology: This disorder presents in the first 1 to 2 weeks of life primarily as intolerance to milk protein secondary to immune complex formation and immediate or delayed hypersensitivity.

b. Symptoms: Range from true anaphylaxis (rare) to vomiting, abdominal pain, diarrhea, urticaria, angioedema, and wheezing. Malabsorption may also occur.

c. Treatment: Although often tried, changing to a soy-based casein-hydrolysate formula is of doubtful benefit. This condition usually resolves spontaneously in the first year of life. Thirty percent of infants with cow's milk protein allergy also suffer from a soy protein allergy and require a more elemental formula.

2. Formula intolerance and colic

a. At some point, most infants have occasional spitting up or vomiting, neither of which is considered formula intolerance. As long as weight gain is maintained and symptoms are not excessive or worrisome, reassurance is the best course of action.

b. Signs and symptoms: Recurrent excessive crying (i.e., colic), some-times associated with abdominal distention, gas, and drawing up of the legs, is occasionally seen after feedings, which suggests milk intolerance.

c. Differential diagnosis: It is important to consider other etiologies for excessive crying, such as intestinal obstruction, overfeeding or underfeeding, hair tourniquet around a digit or penis, hard stools, corneal abrasion, gastroesophageal reflux, or colic associated with psychological stressors in the infant and caretaker. In addition, if the mother consumes large quantities of certain foods (whole milk, spices, caffeine, theobromine) to which the infant is intolerant, colic may occur.

d. Treatment: Elimination of a potentially offensive agent from the maternal diet is often helpful. Formula changes are frequently tried even without good indication. Carrying the infant close to the body, decreasing excessive external stimulation, using comforting motions or sounds, and dealing with mother–baby stressors help as well. Colic generally resolves between 8 and 10 weeks of age.

INTRODUCTION OF SOLID FOODS

1. The physiologically appropriate time to introduce solid foods is between 4 and 6 months. At this age, the extrusion reflex extinguishes, and rhythmic biting movements begin to appear between 7 and 9 months even in the absence of teeth.

2. Schedule

a. 4 to 6 months: Begin with grains (rice cereal, least allergenic) and fruits (bananas, peaches).
   (1) Avoid adding cereal to bottle (does not allow for the normal development of mastication).
   (2) Avoid citrus fruits in the first year.

b. 6 to 9 months: Pureed meats (chicken, veal) and vegetables (yellow-orange to green).

c. Over 9 to 12 months: As teeth emerge and chewing and swallowing boluses develop, introduce different textures, and provide variety. Introduce table foods while avoiding chokeable items.

d. In late infancy, 12 to 30 months: There is a normal physiologic decrease in appetite and lack of interest in food that parallels the decrease in growth rate and concomitant increase in motor and language skills. Pointing out these normal patterns to anxious parents helps them understand why their otherwise healthy toddler "doesn't eat anymore."

2.4 Elimination

1. Caretakers (and many clinicians) are often preoccupied with bladder and bowel habits. Whatever the concern, it is an issue for the primary care provider to address when it becomes a problem for the family.
2. Ask systematically about bladder and bowel habits (i.e., frequency, quantity, quality) during every well-child encounter.
3. Control over defecation generally lags behind bladder control, although some children may achieve bowel control before bladder control.
4. Many behaviorists believe that it is possible to avoid potential toilet-training difficulties by providing detailed anticipatory guidance (at the 1-year visit) about what the caretaker can expect to happen as the child approaches toilet-training readiness. This readiness will depend on not just the age of the child but his or her cognitive and physical readiness.
5. Boxes 2-3 and 2-4 outline the developmental physiology for bladder control and guidelines for determining toilet-training readiness.

2.5 Sleep

Concerns over children's sleeping habits preoccupy adults. Gathering information about napping, bedtime routine, and the duration and quality of sleep is important and will likely elicit concerns in up to 40% of respondents caring for young children (see Chapter 22).

Box 2-3   Developmental Physiology for Bladder Control

1. Neuropsychological maturation
   a. Awareness of bladder fullness: 18 months to 2 years
   b. Retain urine by voluntary conscious control: 2 to 3 years
   c. Voluntary initiation of micturition: 3 to 4 years
   d. Void at will regardless of bladder distention: 6 to 7 years
2. Variations
   a. Birth weight: Infants under 2500 g are slower trainers.
   b. Sex: Girls train before boys.
   c. Race: After 3 years of age, white boys and girls train before black boys.
   d. Differences in sex and race disappear after age 7 years.
3. When dry
   a. Sixty-six percent achieve nighttime dryness by age 3 years; 75%, by age 4; 90%, by age 8.5.
   b. Fifty percent achieve daytime dryness by age 2 years; 90%, by age 4.

Box 2-4   Toilet-Training Readiness

Independent of the child's age, readiness is based on physical and cognitive readiness.
1. Bladder control
   a. Urinates large amounts at once
   b. Dry for several hours at a time
   c. Aware of need to eliminate (i.e., paces, jumps up and down, grabs pants, squats, tells you)
2. Physical readiness
   a. Fine motor coordination
   b. Walking
   c. Helps in dressing and undressing
3. Cognitive readiness
   a. Understands and is responsive to requests
   b. Understands "pee," "poop," "dry," "wet," "clean," "messy," "potty"
   c. Understands what the toilet is for

2.6 Development

1. Basic approach to surveillance of developmental issues
   a. Assume children are normal until proven otherwise.
   b. Approach gathering information in a *proactive* manner.
      (1) Ask open-ended questions for exploration ("Tell me what your 7-month-old child does"), closed-ended ones for specific recognition ("Does he sit up without help?").
      (2) Explore parental concerns; avoid premature closure.
      (3) Foster a sense of confidence in the competence of parents, knowing that they will be more accurate in reporting *current* skills they are likely to observe and track rather than past ones.
   c. Understand the utility and limitations of screening tools.
      (1) History/examination is the most practical "tool" and will be the best entree into potential problems.
      (2) Standardized tests are more structured, but many lack sensitivity in that they tend to undercall problems in difficult or subtle cases. Note that they are *not* tests of intelligence. The routinely used screening tests (i.e., Denver Developmental Assessment II; see Appendix VII) need to be interpreted with an understanding of the larger picture of what the child's world is like (i.e., home environment, education, culture, stressors).
2. Developmental reference skills
   a. Gross motor milestones: Tables 2-1 through 2-5 highlight normal milestones (skills) in each developmental domain and provide key clues to identifying delays or problems (see Chapter 21).

Text continued on page 43

Table 2-1   Gross Motor Milestones

Skill	Age of Acquisition Average Month	Range (mo)	Clues to Delays/Problems
Raises self by arms while lying face down	2	2 wk-5	No head control at 6 mo
Sits alone momentarily	5	4-8	Persistent or prolonged infantile reflexes* (see Appendix VII)
			Obligatory tonic-neck
Rolls from back to stomach	6	4-10	
Sits alone quite steadily for long periods	7	5-9	
Pulls to standing	9	6-12	Unable to sit steadily by 10 mo*
Stands alone	11	9-16	Increased extensor tone on pull to sit/standing*
Walks alone, three steps	12	9-17	Failure to develop protective reflexes at 10 mo*
Walks fast, seldom falls	18	14-24	
Stands on right foot alone	24	16-20	Not walking by 20 mo
Walks up stairs alone with both feet on each step	25	18-30	
Balances briefly on one foot; walks well on toes; jumps from a step	36	17-48	
Hops on one foot	48	23-60	
Goes down stairs, alternating feet	48	23-60	
Throws overhand	48	22+	
Skips on alternating feet; tandem walks backwards	60	48+	
Rides bicycle	60+		

*Suggests cerebral palsy.

Table 2-2 **Fine Motor Milestones**

Skill	Age of Acquisition		Clues to Delays/Problems
	Average Month	Range (mo)	
Reaches	3	2.5-5	Persistent reflexive grasp
Grasps	4	2.5-5	
Retains rattle	4	2.5-6	
Grasps in raking manner	5	4-7.5	
Transfers	6	4.5-7.5	
Radial-palmar grasp	7	5-8	
Radial-digital grasp	9	6-10	
Fine pincer grasp	10	9-12	No pincer by 12 mo
Scribbles spontaneously	15	12-24	
Builds tower of 2-4 blocks; turns 2-3 pages of a book at one time	18	13-20	Consistent handedness before 18 mo
Imitates vertical strokes; turns single pages of book	24	19-36	
Builds tower of 8-10 blocks	30	21+	
Cuts with scissors	36	28+	
Copies circle	36	32+	Inability to copy lines by 3 yr
Opposes thumb to fingers; laces shoes	48	40+	
Copies square	54	48+	
Copies triangle	60	48+	
Draws person with face, arms, legs; ties a knot in a string	60	40+	

Table 2-3   Cognitive Milestones

Skill	Age of Acquisition (Average Month)	Clues to Delays/Problems
Follows a dangling ring to and past midline; facial response to bell ring	2	Limited interest in sights/sounds
Swipes at dangling ring; looks from hand to object	4	
Stares at spot where object disappeared	1-4	
Visually follows dropped object	4-8	
Finds hidden object	9-12	
Recovers hidden object after multiple visible changes of placement of the object	12-18	Mouthing toys at 12 mo
Symbolic play centered on self	12-18	No symbolic play at 24 mo
Understands causal mechanisms	18-24	
Symbolic play directed toward dolls/toys	18-24	
Points to pictures when named	18-24	
Uses magical and egocentric thinking	24-60	
Understands spatial relationships ("in," "on")	36	
Understands "same/different", asks 500 questions	48	
Understands number concepts	60	Inability to follow 3-step instructions at 60 mo
Begins to use concrete operational thinking	60+	Failure to know correct address and phone number
Understands differences between common objects (dog/bird; milk/water)	72	
Uses formal operational thinking	12 yr+	
Considers abstracts and hypotheticals	12 yr+	

Table 2-4 Language Milestones

Skills		Age of Acquisition (Average Month)	Clues to Delays/Problems
Receptive	**Expressive**		
Startles, eyes widen/blink to sound	Range of cries (hunger to pain)	0-3	Not responsive to sounds; hearing problem?
Head turns to sound; raises arms when caregiver says "up"	Babbles, repeats self-initiated sounds	4-9	Not attentive to voices; no vocalizations
Responds to name	Repeats parent-initiated sounds (early babbling)	9-10	Not responsive to own name
Understands and selectively responds to familiar words (e.g., "no")	Complex babbling (jargon)	9-12	Does not notice or care about other people
	First words	9-12	No babbling with consonant sounds
	Symbolic gestures	9-12	
Recognizes body parts and common objects by name; understands up to 50 words	Uses single words (up to 50)	12-18	No pointing; does not understand "baby words"
	Uses words to express needs		
Follows one- or two-step commands	Uses two-word telegraphic sentences ("up," Daddy"); says up to 75 words	18-24	No words at all by 24 mo; does not follow simple request by 24 mo
Points to pictures; comprehends 150 words	Decreased jargon, 2- to 3-word sentences	18-24	
Points to pictures when asked	Begins use of longer (>3-word) sentences; says over 200 words	24	Vowel sounds but no consonants; completely unintelligible to caregivers

Continued

Table 2-4 Language Milestones—cont'd

Skills		Age of Acquisition (Average Month)	Clues to Delays/Problems
Receptive	**Expressive**		
Follows two-step commands	Learns pronouns; articulation: 50% intelligible	24	Fewer than 50 words; no 2-word sentences
Knows color, past/future	Uses longer sentences; articulation: 75% intelligible	36	Many omissions of initial consonants
Can answer questions like "What do we do when sleepy?"	Begins to use negatives Begins to ask questions; may repeat words/phrases (developmental dysfluency)	36	Speech mostly unintelligible to strangers Wants television louder than peers; speech dependent on gestures Stuttering accompanied by facial grimaces
Follows three- to four-step commands; completes opposite analogies ("A brother is a boy; a sister is a ——")	Uses past tense; enjoys exaggerations; articulation: 100% intelligible	48	
Understands all that is within cognitive level ("if," "when," "why")	Has vocabulary of 1500 to 2000 words Uses adult grammatical forms; can tell stories, personal anecdotes; detailed, long-winded descriptions May have persistent difficulties with sounds (r, s, z, ch, sh)	60+	Word endings dropped for plurals, past tense; faulty sentence structure; unusual use of pronouns; abnormal rate, rhythm, articulation, modulation Inability to tell a story about a personal experience suggests potential problems with school readiness

Table 2-5   Social-Emotional Milestones

Domain	Skills	Age of Acquisition (Average Months)	Clues to Delays/Problems
Attachment	Smiles spontaneously but is indiscriminate in social preferences	4-6	No smile by 3 mo
	Recognizes parent	6	Lack of interest in parent or excessive attachment to caregiver or examiner
	Fear of separation	6-8	
	Begins to show differential response to strangers	7-9	No response to parental affection
Social play	Begins exploration further from parents	12	
	Does not want to share	12-15	
	Begins pretend play	15	No imitation by 18 mo
	Displays predominantly parallel play	24	
	Begins interactive imaginative play	36	Overt aggressiveness toward other children/adults
Sense of self	Understands sharing and turn taking	36-48	Inability to form friendships
	Begins to think of rules as fixed	48-60	Difficulty sticking to play activity
	Successfully works in groups	8 yr+	Limited eye contact
	Shows interest (pats) mirror image	6	
	Assumes active role in feeding	6-9	
	Self-feeds	12-15	

Continued

Table 2-5 Social-Emotional Milestones—cont'd

Domain	Skills	Age of Acquisition (Average Months)	Clues to Delays/Problems
Sense of self—cont'd	Happy when mastering a task	18-24	No interest in mastering a task; excessively low threshold for frustration
	Develops autonomy in toileting, dressing, conversing	24-36	
	Knows name	24	
	Assumes greater initiative	36	
	Dresses independently	48	
	Plays collaboratively	48	
	May have imaginary friend	48	
	Develops sense of industry	60	
	Engages in and enjoys competition	8 yr+	No interest in group activity
	Fear of ridicule, failure, catastrophe	6-11 yr	
	Identified with peer groups (prefers friends to family)	10-13 yr	Persistence of imaginary friends
	Concern over physical changes, exclusion from peers, sexual fears	12-17 years	
	Initiates intimate relationships	14-16 yr+	Excessive identification with risk-taking peer group; persistence of concrete thought processes
	Identifies plans for future	16-18 yr+	Vague and unrealistic plan for future

(1) The ontogeny of innate reflexes (Moro, tonic neck, step, walk) leads the way to proper motor development.

(2) Nerve myelination occurs in a cephalic-to-caudal direction; likewise for maturation of motor processes. Note that the development of children's drawings proceeds in a similar manner: Young children draw the head/face as the largest body part; only as they age do body proportion and detail appear in their drawings.

b. Fine motor milestones: A midline-to-distal maturation allows fine-tuning of fine motor skills.

c. Cognitive milestones

(1) Innate visual, auditory, and other sensory capacities evolve and facilitate normal cognitive development.

(2) The Piagetian stages of development underlie the organization of cognition as one moves from sensorimotor (birth to 2 years), to preoperational (2 to 6 years), to concrete operational (6 to 11 years), to abstract (formal operational, 11 years to adult) reasoning.

d. Language milestones

(1) The attention to auditory stimuli and verbal/nonverbal cues prepares for successful language development.

(2) Preverbal communications (pointing, banging) develop into early output restrictions (babbling, jargon, hesitancies) and finally into increasing differentiation (fluent, intelligible speech).

e. Social-emotional milestones

(1) The attention to visual (facial) and auditory cues (reciprocal cooing) creates the framework for social acquisition.

(2) Freudian/neo-Freudian (Erikson) theories of psychodevelopment form an analytic framework for understanding normal and abnormal social interactions.

2.7 Immunizations

RECOMMENDED CHILDHOOD IMMUNIZATION SCHEDULE—UNITED STATES

The Advisory Committee on Immunization Practices (ACIP), the American Academy of Pediatrics (AAP), and the American Academy of Family Physicians (AAFP) have developed a unified childhood immunization schedule (see Appendix VIII-B). Vaccines are listed under the routinely recommended ages. Bars indicate range of acceptable ages for vaccination. Shaded bars indicate catch-up vaccination: at 11 to 12 years of age, hepatitis B vaccine should be administered to children not previously vaccinated. A new tetanus and diphtheria toxoids with acellular pertussis (Tdap [Boostrix]) vaccine is now routinely recommended at the 11- to 12-year-old visit as well. Varicella zoster virus vaccine should be administered to children not previously vaccinated who lack a reliable history of chickenpox.

The meningococcal conjugate vaccine is also recommended at the 11- to 12-year-old visit, the 15-year-old visit, or at college entry. Hepatitis A vaccine is now routinely recommended in most states starting at 12 to 18 months of age, with a booster 6 to 12 months after the first one is given. Visit the Centers for Disease Control and Prevention (CDC) website (www.cdc.gov) for travel information regarding immunizations. Other vaccines, such as human papilloma virus vaccine and rotavirus vaccine, will soon be added to the schedule. Consult the AAP website (www.aap.org) or the latest (2006) edition of the AAP *Red Book* for up-to-date vaccine schedules.

RECOMMENDED ACCELERATED IMMUNIZATION SCHEDULE FOR CHILDREN NOT IMMUNIZED IN THE FIRST YEAR OF LIFE

Appendix VIII-C gives catch-up schedules and minimum intervals between doses. There is no need to restart a vaccine series regardless of the time that has elapsed between doses.

SPECIAL CONSIDERATIONS

1. Hepatitis B vaccine: Infants born to hepatitis B surface antigen–negative mothers should receive the second dose between 1 and 4 months. At least 1 month should have elapsed between the first and second dose. Infants born to hepatitis B surface antigen–positive mothers, or whose mothers' immune status is unknown, should receive both hepatitis B immune globulin 0.5 mL IM within 12 hours of birth and hepatitis B vaccine at a separate site. The second dose should be given at 1 month and the third at 6 months.

2. Diphtheria and tetanus toxoids and acellular pertussis (DTaP): The fourth dose of DTaP may be given at 12 months of age, provided at least 6 months have elapsed since the third dose. Children younger than 7 years of age, in whom pertussis immunization is contraindicated (see Table 2-6 for contraindications), should receive diphtheria-tetanus (DT). Children older than 7 years of age should receive tetanus/diphtheria (Td). After the initial childhood immunizations, Tdap should be administered every 10 years to ensure continued immunity against tetanus, diphtheria, and pertussis. A fifth dose of DTaP is not necessary if the fourth dose was given after the fourth birthday.

3. *Haemophilus influenzae* type b (Hib): Three different Hib vaccines are available. Children who receive the Hib PRP-OMP (meningococcal protein conjugate), manufactured by Merck Sharp & Dohme as Pedvax-HIB, at 2 and 4 months of age do *not* need a third dose at 6 months of age. Only one dose should be given between the ages of 15 and 59 months, even in children who did not complete the initial series. The minimum recommended interval between doses is 2 months, but to "catch up," a minimum interval of 1 month between doses can be used.

4. Inactivated poliovirus vaccine (IPV): The use of oral poliovirus vaccine in the United States has been discontinued because only vaccine-associated cases have been reported in the United States for decades. A minimum of 6 weeks is recommended between doses. When someone is traveling to an area endemic for polio, the schedule can be accelerated by giving doses at 4-week intervals. A fourth IPV is not necessary if the third dose was given after the fourth birthday.

5. Mumps, measles, rubella (MMR): The second dose of MMR should be administered at either 4 to 6 years or 11 to 12 years of age, depending on the state regulations for school entry requirements (see Table 2-6).

The first dose must be given after the first birthday. A minimum interval of 1 month between doses is recommended. A combination vaccine of MMR with varicella vaccine (MMR/V) has been recently approved.

6. Varicella: The live attenuated varicella vaccine was approved in March, 1995 for use in individuals 12 months of age or older who have not had varicella. The AAP currently recommends:

a. One dose at the 12-month-old visit (in combination with MMR or MMR/V)

b. A booster at the 4- to 6-year-old visit (also in combination with MMR or MMRV), or

c. A booster to all children older than 4 years who have already received their second MMR. Recommendations may change.

7. Contraindications to specific vaccines may be found in Table 2-6.

2.8 Accidents and Injury Prevention

Any significant accidents (e.g., burns) or injuries (e.g., fractures), especially those requiring hospitalization, need to be noted. Serious consideration for maltreatment/neglect needs to be entertained whenever a child is encountered with multiple, recurring, or suspect injuries (e.g., unwitnessed injuries in unusual locations).

EPIDEMIOLOGY OF ACCIDENTS AND INJURIES IN CHILDHOOD

1. Before 1 year of age, choking/suffocation accounts for a large portion (73%) of injury-related deaths.

2. After the first year of life, motor vehicle accidents (MVAs) are the leading cause of death in all childhood age groups; almost half of all deaths in children 1 to 14 years of age are due to injuries.

3. MVAs (including pedestrian) account for over 60% of all injury deaths.

4. Before 5 years of age, in addition to MVAs, burns and drownings are significant causes of mortality.

5. Falls, poisonings, tap-water scalds, and sports-related injuries are significant causes of morbidity and result in visits to emergency departments.

6. Intentional or inflicted injury (child abuse, homicide, suicide) may account for up to 25% or more of injury-related deaths in certain populations.

PREVENTION

In 1983, the APP introduced The Injury and Prevention Program (TIPP) to help health care professionals dispense sound safety advice using a minimum of time and expense. The program focuses on developmentally appropriate preventive strategies and is continuously undergoing revisions (see AAP website).

2.9 Screening

The purpose of this section is to familiarize the reader with general principles of health screening and to provide an overview to screening in an outpatient setting for specific pediatric conditions.

Table 2-6 Guide to Contraindications and Precautions to Immunizations

	Contraindications and Precautions	
Vaccine	True (Vaccines May Not Be Given)	Not True (Vaccines May Be Given)
General for all vaccines	Anaphylactic reaction to a vaccine contraindicates further doses of that vaccine	Mild to moderate local reaction (soreness, redness, swelling) after a dose of an injectable antigen
	Anaphylactic reaction to a vaccine constituent contraindicates the use of vaccines containing that substance	Mild acute illness with or without low-grade fever
DTP, DTaP, OPV, IPV, MMR, Hib, HBV, Tdap	Moderate or severe illnesses with or without a fever	Current antimicrobial therapy
		Convalescent phase of illnesses
		Prematurity (same dosage and indications as for normal, full-term infants)
		Recent exposure to an infectious disease
		History of penicillin or other nonspecific allergies or fact that relatives have such allergies
DTP/DTaP	Encephalopathy within 7 days of administration of previous dose of DTP	Temperature of <40.5° C (105° F) after a prior dose of DTP
	Precautions*	Family history of convulsions*
	Fever of ≥40.5° C (105° F) within 48 hr after vaccination with a prior dose of DTP	Family history of sudden infant death syndrome
	Collapse or shocklike state (hypotonic-hyporesponsive episode) within 48 hr of receiving a prior dose of DTP	Family history of an adverse event after DTP administration
	Seizures within 3 days of receiving a prior dose of DTP†	
	Persistent, inconsolable crying lasting ≥3 hr within 48 hr of receiving a prior dose of DTP	

OPV‡	Infection with HIV or a household contact with HIV infection Known altered immunodeficiency (hematologic and solid tumors; congenital immunodeficiency; long-term immunosuppressive therapy) Immunodeficient household contact **Precaution**° Pregnancy	Breast-feeding Current antimicrobial therapy Diarrhea
IPV	Anaphylactic reaction to neomycin or streptomycin **Precaution**° Pregnancy	

This information is based on the recommendations of the Advisory Committee on Immunization Practices (ACIP) and those of the Committee on Infectious Diseases (Red Book Committee) of the American Academy of Pediatrics (AAP), 2006. Sometimes these recommendations vary from those contained in the manufacturers' package inserts. For more detailed information, providers should contact the published recommendations of the ACIP, the AAP, the AAFP, and the manufacturers' package inserts.

*The event or conditions listed as precautions, although not contraindications, should be carefully reviewed. The benefits and risks of administering a specific vaccine to an individual under the circumstances should be considered. If the risks are believed to outweigh the benefits, the immunization should be withheld; if the benefits are believed to outweigh the risks (e.g., during an outbreak or foreign travel), the immunization should be given. Whether and when to administer DTP to children with proven or suspected underlying neurologic disorders should be decided on an individual basis. It is prudent on theoretical grounds to avoid vaccinating pregnant women. However, if immediate protection against poliomyelitis is needed, OPV, not IPV, is recommended.

†Acetaminophen given before administering DTP and thereafter every 4 hr for 24 hr should be considered for children with a personal or family history of convulsions in siblings or parents.

DTaP, diphtheria and tetanus toxoids and acellular pertussis vaccine; DTP, diphtheria, tetanus, pertussis vaccine; HBV, hepatitis B vaccine; Hib, *Haemophilus influenzae* type b vaccine; IPV, inactivated poliovirus vaccine; IVIG, intravenous immune globulin; MMR, measles, mumps, rubella vaccine; OPV, oral poliovirus vaccine; Tdap, tetanus and diphtheria toxoids with acellular pertussis vaccine; VZIG, varicella zoster immune globulin.

Continued

Table 2-6 Guide to Contraindications and Precautions to Immunizations—cont'd

Vaccine	Contraindications and Precautions	
	True (Vaccines May Not Be Given)	Not True (Vaccines May Be Given)
MMR[‡]	Anaphylactic reactions to egg ingestion and to neomycin[§] Pregnancy Known altered immunodeficiency (hematologic and solid tumors; congenital immunodeficiency; long-term immunosuppressive therapy) **Precaution*** Recent (within 3 mo) immune globulin administration	Tuberculosis or positive PPD Simultaneous TB skin testing[¶] Breast-feeding Pregnancy of mother of recipient Immunodeficient family member or household contact Infection with HIV Nonanaphylactic reactions to eggs or neomycin
Hib HBV Varicella	Immunocompromised patients (except patients with cancer under protocol) Pregnancy Anaphylactic reaction to neomycin Active, untreated tuberculosis Any febrile respiratory illness or other active febrile infection Family history of congenital or hereditary immunodeficiency (unless patient's immunocompetence can be demonstrated) **Precautions** Pregnancy should be avoided for 3 mo after vaccination	Pregnancy Immunodeficient or HIV-positive family or household contact Pregnancy of mother of recipient Nonanaphylactic reactions to neomycin

Defer vaccination for at least 5 mo after blood or plasma transfusions, or administration of IVIG or VZIG

IVIG or VZIG should not be given at least 2 mo after vaccination

Lactation

Salicylates should be avoided for 6 wk after vaccination because of the risk of developing Reye's syndrome

Vaccinees in whom a rash develops should avoid contact with immunocompromised susceptible hosts for the duration of the rash

†There is a theoretical risk that administration of multiple live virus vaccines (OPV and MMR) within 30 days of one another if not given on the same day will result in a suboptimal immune response. There are no data to substantiate this.

§Persons with a history of anaphylactic reactions after egg ingestion should be vaccinated only with extreme caution. Protocols have been developed for vaccinating such persons and should be consulted (J Pediatr 102:196-199, 1983; J Pediatr 113:504-506, 1988).

¶Measles vaccination may temporarily suppress tuberculin reactivity. If testing can not be done the day of MMR vaccination, the test should be postponed for 4-6 weeks.

Used with permission of the American Academy of Pediatrics. Pickering LK, Baker CJ, Long SS, McMillan JA (eds): Red Book: 2006 Report of the Committee on Infectious Diseases, 27th ed. Elk Grove, Ill, American Academy of Pediatrics, 2006.

OVERALL GOAL OF HEALTH SCREENING

1. Purpose: The primary purpose is to screen *asymptomatic* patients and to detect diseases/disorders/conditions whose morbidity and mortality can be reduced by early detection and treatment.
2. Health screening measures for specified conditions: Box 2-5 lists conditions that are under the screening purview of the pediatric primary care provider.

SCREENING FOR METABOLIC CONDITIONS IN NEONATES

1. Who to screen: In addition to routine neonatal screening (as outlined in Chapter 5), consider metabolic screening in any newborn with the following conditions:
   a. Vomiting, lethargy, poor feeding
   b. Apparent sepsis
   c. Apparent cardiac disease
   d. Seizures
   e. Hypoglycemia
   f. Jaundice
   g. Acidosis/ketonuria
   h. Dysmorphism
   i. Unusual odors
2. If an infant has hyperammonemia as well as acidosis, think of *organic acidemias* (methylmalonic acidemia); if hyperammonemia alone (i.e., without acidosis/ketosis), think of an *inborn error of ureagenesis* (ornithine transcarbamylase deficiency, citrullinemia).

VISION SCREENING

1. Purposes of vision screening are to detect:
   a. Correctable eye problems that could lead to blindness or interfere with appropriate development and education.
   b. Potential systemic/organic condition (e.g., central nervous system lesions).
   Note: All children should be screened at birth, during the first year of life, then every 2 to 3 years thereafter.
2. Vision screening in newborns/infants
   a. Examination: Attempt to assess the following:
      (1) Red reflex: To rule out cataracts, retinoblastoma (leukokoria, so-called "cat's eye"), and optic nerve problems
      (2) Fixation
         (a) Position of corneal light reflex in reference to center of cornea
         (b) With alternating eyes occluded (cover test)
         (c) With both eyes open
      (3) Following
         (a) Monocular, then binocular movement
         (b) Right eye by infants with esotropia to fixate and follow objects in left visual field, and vice versa
      (4) Acuity/alignment: Intermittent esotropia is quite common in the newborn infant. If not intermittent or persistent after 6 weeks of age, refer to ophthalmologist.

Box 2-5   Conditions Screened by the Pediatric Care Provider

By Physical Examination

Cataracts
Developmental dislocation of the hip
Congenital or acquired heart disease
Cryptorchidism
Dental problems
Genetic syndromes
Glaucoma
Growth failure/acceleration
Lymphadenopathy
Scoliosis/musculoskeletal problems
Strabismus
Tumors (benign and malignant)

By Laboratory Investigation

Anemia
Hypothyroidism
Branched-chain ketoaciduria
Phenylketonuria
Homocystinuria   } Newborn screen
Cystic fibrosis
Galactosemia
Tyrosinemia
Hypercholesterolemia
Neuroblastoma
Methylmalonic aciduria
Glucose-6-phosphate dehydrogenase (G-6-PD) deficiency
Lead intoxication
Tay-Sachs disease
Sickle cell anemia
Thalassemia
Bacteriuria
Hematuria
Proteinuria

By In-Office Procedures

Height and weight (head circumference in infants)
Blood pressure
Auditory screening/middle ear disease
Vision screening (visual acuity)
Developmental assessments (include language and speech)
Tuberculin skin testing

(a) Difficult to assess in infancy; usually accomplished by assessing fixation (alignment) pattern

(b) Pupillary constriction and blinking/closing to bright light (suggests an intact pathway to the visual cortex)

(c) Possible problem indicated by induced nystagmus (by rotating the infant) that does not abate within 15 to 30 seconds

b. Guidelines for referral of newborns/infants

(1) Presence of risk factors (family history of retinoblastoma, congenital cataracts, genetic/metabolic disease)

(2) Abnormal/unobtainable red reflex at any age

(3) Nystagmus at birth

(4) Lack of response (constriction, blinking) to bright light in infancy

(5) Inability to fixate steadily in one or both eyes by 3 to 4 months

(6) Objection to occlusion of one eye (i.e., poor vision in the non-occluded eye will make the infant anxious)

(7) Any parental concern

3. Vision screening in preverbal children

a. Examination: The purpose of the examination in this age group is to detect amblyopia (diminished vision from suppression of images) or problems that lead to amblyopia (i.e., strabismus—see later discussion). By 6 months of age, fixation and following are well developed.

b. Procedures

(1) Attempt to compare visual acuity of one eye with other eye (have child fix on toys, first at a distance, then nearby with each eye separately).

(2) Screen at least once in first year of life.

(3) Diagnostic procedures

(a) Corneal light reflex test

(i) Child fixated on light

(ii) Light reflected off of cornea

(iii) Normally, light aligned symmetrically in both pupils

(iv) Esotropia: Light reflex deviated temporally away from pupil in deviated eye; exotropia: reflex displaced nasally in deviated eye

(b) Cover test (Fig. 2-3): Diagnostic for tropias and phorias

c. Strabismus (squint): The most common clinical finding

(1) Affects 4% of children younger than 6 years; 30% to 50% have secondary visual problems.

(2) Misalignment results in amblyopia, impaired depth perception (loss of fusion), and poor cosmetic appearance.

(3) Can be almost latent (phoria) or constantly present (tropia)

(4) Types (Fig. 2-4)

(a) Esotropia (inward deviation)

(i) Represents 50% to 75% of all cases of strabismus

(ii) Congenital/infantile, before 6 months

(iii) Alternate fixation: Each eye takes turn in deviating; less likely to develop amblyopia

(iv) Constant fixation: One eye always turned in; associated with amblyopia

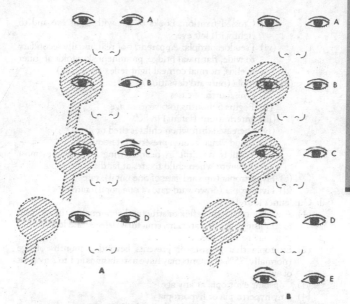

Figure 2-3 **A,** Cover test demonstrating a tropia. *A,* Right eye fixating and an esotropia is present on left. *B,* Bring cover in front of right eye. *C,* Left eye makes a refixation movement outward to maintain fixation on object. *D,* If right eye is the preferred eye for fixation, as cover is removed it will straighten out and left eye will turn in. **B,** Cover test demonstrating a phoria. *A,* Eyes are straight. *B,* Bring cover in front of right eye. *C,* Fusion is disrupted, and right eye drifts outward under cover (exophoria). *D,* Binocularity is reestablished when cover is removed. *E,* A refixation movement inward to maintain fusion and ocular alignment is quickly made by the exophoric eye. Eyes are straight. (Adapted from Magramm I: Amblyopia: Etiology, detection, and treatment. Pediatr Rev 13:7-14, 1992. Elk Grove Village, Ill, American Academy of Pediatrics, 1992.)

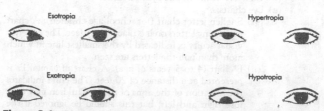

Figure 2-4 Types of strabismus. Note displaced corneal light reflex in misaligned eye. (Adapted from Magramm I: Amblyopia: Etiology, detection, and treatment. Pediatr Rev 13:7-14, 1992. Elk Grove Village, Ill, American Academy of Pediatrics, 1992.)

      (v) Crossed fixation: Looks to left with right eye and to right with left eye

      (vi) Pseudoesotropia: Apparent, not real, usually secondary to wide, flat nasal bridge, prominent skin folds at inner eyelids; normal corneal light reflex (centered)

    (b) Exotropia (outward deviation)

      (i) One fourth of cases

      (ii) Begins 6 months to 6 years of age

      (iii) Intermittent (latent) in 80%

      (iv) Increased drift when child is tired or ill

      (v) Good visual acuity; preserved stereovision

      (vi) Possibly no drift in near viewing but becomes most apparent when child fixates at far distance

    (c) Hypertropia (upward gaze of one pupil): rare

    (d) Hypotropia (downward gaze of one pupil): rare

  d. Guidelines for referral

    (1) Any abnormal light reflex or structural abnormality (in addition to strabismus, subtle cataracts, structural defects, and leukokoria) that may be identified

    (2) Esotropia that persists or presents beyond 3 months of age (normally, 75% of infants may have a strabismus at 1 to 2 months of age)

    (3) Constant exotropia at any age

    (4) Any hypertropia or hypotropia

4. Vision screening in preschool/school-age children

  a. Examination: The purpose of the examination in this age group is to identify amblyopia (in this age group, it is likely to be secondary to refractive or focusing errors). Three major types of problems are possible:

    (1) Myopia (near-sightedness—main reason that children fail vision test)

    (2) Hyperopia (far-sightedness)

    (3) Astigmatism: Light rays in two medians out of focus

  b. Diagnostic tests

    (1) Tests for acuity

      (a) Acuity screening should begin by age 3 years.

      (b) Compare acuity in one eye at a time.

      (c) Eye charts:

        (i) Snellen letter chart (for school-age children): A chart with many letters on it is placed at 20 feet. The patient's visual acuity is indicated by the smallest line in which more than half the letters are seen.

        (ii) E chart (4 to 5 years of age): A chart of capital Es is presented at a distance of 20 feet. The child indicates the direction of the arms of the E. Children may confuse right and left, but this should be ignored if the child can accurately and easily distinguish the horizontal Es from the vertical ones.

        (iii) HOTV chart (3 to 5 years of age): A chart with a combination of different-sized letters limited to H, O, T,

and V is presented 10 feet from the child while the child holds a card with the letters H, O, T, and V printed on it. The child is asked to match the letter pointed at by the examiner to the corresponding card held by the child.
  (iv) Picture recognition (2.5 to 3 years of age): A chart (Allen card) with pictures is held at 16 inches or projected over a known distance.

> Tips: Younger children often have difficulty concentrating at 20 feet, so bring the chart closer. The only disadvantage is that near vision is always better than distance, even with an impairment. Be certain that the untested eye is well covered: otherwise the test will not pick up the amblyopia because the child will peek to see better and to please the examiner.

  (2) Tests for stereoacuity: May be performed in children 4 years of age and older, although full maturity of stereopsis does not occur until about 6 years.
  c. Guidelines for referral of older children:
    (1) Decrease in vision (20/40 or less) in one or both eyes
    (2) Any decrease in both distance and near acuity (suggests astigmatism or organic problem)
    (3) Persistent or difficult-to-treat "pink eye" (suggests uveitis)
    (4) Photophobia (uveitis)
    (5) Excessive tearing, dry eyes
    (6) Droopy or malpositioned lids
    (7) Suspect lesions around the eyes
    (8) Change in color, size, shape of pupil
    (9) Hazy, blurred, double vision, or floating objects
Note: Wearing glasses neither prevents nor hastens the development of myopia—it only allows the child to see better.

AUDITORY SCREENING

1. Purpose of hearing screening: To detect hearing loss that will interfere with the normal development of speech and oral language. A hearing loss of 30 dB or more in the frequency range for speech recognition (500 to 4000 Hz) will interfere with normal development.
2. Etiologies: Two basic etiologies are associated with hearing loss in children: sensorineural hearing loss and conductive hearing loss.
  a. Sensorineural hearing loss (SNHL)
    (1) Major forms
      (a) Congenital (detected at birth or later): 1.5 to 6.0 per 1000 births
        (i) Genetic: 50% of all SNHL, usually autosomal recessive, or secondary to syndromes (e.g., neurofibromatosis)
        (ii) Nongenetic: Secondary to effects on maternal/fetal environment (e.g., cytomegalovirus [CMV] infection, rubella, ototoxic drugs, anoxia, prematurity)
      (b) Acquired after birth: Usually not associated with anomalies and can have multiple etiologies:
        (i) Bacterial infection (e.g., meningitis—SNHL can occur in 20% of cases)

    (ii) Viral infection (e.g., mumps, labyrinthitis)
    (iii) Ototoxic drugs
    (iv) Trauma (rock concerts at 110 dB)
    (v) Metabolic disorders (renal disease, hypothyroidism)
    (vi) Autoimmune/neoplastic disorders
   (2) Most children born with SNHL have no associated defects
  b. Conductive hearing loss (CHL): By 2 years of age, 1 child in 25 will have mild to moderate (i.e., 15 to 20 dB) loss. Causes:
   (1) Middle ear disease (acute otitis media; otitis media with effusion [OME])
   (2) Foreign body (cerumen)
 3. Universal hearing screening is now provided for all neonates in the United States.
  a. Infants and children (29 days through 2 years of age) when *certain health conditions* occur should undergo rescreening. These include:
   (1) Parent/caregiver concern
   (2) Bacterial meningitis and other infections associated with SNHL
   (3) Head trauma (loss of consciousness or skull fracture)
   (4) Stigmata associated with syndromes known to include SNHL or CHL
   (5) Ototoxic medications (chemotherapeutic agents, aminoglycosides, loop diuretics)
   (6) Recurrent or persistent otitis media with effusion for at least 3 months
  b. Infants and children (20 days through 3 years of age) who require *periodic monitoring* of hearing to detect delayed-onset SNHL or CHL. Infants and children with these indicators require hearing evaluation at least every 6 months until 3 years of age and at appropriate intervals thereafter. Indicators associated with delayed-onset SNHL include the following:
   (1) Family history of hereditary childhood hearing loss
   (2) In utero infection (CMV, rubella, syphilis, herpes, toxoplasmosis)
   (3) Neurofibromatosis type II and neurodegenerative disorders
  c. Indicators associated with CHL
   (1) Recurrent or persistent OME
   (2) Anatomic deformities and other disorders that affect eustachian tube function
   (3) Neurodegenerative disorders
 4. Screening and diagnostic techniques
  a. Infants
   (1) Careful observation: Along with asking the caretaker directly if the infant hears, observation is the most practical method with which to screen for adequate hearing in infancy. One can observe the infant's head turning or body startling to a bell or other loud noise; this will usually detect only severe (70 dB or more) loss.
   (2) Otologic examination: In young infants it is difficult to obtain adequate visualization.
   (3) Brain stem evoked auditory response

(a) This state-of-the-art technique assesses the integrity of the eighth cranial nerve and brain stem auditory pathways by measuring stimulus-contingent, synchronous discharges of auditory neurons.

(b) It does not give frequency-specific threshold information but provides a reasonable estimate of hearing sensitivity in the frequencies normally associated with human speech (2 to 4 kHz).

b. Toddlers
  (1) Pneumo-otoscopic examination: Carefully performed, pneumatic otoscopy is the standard for screening and diagnosing middle-ear disease in this and older age groups.
  (2) Tympanometry/impedance audiometry
    (a) Most reliable in children older than 12 months of age and an important adjunct to otoscopy
    (b) Quantifies middle-ear pressure, tympanic membrane and ossicular mobility, eustachian tube function, acoustic and tactile stapedius muscle reflexes, and tensor tympani muscle reflex
    (c) Using the acoustic reflex, a 70- to 90-dB pure tone stimulation is provided to the cochlear nerve (cranial nerve VIII), which leads to reflex contraction of the stapedial muscle (cranial nerve VII), which in turn causes stiffening of the tympanic membrane.
    (d) *Not* a hearing test, but "hearing" (i.e., conductive hearing) can be extrapolated from the response. Tympanometry will detect 93% of severe cases and 50% of moderate cases of SNHL.
    (e) Most advantageous for the diagnosis of middle-ear effusion (85% or higher specific)—that is, children who have or have had chronic/persistent otitis media or OME.
    (f) Figure 2-5 illustrates the three basic types of curves generated by the tympanogram and how to interpret the curves when evaluating a child.
c. Preschool/school-age: The goal in this age group (and older) is to detect even mild (15- to 20-dB) hearing loss.
  (1) Pneumo-otoscopic examination
  (2) Tympanometry/impedance audiometry
  (3) Pure tone audiometry—can be performed in schools and office settings

5. Guidelines for referral for formal audiologic evaluation
a. Parental/health professional concern
b. High-risk infants (as noted earlier)
c. Older children
  (1) Failure to hear stimulus at two different frequencies in one ear at 25 dB
  (2) Failure to respond to 1 or 2 kHz or two of the three higher frequencies
d. Persistently abnormal tympanogram (flat or abnormal curves that are present on serial evaluations over 2 to 3 months, especially if

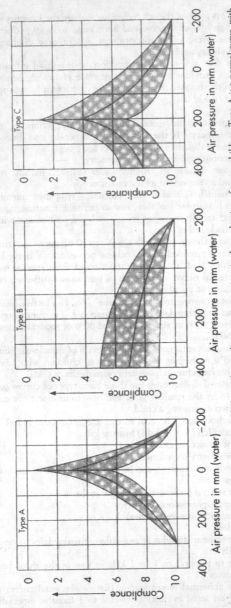

Figure 2-5 Use of impedance audiometry to help confirm audiometric impressions in the evaluation of young children. Type A is a normal curve, with normal tympanic membrane compliance. Type B is a curve showing middle ear effusion, consistent with acute otitis media or otitis media with effusion (OME). Type C is a curve showing normal to slight effusion, consistent with resolving OME. (Adapted from Frankenburg WK: Screening: General considerations. In Hoekelman RA [ed]: Pediatric Care. St. Louis, Mosby, 1987.)

abnormality is bilateral, in a child 24 months of age or younger) or an elevated threshold (100 dB or more) of the acoustic reflex response
    e. Abnormal language development (especially receptive)
    f. Poor behavioral/socialization skills
    g. Poor school performance (e.g., attention deficit hyperactivity disorder)

ANEMIA

1. Purpose of screening for anemia: to detect
    a. Correctable nutritional anemias (e.g., iron deficiency)
    b. Genetically determined anemias (hemoglobinopathies)
    c. Anemias secondary to generalized/systemic disorders. The work-up, differential diagnosis, and management of anemia are discussed in Chapter 14.
2. Caveats on anemia and screening tests
    a. In infancy, there exists a normal physiologic nadir of hemoglobin (Hb) secondary to normal red cell death, termed *physiologic anemia of infancy*. It occurs at:
       (1) 8 to 12 weeks in full-term infants (Hb = 10 g/dL)
       (2) 6 to 8 weeks in premature infants (Hb = 8 g/dL)
    b. Most pediatric anemia is microcytic (to determine the lower limit of the mean corpuscular volume [MCV], add 70 to the age of child after 2 years of age).
    c. Iron deficiency (Fe def) and thalassemia trait are the most common pediatric anemias.
    d. Mentzer index: (MCV ÷ red blood cell count) > 13 = Fe def; < 11 = thalassemia minor
    e. Free erythrocyte protoporphyrin is elevated (>50 µg/dL whole blood) in Fe def (and very elevated in significant lead intoxication).
    f. Red cell distribution width, calculated as (standard deviation of MCV × 100)/MCV, is elevated (>15%) in Fe def, normal (11% to 14%) in thalassemia minor.
3. When/whom to screen
    a. Toddlers who preferentially prefer iron-poor cow's milk to iron-enriched solid foods
    b. Infants with history of significant jaundice in newborn period (suggests hemolytic anemia)
    c. Infants with an abnormal result on newborn screen for possible hemoglobinopathies (at 6 months of age)
    d. Healthy infants at 9 to 12 months of age; rapid growth and increased hemoglobin mass can outstrip iron intake. At this time, lead is also checked when indicated.
    e. Premature infants before 6 to 9 months of age
    f. Adolescents (pubertal growth spurt, menses). In girls, screen once at least 1 year after the onset of menses.
    g. Positive family history for hemoglobinopathies or hemolytic anemias (if the child is of Asian or European extraction, consider hemoglobin electrophoresis in parents).
    h. Immigrant children and those with special needs
4. Guidelines for referral, based on:
    a. Degree/type of anemia

    b. Lack of response to standard iron therapy for suspected Fe def
    c. Any anemia associated with pancytopenia, significant neutropenia, or thrombocytopenia or bleeding disorder
    d. Suspected underlying or systemic condition with an anemia out of proportion to expected

SCREENING FOR LEAD EXPOSURE

1. Purpose of lead screening: The purpose of screening for lead exposure is to identify (as early as possible) and follow up on children with a significant lead burden that, if untreated, may place them at risk for physiologic and neurocognitive sequelae. The treatment of lead exposure is discussed in Chapter 24.
2. Caveats
    a. A blood level of 0 to 9 µg/dL is considered normal.
    b. A blood level of 10 µg/dL or more is concerning and suggests lead exposure.
    c. Adverse effects (neurobehavioral disturbances) can occur at blood lead levels of 10 µg/dL or more. These include subtle delays in cognitive and behavioral development such as distractibility, impulsiveness, hyperactivity, and sleep disturbances.
    d. Lead interferes with heme synthesis; at a level of 15 to 25 µg/dL or more, anemia (secondary iron deficiency) may develop and precipitate symptoms.
    e. Encephalopathy may develop with a blood lead level of 55 µg/dL or more.
3. Screening
    a. Age range to consider lead screening: 9 months to 3 years (and older if at high risk for significant exposure)
    b. Free-flowing, venous blood sample ideal; finger-stick acceptable but subject to contamination. An elevated level needs to be confirmed by a venous blood sample.
    c. Screening should begin at 9 to 12 months and be repeated again at 24 months, unless risk assessment is positive, in which case it should be performed more frequently.
    d. In conducting a risk assessment for significant exposure, ask parents:
        (1) Does your child:
            (a) Live in or regularly visit a house (e.g., day care center, preschool, the home of a babysitter or a relative) with peeling or chipping paint built before 1960?
            (b) Live in or regularly visit a house built before 1960 with recent, ongoing, or planned renovation or remodeling?
            (c) Have a brother or sister, housemate, or playmate being followed up or treated for lead poisoning (i.e., blood level of 10 µg/dL or more)?
            (d) Live with an adult whose job or hobby involves exposure to lead?
            (e) Live near an active lead smelter, battery recycling plant, or other industry likely to release lead?
        (2) A positive response to any question suggests the need for screening as frequently as *every 3 months* for some children depending

on risk and lead levels until 6 years of age. Symptomatic children require immediate diagnostic testing.
4. Recommended actions for child with lead poisoning (Table 2-7): Contacting state lead poison control can provide referral to a lead clinic; medical consultation; discharge planning; educational materials; nutrition information; and environmental inspections.

SCREENING FOR TUBERCULOSIS

1. Purposes of tuberculosis (TB) screening: To diagnose TB *infection* in asymptomatic individuals and to reduce the number of cases of symptomatic TB *disease*. The treatment of TB is discussed in Chapter 19.
2. Indications for testing and risk factors for the development of TB infection in children:
   a. Contacts with adults who have confirmed infectious TB (test immediately)
   b. Children immigrating from endemic areas (e.g., Asia, Middle East, Africa, Latin America) (test immediately)
   c. Any child with a clinical illness or an abnormality on a chest radiograph suggestive of TB (test immediately)
   d. Children who have spent more than 3 months traveling in endemic countries (test as soon as possible)
   e. Children with immunosuppressive conditions (cancer, HIV; test annually)
   f. Children with other medical risk factors (diabetes mellitus, chronic renal failure, malnutrition; test annually)
   g. Incarcerated adolescents (test annually)
   h. Children frequently exposed to high-risk adults (i.e., who have HIV infection or are homeless, users of intravenous and other street drugs, poor and medically indigent residents of nursing homes, migrant farm workers; test annually)
3. Recommendations for tuberculin skin test (TST)
   a. The recommended test is the Mantoux test, five tuberculin units of purified protein derivative (PPD).
   b. Routine annual TB testing of children with no risk factors in low-prevalence communities is not indicated. Alternative strategies are to test three times during childhood: 12 to 15 months, 4 to 6 years, and 14 to 16 years. This would especially apply to children who are at risk for progression of TB *infection* to TB *disease*. Examples include children with illness (e.g., diabetes, renal failure) or those on immunosuppressive medication.
   c. An initial TST should be performed on all children before initiation of immunosuppressive therapy (including prolonged steroid therapy).
   d. Children at high risk should be tested annually.
4. Interpretation of Mantoux test (Box 2-6)
   a. The test should be read by qualified medical personnel; parental interpretations may be inaccurate.
   b. Initial TB skin testing is usually done between 12 and 15 months of age, at the same time the MMR vaccine is given. If not done concurrently

Action	Blood Lead Levels			
	15-19 µg/dL	20-44 µg/dL	45-69 µg/dL	≥70 µg/dL
Venous confirmation		X	Urgent*	Emergency* during chelation
Medical treatment		X	Contraindicated therapy	
Consider iron supplements	X	X		X
Education and nutritional counseling	X	X	X	Emergency*
Environmental investigation and abatement	X†	X	Urgent	

*Recommended treatment at an experienced lead-poisoning clinic. Venous lead blood level ≥70 µg/dL requires inpatient chelation therapy. Inpatient therapy may also be needed for a blood level <70 µg/dL, if child has pica and environment unsafe or unknown.

For blood levels 15 to 19 µg/dL, environmental inspection and abatement should be conducted if resources permit.

†When consecutive tests obtained 3 to 4 mo apart are 15 to 19 µg/dL, environmental inspection and abatement should be conducted if resources permit.

> ### Box 2-6   Definition of Positive Tuberculin Skin Test (TST)
>
> *Results in Infants, Children, and Adolescents**
>
> - Induration ≥5 mm
>
> Children in close contact with known or suspected contagious cases of tuberculosis disease
>
> Children suspected to have tuberculosis disease:
>
> Findings on chest radiograph consistent with active or previously active tuberculosis
>
> Clinical evidence of tuberculosis disease[†]
>
> Children receiving immunosuppressive therapy[‡] or with immunosuppressive conditions, including HIV infection
>
> - Induration ≥10 mm
>
> Children at increased risk of disseminated disease:
>
> Those younger than 4 years of age
>
> Those with other medical conditions, including Hodgkin's disease, lymphoma, diabetes mellitus, chronic renal failure, or malnutrition
>
> Children with increased exposure to tuberculosis disease:
>
> Those born, or whose parents were born, in high-prevalence regions of the world
>
> Those frequently exposed to adults who are HIV infected, homeless, users of illicit drugs, residents of nursing homes, incarcerated or institutionalized, or migrant farm workers
>
> Those who travel to high-prevalence regions of the world
>
> - Induration ≥15 mm
>
> Children 4 years of age or older without any risk factors

*These definitions apply regardless of previous bacillus Calmette-Guérin (BCG) immunization; erythema at TST site does not indicate a positive test result. TSTs should be read at 48 to 72 hours after placement.

[†]Evidence by physical examination or laboratory assessment that would include tuberculosis in the working differential diagnosis (e.g., meningitis).

[‡]Including immunosuppressive doses of corticosteroids.

HIV, human immunodeficiency virus.

with MMR, testing should be postponed 4 to 6 weeks after MMR vaccination to prevent a false-negative result because the measles vaccine can temporarily suppress tuberculin reactivity.

SCREENING FOR CHOLESTEROL

1. Purpose: To identify individuals with elevated cholesterol levels—a potential risk factor for coronary heart disease. Low-density lipoproteins (LDL) have been associated with atherosclerotic heart disease in adults. Screening in this case is done to identify a risk factor, not a disease or condition. Elevated cholesterol (or LDL) may predispose to atherosclerosis, which in turn may cause coronary artery disease.

2. Ensure test accuracy with the following measures.
   a. Make sure the child is sitting up. Lying down for more than a few minutes can falsely lower the lipid and lipoprotein results.
   b. Instruct the child to fast for 12 hours (nothing to eat or drink except water) before a lipoprotein analysis or triglyceride determination. Fasting is not necessary for total blood cholesterol measurement.
   c. Do not test a child who is actively ill or has an infectious disease.
   d. Do not test pregnant adolescents.
   e. Evaluate adolescents for possible medication such as oral contraceptives, steroids, isotretinoin (Accutane), or phenobarbital, which can alter cholesterol levels.
   f. Use a well-standardized laboratory.
3. Cholesterol classification levels in children (Table 2-8)
4. Decision trees for risk assessment and clinical evaluation
   a. Risk assessment decision tree: Family history is a key factor in deciding when and whom to screen. Use the algorithm in Figure 2-6 to determine first whether the child (family) is at risk for hypercholesterolemia, then perform blood cholesterol.
   b. Clinical evaluation decision tree: Figure 2-7 provides guidelines on managing the patient if a lipoprotein analysis is obtained because of either positive family history or elevated blood cholesterol, or both.

2.10 Anticipatory Guidance

At each visit, the pediatrician should discuss with caretakers certain age-appropriate topics to prepare them in the months to come on what to expect from their child. These issues include physical and emotional changes, nutritional counseling, and safety concerns. The AAP has developed some guidelines to help clinicians cover these issues at every health maintenance visit (see AAP website). The following are *key* anticipatory guidance issues to cover at *each* visit. Note that issues such as nutrition, safety, and development are essential elements of every well-child visit.

PRENATAL VISIT

At this visit, you should discuss:
1. Feeding methods: Breast versus bottle
2. Effects of smoking, drugs, and alcohol on pregnancy and newborn

	Acceptable (75% of Children Screened)	Borderline (20%)	High (5%)
Total	<170 mg/dL	170-199 mg/dL	≥200 mg/dL
LDL	<110 mg/dL	110-129 mg/dL	≥130 mg/dL

LDL, low-density lipoprotein.

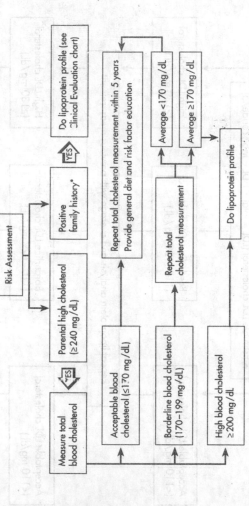

Figure 2-6   Hypercholesterolemia risk assessment in the child.
*Defined as a history of premature (before age 55) cardiovascular disease in a parent or grandparent.
(Adapted from National Cholesterol Education Program: Report of the Expert Panel on Blood Cholesterol Levels in Children and Adolescents. NIH publication no. 91-2732. Bethesda, Md, Department of Health and Human Services, Public Health Service, National Institutes of Health, National Heart, Lung, and Blood Institute, 1991.)

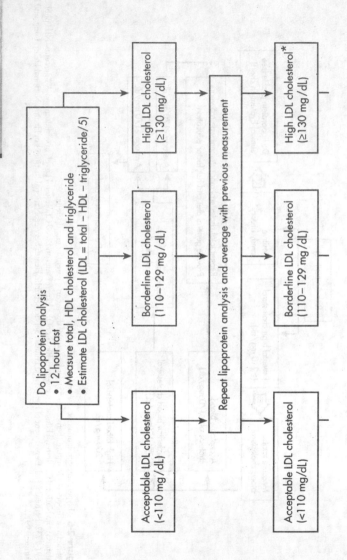

Do lipoprotein analysis
- 12-hour fast
- Measure total, HDL cholesterol and triglyceride
- Estimate LDL cholesterol (LDL = total − HDL − triglyceride/5)

Acceptable LDL cholesterol (<110 mg/dL)

Borderline LDL cholesterol (110–129 mg/dL)

High LDL cholesterol (≥130 mg/dL)

Repeat lipoprotein analysis and average with previous measurement

Acceptable LDL cholesterol (<110 mg/dL)

Borderline LDL cholesterol (110–129 mg/dL)

High LDL cholesterol* (≥130 mg/dL)

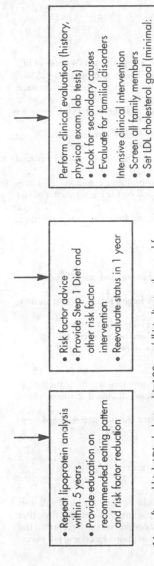

Repeat lipoprotein analysis within 5 years
- Provide education on recommended eating pattern and risk factor reduction

- Risk factor advice
- Provide Step 1 Diet and other risk factor intervention
- Reevaluate status in 1 year

Perform clinical evaluation (history, physical exam, lab tests)
- Look for secondary causes
- Evaluate for familial disorders

Intensive clinical intervention
- Screen all family members
- Set LDL cholesterol goal (minimal: <130 mg/dL; ideal: <110 mg/dL)
- Prescribe Step 1 (then Step 2) Diet

*A confirmed high LDL cholesterol (≥130 mg/dL) indicates the need for further evaluation and intensive clinical intervention, which includes evaluation for secondary and familial disorders, professional dietary counseling, and regular follow-up. A child sometimes may have an initial high LDL cholesterol but, when retested, may have a level of <110 mg/dL. Such discrepant analyses may be related to laboratory variability, a drastic change in intake of saturated fat and cholesterol, or weight loss. Based on the circumstances you will need to decide whether a third baseline LDL value is indicated. If the average of the child's LDL cholesterol level is ≥130 mg/dL, look for secondary causes of hypercholesterolemia.

Figure 2-7 Patient management based on results of lipoprotein analysis. HDL, high-density lipoprotein; LDL, low-density lipoprotein. (Adapted from National Cholesterol Education Program: Report of the Expert Panel on Blood Cholesterol Levels in Children and Adolescents. NIH publication no. 91-2732. Bethesda, Md, Department of Health and Human Services, Public Health Service, National Institutes of Health, National Heart, Lung, and Blood Institute, 1991.)

3. Sibling reactions to the new baby
4. Circumcision: Pros and cons

NEWBORN VISIT

This visit usually takes place in the hospital within the first 24 hours of life. The parents are concerned mainly with whether their baby is normal, and they may not be ready for a lengthy discussion. There are, however, some very important aspects of newborn care to discuss:

1. Umbilical cord care (apply alcohol with swab once or twice a day for 5 days)
2. Penile care (petroleum jelly [Vaseline] after circumcision: Gentle cleansing, no retraction of foreskin on uncircumcised boy)
3. Sleeping patterns and infant positioning (i.e., infant should be placed on back or on side, not prone or on belly).
4. Breast-feeding advice (technique, positioning, common complications, maternal diet, number of stools and consistency, number of wet diapers)
5. Bottle feeding advice (types of bottles and formulas, how to prepare, normal amounts)
6. Feeding, burping techniques, and spitting up
7. Stools
8. Pacifiers/self-soothing techniques
9. Postpartum adjustment: Mother's mood swings and question of depression, father's role, and siblings' reactions
10. Injury prevention (see previous). Don't forget: Infant car seat in rear-facing position on back (middle) seat.
    a. Choking; no necklace/strings around baby's neck
    b. *Never* leave unattended in a place where he or she can fall.
    c. *Never* leave alone with young siblings or pets.

TWO-WEEK VISIT

At this time, caretakers usually have many questions regarding their newborn, and readdressing some of the same issues discussed at the newborn visit is necessary.

1. Nutrition (check weight gain): The infant should have regained birth weight or be above it.
2. Bladder and bowel habits
3. Crying
4. Parental support (ask how mother is doing, extra help)

TWO-MONTH VISIT

1. Injury prevention: Discuss falls in particular because the child will start rolling over very soon. Also instruct parents on selecting toys that cannot break, are too big to swallow, and contain no small parts that the infant could detach. The infant will start to grasp objects and put everything into his or her mouth.
2. Nutrition
   a. Do not start solids until 4 to 6 months of age.
   b. Do not give more than 1 to 2 oz of water a day, if any (remind them that breast milk and formula are 80% water).

FOUR-MONTH VISIT

1. Injury prevention: Discourage the use of an infant walker (explain high incidence of head injuries and no advantage to earlier ambulation).
2. Nutrition
   a. Discourage bottle propping.
   b. No bottle in bed (explain high incidence of dental caries and ear infections)
   c. Introduction of solids and juices

SIX-MONTH VISIT

1. Injury prevention
   a. Discuss home hazards extensively because the infant is now much more active and soon will be able to start crawling (e.g., cabinets, table edges, small objects, electrical cords and sockets, tablecloths, lamps).
   b. Discuss the use of gates on stairs and the playpen as a safe area to be in while unattended.
   c. Discuss water safety (temperature, bathtub, pools).
   d. Give poison control sticker/number.
2. Nutrition: Discuss introduction of solids, water and juices, vitamins/fluoride/iron.
3. Sleep habits: Address separation anxiety and use of transitional object.

NINE-MONTH VISIT

1. Injury prevention: Same as previous visit.
2. Car safety: Remind parents that their infant should still be facing the back of the car until 1 year of age, even if the infant's weight exceeds 20 lb.
3. Nutrition
   a. Encourage the use of a training cup.
   b. Discuss the normal decrease in appetite by the end of the first year.
   c. Give toast or crackers for self-feeding/introduction of safe table foods.
4. Discuss sleep disturbances: Normal night wakening, nightmares versus night terrors.

TWELVE-MONTH VISIT

1. Injury prevention: Same as previous visit.
2. Discuss car safety: Car seat should be upgraded to a toddler seat once infant's weight exceeds 20 lb. Car seat can now be placed facing the front, but still should be in the back seat. Manufacturer's instructions should be followed closely.
3. Nutrition: Increase the variety of table foods; discuss foods to avoid because of risk of aspiration (e.g., raisins, peanuts, grapes, hard candy, hot dogs).

FIFTEEN-MONTH VISIT

1. Injury prevention: Same as previous visit.
2. Nutrition: Discuss normal decrease in appetite, weaning from a bottle, use of cup and spoon, finger feeding.
3. Development: Discuss increase in independence, oppositional behavior, temper tantrums. Discuss limit setting, discipline techniques, use of positive reinforcement, importance of consistency among parents/caretakers.

Advise caretakers about age-appropriate play, language development, social interactions.

EIGHTEEN-MONTH AND TWO-YEAR-OLD VISITS

1. Injury prevention: Same as previous visit.
2. Development
   a. The importance of reading to enhance language skills
   b. Parallel play and age-appropriate toys and games
   c. Self-comforting behaviors
3. Nutrition: Loss of appetite, avoiding meal struggles, weaning from bottle. Discourage juice, soda, and flavored drinks.
4. Toilet training: Discuss readiness for training and letting child dictate training.
5. Sleep habits: Discuss changing to a bed, particularly if the child can climb out of the crib.

THREE- TO FIVE-YEAR-OLD VISITS

1. Injury prevention
   a. Car safety: A regular seat belt can be used when the child weighs 80 lb or more. A booster seat should be used in children who weigh between 40 and 80 lb.
   b. Street safety
   c. Bicycle safety: Encourage the use of a helmet.
   d. Firearms
2. Development
   a. The importance of communication with child-shared play
   b. Speech dysfluency/stuttering
   c. Discipline
   d. Toilet training
   e. School readiness
   f. Strangers; good touch versus bad touch
3. Nutrition: Discourage foods high in cholesterol and salt as well as junk food. Discourage juice/soda.
4. Dental care: Children may begin to see a dentist at this time.

SIX- TO TEN-YEAR-OLD VISITS

1. Injury prevention: Same as previous visit
2. Nutrition: Same as previous visit
3. Development
   a. Relationships with peers/peer pressure will be forming.
   b. Limit television watching/video games.
   c. Sports/physical activities are necessary.
   d. Child should know home address and phone number.
4. School issues (grades, relationships with teachers and peers, discipline/behavioral problems, attention span, organizational skills)

ELEVEN- TO EIGHTEEN-YEAR-OLD VISITS

See Chapter 6.

SUGGESTED READING

Pickering, LK, Baker CJ, Long SS, McMillan JA (eds): Red Book: 2006 Report of the Committee on Infectious Diseases, 27th ed. Elk Grove, Ill, American Academy of Pediatrics, 2006.

American Academy of Pediatrics, Committee on Environmental Health: Lead poisoning: From screening to primary prevention. Pediatrics 92:176-183, 1993.

American Academy of Pediatrics, Committee on Nutrition: Statement on cholesterol. Pediatrics 90:469-473, 1992.

American Academy of Pediatrics, Joint Committee on Infant Hearing: 1994 Position statement. Pediatrics 95:152-156, 1995.

Asher MA: Screening for congenital dislocation of the hip, scoliosis, and other abnormalities affecting the musculoskeletal system. Pediatr Clin North Am 33:1335-1353, 1986.

Dixon SD, Stein MT: Encounters with Children: Pediatric Behavior and Development. St. Louis, Mosby, 1987.

Epstein S, Reilly JS: Sensorineural hearing loss. Pediatr Clin North Am 36:1501-1520, 1989.

Frankenburg WK: Screening-general considerations. In Hockelman RA (ed): Primary Pediatric Care. St. Louis, Mosby, 1987.

Friendly DS: Development of vision in infants and young children. Pediatr Clin North Am 40:693-703, 1993.

Green M, Haggerty RJ: Ambulatory Pediatrics IV, 4th ed. Philadelphia, WB Saunders, 1990.

Illingsworth RS: Development of the Infant and Young Child, Normal and Abnormal, 9th ed. London, Churchill Livingstone, 1987.

Irons M: Screening for metabolic disorder: How are we doing? Pediatr Clin North Am 40:1073-1085, 1993.

Johnson KB (ed): The Harriet Lane Handbook: A Manual for Pediatric House Officers, 13th ed. St. Louis, Mosby, 1993.

Johnson TR, Moore WM, Jeffries JS: Children Are Different: Developmental Physiology, 2nd ed. Columbus, Ohio, Ross Laboratories, 1978.

Katcher AL, Haber JS: The pediatrician and early intervention for the developmentally disabled or handicapped child. Pediatr Rev 12:305, 1991.

Lowrey GH: Growth and Development of Children, 8th ed. St. Louis, Mosby, 1986.

National Cholesterol Education Program: Report of the Expert Panel on Blood Cholesterol Levels in Children and Adolescents. NIH publication no. 91-2732. Bethesda, Md, Department of Health and Human Services, Public Health Service, National Institutes of Health, National Heart, Lung, and Blood Institute, 1991.

Scoles PV: Pediatric Orthopedics in Clinical Practice, 2nd ed. St. Louis, Mosby, 1992.

Sinclair D: Human Growth after Birth, 5th ed. Oxford, Oxford University Press, 1989.

WEBSITES

American Academy of Family Physicians: www.aafp.org
American Academy of Pediatrics: www.aap.org
Centers for Disease Control and Prevention: www.cdc.gov/nip

Differential Diagnoses

3

Anthony J. Alario and
Jonathan D. Birnkrant

The following is a compendium of differential diagnostic possibilities by age group, given a symptom. Those in bold represent emergency conditions that need to be ruled out first. Other differential diagnoses are covered in separate chapters under their respective organ systems and associated conditions.

Abdominal Pain, Chronic/Recurrent

	Infant (0–1 yr)	Child (1–12 yr)	Adolescent (12–18 yr)
Volvulus	✓		
Child abuse trauma	✓		
Posterior urethral valves	✓		
Intussusception	✓	✓	
Urinary tract infection	✓	✓	✓
Constipation	✓	✓	✓
Intestinal obstruction	✓	✓	✓
Henoch-Schönlein purpura	✓	✓	✓
Recurrent abdominal pain syndrome		✓	
Sexual abuse		✓	
Chronic lead poisoning	✓	✓	
Abdominal migraine		✓	✓
Pancreatitis		✓	✓
Renal calculi		✓	✓
Inflammatory bowel disease (Crohn's/colitis)		✓	✓
Sickle cell anemia	✓	✓	✓
Gastroesophageal reflux disease	✓	✓	✓
Dysmenorrhea			✓

Abdominal Pain, Generalized/Periumbilical

	Infant (0–1 yr)	Child (1–12 yr)	Adolescent (12–18 yr)
Necrotizing enterocolitis	✓		
Intussusception	✓	✓	
Gastroenteritis	✓	✓	✓
Constipation	✓	✓	✓
Urinary tract infection	✓	✓	✓
Intestinal parasites	✓	✓	✓
Lactose intolerance	✓	✓	✓
Testicular torsion	✓	✓	✓
Intestinal obstruction	✓	✓	✓
Pseudomembranous colitis	✓	✓	✓
Volvulus		✓	
Encopresis		✓	
Irritable bowel syndrome		✓	✓
Psychosomatic		✓	✓
Diabetic ketoacidosis		✓	✓
Sickle cell anemia		✓	✓
Peritonitis		✓	✓
Peptic ulcer		✓	✓
Abdominal abscess		✓	✓
Cholecystitis		✓	✓

Alopecia

	Infant (0–1 yr)	Child (1–12 yr)	Adolescent (12–18 yr)
Hypothyroidism	✓		
Ectodermal dysplasia	✓		
Seborrheic dermatitis	✓	✓	✓
Child abuse	✓	✓	
Tinea capitis	✓	✓	
Nutritional deficiencies	✓	✓	✓
Psoriasis	✓	✓	✓
Trauma	✓	✓	✓
Burns	✓	✓	✓
Drug reaction	✓	✓	✓
Alopecia areata		✓	✓
Trichotillomania		✓	✓
Anorexia nervosa			✓

3—Differential Diagnoses

Amenorrhea, Secondary

	Infant (0–1 yr)	Child (1–12 yr)	Adolescent (12–18 yr)
Pregnancy			✓
Oral contraception			✓
Ectopic pregnancy			✓
Stress			✓
Hypothyroidism			✓
Polycystic ovarian disease			✓
Drug reaction			✓
Anorexia nervosa			✓
Ruptured/hemorrhagic ovarian cyst			✓
Functional benign ovarian tumor			✓
Thyroiditis			✓
Pituitary adenoma			✓
Hypopituitarism			✓

Anxiety

	Infant (0–1 yr)	Child (1–12 yr)	Adolescent (12–18 yr)
Autism	✓	✓	
Drug withdrawal	✓	✓	
Depression		✓	✓
Post-traumatic stress disorder		✓	✓
Delirium		✓	✓
Obsessive-compulsive disorder		✓	✓
Anorexia nervosa		✓	✓
Panic disorder		✓	✓
Phobia		✓	✓
Hyperthyroidism		✓	✓
Diabetic hypoglycemia		✓	✓
Hepatic encephalopathy		✓	✓
Chronic fatigue syndrome			✓

Arthralgia

	Infant (0–1 yr)	Child (1–12 yr)	Adolescent (12–18 yr)
Rheumatic fever		✓	
Fifth disease		✓	
Trauma		✓	✓
Viral infection		✓	✓
Septic arthritis		✓	✓
Hemarthrosis		✓	✓
Serum sickness		✓	✓
Lyme disease		✓	✓
Juvenile idiopathic arthritis		✓	✓
Henoch-Schönlein purpura		✓	✓
Avascular necrosis		✓	✓
Connective tissue disorder		✓	✓

Arthritis, Monoarticular

	Infant (0–1 yr)	Child (1–12 yr)	Adolescent (12–18 yr)
Septic arthritis	✓	✓	✓
Tuberculosis	✓	✓	✓
Lyme disease	✓	✓	✓
Juvenile idiopathic arthritis	✓	✓	✓
Rheumatic fever	✓	✓	✓
Henoch-Schönlein purpura	✓	✓	✓
Kawasaki's disease	✓	✓	✓
Sickle cell anemia	✓	✓	✓
Acute leukemia	✓	✓	✓
Connective tissue disease	✓	✓	✓
Inflammatory bowel disease (Crohn's/colitis)		✓	✓

Ascites

	Infant (0–1 yr)	Child (1–12 yr)	Adolescent (12–18 yr)
Congenital abnormality of lymphatics	✓		
Portal hypertension	✓	✓	✓
Portal vein thrombosis	✓	✓	✓
Hypoalbuminemia	✓	✓	✓
Acute pancreatitis	✓	✓	✓
Mesenteric adenitis	✓	✓	✓
Peritonitis	✓	✓	✓
Tuberculosis	✓	✓	✓
Cardiomyopathy		✓	✓
Budd-Chiari syndrome			✓
Alcoholic hepatitis			✓

Azotemia

	Infant (0–1 yr)	Child (1–12 yr)	Adolescent (12–18 yr)
Acute glomerulonephritis	✓	✓	✓
Acute renal failure	✓	✓	✓
Bladder trauma	✓	✓	✓
Acute tubular necrosis	✓	✓	✓
Rocky Mountain spotted fever	✓	✓	✓
Chronic renal failure	✓	✓	✓
Dehydration	✓	✓	✓
Rhabdomyolysis		✓	✓
Pelvic tumor		✓	✓

Bleeding from Anus

	Infant (0–1 yr)	Child (1–12 yr)	Adolescent (12–18 yr)
Anal fissure	✓	✓	✓
Constipation	✓	✓	
Child abuse	✓		
Milk allergy	✓		
Sigmoid/rectal prolapse	✓	✓	
Enterocolitis	✓	✓	✓
Meckel's diverticulum	✓	✓	✓
Hemangioma	✓	✓	✓
Juvenile polyps		✓	
Intussusception		✓	
Crohn's disease		✓	✓
Hemorrhoids			✓
Ulcerative colitis			✓

Chest Pain, Acute

	Infant (0–1 yr)	Child (1–12 yr)	Adolescent (12–18 yr)
Cardiac tamponade		✓	✓
Bacterial pneumonia		✓	✓
Viral pneumonia		✓	✓
Costochondritis		✓	✓
Pneumothorax		✓	✓
Asthma		✓	✓
Trauma		✓	✓
Pericarditis		✓	✓
Muscular strain		✓	✓
Panic disorder		✓	✓
Recreational drug abuse		✓	✓
Gastroesophageal reflux disease		✓	✓
Foreign body		✓	
Sickle cell anemia		✓	✓
Pulmonary thromboembolism			✓
Biliary tract disease			✓

3—Differential Diagnoses

Convulsions

	Infant (0–1 yr)	Child (1–12 yr)	Adolescent (12–18 yr)
Febrile seizure	✓		
Diabetic hypoglycemia	✓		
Viral infection	✓		
Chronic lead poisoning	✓	✓	
Epilepsy	✓	✓	✓
Hypothermia	✓	✓	✓
Poisoning	✓	✓	✓
Encephalitis	✓	✓	✓
Bacterial meningitis	✓	✓	✓
Viral meningitis	✓	✓	✓
Trauma	✓	✓	✓
Hypercapnia	✓	✓	✓
Metabolic encephalopathy	✓	✓	✓
Primary intracerebral hemorrhage/stroke	✓	✓	✓
Subarachnoid hemorrhage and cerebral aneurysm	✓	✓	✓
Brain tumor	✓	✓	✓
Breath-holding spell		✓	✓
Diabetic ketoacidosis		✓	✓
Brain abscess			✓
Alcohol abuse/drugs			✓

Delirium

	Infant (0–1 yr)	Child (1–12 yr)	Adolescent (12–18 yr)
Chronic lead poisoning	✓		
Postictal/postseizure phase	✓	✓	✓
Sepsis/fever	✓	✓	✓
Hyponatremia	✓	✓	✓
Bacterial meningitis	✓	✓	✓
Hypoxia	✓	✓	✓
Hypercapnia	✓	✓	✓
Hyperthyroidism	✓	✓	✓
Acute renal failure	✓	✓	✓
Hypothermia	✓	✓	✓
Carbon monoxide poisoning		✓	✓
Postconcussive syndrome		✓	✓
Diabetic hypoglycemia		✓	✓
Recreational drug abuse		✓	✓
Heat stroke and heat exhaustion		✓	✓
Encephalitis		✓	✓
Hypercalcemia		✓	✓

Dysphagia

	Infant (0–1 yr)	Child (1–12 yr)	Adolescent (12–18 yr)
Achalasia	✓	✓	
Gastroesophageal reflux disease	✓	✓	✓
Primary intracerebral hemorrhage/stroke	✓	✓	✓
Foreign body	✓	✓	✓
Gastritis	✓	✓	✓
Epiglottitis	✓	✓	✓
Tonsillitis		✓	✓
Transient ischemic attack		✓	✓
Esophagitis		✓	✓
Thyroiditis		✓	✓

Dysuria

	Infant (0–1 yr)	Child (1–12 yr)	Adolescent (12–18 yr)
Urethritis		✓	
Prepubescent vulvovaginitis		✓	
Urinary tract infection		✓	✓
Pyelonephritis		✓	✓
Cystitis		✓	✓
Chemical irritant		✓	✓
Genital herpes		✓	✓
Balanitis	✓	✓	✓
Mucocutaneous candidiasis			✓
Bacterial vulvovaginitis			✓
Genital warts			✓
Sexually transmitted diseases (*Chlamydia trachomatis*, gonorrhea, lymphogranuloma venereum, syphilis)			✓

Edema

	Infant (0–1 yr)	Child (1–12 yr)	Adolescent (12–18 yr)
Hypothyroidism	✓		
Congestive heart failure	✓	✓	
Drug reaction	✓	✓	✓
Hypoalbuminemia	✓	✓	✓
Kawasaki's disease	✓	✓	
Cellulitis	✓	✓	✓
Cardiomyopathy	✓	✓	✓
Lymphatic obstruction	✓	✓	✓
Nephrotic syndrome	✓	✓	✓
Nephritic syndrome	✓	✓	✓
Thoracic outlet syndrome		✓	✓
Nutritional deficiencies	✓	✓	✓
Myxedema	✓	✓	✓
Venous obstruction	✓	✓	✓
Allergic reactions and anaphylaxis	✓	✓	✓
Acute glomerulonephritis		✓	✓
Pericarditis		✓	✓
Superior vena cava syndrome		✓	✓
Stevens-Johnson syndrome		✓	✓

Facial Paralysis

	Infant (0–1 yr)	Child (1–12 yr)	Adolescent (12–18 yr)
Congenital facial palsy	✓		
Trauma	✓	✓	✓
Cavernous sinus thrombosis	✓	✓	✓
Lyme disease	✓	✓	✓
Bell's palsy (postviral)		✓	✓
Dental infection		✓	✓
Mastoiditis		✓	✓
Mumps		✓	✓
Sarcoidosis			✓

Gynecomastia

	Infant (0–1 yr)	Child (1–12 yr)	Adolescent (12–18 yr)
Maternal estrogen	✓		
Klinefelter's syndrome		✓	✓
Chronic renal failure		✓	✓
Testicular malignancy			✓
Recreational drug abuse			✓
Normal variant			✓

Hematemesis/Upper Gastrointestinal Bleeding

	Infant (0–1 yr)	Child (1–12 yr)	Adolescent (12–18 yr)
Swallowed maternal blood	✓		
Hemorrhagic disease of newborn	✓		
Volvulus	✓		
Gastroesophageal reflux disease	✓	✓	✓
Drug reaction	✓	✓	✓
Gastritis		✓	✓
Peptic ulcer		✓	✓
Acute iron toxicity		✓	✓
Esophageal varices		✓	✓
Mallory-Weiss tear			✓

Hematuria

	Infant (0–1 yr)	Child (1–12 yr)	Adolescent (12–18 yr)
Nephroblastoma (Wilms' tumor)	✓		
Urinary tract infection	✓	✓	✓
Acute glomerulonephritis	✓	✓	✓
Trauma	✓	✓	✓
Sickle cell anemia	✓	✓	✓
Hemophilia A	✓	✓	✓
Drug reaction	✓	✓	✓
Urethritis			✓
Renal calculi			✓

Hemoglobinuria

	Infant (0–1 yr)	Child (1–12 yr)	Adolescent (12–18 yr)
Hemolysis	✓	✓	✓
Henoch-Schönlein purpura	✓	✓	✓
Trauma	✓	✓	✓
Hemolytic disease of the newborn (erythroblastosis fetalis)	✓		
Malaria	✓	✓	✓
Hemolytic-uremic syndrome		✓	✓
Disseminated intravascular coagulation		✓	✓
Drug reaction		✓	✓
Snake and reptile bites		✓	✓
Prosthetic cardiac valve		✓	✓
Paroxysmal hemoglobinuria after exercise		✓	
Paroxysmal nocturnal hemoglobinuria			✓

Hemoptysis

	Infant (0–1 yr)	Child (1–12 yr)	Adolescent (12–18 yr)
Ulcerative colitis		✓	
Epistaxis	✓	✓	✓
Arteriovenous malformation	✓	✓	✓
Thrombotic thrombo-cytopenic purpura	✓	✓	✓
Acute leukemia	✓	✓	✓
Pulmonary hemosiderosis	✓	✓	✓
Trauma		✓	✓
Bacterial pneumonia		✓	✓
Foreign body		✓	✓
Cystic fibrosis		✓	✓
Tuberculosis			✓

Hepatomegaly

	Infant (0–1 yr)	Child (1–12 yr)	Adolescent (12–18 yr)
Hemolytic disease of the newborn (erythroblastosis fetalis)	✓		
Congestive heart failure	✓	✓	✓
Viral hepatitis	✓	✓	✓
Sickle cell anemia	✓	✓	✓
Thalassemia	✓	✓	✓
Bartonella infection (cat-scratch disease)	✓	✓	✓
Cytomegalovirus	✓	✓	✓
Mononucleosis	✓	✓	✓
Mucopolysaccharidosis	✓	✓	✓
Neuroblastoma	✓	✓	✓
Acute leukemia	✓	✓	✓
Hepatoma		✓	✓
Sickle cell trait		✓	✓
Crohn's disease		✓	✓

Hyperhidrosis

	Infant (0–1 yr)	Child (1–12 yr)	Adolescent (12–18 yr)
Heat stroke and heat exhaustion	✓	✓	✓
Hypothyroidism	✓	✓	✓
Insect and spider bites and stings	✓	✓	✓
Infective endocarditis	✓	✓	✓
Malaria	✓	✓	✓
Orthostatic hypotension		✓	✓
Anxiety		✓	✓
Hyperthyroidism		✓	✓
Congestive heart failure		✓	✓
Pheochromocytoma		✓	✓
Recreational drug abuse		✓	✓
Familial dysautonomia		✓	✓
Drug reaction		✓	✓

Hyperpigmentation

	Infant (0–1 yr)	Child (1–12 yr)	Adolescent (12–18 yr)
Neurofibromatosis	✓	✓	✓
Melanoma	✓	✓	✓
Addison's disease		✓	✓
Scarlet fever		✓	✓
Cushing's syndrome		✓	✓
Hemochromatosis		✓	✓
Peutz-Jeghers syndrome (freckles, nailbeds)		✓	✓

Hypertension

	Infant (0–1 yr)	Child (1–12 yr)	Adolescent (12–18 yr)
Classic congenital adrenal hyperplasia	✓		
Essential hypertension	✓	✓	
Renal artery stenosis	✓	✓	✓
Coarctation of the aorta	✓	✓	✓
Nephroblastoma (Wilms' tumor)	✓	✓	✓
Malignant hypertension	✓	✓	✓
Pheochromocytoma	✓	✓	✓
Cushing's syndrome	✓	✓	✓
Chronic renal failure	✓	✓	✓
Systemic lupus erythematosus		✓	✓
Acute glomerulonephritis		✓	✓
Polycystic kidney disease		✓	✓
Pregnancy-induced hypertension			✓
Nephritic syndrome			✓

Hypotonia

	Infant (0–1 yr)	Child (1–12 yr)	Adolescent (12–18 yr)
Sepsis	✓		
Bacterial meningitis	✓		
Muscular dystrophy	✓		
Viral meningitis	✓		
Mucopolysaccharidosis	✓	✓	
Hyponatremia	✓	✓	✓
Inborn errors of metabolism	✓	✓	
Hypothyroidism	✓	✓	✓
Cerebral palsy	✓	✓	✓
Down syndrome	✓	✓	✓
Prader-Willi syndrome	✓	✓	✓
Marfan's syndrome	✓	✓	✓
Celiac disease	✓	✓	✓
Myotonic dystrophy	✓	✓	✓
Spinal muscular atrophy	✓	✓	✓
Guillain-Barré syndrome (acute infective polyneuritis)		✓	✓
Myasthenia gravis		✓	✓

Lightheadedness

	Infant (0–1 yr)	Child (1–12 yr)	Adolescent (12–18 yr)
Panic disorder		✓	
Anxiety		✓	✓
Syncope		✓	✓
Orthostatic hypotension		✓	✓
Hyperventilation		✓	✓
Anemia		✓	✓
Chronic fatigue syndrome		✓	✓
Conversion disorder		✓	✓
Atrioventricular block		✓	✓
Carbon monoxide poisoning		✓	✓
Alcohol abuse			✓

Melena, Lower Gastrointestinal Bleeding

	Infant (0–1 yr)	Child (1–12 yr)	Adolescent (12–18 yr)
Volvulus	✓		
Hemolytic disease of the newborn (erythroblastosis)	✓		
Anal fissure	✓	✓	✓
Intussusception	✓	✓	✓
Salmonella infection	✓	✓	✓
Campylobacter infection	✓	✓	✓
Malignancy	✓	✓	✓
Ischemic bowel	✓	✓	✓
Ulcerative colitis	✓	✓	✓
Liver cirrhosis		✓	✓
Meckel's diverticulum		✓	✓
Peptic ulcer		✓	✓
Crohn's disease		✓	✓
Hemorrhoids			✓
Mallory-Weiss tear			✓

Neck Mass

	Infant (0–1 yr)	Child (1–12 yr)	Adolescent (12–18 yr)
Branchial cyst	✓	✓	✓
Thyroglossal duct cyst	✓	✓	✓
Skin abscess	✓	✓	✓
Thyroiditis	✓	✓	✓
Parotitis	✓	✓	✓
Malignancy	✓	✓	✓
Laryngeal cancer		✓	✓
Lymphadenopathy		✓	✓
Hodgkin's disease		✓	✓
Non-Hodgkin's lymphoma		✓	✓

Pancytopenia

	Infant (0-1 yr)	Child (1-12 yr)	Adolescent (12-18 yr)
Parvovirus B19 infection	✓	✓	✓
Drug reaction	✓	✓	✓
Acute leukemia	✓	✓	✓
Neuroblastoma	✓	✓	✓
Myelodysplastic syndromes	✓	✓	✓
Intestinal parasites	✓	✓	✓
Fanconi's syndrome	✓	✓	✓
Primary human immuno-deficiency virus infection	✓	✓	✓
Chronic lymphocytic leukemia	✓	✓	✓
Connective tissue disease (systemic lupus erythematosus)		✓	✓
Babesiosis		✓	✓

Papilledema

	Infant (0–1 yr)	Child (1–12 yr)	Adolescent (12–18 yr)
Trauma/child abuse	✓		
Cavernous sinus thrombosis	✓	✓	✓
Raised intracranial pressure	✓	✓	✓
Hydrocephalus	✓	✓	✓
Brain tumor	✓	✓	✓
Intracranial hemorrhage	✓	✓	✓
Encephalitis	✓	✓	✓
Encephalopathy	✓	✓	✓
Cerebral edema	✓	✓	✓
Brain abscess		✓	✓
Benign intracranial hypertension (pseudotumor cerebri)		✓	✓

Pelvic Pain

	Infant (0–1 yr)	Child (1–12 yr)	Adolescent (12–18 yr)
Prepubescent vulvovaginitis		✓	
Urinary tract infection		✓	✓
Phimosis and paraphimosis		✓	✓
Dysmenorrhea		✓	✓
Renal calculi		✓	✓
Pregnancy			✓
Benign ovarian tumor			✓
Ruptured/hemorrhagic ovarian cyst			✓
Ectopic pregnancy			✓
Pelvic inflammatory disease			✓
Ovarian torsion			✓
Chlamydia trachomatis infection			✓

Peripheral Neuropathy

	Infant (0–1 yr)	Child (1–12 yr)	Adolescent (12–18 yr)
Carbon monoxide poisoning	✓	✓	✓
Lyme disease	✓	✓	✓
Guillain-Barré syndrome		✓	✓
Chronic lead poisoning		✓	
Chemical/pesticide poisoning		✓	✓
Diabetes		✓	✓
Chronic renal failure		✓	✓
Primary human immunodeficiency virus infection			

Petechiae

	Infant (0–1 yr)	Child (1–12 yr)	Adolescent (12–18 yr)
Disseminated intravascular coagulation	✓		
Osteogenesis imperfecta	✓		
Viral infection	✓	✓	✓
Sepsis	✓	✓	✓
Drug reaction	✓	✓	✓
Meningococcemia	✓	✓	✓
Idiopathic thrombocytopenic purpura	✓	✓	✓
Bacterial meningitis	✓	✓	✓
Viral meningitis	✓	✓	✓
Henoch-Schönlein purpura	✓	✓	✓
Aplastic anemia	✓	✓	✓
Acute leukemia	✓	✓	✓
Idiopathic thrombocythemia	✓	✓	✓
Myelodysplastic syndromes		✓	✓

Pleural Effusions

	Infant (0–1 yr)	Child (1–12 yr)	Adolescent (12–18 yr)
Bacterial pneumonia	✓	✓	✓
Congestive heart failure	✓	✓	✓
Nephrotic syndrome	✓	✓	✓
Liver failure	✓	✓	✓
Empyema	✓	✓	✓
Protein-losing enteropathy		✓	✓
Tuberculosis		✓	✓
Fluid overload		✓	✓
Malignancy		✓	✓

Polyarticular Arthritis

	Infant (0–1 yr)	Child (1–12 yr)	Adolescent (12–18 yr)
Fifth disease		✓	✓
Kawasaki's disease	✓	✓	✓
Chlamydia pneumoniae infection		✓	✓
Septic arthritis		✓	✓
Rheumatic fever		✓	✓
Juvenile idiopathic arthritis		✓	✓
Viral infection		✓	✓
Henoch-Schönlein purpura		✓	✓
Connective tissue disease		✓	✓
Lyme disease		✓	✓
Sickle cell anemia		✓	✓
Inflammatory bowel disease (Crohn's disease, ulcerative colitis)		✓	✓
Acute leukemia		✓	✓

Proteinuria

	Infant (0–1 yr)	Child (1–12 yr)	Adolescent (12–18 yr)
Urinary tract infection	✓	✓	✓
Nephrotic syndrome	✓	✓	✓
Henoch-Schönlein purpura	✓	✓	✓
Nephritic syndrome	✓	✓	✓
Diabetes		✓	✓
Orthostatic hypotension		✓	✓
Systemic lupus erythematosus		✓	✓
Acute glomerulonephritis		✓	✓
Pregnancy-induced hypertension			✓

Pruritus, Generalized

	Infant (0–1 yr)	Child (1–12 yr)	Adolescent (12–18 yr)
Atopic dermatitis	✓	✓	✓
Contact dermatitis	✓	✓	✓
Allergic reactions and anaphylaxis	✓	✓	✓
Herpes zoster, shingles	✓	✓	✓
Psoriasis	✓	✓	✓
Chickenpox	✓	✓	✓
Urticaria	✓	✓	✓
Scabies	✓	✓	✓
Body lice	✓	✓	✓
Liver failure		✓	✓
Head lice		✓	✓
Photodermatitis		✓	✓
Fungal infection		✓	✓
Pityriasis rosea		✓	✓
Folliculitis		✓	✓
Pubic lice		✓	✓

Ptosis

	Infant (0–1 yr)	Child (1–12 yr)	Adolescent (12–18 yr)
Congenital facial palsy	✓		
Trauma	✓	✓	✓
Cavernous sinus thrombosis	✓	✓	✓
Turner's syndrome	✓	✓	✓
Myasthenia gravis	✓	✓	✓
Botulism	✓	✓	✓
Lyme disease		✓	✓
Cluster headache		✓	✓
Horner's syndrome		✓	✓

Purpura

	Infant (0–1 yr)	Child (1–12 yr)	Adolescent (12–18 yr)
Child abuse	✓	✓	
Meningococcemia	✓	✓	✓
Trauma	✓	✓	✓
Erythema multiforme	✓	✓	✓
Bacterial meningitis	✓	✓	✓
Vitamin K deficiency	✓	✓	✓
Henoch-Schönlein purpura	✓	✓	✓
Idiopathic thrombocytopenic purpura	✓	✓	✓
Thrombotic thrombocytopenic purpura			✓

Pyuria

	Infant (0–1 yr)	Child (1–12 yr)	Adolescent (12–18 yr)
Urinary tract infection	✓	✓	✓
Polycystic kidney disease	✓	✓	✓
Kawasaki's disease	✓	✓	
Urethritis		✓	✓
Tuberculosis		✓	✓
Renal calculi		✓	✓
Acute appendicitis		✓	✓
Prostatitis			✓

Scrotal Pain

	Infant (0–1 yr)	Child (1–12 yr)	Adolescent (12–18 yr)
Hair tourniquet	✓		
Hydrocele	✓	✓	✓
Inguinal hernia	✓	✓	✓
Trauma	✓	✓	✓
Testicular torsion	✓	✓	✓
Orchitis	✓	✓	✓
Epididymitis		✓	✓
Testicular malignancy		✓	✓
Prostatitis			✓
Varicocele (swelling mostly)			✓

Syncope

	Infant (0–1 yr)	Child (1–12 yr)	Adolescent (12–18 yr)
Breath-holding	✓		
Febrile seizure	✓	✓	
Congenital heart disease	✓	✓	
Epilepsy	✓	✓	✓
Vasovagal response	✓	✓	✓
Paroxysmal atrial tachycardia	✓	✓	✓
Cardiomyopathy	✓	✓	✓
Ventricular tachycardia	✓	✓	✓
Atrioventricular block	✓	✓	✓
Hyperventilation		✓	✓
Conversion disorder		✓	✓
Orthostatic hypotension		✓	✓
Diabetic hypoglycemia		✓	✓
Marfan's syndrome		✓	✓
Carbon monoxide poisoning		✓	✓
Aortic stenosis		✓	✓

Thrombocytopenia

	Infant (0–1 yr)	Child (1–12 yr)	Adolescent (12–18 yr)
Thrombocytopenia–absent radius syndrome	✓		
Congenital rubella syndrome	✓		
Sepsis	✓	✓	✓
Birth asphyxia	✓		
Idiopathic thrombocytopenic purpura	✓	✓	✓
Drug reaction	✓	✓	✓
Aplastic anemia	✓	✓	✓
Acute leukemia	✓	✓	✓
Hemolytic-uremic syndrome	✓	✓	✓
Malaria	✓	✓	✓
Systemic lupus erythematosus		✓	✓
Megaloblastic anemias		✓	✓
Thrombotic thrombocytopenic purpura		✓	✓
Fanconi's anemia		✓	✓
Myeloproliferative disorders		✓	✓

Tinnitus

	Infant (0–1 yr)	Child (1–12 yr)	Adolescent (12–18 yr)
Impacted cerumen		✓	✓
Acute otitis media		✓	✓
Chronic otitis media		✓	✓
Ossicular trauma		✓	✓
Salicylate poisoning		✓	✓
Migraine headache		✓	✓
Temporomandibular joint syndrome		✓	✓
Acoustic neuroma			✓
Eustachian tube dysfunction		✓	✓
Arteriovenous malformation		✓	✓
Vascular aneurysm		✓	✓

Tremor

	Infant (0–1 yr)	Child (1–12 yr)	Adolescent (12–18 yr)
Nondiabetic hypoglycemia	✓		
Cerebral palsy	✓	✓	✓
Charcot-Marie-Tooth disease	✓	✓	✓
Diabetic hypoglycemia	✓	✓	✓
Hepatic encephalopathy		✓	✓
Anxiety		✓	✓
Hyperthyroidism		✓	✓
Wilson's disease		✓	✓
Benign essential/familial tremor syndrome			✓
Alcohol abuse			✓

Urethral Discharge

	Infant (0–1 yr)	Child (1–12 yr)	Adolescent (12–18 yr)
Foreign body	✓	✓	✓
Cystitis	✓	✓	✓
Urethral prolapse	✓	✓	✓
Sexual abuse	✓	✓	✓
Urethritis		✓	✓
Balanitis and balanoposthitis		✓	✓
Gonorrhea		✓	✓
Chlamydia trachomatis infection		✓	✓
Syphilis		✓	✓
Reiter's syndrome		✓	✓

3—Differential Diagnoses

Vaginal Bleeding, Abnormal

	Infant (0–1 yr)	Child (1–12 yr)	Adolescent (12–18 yr)
Maternal estrogen	✓		
Trauma/sexual abuse	✓		
Foreign body	✓	✓	✓
Chlamydia trachomatis infection		✓	✓
Precocious puberty		✓	
Trauma		✓	✓
Cystitis		✓	✓
Bacterial vulvovaginitis		✓	✓
Ruptured/hemorrhagic ovarian cyst		✓	✓
Genital warts		✓	✓
Idiopathic thrombocytopenic purpura		✓	✓
Oral contraception			✓
Dysfunctional uterine bleeding			✓
Iron-deficiency anemia			✓
Ovulatory bleeding			✓
Hypothyroidism			✓
Vaginal bleeding during pregnancy			✓
Pelvic inflammatory disease			✓
Miscarriage			✓
Ectopic pregnancy			✓

Vaginal Discharge

	Infant (0–1 yr)	Child (1–12 yr)	Adolescent (12–18 yr)
Physiologic	✓	✓	✓
Mucocutaneous candidiasis	✓	✓	✓
Foreign body	✓	✓	✓
Sexual abuse	✓	✓	✓
Chlamydia trachomatis infection		✓	✓
Bacterial vulvovaginitis		✓	
Prepubescent vulvovaginitis		✓	
Urethritis		✓	
Gonorrhea		✓	✓

Vertigo

	Infant (0–1 yr)	Child (1–12 yr)	Adolescent (12–18 yr)
Temporal lobe epilepsy	✓	✓	✓
Trauma	✓	✓	✓
Brain tumor	✓	✓	✓
Drug reaction	✓	✓	✓
Cholesteatoma	✓	✓	✓
Labyrinthitis		✓	✓
Benign paroxysmal positional vertigo		✓	✓
Hyperventilation		✓	✓
Migraine headache		✓	✓
Acoustic neuroma		✓	✓
Arnold-Chiari malformation		✓	✓
Multiple sclerosis			✓

Wheezing

	Infant (0–1 yr)	Child (1–12 yr)	Adolescent (12–18 yr)
Bronchiolitis	✓	✓	✓
Asthma	✓	✓	✓
Cystic fibrosis	✓	✓	✓
Gastroesophageal reflux disease	✓	✓	✓
Foreign body	✓	✓	✓
Congenital heart disease	✓	✓	✓
Bacterial pneumonia	✓	✓	✓
Viral pneumonia	✓	✓	✓
Allergic reactions and anaphylaxis	✓	✓	✓
Angioedema	✓	✓	✓
Drug reaction	✓	✓	✓
Mycoplasmal pneumonia		✓	✓

Dysmorphology and Common Syndromes

4

Dianne N. Abuelo

4.1 Dysmorphology and Approach to the Dysmorphic Infant or Child

1. Introduction: Dysmorphology is the study of the abnormal development of tissue.
   a. *Major* congenital anomalies: These are abnormalities of major surgical or cosmetic significance, such as congenital heart disease, spina bifida or other neural tube defects, and cleft lip or palate. They are present in about 3% of newborns. Other conditions may not become apparent until later in life, raising the total to 5% to 6%. Recurrence risk in additional children is approximately 3% to 5%. For neural tube defects, the risk can be decreased by prenatal folic acid supplementation.
   b. *Minor* congenital anomalies: Unusual morphologic features not of serious medical or cosmetic significance can be present in about 15% of otherwise normal infants. If a child has three or more minor anomalies, he or she should be examined carefully to look for a more serious defect. Some of these are familial and may or may not be clinically significant. Minor anomalies include the following:
      (1) Epicanthal folds
      (2) Clinodactyly of the fifth fingers
      (3) Single or bridged horizontal palmar creases
      (4) Preauricular ear pits
      (5) Syndactyly of the second and third toes
2. Pathophysiology
   a. Malformation: A morphologic defect of an organ, part of an organ, or a larger region that results from an intrinsically abnormal developmental process
   b. Deformation: An abnormal shape or position caused by mechanical forces (e.g., club foot secondary to oligohydramnios). Many deformations are produced by intrauterine constraint in an otherwise normal fetus. Some deformations are associated with an underlying abnormality that causes susceptibility to mechanical forces (e.g., club foot deformation in infants with spina bifida or myotonic dystrophy).
   c. Disruption: A morphologic defect of an organ or a larger region resulting from the extrinsic breakdown of, or interference with, an originally normal developmental process (e.g., amniotic band syndrome)

Table 4-1 **Identification of Patterns of Malformation**

Type	Definition	Examples
Syndrome	A pattern of anomalies due, or thought to be due, to a single, specific cause	Marfan's, Down, fetal alcohol syndromes
Sequence	An underlying anomaly giving rise to a cascade of secondary problems	Pierre Robin sequence (micrognathia, leading to defect in tongue descent, leading to cleft palate)
Association	A nonrandom combination of anomalies that occur together more frequently than expected by chance	VACTERL (vertebral, anal, cardiac, tracheoesophageal, renal, limb anomalies)

3. Patterns of malformations: Most malformations occur as isolated defects, but some infants have multiple abnormalities that may correspond to certain patterns. Identification of these patterns enables more accurate prediction of natural history, type of inheritance if any, and recurrence risk for family members (Table 4-1).

4. Clinical features
   a. History: A complete history, with details of the pregnancy, delivery, and neonatal course and the subsequent medical, developmental, and family history, should be obtained.
   b. Physical examination: The dysmorphology examination is a careful visual inspection of the entire body surface. In addition to routine measurements of height, weight, and head circumference, other measurements (e.g., interpupillary distance) may be appropriate in certain patients.

5. Diagnosis
   a. Table 4-2 provides examples of dysmorphic features and associated conditions. For example, the syndrome that would best fit a child who has a cleft palate, upturned nose, hypospadias, and syndactyly of the second and third toes is Smith-Lemli-Opitz syndrome.
   b. Additional resources: A useful listing of dysmorphic features and the syndromes in which they occur can be found in *Smith's Recognizable Patterns of Human Malformation*; if one cannot make a definitive diagnosis easily, databases such as the *London Dysmorphology Database* can provide a list of possibilities.

4.2 Common Congenital Syndromes

1. Marfan's syndrome
   a. For a clinical diagnosis of Marfan's syndrome, there should be involvement of the skeleton and two other systems, including one

Table 4-2   Dysmorphic Features in Relation to Clinical Conditions

Body Part	Anomaly	Condition
Face	Flat profile	Down syndrome
	Prominent forehead	Achondroplasia
Eyebrows	Synophrys	Cornelia de Lange syndrome
Eyes	Stellate pattern of iris	William's syndrome
	Coloboma or iris	CHARGE association
	Hypertelorism	Aarskog's syndrome
	Hypotelorism	Holoprosencephaly
	Narrow palpebral fissures	Fetal alcohol syndrome
Ears	Low-set	Noonan's syndrome
	Overhanging helix	Down syndrome
	Protuberant	Fragile X syndrome
Nose	Upturned	Smith-Lemli-Opitz, Cornelia de Lange syndromes
Lip	Cleft	Trisomy 13
Mouth	Downturned	Prader-Willi syndrome
Palate	Cleft	Smith-Lemli-Opitz, 22q11 deletion syndromes
Tongue	Large	Beckwith-Wiedemann syndrome
Chin	Micrognathia	Pierre Robin sequence
Philtrum	Long, flat	Fetal alcohol syndrome
	Short	22q11 deletion syndromes

Continued

Table 4-2 **Dysmorphic Features in Relation to Clinical Conditions—cont'd**

Body Part	Anomaly	Condition
Neck	Webbed	Turner's, Noonan's syndromes
	Increased posterior tissue	Down syndrome
Chest	Pectus deformity	Marfan's, Noonan's syndromes
Genitalia	Hypospadias	Smith-Lemli-Opitz syndrome
	Shawl scrotum	Aarskog's syndrome
	Hypogonadism	Prader-Willi syndrome
	Ambiguous	Chromosome anomalies, congenital adrenal hyperplasia
Extremities	Small hands and feet	Prader-Willi syndrome
	Long fingers	Marfan's syndrome
	Syndactyly of toes 2 and 3	Smith-Lemli-Opitz syndrome

major manifestation. If there is a definitely affected first-degree relative, then involvement of two systems is required (a major manifestation preferred).

(1) Major manifestations:
  (a) Aortic dilation or dissection
  (b) Ectopic lens
(2) Other findings include:
  (a) Pectus excavatum or carinatum
  (b) Arachnodactyly
  (c) Tall stature, scoliosis
  (d) Joint hypermobility
  (e) Mitral valve prolapse
  (f) Skin striae
  b. Management: Close monitoring by cardiology, orthopedics, and ophthalmology, as appropriate. Prohibition of heavy contact sports.
2. Neurofibromatosis type 1 (NF-1): Of the following six findings, two or more must be present to establish a clinical diagnosis of NF-1:
  a. Six or more café au lait macules, greatest diameter more than 5 mm in prepubertal patients and more than 15 mm in postpubertal patients
  b. Two or more neurofibromas of any type, or one plexiform neurofibroma
  c. Freckling in the axillary or inguinal region
  d. Optic glioma
  e. Two or more Lisch nodules (hamartomas of iris)
  f. A distinctive osseous lesion such as sphenoid dysplasia or pseudoarthrosis
3. Trinucleotide repeat syndromes: Caused by repetition or expansion of certain nucleotide triplets, which leads to instability of the DNA and abnormal expression of the involved genes. Examples include myotonic dystrophy, Huntington's disease, and fragile X syndrome.
  a. Fragile X: The most common inherited cause of mental retardation. Clinical features include:
    (1) Long face
    (2) Large testes
    (3) Prominent ears
    (4) Aversive gaze, hand flapping
    (5) Mental retardation
    (6) Positive family history
4. Chromosome anomalies
  a. Trisomies: Rather than the normal two sets, there are three full sets (or parts) of chromosomes. Examples include Down syndrome (trisomy 21), trisomy 13, and trisomy 18.
    (1) Down syndrome: clinical features
      (a) Flat facies, protruding tongue
      (b) Brachycephaly (flat back of head)
      (c) Epicanthal folds
      (d) Small pinnae, overfolded helix
      (e) Congenital heart disease (about 50%)
      (f) Upward-slanting palpebral fissures
      (g) Short neck, increased posterior tissue

   (h) Short fingers, hypoplastic middle phalanx of fifth finger
   (i) Single horizontal palmar crease
   (j) Hypotonia
   (2) Trisomies 13 and 18: clinical features shown in Box 4-1.
b. Microdeletion syndromes: Deletion of parts of a chromosome. Syndromes include Prader-Willi (deletion of paternal chromosome 15) and Angelman's (deletion of maternal chromosome 15).
   (1) Prader-Willi syndrome: Clinical features
      (a) Hypotonia in infancy, feeding problems
      (b) Obesity developing between 1 and 6 years of age
      (c) Small hands and feet
      (d) Hyperphagia
      (e) Mild facial dysmorphism
      (f) Hypogonadism, genital hypoplasia
      (g) Mild to moderate mental retardation
      (h) Behavior problems

Box 4-1   Clinical Features of Trisomies 13 and 18

Both 13 and 18

Poor survival
Facial dysmorphism
Abnormal pinnae
Micrognathia
Congenital heart disease
Abnormal hands
Cryptorchidism
Profound mental retardation

More Common in 13

Sloping forehead
Eye defects, microphthalmia
Cleft lip/palate
Scalp defects
Polydactyly
Seizures, apnea
Holoprosencephaly

More Common in 18

Low birth weight, intrauterine growth retardation
Narrow palpebral fissures
Small facial features
Prominent occiput
Clenched hand with index finger overlapping third, and fifth overlapping fourth
Hypertonia
Rocker-bottom feet

4—Dysmorphology

    (2) Angelman's syndrome: Clinical features
       (a) Frequent smiling or laughter
       (b) Ataxic gait and movements
       (c) Severe mental retardation, nonverbal
       (d) Large mouth, protruding tongue
       (e) Seizures
  c. Sex chromosome anomalies: Mosaicism is common. (Major congenital malformations are less common than with disorders of the autosomes.) Examples include Turner's (missing or abnormal X chromosome) and Klinefelter's syndromes (extra X chromosome [47, XXY]).
    (1) Turner's syndrome: Clinical features
       (a) Short stature
       (b) Congenital lymphedema
       (c) Short or webbed neck
       (d) Cardiovascular malformation (e.g., coarctation)
       (e) Primary amenorrhea
       (f) Ovarian dysgenesis
       (g) Prominent or anomalous ears
       (h) Normal IQ: Performance below verbal
       (i) Renal malformation (e.g, horseshoe kidney)
    (2) Klinefelter's syndrome: clinical features
       (a) Some have slightly lowered IQ
       (b) Small testes, infertility
       (c) Long legs
       (d) Some have behavior problems
       (e) Gynecomastia in 40%

SUGGESTED READING

Baraitser M, Winter RM: London Dysmorphology Database. Oxford, Oxford University Press, 1993.
Jones KL (ed): Smith's Recognizable Patterns of Human Malformation, 6th ed. Philadelphia, Elsevier, 2005.

WEBSITES

Gene tests: www.genetests.org
Genetics Home Reference: http://ghr.nlm.nih.gov/
Online Mendelian Inheritance in Man: www.ncbi.nlm.nih.gov/omim

The Newborn Infant

5

William J. Cashore

5.1 Approach to the Newborn Infant

BASIC NEONATAL ADAPTATION AND DEVELOPMENTAL PHYSIOLOGY

1. At birth, the infant must stabilize temperature and independently assume respiratory, nutritional, and excretory functions previously performed by the placenta. A brief listing of these adaptations and the accompanying physiologic changes is appropriate.
   a. Respiratory: Initiated by chemical, thermal, and tactile stimulation. Thoracic compression and recoil during birth partly clear the upper airway and expand the chest. Some residual lung fluid may persist for several hours in normal newborns. Crying helps to sustain positive end-expiratory pressure and distal airway expansion.
   b. Temperature stabilization:
      (1) Newborns generate heat by lipolysis of brown fat, and respond to hyperthermia by increasing cardiac output and insensible water loss.
      (2) Maternal fever increases fetal/neonatal core temperature by about 0.5° C. Fever often causes fetal tachycardia before delivery and neonatal tachycardia after delivery.
      (3) The "thermal neutral zone" is the gradient between environmental and body temperature at which the newborn consumes the least energy to maintain thermal stability.
         (a) Term infants can conserve heat by skin-to-skin contact, light clothing (including a cap), and avoidance of environmental cold spots.
         (b) Preterm infants may need external heat.
      (4) Cold exposure consumes energy that is thereby unavailable to sustain growth.
   c. Cardiovascular adaptation:
      (1) In utero
         (a) The pulmonary vascular bed is high resistance, and substantially bypassed.
         (b) The right ventricle provides substantial systemic flow by shunting umbilical venous blood arriving through the lower right atrium across the ductus arteriosus.

(c) The placenta, supplied by the left-sided circulation, is a high-flow, low-resistance organ serving physiologic functions of gas exchange, nutrition, and excretion.

(2) At birth, the relationship of ventricular outputs changes.

(a) The pulmonary capillary bed expands.

(b) Right atrial and ventricular pressures fall.

(c) As systemic resistance increases, left atrial and ventricular pressures rise.

(d) An increase in left atrial pressure closes the foramen ovale.

(e) Umbilical arteries, ductus venosus, and ductus arteriosus constrict in response to increased O_2 tension.

d. Renal adaptation: Compared with older infants, the newborn has decreased glomerular filtration and tubular reabsorption, slightly increased fractional Na^+ excretion, and decreased concentrating ability (600 to 650 mOsm/L versus 1400 to 1500 mOsm/L in adults).

(1) Neonatal feedings should provide ample free water.

(2) Formula feeding may require more free water than breast-feeding.

(3) Do not feed infants water; free water fraction should be obtained through breast or formula feeding.

2. Newborn physiology.

a. Early transitional physical findings include transient rales and rhonchi, low-intensity heart murmurs, and facial cyanosis during crying or feeding.

b. Normal vital signs in the newborn are shown in Table 5-1.

FETAL AND NEONATAL GROWTH

1. Fastest fetal growth velocity is at 24 to 36 weeks of gestational age.

2. Mean (50th percentile) weights are approximately

a. 1000 g at 27 weeks

b. 1500 g at 31 weeks

c. 2550 g at 35 weeks

d. 2800 g at 36 to 37 weeks

3. By weight for gestational age, newborns may be classified as small for gestational age (SGA, <10th percentile), appropriate for gestational age (AGA, 10th to 90th percentile), or large for gestational age (LGA, >90th percentile). Many cases of SGA and LGA infants do not have a recognizable cause, but some known causes include:

a. SGA: Known causes of intrauterine growth restriction include maternal hypertensive disorders, malnutrition, and congenital viral infections.

Table 5-1   **Normal Vital Signs in the Newborn Period**

Sign	Rate
Heart rate	90–140/min
Respirations	30–60/min
Temperature	36.5° C–37.0° C (97.8° F–98.6° F)
Mean blood pressure*	40–55 mm Hg

*In many nurseries, this is not routinely done.

Table 5-2 Nutrient Requirements for Newborn Infants	
Nutrient	**Unit**
Water	150–180 mL/kg/day
Calories	100–120 kcal/kg/day
Protein	2–3 g/kg/day
Carbohydrate	15–16 g/kg/day
Fat	3–4 g/kg/day

    b. LGA: Causes of macrosomia (i.e., infants ≥4 kg birth weight) include familial large size and gestational glucose intolerance.

NUTRITION

Nutrient requirements for newborn growth are summarized in Table 5-2. Also see Chapter 2.

1. Breast milk
   a. Adequate for at least 6 to 9 months. After postnatal day 2 or 3, neonatal suckling and maternal endocrine changes sustain milk production.
   b. Nutrients are adequate and biologically available, with the possible exception of vitamin K in the newborn period and fluoride during the first year.
   c. Iron and calcium absorption from breast milk are usually adequate.
2. Formula: Modern formulas are nutritionally adequate, but differ substantially in composition from both human milk and whole cow's milk. Always prescribe *formula with iron*.
3. Feeding intolerance: Common question
   a. Postprandial spitting is normal. Consider "reflux" only if an infant is hard to feed or recurrently distressed during and after feeding.
   b. "Lactose intolerance" is rare in newborns and usually associated with lower gastrointestinal manifestations rather than with regurgitation or spitting.
4. An appropriate age to start solid foods is with the appearance of teeth.

HOSPITAL DISCHARGE

1. Standard length of stay: For many hospitals, physician groups, and insurance plans, 48 hours is now the standard length of stay for a vaginal delivery (local practices may vary). In general, neonatal mortality, morbidity, and readmissions have not increased in the 10 to 15 years since the "standard" maternal/neonatal length of stay was reduced to 48 hours. The most favorable outcomes have been reported by organizations with standardized approaches and record keeping and substantial control over their medical services.
2. Early discharge: "Early" neonatal discharge is an imprecise term, but understood by many to mean a maternal and neonatal hospital stay of less than 48 hours. The following criteria should be considered for early discharge:
   a. Maternal: The mother should be medically stable. The family's competence to care for a newborn should be established by suitable screens.

Box 5-1   Medical Criteria for Neonatal Early Discharge

Gestation >35 wk and weight >2000 g
Vital signs stable × 12 hr or more:
    Respiratory rate <60/min
    Heart rate 90 to 140/min
    Axillary temperature 97° to 99.6° F
Examined by physician and discharge order written
No abnormal cardiorespiratory findings
No significant jaundice
Cord drying and clean
Circumcision healing and not bleeding
Hearing screen performed or arranged
No unresolved medical issues
Laboratory screens
Maternal/fetal group B *Streptococcus* status and treatment resolved
Initial metabolic screen is drawn
No significant blood group incompatibilities
Appropriate medications given
Eye prophylaxis
Vitamin K
Hepatitis vaccine/hepatitis B immune globulin if routine or if mother
    is high risk
Voided and stooled at least once
Feeding pattern
Adequate latch-on behavior if breast-feeding
Suck/swallow coordination
Successful feeding at least twice
No significant vomiting
Short term follow-up arrangements: prearranged at time of discharge
Notify primary physician
Call by home-care nurse 24 to 48 hours postdischarge
House or office visit 48 to 72 hours postdischarge

 b. Neonatal: Specific criteria and findings suitable for "early" discharge
  are listed in Box 5-1.
 c. Common problems with "early" discharge:
  (1) Inadequate breast-feeding
  (2) Unrecognized hyperbilirubinemia
  (3) Missed or late follow-up appointments
  (4) Need to repeat some screening tests

NEWBORN SCREENING

See also Chapter 2.
1. Assessments performed to determine and ensure physiologic stability:
 a. Initial nursing assessment
 b. Regular vital signs, assessment of early jaundice
 c. Physician examinations and discharge planning

2. Performed for specific conditions:
   a. Hearing screen: Mandated by most states before discharge.
   b. Metabolic screening: Mandated by all states for rare but treatable conditions that are asymptomatic in the newborn period. Neonatal screens are not generally used for untreatable disorders or for conditions not needing treatment until their clinical onset later in life. With some variations depending on the state, a sample list of screening tests is shown in Table 5-3.

5.2 Diseases and Disorders of the Newborn

The most common neonatal disorders of term infants requiring medical attention are jaundice and respiratory distress. Although bacterial sepsis is actually a low-frequency event (about 1 or 2/1000) in term newborns, a high level of suspicion needs to be maintained, along with a low threshold for diagnostic evaluation with appropriate therapeutic intervention.

RESPIRATORY DISORDERS

1. Clinical features: Newborns with respiratory disorders may present with the following clinical features:
   a. Tachypnea: Respiratory rates ≥60/min to 65/min. This is the most common clinical finding in respiratory disorders (if respiratory rate is decreased, it could signal exhaustion and impending respiratory collapse).
   b. Chest wall: Retractions with or without an expiratory "grunting"
   c. Auscultation: Rales or rhonchi
   d. Skin: Cyanosis in room air
2. Transient tachypnea of the newborn
   a. Etiology and pathophysiology: Rapid, nondistressed breathing caused by alveolar retention of amniotic fluid. More common with maternal glucose intolerance or delivery by cesarean section.
   b. Clinical features: O_2 requirement is minimal, if any, and stable (usually ≤25% to 35% inspired oxygen concentration). Can be precipitated or aggravated by cold stress.
   c. Radiologic findings: Chest radiograph is "streaky" with clear parenchyma.
   d. Management: Usually resolves within 24 to 72 hours (Table 5-4).
3. Respiratory distress syndrome
   a. Etiology and pathophysiology: Usually in preterm infants (but not always!), it is a disorder of surfactant deficiency (responds to surfactant replacement).
   b. Clinical features (see Table 5-4)
   c. Radiologic findings: Chest radiograph
      (1) Low lung volumes with generalized atelectasis
      (2) Uniform opaque "ground-glass" appearance
   d. Management: Table 5-4 lists criteria for evaluation, O_2 administration, and assisted ventilation in neonatal respiratory distress.
      (1) Clinical course of neonatal respiratory distress syndrome: O_2 requirement progresses for 1 to 3 days, slowly resolving with supportive management or assisted ventilation.

Table 5-3 Neonatal Metabolic Screening Tests

Disorder[a]	Consequences	Metabolic Screening Test
Hypothyroidism	Delayed growth and development (weight > length)	Thyroxine (T_4), thyroid-stimulating hormone
Phenylketonuria (PKU)	Severe retardation Vomiting, lethargy Eczematoid rash Musty/mousy odor	Phenylalanine
Galactosemia	Acidosis Growth failure Sepsis (E. coli) Cataracts Liver dysfunction	Galactose-1-p Uridyl transferase
Congenital adrenal hyperplasia	Virilization Salt-losing crises	17-OH progesterone
Maple syrup urine disease	Acidosis Hypoglycemia Seizures	Leucine
Sickle cell disease, thalassemia	Anemia Early overwhelming infections	Hemoglobin electrophoresis
Homocystinuria	Acidosis Delayed growth and development Vascular thrombosis Lens dislocation	Homocystine
Biotinidase deficiency	Defective metabolism of amino acids and neurotransmitters	Biotinidase

[a]Screens listed are routine in 15 or more states. In addition, two to four states screen for tyrosinemia, cystic fibrosis, or toxoplasmosis.

    (2) Exogenous surfactant administration usually shortens the course.

    (3) Some cases progress to severe respiratory failure with apnea and extensive pulmonary collapse, especially in very premature infants, requiring assisted ventilation.

4. Bacterial pneumonia and sepsis: May occur by aspiration or infiltration of infected amniotic fluid, or by hematogenous spread

   a. Etiology and pathophysiology: More frequent in premature than in term infants, most cases are caused by maternal group B *Streptococcus* (GBS). Maternal GBS screening and prophylaxis have reduced the incidence and mortality of neonatal GBS sepsis.

   b. Clinical features

    (1) Early onset: 6 to 12 hours of respiratory distress and pulmonary infiltrates

    (2) In addition to respiratory distress, septic infants often have a shocklike appearance, falling white count, and temperature instability (usually low).

   c. Management (see Table 5-4)

    (1) Antibiotics: Ampicillin and gentamicin

    (2) Neonatal sepsis can be fatal despite prompt intervention.

5. Meconium aspiration

   a. Etiology and pathophysiology

    (1) Considered a response to fetal distress that may not have been detected by fetal cardiac monitoring. Viscous meconium forms plugs in small airways. Bacterial contamination may worsen meconium aspiration.

    (2) Meconium staining without distress or aspiration is also common, occurring in 10% to 15% of vaginal deliveries.

   b. Clinical features: Examination and radiographs often show air trapping, hyperinflation, or localized small infiltrates.

   c. Management (see Table 5-4): Intrapartum management to decrease morbidity includes upper airway suctioning upon delivery of the head (10 to 20 seconds) and while body is still intravaginal, inhibiting reflex lung expansion and therefore aspiration. At delivery, a pediatric provider skilled in resuscitation should

    (1) Quickly examine the infant.

    (2) Inspect and suction the upper airway for meconium.

    (3) If the infant has respiratory depression, perform direct laryngoscopy to suction meconium from the upper airway and trachea. Routine intubation by pediatrician to suction meconium from vigorous infants with good Apgar scores is not necessary.

6. Pneumothorax

   a. Etiology and pathophysiology: may be spontaneous or associated with the conditions listed above (especially meconium aspiration syndrome)

   b. Clinical features: May be associated with non-distressed tachypnea

    (1) Examination: Decreased breath sounds with or without mediastinal shift

    (2) Radiologic findings: Chest radiograph shows a clear area with distinct margin and absent lung markings.

Table 5-4 Evaluation and Management of Neonatal Respiratory Distress

Problems	Response
Tachypnea (respiratory rate persists ≥60/min)	Examination Chest radiography Pulse oximetry Arterial blood gases, if tachypnea or lowered O_2 saturation persists
Pao_2 ≤45 mm Hg, or Sao_2 ≤85%	Supplement O_2 to maintain $Paco_2$ 45-75 mm Hg, and Sao_2 85%-95%*
Respiratory distress syndrome with hypoxemia (based on clinical findings and chest radiograph)	O_2 ± CPAP, if Pao_2 is ≤35-55 mm Hg
Pco_2 ≥60 mm Hg	Intubate and ventilate†
Apnea Recurrent, or profound Periodic breathing of prematurity	Intubate and ventilate Methylxanthines, ± CPAP

*Unless patient has duct-dependent congenital heart disease.
†Maintain pH ≥7.25, Pao_2 45-75 mm Hg, Pco_2 35-50 mm Hg.
CPAP, continuous positive airway pressure.

   c. Management (see Table 5-4)
      (1) Nontension pneumothorax: May not require specific treatment
      (2) Tension pneumothorax: May require thoracentesis or chest tube
      (3) "O_2 washout" of air leaks is of doubtful value.
7. Congenital malformations
   a. Etiology and pathophysiology: Respiratory distress caused by upper airway obstruction or pulmonary compromise due to malformations. Examples include
      (1) Choanal atresia or stenosis
      (2) Micrognathia/retroglossia, especially with cleft palate
      (3) Congenital laryngeal or tracheal stenosis, or tracheomalacia
      (4) Tracheoesophageal fistula
      (5) Diaphragmatic hernia
      (6) Pulmonary cystadenomatoid malformations
      (7) Pulmonary hypoplasia
   b. Clinical features: These often present with dyspnea, retractions, and decreased air exchange.
   c. Diagnosis: Evaluation should include
      (1) Nostrils: Passage of a *soft* catheter or auscultation of the nostrils (rules out choanal atresia)
      (2) Oropharynx: Thorough examination
      (3) Neck and larynx: Auscultation
      (4) Chest: Special attention to uneven breath sounds and adventitious sounds
      (5) Abdomen: A scaphoid abdomen with bowel sounds in the left chest suggests a diaphragmatic hernia.
      (6) Radiologic: Chest radiograph, including upper airway soft tissues and air column
      (7) Consultation: Evaluation of severe upper airway malformations may require consultation for fiberoptic laryngoscopy and bronchoscopy.

JAUNDICE AND HEMOLYSIS

1. Introduction: Screening of newborn infants for early hyperbilirubinemia is recommended by the Joint Commission on the Accreditation of Health Care Organizations (JCAHO) and as a clinical management guideline by the American Academy of Pediatrics (AAP). Most cases of neonatal jaundice are mild, idiopathic, and benign. However, hemolytic causes of hyperbilirubinemia, as well as idiopathic or "breast-feeding" jaundice, can be associated with clinically significant jaundice. See Table 5-5 and Box 5-2 for management guidelines.
2. Rhesus factor (Rh) incompatibility
   a. Etiology and pathophysiology: Antenatal sensitization of an Rh-negative mother to Rh-positive fetal red blood cells (RBCs). Maternal anti-Rh antibody crosses the placenta and attacks fetal RBCs. Hemolysis results in fetal anemia and jaundice, persisting after birth.
   b. Management: Mothers are screened for Rh type and anti-Rh antibodies.

Table 5-5 Suggested Guidelines for Management of Hyperbilirubinemia

Weight (g)	Do First Bilirubin	Phototherapy	Exchange Transfusion
≤750	Day 1	~5 mg/dL	>10 mg/dL
≤1000	Day 1	5–6 mg/dL	>10–12 mg/dL
≤1250	Day 1	6–8 mg/dL	>12–15 mg/dL
≤1500	Day 1 or 2	8–10 mg/dL	>15 mg/dL
≤1750	Day 2 or when jaundiced	10–12 mg/dL	>16–20 mg/dL
≤2000	When jaundiced	>12 mg/dL	~20 mg/dL
≤2500	When jaundiced	14–17 mg/dL	20–25 mg/dL
>2500	When jaundiced	18–20 mg/dL	22–25 mg/dL

> ### Box 5-2   Anticipatory Management of Neonatal Jaundice
>
> Know maternal blood type
> Know infant's blood type if mother is Rh negative
> Identify jaundice (especially if early onset)
>   Visual assessment with each set of vital signs, or
>   Skin reflectance for jaundice, or
>   Serum total bilirubin with metabolic screen
> Laboratory assessment for early jaundice
>   Serum bilirubin (repeat as needed)
>   Neonatal blood type and antibody screen
>   Hemoglobin, hematocrit, red blood cell indices and morphology
>   Additional tests (e.g., for liver function or infection) according to
>   the clinical presentation and subsequent course
> Management
>   Estimate hour-specific rate of increase in bilirubin
>   Arrange early follow-up (≤48 hr) if infant is discharged
> Interventions
>   Continued observation,
>   Phototherapy, or
>   Exchange transfusions (see Box 5-3) as indicated by clinical diag-
>   nosis and specific rate of increase

   (1) Antibody screen negative: The mother is given anti-Rh immune
       globulin at 28 weeks and at parturition. (Prophylaxis is highly
       effective.)
   (2) Antibody screen positive
       (a) Antibody titer is monitored during pregnancy.
       (b) Affected fetuses are followed with ultrasonography, amnio-
           centesis, and sometimes intrauterine transfusions.
       (c) Affected newborns need correction of anemia and treat-
           ment for jaundice of hemolytic origin (which is sometimes
           severe and may require exchange transfusion; see Table 5-5
           and Box 5-3).
3. A-B-O incompatibility
   a. Etiology and pathophysiology
       (1) There is a potential A-B-O mismatch in 20% to 25% of preg-
           nancies.
       (2) Group O mothers have preformed anti-A and anti-B antibodies;
           however, about 90% of susceptible group A or B fetuses are unaf-
           fected or mildly affected.
       (3) Those severely affected have early jaundice and mild anemia.
   b. Diagnosis: Maternal and neonatal antibody screens are of limited
      sensitivity and specificity; look for early jaundice, family history,
      enlarged spleen, and mild anemia. Test bilirubin on basis of early
      jaundice.

Box 5-3   Exchange Transfusion

Criteria

Cord hemoglobin <10 g/dL
Postnatal increase in bilirubin >1 mg/dL/hr
Anemia (hemoglobin <10–12 g/dL) plus postnatal increase in bilirubin >0.5 mg/dL/hr
Postnatal increase in bilirubin >20 mg/dL

Technique

Reconstituted whole blood, 160–170 mL/kg
Umbilical vein catheter (or continuous vein-artery technique)
Aliquots: withdraw/infuse 5 mL/kg/min
Operating time: 60–90 min
Continuous monitoring of heart rate and O_2 saturation
Replace Ca^{2+}; 100 mg Ca^{2+} gluconate per 100 mL blood exchanged
No oral intake 1 hr before and 5–6 hours after procedure

Results

Plasma bilirubin decreases by 45%–50%, with "rebound" up to 25% of the difference within 1–2 hr (usually about 10%)
Decrease in tissue bilirubin: re-equilibration with plasma
Decrease in circulating antibody
Replacement of susceptible red blood cells
Partial correction of blood volume and decreased red blood cell mass

Complications

Embolism
Unstable cardiac output and blood pressure
Ruptured spleen/liver
Electrolyte imbalance
Hyperglycemia→hypoglycemia
Metabolic acidosis
Infection
Transfusion reaction

Nonhemolytic causes of jaundice
a. "Physiologic" delay in bilirubin excretion: sometimes related to
   (1) Prematurity
   (2) Minor polymorphisms in the conjugating enzyme
b. Inadequate milk intake
c. Breast-feeding (cause is unknown)
d. Bruising during delivery
e. Internal hemorrhage
f. Polycythemia (e.g., from chronic hypoxia or placental transfusion)
g. Hepatobiliary disease
h. Infection (hepatitis or bacterial sepsis)

5. Kernicterus
   a. Etiology and pathophysiology: Kernicterus is a type of choreoathetoid, dystonic cerebral palsy caused by bilirubin intoxication of the central nervous system.
   b. Clinical features
      (1) Early signs: Lethargy, poor feeding, opisthotonus, and a high-pitched cry
      (2) Later signs: Choreoathetosis, involuntary movements, and cranial nerve dysfunction including central hearing loss
   c. Diagnosis
      (1) The risk for kernicterus in "normal" term infants is increased when serum indirect bilirubin is 25 to 30 mg/dL or higher.
      (2) Premature infants and infants with Rh hemolytic disease have increased risk for kernicterus at about 20 mg/dL.
   d. Management (see Boxes 5-2 and 5-3)
      (1) Phototherapy requires
         (a) Adequate light source (10 to 30 μW/cm²/nm)
         (b) A large surface area of exposed skin: Undress infant except for eye patches and a small diaper.
         (c) Multidirectional light sources
         (d) Limited, brief interruptions (i.e., time out of lights is ≤30 minutes for feeding, changes)
         (e) "Intensive" phototherapy at 20 to 50 μW/cm²/nm while preparing for exchange transfusion

ANTENATAL MATERNAL DRUG EXPOSURE

1. Drug exposure
   a. Cannabis: Neonatal effects, if any, are minimal and subtle.
   b. Cocaine: Premature labor; low birth weight; anecdotal reports of fetal vascular injury; no characteristic withdrawal syndrome
   c. Opiates (e.g., heroin, oxycodone [OxyContin])
      (1) Associated with low birth weight, secondary to prematurity, and intrauterine growth restriction
      (2) Neonatal withdrawal: Often takes 1 to 2 weeks or longer for recovery
      (3) Methadone maintenance may be associated with more normal birth weights, but with a longer withdrawal time (i.e., 2 to 4 weeks) than heroin and more severe symptoms.
      (4) Management: Use an oral morphine preparation to control severe withdrawal signs and symptoms. Consult the hospital pharmacy as to the exact preparation, strength, and dosing schedule. ("Dilute tincture of opium" is a misnomer and should not be ordered as such.) Low-dose phenobarbital (3 to 5 mg/kg orally daily) may reduce the morphine dose and duration of symptomatic withdrawal
      (5) History of intravenous drug use raises suspicion of human immunodeficiency virus exposure.
   d. Maternal antidepressant use (especially sustained serotonin reuptake inhibitors) may be associated with a brief (1- to 3-day) period of neonatal instability or periodic breathing.

2. Diagnosis: Test urine and meconium.
3. Management
   a. Reportable to child welfare services in some states
   b. Work with appropriate hospital and state agencies in making discharge plans for drug-exposed infants.

NEONATAL HYPOGLYCEMIA

1. Etiology and pathophysiology: often associated with intrauterine growth restriction (decreased stores), macrosomia (hyperinsulinemia), or cold stress (increased consumption)
2. Normal plasma glucose values:
   a. Term, 40 to 80 mg/dL
   b. Preterm, 35 to 70 mg/dL
3. Management
   a. Bedside screening of at-risk infants every 1 to 2 hours until stable or fed
   b. Confirm low bedside results with a stat laboratory value.
   c. Maintenance glucose: 6 mg/kg/min as 10% glucose (~80 mL/kg/day)
   d. "Mini bolus"—100 mg/kg as 10% glucose over 5 to 10 minutes
   e. Severe hypoglycemia may require hypertonic glucose by central line.
   f. Start regular feedings as soon as the infant is ready.

APNEA/PERIODIC BREATHING OF PREMATURITY

1. Diagnosis: All newborns have periodic breathing. Clinically significant apnea is a pause of 20 seconds or more, associated with a change in heart rate or oxygenation.
2. Management: An incremental approach to apnea of prematurity
   a. Gently stimulate for short apneic pauses.
   b. Reposition for airway patency, especially after feeding.
   c. Rearrange schedule to cluster "stressful" events.
   d. Caffeine at 20 mg/kg loading dose and 8 to 10 mg/kg/day
   e. Low-flow nasal cannula, nasal continuous positive airway pressure, or even assisted ventilation may be needed for severe recurrent apnea.
   f. Frequency and severity of apnea are only weakly associated with anemia or with gastroesophageal reflux. However, worsening or de novo apnea may be a sign of sepsis. Individualize evaluation and treatment for these conditions.

ANEMIA

1. Term infants: The most common causes of acute anemia are perinatal hemorrhage (may be transplacental) and hemolysis due to maternal blood group antibodies. Management includes the following:
   a. Check antibody screens, reticulocyte count, RBC indices, and RBC morphology in addition to hemoglobin (Hgb) and hematocrit (Hct).
   b. Hemoglobins in the range of 8 to 10 g/dL are often well tolerated.
   c. Transfuse for acute volume loss or persistent hemolysis.
2. Preterm infants: Anemia of prematurity results from sampling losses, prolonged suppression of erythropoiesis, and inadequate nutrient stores (e.g., iron and vitamin E). Management includes the following:
   a. Follow reticulocyte counts as well as Hgb and Hct.
   b. Individualize transfusion decisions; transfusion "per protocol" for low Hct may prolong suppression of erythropoiesis.

   c. Recombinant erythropoietin is of some benefit, but not uniformly effective.

NEONATAL SEIZURES

1. Etiology and pathophysiology
   a. Intracranial or intraventricular hemorrhage
   b. Hypoxic-ischemic encephalopathy
   c. Parenchymal or vascular central nervous system malformations
   d. Antenatal insults not related to perinatal events (e.g., cortical infarction)
   e. Bacterial or viral infections
   f. Intoxication or opiate withdrawal
   g. Metabolic (hypoglycemia, hypocalcemia)
2. Clinical features: Stereotyped, "slow/fast" movements unrelated to stimulus or comfort measures. Rapid, stimulus-sensitive tremors are usually not seizures.
3. Diagnosis: Confirmation by electroencephalography. Also perform lumbar puncture and imaging studies as clinically indicated.
4. Management: A qualified pediatric neurologist should supervise and monitor evaluation and treatment. For emergent treatment, consider diazepam (0.2 to 0.5 mg/kg intravenously (IV) or 0.5 mg/kg rectally) or lorazepam (0.05 to 0.1 mg/kg IV). For chronic treatment, phenobarbital is the monotherapy of choice (loading dose 20 mg/kg and daily 2 to 3 mg/kg/day). See also Chapter 20.

NEONATAL SEPSIS AND INFECTION

1. Etiology and pathophysiology
   a. Perinatal: Most intrauterine or intrapartum neonatal infections present clinically within 12 to 24 hours after birth. GBS is the most common cause of neonatal bacteremia and meningitis. Maternal screening and intrapartum penicillin prophylaxis have decreased neonatal mortality and attack rates from GBS disease. Other causes of perinatal sepsis include *Listeria monocytogenes*, Gram-negative rods (*Escherichia coli, Klebsiella*), and *Staphylococcus* species.
   b. Nosocomial infections are usually superficial and mild if the nursery stay is short.
   c. Neonatal intensive care unit infections are most frequent in infants with extremely low birth weight, and are often opportunistic infections (*Staphylococcus epidermidis, Enterococcus, Candida* species, and methicillin-resistant *Staphylococcus aureus*).
2. Clinical features: Look for clinical symptoms suggesting sepsis, including temperature instability (often low), poor feeding, apnea, or desaturation.
3. Diagnosis
   a. Laboratory: Blood culture, complete blood count with white blood cell differential
   b. Urine cultures by catheter are often "false positive." They are reliable if obtained by bladder tap, or a high colony count for a single organism is identified.
   c. Procedures: Lumbar puncture and cerebrospinal fluid culture in many cases, especially if infant is >12 hours old
   d. Radiologic: Chest radiograph for infants with respiratory distress

Box 5-4 Antibiotics Commonly Used in Newborn Infants

Ampicillin
Penicillin
Gentamicin*†
Cefotaxime
Oxacillin
Vancomycin*†

*Lower dose and longer dose intervals for low–birth-weight infants.
†Follow peak/trough blood levels and serum creatinine.

4. Management
   a. Antibiotics commonly given to newborns are shown in Box 5-4
   b. Empirical treatment begins with ampicillin and gentamicin (which covers the most common organisms, including GBS). Avoid empirical use of vancomycin and cephalosporins.

5.3 Water and Electrolytes

See also Chapter 9.

1. Introduction: The size of newborns means that even small adjustments in fluids and electrolytes account for a larger percentage of overall change. Therefore, for the infant who needs resuscitation or cannot or should not be fed (e.g., because of sepsis or seizure work-up), calculations of water and electrolytes are critical.
2. Provide short-term IV support to larger infants with 5% to 10% dextrose at 60 to 80 mL/kg/day during the first 1 to 2 days.
3. Add Na 3 to 4 mEq/kg/day after day 2, and potassium chloride (KCl) 1 to 2 mEq/kg/day if serum K^+ is normal (catabolism and stress may increase serum K^+).
4. Small premature infants have high insensible water losses and require a higher volume per kilogram of free water than larger infants. Watch low–birth-weight infants for inappropriate weight loss accompanied by decreased urine output and hypernatremia.
5. If after the initial day of stabilization of fluid and electrolyte the newborn infant continues NPO, IV protein (amino acids) and fat should be added for nutritional supplement.
6. Monitor glucose intolerance by regular determinations of plasma and urine glucose.

SUGGESTED READING

American Academy of Pediatrics, Subcommittee on Hyperbilirubinemia: Clinical practice guideline: Management of hyperbilirubinemia in the newborn infant of 35 or more weeks of gestation. Pediatrics 114:297-316, 2004.
Bhat DR, Reber DJ, Wirtschafter DD, et al: Neonatal Drug Formulary, 3rd ed. Los Angeles, Neonatal Drug Formulary, 1993.

Cashore WJ: Care of the newborn. In Coustan DR, Haning RV, Singer DB (eds): Human Reproduction, Growth, and Development. Boston, Little, Brown, 1995.

Cashore WJ: Neonatal adaptation. In Coustan DR, Haning RV, Singer DB (eds): Human Reproduction, Growth, and Development. Boston, Little, Brown, 1995.

Cashore WJ, Peter G: Infections acquired in the nursery: Epidemiology and control. In Remington JS, Klein JO (eds): Infectious Diseases of the Fetus and Newborn Infant, 4th ed. Philadelphia, WB Saunders, 1995.

Cochran WD: Management of the normal newborn. In Oski FA, DeAngelis CD, Feigin RD, et al (eds): Principles and Practice of Pediatrics, 2nd ed. Philadelphia, JB Lippincott, 1994.

Schreiner RL: Physical examination. In Schreiner RL, Bradburn NC (eds): Care of the Newborn, 2nd ed. New York, Powers, 1988.

Serwer GA: Postnatal circulatory adjustments. In Polin RA, Fox WW (eds): Fetal and Neonatal Physiology. Philadelphia, WB Saunders, 1992.

Adolescent Medicine 6

Patricia Flanagan, Suzanne Riggs,
and Zeev Harel

6.1 Introduction

1. Age: Adolescence is defined as the period between childhood and adulthood, starting at about 10 or 12 years and ending at about 25 years of age.
2. Physiology: A rapid growth phase and development of secondary sex characteristics (defined by the Tanner stages) mark this period (see Chapters 2 and 7, and Appendix V).
3. Cognitive development
   a. Concrete thought (early adolescence)
   b. Abstract thought (middle to late adolescence): The development of abstract thought allows adolescents to formulate hypotheses, consider complex interactions, and understand the maintenance of social order.
4. Psychological development: Three major categories
   a. Establishment of autonomy: Peer groups becoming the major primary social support beginning around 15 to 17 years. This is a peak period for family conflict.
   b. Psychosocial and psychosexual development
      (1) Acceptance of physical change
      (2) Establishment of peer relations: Same-sex peers in early adolescence and dating later in adolescence
      (3) The development of responsible behavior (e.g., work, camp counselor)
      (4) The evolution of personal values (e.g., taking sides on social/moral issues—politics, religion, etc.)
   c. Future orientation
      (1) Largely a task of later adolescence (18 to 21 years)
      (2) Decisions regarding vocational and social/relationship choices
5. Behavior: Adolescence is a relatively healthy stage of life in which much health risk, morbidity, and mortality are associated with behavioral decision making.

6.2 Adolescent Health Maintenance

1. Optimizing the encounter
   a. Trust and confidentiality: Establishing trust and preserving confidentiality are important to adolescents. Always be up-front: let them know what will, and what won't, be confidential. After the fact is too late!
   b. Autonomy: Nurturing their struggle by providing an open, trusting environment and by giving them opportunities to express themselves in their own words.
2. The office visit: Normal health screening
   a. Frequency: Adolescents should have full physical examinations at least every 2 years (every year is highly recommended, primarily to monitor psychosocial changes and deliver prevention messages).
   b. History: An acronym for the adolescent interview is HEADSS:

Home: Who lives with you, what are your relationships like, is there any domestic violence

Education: School progress, attendance, grades, connections, vocation

Activities: Friends, hobbies, sports, interpersonal violence, weapons carrying

Drugs: Tobacco, alcohol, marijuana, other drugs, how often, with whom

Sexuality: Sexual experiences, orientation, sexual intercourse, partners, sexually transmitted infections (STIs), contraception

Suicide/depression: Feelings, sadness, sleep, history of mental health issues, suicidal thoughts, plans, prior attempts

   c. Physical examination: Areas of special focus in adolescents can be found in Table 6-1.
3. The office visit: Selected adolescent issues and disorders to consider during the health maintenance encounter
   a. Genitourinary (for gynecologic disorders, see Section 6.3)
      (1) Urinary infections (see Chapter 18)
      (2) STIs
         (a) Etiology: Important infections in adolescents include *Chlamydia trachomatis*, gonorrhea, herpes simplex virus (HSV), *Trichomonas*, condyloma acuminatum (human papilloma virus [HPV]), *Gardnerella*, and human immunodeficiency virus (HIV).
         (b) Diagnosis: Screen sexually active youth at least annually; urine tests are sensitive and specific for *Chlamydia* and gonococcus.
         (c) Treatment: By law, adolescents may be treated for STIs without parental permission in all states.
         (d) Note: Any STI in a patient younger than 12 years of age must be reported as possible child abuse.
      (3) See Section 6.3 for vaginitis, pelvic inflammatory disease (PID), and toxic shock syndrome.
   b. Breast masses
      (1) Asymmetry is common and usually resolves.
      (2) Fibrocystic disease and fibroadenoma are the most common masses.

Table 6-1 Guidelines for Adolescent Health Supervision Visits

Early Adolescent (10–14 yr)	Middle Adolescent (15–16 yr)	Late Adolescent (17–20 yr)
Interview with Parent/Patient		
General questions or concerns		
Family stresses and communication		Interview teen alone, if possible
Schoolwork and friends		
Assess for mood, attitude, school performance	Dating, discipline, school performance	
Health concerns		
Sports, hobbies		
Junior high school adjustment		
		Future goals, work, or plans after graduation
Friends/dating		
Home environment		
Sexuality		
Tobacco, drugs, alcohol		
Feelings: worry, sadness		

Continued

Table 6-1   Guidelines for Adolescent Health Supervision Visits—cont'd

Physical Examination (Patient alone; chaperone may be indicated for younger patients or opposite sex)

Height/weight plotted; calculate body mass index
Vision/hearing screening
Blood pressure
Tanner stage/external genital examination
Gynecomastia/breast asymmetry
Scoliosis screen
Skinfold thickness, acne
Self-examination of breast/testes, if mature
Sports fitness screening
(3-minute orthopedic examination)

Pelvic examination (and Pap smear) if menstrual problems or sexually active for ≥3 yr

Pelvic examination (and Pap smear) if menstrual problems or sexually active for ≥3 yr

Procedures

Hematocrit

Hematocrit (optional)

Hematocrit

Tuberculin if indicated
Rubella titer if none previously
If sexually active, screen for gonorrhea, syphilis, and chlamydia

STI screen, Pap smear if sexually active ≥3 yr

Cholesterol/triglycerides in high-risk individuals

Immunizations

Immunization status

Mumps, measles vaccine if none previously

Rubella vaccine for nonimmune female patients if not pregnant; varicella vaccine if indicated

Newer vaccines: meningococcal vaccine, human papilloma virus vaccine (see latest *AAP Red Book* for current recommendations)

Tetanus-diphtheria (Td) booster every 10 yr; or new DTaP vaccine

Mumps, measles vaccine if none previously

Td booster every 10 yr

Anticipatory Guidance

Health habits (smoking, diet, safety, substance use)

Social interaction

Academic activities

Interaction with parents

Health habits (smoking, diet, auto safety, substance use, STI/pregnancy prevention)

Interaction with parents/adults

Independent adult lifestyle

STI, sexually transmitted infection.

Modified from American Academy of Pediatrics: *Guidelines for health supervision II*, Elk Grove Village, Ill., 1983, American Academy of Pediatrics.

    (3) Male gynecomastia is common and can last 6 months to 2 years; if present after Tanner stage 5, may need surgical opinion.

c. Testicular and scrotal disorders

    (1) Varicocele is the dilatation of vessels in the spermatic cord.

        (a) Occurs in 15% of male adolescents, usually on left because of relative obstruction of spermatic veins, feels like "bag of worms"

        (b) Can reduce fertility if extensive, refer to urologist if there is size discrepancy in testicles

    (2) Inguinal hernias

    (3) Hydrocele: Fluid-filled cavity in the sac that transilluminates and does not reduce (as a hernia does if it is not strangulated)

    (4) Spermatocele: Fluid-filled cyst of epididymis that transilluminates (smaller than hydrocele, it is nodular)

    (5) Testicular torsion (incidence, 1:4000; see also Chapter 18)

d. Reproductive health issues: See Section 6.4 for contraception and pregnancy issues (including elective termination).

e. Mental health issues

    (1) Depression: Signs such as recurrent somatic complaints, fatigue, changing peer relationships, poor school performance or attendance, recent loss, excessive sleepiness/insomnia may indicate depression.

    (2) Suicide

        (a) Girls make more attempts, but boys are more often successful.

        (b) Third most common cause of death in adolescents and young adults

        (c) Be aware! Suicide is frequently associated with a recent loss or stressors, such as conflict with family, friends, or boyfriend/girlfriend.

        (d) Methods in order of frequency include cutting, firearms, hanging, and drug overdoses.

        (e) Some of the psychiatric medications for depression have been associated with an increase in adolescent suicide.

    (3) Delinquency

    (4) Eating disorders (see Section 6.5)

    (5) Sexual abuse (Fig. 6-1)

        (a) Rape: Teenagers make up half of all rape victims.

        (b) Incest: Most commonly it occurs between father or stepfather and daughter.

    (6) Substance abuse

        (a) See Box 6-1 for stages of substance abuse.

        (b) Commonly abused substances: Tobacco, alcohol (most common), and marijuana. Recently there has been increased use of amphetamines and prescription medications.

        (c) Substance abuse screening: RAFFT (Box 6-2)

f. Dermatologic problems

    (1) Acne is the major skin problem in adolescents and a source of stress because of their preoccupation with appearance.

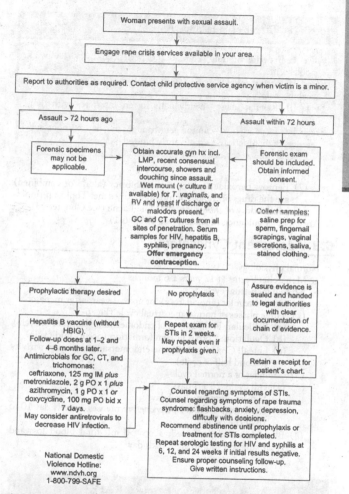

Figure 6-1   Approach to the sexual assault victim. CT, *Chlamydia trachomatis*; GC, gonococcus; HBIG, hepatitis B immune globulin; HIV, human immunodeficiency virus; LMP, last menstrual period; STI, sexually transmitted infection. (Adapted from Hatcher RA, Nelson A, Zieman M, et al: Pocket Guide to Managing Contraception. Tiger, Ga, Bridging the Gap Foundation, 2002, p A25.)

Box 6-1   Stages of Substance Abuse

Stage I: Experimentation—common, experienced by virtually all adolescents
Stage II: Stress relief—an attempt at self-medication instead of seeking help
Stage III: Regular abuse—nearly daily, often interferes with daily function
Stage IV: Dependence—cannot get through the day without substance, daily function is significantly limited

      (2) Benzoyl peroxide and topical antibiotics (alone or combined) are the drugs of choice for inflammatory acne. Topical retinoids are the drug of choice for comedonal acne (see Chapter 13).
  4. Anticipatory guidance/education (see Table 6-1)

6.3 Adolescent Gynecology

1. Normal physiology
   a. Menarche: Begins at 12 years ± 6 months
   b. Normal menstrual cycle
      (1) Often irregular (anovulatory) for up to 2 years after menarche
      (2) Three phases of normal menstrual cycle (Fig. 6-2)
         (a) Follicular: Proliferation of endometrium (first half of cycle)
         (b) Ovulation: Corpus luteum formation (occurs mid-cycle)
         (c) Luteal: Change within the endometrium, secretory activity (second half of cycle)
      (3) Calendar of a normal cycle
         (a) Full cycle: 28 ± 7 days
         (b) Menses duration: 4 ± 2 days
         (c) Ovulation: Occurs 14 days before menses, usually day 10 to 18 of the cycle
      (4) Blood loss and pads used: 30 to 50 mL total blood loss and approximately four to eight pads/day

Box 6-2   Assessing Substance Abuse: RAFFT

R: Do you smoke marijuana or do drugs to **relax** or **relieve** stress?
A: Do you ever smoke marijuana or do drugs **alone** (e.g., alone in your room)?
F: Does anyone in your **family** have an alcohol or drug problem?
F: Do any of your **friends** smoke marijuana or do drugs?
T: Have you ever gotten into **trouble** with police or the law for using drugs?

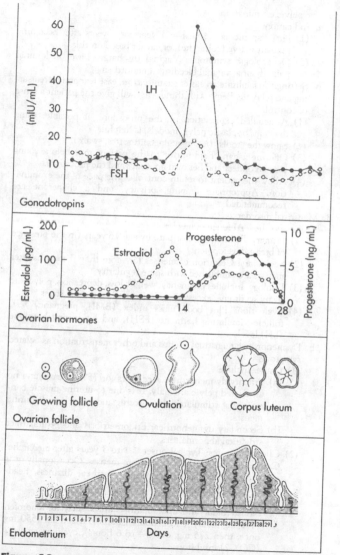

Figure 6-2 Physiology of the normal ovulatory menstrual cycle: gonadotropin secretion, ovarian hormone production, follicular maturation, and endometrial changes during one cycle. (From Emans SJ, Laufer M, Goldstein DP [eds]: Pediatric and Adolescent Gynecology, 5th ed. Philadelphia, Lippincott Williams & Wilkins, 2005.)

2. The pelvic examination
   a. Indications
      (1) First Papanicolaou smear—21 years or 3 years after becoming sexually active (coitarche), or earlier based on risk
      (2) Gynecologic symptoms: Vaginal discharge; lower abdominal pain; dysuria; vaginal bleeding; amenorrhea
   b. Setting: To facilitate an easier examination, ease fear and be reassuring and relaxing. Begin with things that will give the patient a sense of control.
      (1) A detailed explanation of the procedure, if possible, using diagrams or plastic pelvic models, is helpful.
      (2) Show the "tools" (i.e., specula, culturettes, swabs).
      (3) Offering a hand-held mirror to the patient may help a young woman understand her own anatomy and the procedure.
      (4) Allow the patient to retain control of the pace of the examination. Appropriate draping, privacy, and a chaperone are recommended
3. Menstrual disorders
   a. Amenorrhea: Absence of menses
      (1) Primary: Failure to menstruate by age 16 years (in the presence of breast development)
      (2) Secondary: Cessation of menses for more than 3 months after menses are established with some regularity
      (3) Etiology: Includes pregnancy, weight loss, depression, polycystic ovary syndrome, excessive exercise, and emotional stress
      (4) Evaluation: Plot body mass index (BMI), pregnancy test, follicle-stimulating hormone (FSH), and luteinizing hormone (LH) levels
   b. Dysmenorrhea: menstrual cramps and other menstruation associated symptoms
      (1) Causes include
         (a) Primary dysmenorrhea: Accounts for 75% of cases and no associated pelvic anomaly. It is due to uterine muscle contractions stimulated by prostaglandins released during menses.
         (b) Secondary dysmenorrhea: Endometriosis and genital tract structural abnormalities
      (2) Clinical features: Typical onset is 1 to 3 years after menarche. Cramps may start 1 to 4 days before menses. Occasionally, it is accompanied by nausea, vomiting, diarrhea, dizziness, headaches, and facial blemishes.
      (3) Management
         (a) Nonsteroidal anti-inflammatory drugs such as ibuprofen (400 mg, every 4 to 6 hours), naproxen sodium (550 mg once, then 275 mg, every 4 to 6 hours), cyclooxygenase-2 (COX-2) inhibitors
         (b) Oral contraceptives for 3 to 6 months
         (c) Increasing omega-3 fatty acids intake leads to production of less potent prostaglandin and leukotrienes and may ameliorate dysmenorrhea symptoms.

c. Dysfunctional uterine bleeding (DUB)
  (1) Pathophysiology: DUB is associated with anovulation and with no underlying pathologic process (lack of progesterone with anovulation leads to unopposed estrogen stimulation of endometrium and unpredictable bleeding).
  (2) Patterns of DUB
    (a) Polymenorrhea: Interval between menses less than 21 days
    (b) Menorrhagia (hypermenorrhea): Prolonged (>7 days) and heavy (over 80 mL/period; 8 to 14+ pads/day) at regular intervals
    (c) Metrorrhagia: Prolonged and excessive bleeding at irregular intervals
    (d) Oligomenorrhea: Infrequent bleeding at intervals longer than 35 days
  (3) Management: Depends on the severity
    (a) Mild: Normal hemoglobin. Treatment may be observation or, if agreeable, oral contraceptive pills (OCPs) to regulate cycles.
    (b) Moderate: Mild anemia, Monophasic combination OCP (e.g., Ovral), one tablet twice a day for 3 to 4 days usually stops active bleeding; then one tablet for 21 days, and iron supplementation.
    (c) Severe bleeding
      (i) Admit/stabilize if orthostatic or showing signs of acute blood loss.
      (ii) Combination OCP (e.g., Ovral) 1 tablet every 6 hours until bleeding stops (usually within first 24 hours), then twice a day for 21 days.
      (iii) Alternate therapy for acute hemorrhage: estrogen 25 mg intravenously (IV) every 4 hours, two to three doses
d. Etiologic diagnosis of abnormal menstrual bleeding
  (1) Pregnancy: Ectopic pregnancy, spontaneous abortion, molar pregnancy
  (2) Clotting abnormality: Von Willebrand's disease (especially if present from first menses)
  (3) Endocrine: Hyperthyroid or hypothyroid disease, adrenal disease, diabetes mellitus, hyperprolactinemia, polycystic ovary syndrome
  (4) Medications: Progestin—only hormonal contraceptives (e.g., Depo-Provera), anticoagulants, platelet inhibitors
  (5) Foreign body: Commonly, retained tampons; trauma
  (6) Infection: PID (salpingitis/endometriosis), cervicitis
  (7) Anatomical: Cervical polyps, uterine myoma, endometriosis
  (8) Systemic illness: Lupus erythematosus, iron deficiency
e. Laboratory evaluation of menstrual disorders
  (1) Complete blood cell count, beta-human chorionic gonadotropin (hCG; pregnancy test), screen urine or cervix for *Neisseria gonorrhoeae* and *Chlamydia*, and plot BMI
  (2) Depending on specific symptoms, examination results, and suspected etiology, consider LH/FSH levels (especially for amenorrhea), thyroid function tests, von Willebrand's disease screen,

clotting/bleeding studies, levels of prolactin and testosterone, and ultrasonography of pelvis.

 f. Management: Specific to the diagnosis (see Etiologies, previously)

4. Infections (see also Chapter 19)

 a. STIs (see Section 6.2)

 b. Vaginitis

  (1) *Candida albicans* infections are the most common cause of vaginitis in adolescents.

  (2) Bacterial vaginosis

 c. PID: Most commonly caused by recurrent or untreated chlamydial infection or gonorrhea, may be polymicrobial (for treatment guidelines, see Chapter 19)

 d. Toxic shock syndrome: Acute illness caused by *Staphylococcus aureus* toxin and associated with tampon and menses, among other causes. Clinical features include sudden onset of fever, sunburn rash, headache, vomiting, and diarrhea; may quickly progress to hypotensive shock. Management includes IV antistaphylococcal antibiotics and fluid resuscitation; steroids and pressors may be needed.

6.4 Reproductive Health: Adolescent Contraception and Pregnancy

CONTRACEPTION

1. Provide contraception information; have reading material available.

 a. Assess motivation not to become pregnant, which is very important in determining the success of any contraceptive method.

 b. There are no specific laws in many states regarding the distribution of contraceptives; know your state's regulations.

2. Methods to prevent pregnancy

 a. Abstinence: Safest method. Discuss refusal skills with every adolescent. Oral and anal sex should also be discussed because many teens who engage in these behaviors consider themselves abstinent.

 b. Hormonal: Recently there has been an increased use of hormonal patches (Ortho Evra), injections (Depo-Provera), and vaginal rings (NuvaRing; see Tables 6-2 and 6-3 regarding contraceptives).

  (1) OCPs: the most common form of contraception used by adolescents

   (a) Types

    (i) Combination: estrogen and progestins (Table 6-2)

    (ii) Minipill: progestin alone (for breast-feeding women)

   (b) Action

    (i) Suppress ovarian-hypothalamic axis, inhibit ovulation

    (ii) Alter endometrium to decrease likelihood of implantation

    (iii) Increase viscosity of cervical mucus ("hostile mucus")

   (c) Choosing a pill depends on the patient. Tailor OCP to patient (Box 6-3).

   (d) Possible side effects

    (i) Nausea

Name	Progestin (mg)	Estrogen (µg)	Manufacturer
Monophasic			
Alesse	Levonorgestrel (0.1)	Ethinyl estradiol (20)	Wyeth
Desogen	Desogestrel (0.15)	Ethinyl estradiol (30)	Organon
Ovral	Norgestrel (0.5)	Ethinyl estradiol (50)	Wyeth
Yasmin*	Drospirenone (3.0)	Ethinyl estradiol (30)	Berlex
Multiphasic			
Ortho Tri-Cyclen	Norgestimate (0.180[7])	Ethinyl estradiol (35[7])	Ortho
Ortho Tri-Cyclen Lo*	Norgestimate (0.180[7])	Ethinyl estradiol (25[7])	Ortho
Tri-Norinyl	Norethindrone (0.5[7])	Ethinyl estradiol (35[7])	Syntex
Progestin Only			
Ovrette	Norgestrel (0.075)	None	Wyeth
Extended (Trimonthly)			
Seasonale* (84 active pills + 7 placebos; menses every 3 mo, i.e., 1 time/season)	Levonorgestrel (0.15)	Ethinyl estradiol (30)	Barr Laboratories

*New oral contraceptive pill.

Box 6-3   Choosing an Oral Contraceptive Pill

Women with no problems should be prescribed a low dose OCP (monophasic or triphasic).

Prescribe OCP with a potent progestin (such as norgestrel or levonorgestrel) to

Women with heavy menstrual bleeding

Women with severe dysmenorrhea

Women with signs of fluid retention (bloating)

Prescribe OCP with a less androgenic progestin (such as norgestimate, desogestrel, or drospirenone) to

Women with severe acne

Women with hirsutism

Women with polycystic ovary disease

Women who are overweight

       (ii) Weight gain

     (iii) Breakthrough bleeding

     (iv) Headaches

      (v) Hypertension

     (vi) Vascular thrombosis

  (2) Medroxyprogesterone: Depo-Provera Injectable, 150 mg intramuscularly or Depo-subq Provera 104 mg SC every 12 weeks; suppresses hypothalamic-ovarian axis; prevents mid-cycle LH surge. Possible side effects include

    (a) Irregular bleeding

    (b) Amenorrhea

    (c) Weight gain

    (d) Risk for osteopenia

  (3) Intrauterine contraceptives: Prevent impregnation by changes in endometrial environment as well as changes in cervical mucus

    (a) Types

      (i) Mirena: Levonorgestrel-releasing intrauterine system, lasts 5 years

     (ii) ParaGard: Copper-containing, lasts 10 years

    (b) Possible side effects

      (i) Vaginal discharge

     (ii) Cramping on insertion

 c. Male condoms

  (1) *Encourage condom use in conjunction with any other contraceptive method to protect against STIs such as HIV, HPV, gonorrhea, and chlamydia.*

  (2) Proper use of condoms and their application must be explained, even demonstrated on a model.

  (3) Do not use petroleum jelly or other oil-based products with latex condoms.

Type of Contraceptive	Pregnancy Rate
Oral contraceptives	
Combination	0.3–0.7
Minipill	1.5–3.0
Intrauterine devices	
Progestasert	2.1
Copper	1.0
Condom and foam	2–10
Condom	2–20
Diaphragm and contraceptive cream	2.5–23
Cervical cap	6–17
Contraceptive sponge	13–28
Contraceptive foams and suppositories	3–30
Depo-Provera	0.4
Norplant	0.3–0.7

From Emans TJH, Goldstein DP (eds): Pediatric and Adolescent Gynecology, 3rd ed. Boston, Little, Brown, 1990.

    (4) Discuss the availability of polyurethane condoms with patients allergic to latex.
    (5) Note: Couples who choose to use condoms for pregnancy protection should be reminded about emergency contraception.
  d. See Table 6-3 for pregnancy rates with different contraceptives.
  e. Emergency contraception: High-dose hormonal contraception can reduce risk of pregnancy after unprotected intercourse. All adolescents should be aware of emergency contraception as well as how and when to access it. *Emergency contraception prevents pregnancy; it will not abort an established pregnancy.*
    (1) Give within 120 hours (preferably within 24 to 48 hours) of unprotected intercourse.
    (2) Plan B (progestin only)
      (a) One tablet (levonorgestrel 750 µg) to be taken as soon as possible after intercourse, one additional tablet to be taken 12 hours after the first dose. Alternatively, can safely give two pills at same time.[3]
      (b) Prevents 80% of pregnancies that might have occurred without treatment.
      (c) Nausea/vomiting are the most common side effects (23%/6% Plan B). If vomiting is a problem, consider giving both pills intravaginally.[2]
    (3) If possible, do a pregnancy test first to rule out preexisting pregnancy.

PREGNANCY

1. Epidemiology: Despite a decline in the rate of teenage pregnancy, more than 800,000 teenagers become pregnant each year; repeat pregnancies occur in 20% to 40% of adolescents within 2 years.

2. Clinical features: symptoms
   a. Amenorrhea or light/short/late bleeding
   b. Nausea/vomiting
   c. Urinary frequency
   d. Breast tenderness/fullness
   e. Abdominal fullness
   f. Weight gain/weight loss
3. Clinical features: signs
   a. Lower abdominal fullness
   b. Cervical changes (blue, soft)
   c. Pigment changes associated with hormonal change ("mask of pregnancy"/linea nigra)
4. Laboratory findings: hCG
   a. Urine hCG is usually positive before a missed period (2 to 4 days postconception); specifics vary with the test. It may be negative late in the pregnancy.
   b. Serum beta-hCG begins to be detectable 48 hours postconception and climbs (doubles every 2 to 3 days) through the first trimester, and peaks at 12 weeks (about 100,000 mIU). It will remain positive, but falls 1 to 2 weeks after miscarriage or termination.
5. Complications
   a. Ectopic pregnancy: Amenorrhea, abdominal pain, vaginal bleeding
      (1) Factors increasing risk
         (a) Previous ectopic pregnancy
         (b) Previous PID
         (c) Intrauterine device used as contraceptive
         (d) Progestin-only contraceptives used
      (2) Management
         (a) Consideration should prompt obstetrics/gynecology consult
         (b) Quantitative beta-hCG
         (c) Sonogram, especially with transvaginal probe
   b. Threatened or spontaneous abortion: Vaginal bleeding or abdominal cramping with positive beta-hCG (or known pregnancy) requires immediate obstetrics/gynecology consult because of risk of miscarriage.
6. Management
   a. Options counseling: Provide information regarding legally available choice.
      (1) Carry to term/parenting
      (2) Elective termination
      (3) Adoption
   b. Elective termination
      (1) Epidemiology: There are about 300,000 teenage abortions each year (30% of the total). Women from low-income families choose abortion 50% less often than those from middle- and upper-income families.
      (2) Legal: Restrictions on abortions for minors varies from state to state; know your state laws. *No minor can be forced to undergo an abortion regardless of her maturity or the wishes of her parents.*
      (3) The procedure varies according to gestation.

    (a) Surgical
      (i) Early (before 13 weeks): Most commonly suction curettage
      (ii) After 13 weeks: Procedure limited to 20 weeks maximum in most states
      (iii) Dilation and evacuation
      (iv) Prostaglandin-induced labor
    (b) Medical: Early in gestation and in appropriate settings, oral agents are being used to induce abortion.
      (i) RU486
      (ii) Methotrexate (now more commonly used for ectopic pregnancy)

7. Special consideration for adolescent pregnancies
   a. Greater risk than adults for delivering small or preterm infants
   b. Need for early and continuous prenatal care
   c. Risk for inadequate weight gain, anemia, STIs, substance abuse

6.5 Eating Disorders in Children and Adolescents

1. Definitions and diagnostic criteria
   a. Introduction: Although eating disorders *primarily* affect adolescents and young adults, usually girls, even younger patients and boys are at risk; and their numbers are growing. Eating problems range from mild (subclinical) to severe. Much of the literature fails to recognize the unique physiologic, psychological, and developmental issues related to young patients suffering from eating disorders.
   b. Anorexia nervosa (AN)
     (1) Definition: *Anorexia nervosa* is a syndrome in which caloric intake is insufficient to maintain weight or normal growth and is associated with a delusion of being fat and an obsession to be thinner; neither the delusion nor the obsession diminishes with weight loss.[1]
     (2) Diagnostic criteria
       (a) Refusal to maintain body weight at or above minimal weight for height (i.e., weight loss of over 15% from ideal body weight or failure to gain weight in a prepubertal patient)
       (b) Intense fear of gaining weight
       (c) Disturbed weight/shape perception
       (d) Secondary amenorrhea
   c. Bulimia nervosa (BN)
     (1) Diagnostic criteria
       (a) Recurrent episodes of binge eating
       (b) Recurrent inappropriate compensatory behaviors to prevent weight gain (i.e., self-induced vomiting, use of laxatives, diuretics, other medications, enemas, or simply fasting or excessive exercise)
       (c) Binge eating and compensating behaviors occurring two times per week for 3 months
       (d) Self-evaluation unduly influenced by weight/shape
       (e) Does not occur exclusively during episodes of AN

(2) Binge eating
  (a) Food is eaten quickly, swallowed without chewing.
  (b) Quantity of food eaten is large, with potentially thousands of calories consumed.
  (c) Food is eaten alone and secretively.
  (d) There is a frenzied quality to the bingeing.
  (e) Depression, anxiety, and guilt follow the binges.
(3) BN compared with AN (Fig. 6-3): BN has

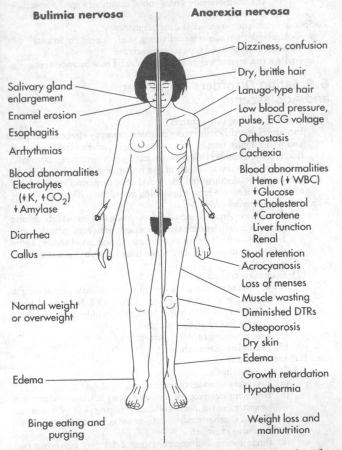

Bulimia nervosa

Salivary gland enlargement
Enamel erosion
Esophagitis
Arrhythmias
Blood abnormalities
Electrolytes
($\downarrow$K, $\uparrow$CO$_2$)
$\downarrow$Amylase
Diarrhea
Callus
Normal weight or overweight
Edema
Binge eating and purging

Anorexia nervosa

Dizziness, confusion
Dry, brittle hair
Lanugo-type hair
Low blood pressure, pulse, ECG voltage
Orthostasis
Cachexia
Blood abnormalities
Heme ($\downarrow$WBC)
$\downarrow$Glucose
$\uparrow$Cholesterol
$\uparrow$Carotene
Liver function
Renal
Stool retention
Acrocyanosis
Loss of menses
Muscle wasting
Diminished DTRs
Osteoporosis
Dry skin
Edema
Growth retardation
Hypothermia
Weight loss and malnutrition

Figure 6-3 Medical complications of eating disorders. DTR, deep tendon reflex; ECG, electrocardiogram; WBC, white blood cell count. (Based on data from Comerci GH: Eating disorders in adolescents. Pediatr Rev 10[2]:37–47, 1988.)

          (a) More psychiatric disturbance
          (b) More premorbid obesity
          (c) More food faddishness
          (d) More drug/alcohol problems
          (e) More legal/school problems
          (f) More sexual promiscuity
          (g) More self-mutilation/self-harm behavior
        (4) Eating disorder not otherwise specified
          (a) Mildly distorted body image
          (b) Weight 90% or less of average for height
          (c) Use of potentially harmful weight control methods or strong drive to lose weight

2. Epidemiology of eating disorders
  a. More than 90% are female.
  b. More than 95% are white.
  c. More than 75% are adolescent when the eating disorder is first diagnosed.
  d. AN develops in 1% of teenage girls.
  e. BN develops in 5% of older adolescent/young adult women.
  f. Subclinical eating disorders develop in 10% of postpubertal girls/young adult women.
  g. Incidence rates for AN have steadily increased from 1955 to the 2000s among 10- to 19-year-olds, but not among adults.
  h. The prevalence rate for AN in 15- to 19-year-old women is 0.48% (in the United States), making AN the third most common chronic condition after obesity and asthma.

3. Pathogenesis
  a. Predisposing and precipitating factors include
    (1) Female sex
    (2) Perfectionist and eager to please
    (3) Difficulty communicating negative emotions (anger, sadness, fear)
    (4) Difficulty resolving conflict
    (5) Low self-esteem
    (6) Fears of maturation and sexual development
    (7) Ambivalence about growing up
    (8) Previous or current history of sexual abuse
  b. Perpetuating factors
    (1) Biologic: Starvation reinforces starvation.
    (2) Psychological: The eating disorder helps the youngster in coping with the turbulent issues of adolescence; both patient and family are ambivalent about getting better.
  c. Family characteristics
    (1) Enmeshment—parents overly involved with children who should be exploring independence
    (2) Protectiveness (i.e., from negative emotions)
    (3) Lack of conflict resolution
    (4) Poor communication
    (5) Eating disorder as a way for homeostatic balance in family interaction

4. Differential diagnosis of eating disorders
   a. Psychiatric: Obsessive-compulsive disorder, affective disorders, thought disorders
   b. Neurologic: Midline central nervous system tumors, especially in male patients
   c. Gastrointestinal: Inflammatory bowel disease, achalasia, neoplasm
   d. Endocrine: Panhypopituitarism, hypothyroidism or hyperthyroidism, diabetes mellitus
5. Outpatient evaluation of weight loss
   a. Initial assessment
      (1) Is weight loss intentional and desired?
      (2) Is weight goal realistic and healthy?
      (3) Is there any purging behavior?
      (4) Is dieting or exercise excessive?
      (5) Is pursuit of thinness an overriding concern?
   b. Symptoms of malnutrition
      (1) Physical
         (a) Amenorrhea
         (b) Cold hands and feet (may present with diagnosed Raynaud's phenomenon)
         (c) Constipation, dry skin, dry hair
         (d) Headaches, fainting, dizziness
         (e) Lethargy
         (f) Anorexia
      (2) Mental/emotional
         (a) Difficulty concentrating
         (b) Difficulty making decisions
         (c) Irritability
         (d) Depression
         (e) Social withdrawal
         (f) Food obsessions
6. Management
   a. Overview
      (1) Make initial assessment, with purpose of developing a plan to help patients feel better and not specifically to "rule out" eating disorder.
      (2) Educate the patient and demystify the illness.
      (3) Set weight goals and visit frequency.
      (4) Arrange nutritional consultation to establish caloric and weight goals.
      (5) Make referral for individual, family, group counseling.
      (6) Avoid becoming part of any dysfunctional family dynamics.
      (7) Determine need for hospitalization.
   b. Indications for hospitalization
      (1) Severe malnutrition
         (a) Weight below 75% of ideal body weight
         (b) Weight below 15% BMI
      (2) Dehydration
      (3) Physiologic instability (bradycardia, hypotension, hypothermia, orthostasis)

   (4) Arrested growth and development

   (5) Failure of outpatient treatment

   (6) Uncontrollable bingeing and purging

   (7) Acute food refusal

   (8) Acute medical complications of malnutrition (syncope, seizures, cardiac failure, pancreatitis)

   (9) Acute psychiatric emergencies (suicidal ideation, acute psychosis)

   (10) Comorbid diagnosis that interferes with treatment (severe depression, obsessive-compulsive disorder, severe family dysfunction)

   (11) If hospitalization warranted, close collaboration with nutrition and medical team to avoid complications such as cardiac and refeeding syndromes

  c. Role of the primary care provider

   (1) Early, identification (i.e., check BMI, discuss possibility of an eating disorder with patient once suspected)

   (2) Initiation of effective intervention, referral as needed

   (3) Medical follow-up, including amenorrhea and screening for osteoporosis

  d. Principles for successful care

   (1) Proposed by Comerci

    (a) Establishment of trust

    (b) Involvement of family and treatment

    (c) Early restoration of normal nutritional and physiological state

    (d) Team approach–therapeutic partnership formation (e.g., pediatrician, social worker, nutritionist, psychologist)

7. Outcome

 a. This is a chronic illness. Approximately 70% of adolescent patients "recover"; 15% to 25% of adolescents "relapse."

 b. Mortality: With treatment, the mortality rate is under 5%; the most common cause of death is suicide.

 c. Prognosis

  (1) AN

   (a) Good indicators

    (i) Early age of onset

    (ii) Aggressive, early treatment

   (b) Poor indicators

    (i) Disturbed parent–child relationships

    (ii) Long duration of illness or later onset illness

    (iii) Concomitant personality disorder

    (iv) Presence of vomiting and so forth

  (2) BN

   (a) Poor indicators

    (i) Presence of significant depression

    (ii) Comorbidity with substance abuse

    (iii) Coexistent personality disorder

    (iv) History of sexual abuse

REFERENCES

1. Kreipe R: Eating disorders among children and adolescents. Pediatr Rev 16: 370-379, 1995.
2. Mor E, Saadat P, Kives S, et al: Comparison of vaginal and oral administration of emergency contraception. Fertil Steril 84:40-45, 2005.
3. Von Hertzen H, Piaggio G, Ding J, et al: Low dose mifepristone and two regimens of levonorgestrel for emergency contraception: A WHO multicentre randomized trial. Lancet 360:1803-1810, 2002.

SUGGESTED READING

Comerci GD: Eating disorders in adolescents. Pediatr Rev 10(2):1-11, 1988.
Dias P: Adolescent substance abuse: Assessment in the office. Pediatr Clin North Am 49:269-300, 2002.
Emans SJ, Laufer M, Goldstein DP (eds): Pediatric and Adolescent Gynecology, 5th ed. Philadelphia, Lippincott Williams & Wilkins, 2005.
English A, Matthews M, Extavour K, et al: State Minor Consent Statutes: A Summary Prepared by the National Center for Youth Law. San Francisco, National Center for Youth Law, 1995.
Hampton HL: Examination of the adolescent patient. Obstet Gynecol Clin North Am 27:1-18, 2000.
Neinstein L: Adolescent Health Care: A Practical Guide, 4th ed. Philadelphia, Lippincott Williams & Wilkins, 2002.

WEBSITES

National Center for Youth Law: www.youthlaw.org
MMWR Sexually Transmitted Disease Treatment Guidelines 2002: www.CDC.gov/STD/treatment

Endocrinologic Disorders

7

Cynthia H. Meyers-Seifer, Rebecca R. McEachern, and Philip A. Gruppuso

7.1 Growth Disorders

GENERAL PRINCIPLES OF GROWTH

The range of normal growth varies with age (see also Chapter 2 and Appendix II). Normal growth requires adequate nutrition and appropriate levels of thyroid hormone, growth hormone (GH), and sex steroids. Chronic systemic illness or environmental deprivation may impair growth.

SHORT STATURE/GROWTH FAILURE

1. Definition: Short stature is defined as length or height below the third percentile for age, or below the third percentile for the mid-parental target height. Growth failure indicates a growth velocity below the fifth percentile for age.
2. Etiology and pathophysiology
   a. Nonendocrine causes of short stature vastly outnumber endocrine causes, the latter being relatively rare (Boxes 7-1 and 7-2).
   b. Familial short stature and constitutional delay are normal variants presenting in healthy short children. In both situations growth velocity is within normal limits.
      (1) Familial short stature: Skeletal age (see later) is equal to the chronologic age.
      (2) Constitutional delay: Skeletal age is delayed and often approximates the height age (age at which the height would be at the 50th percentile).
   c. GH deficiency is most commonly idiopathic but may be associated with midline facial or central nervous system (CNS) defects, trauma (including birth), infection or inflammation, irradiation or chemotherapy, and hypothalamic or pituitary tumors.
3. Evaluation
   a. History
      (1) Important historical topics include pregnancy, labor, and delivery; birth weight and length; trauma; chronic illness; nutrition; family heights and pubertal timing; complete review of systems; and growth velocity from previous records.

Box 7-1   Non-endocrine Causes of Short Stature

Familial short stature
Constitutional delay
Skeletal dysplasias (osteochondrodysplasias and dysostoses)
Chromosomal abnormalities
Miscellaneous syndromes characterized by short stature
Intrauterine growth retardation
Undernutrition
Chronic systemic disease
    Bowel disorders (including celiac disease, inflammatory bowel disease)
    Kidney disorders (including renal tubular acidosis)
    Cardiovascular disorders
    Metabolic disorders
    Hematopoietic disorders
    Pulmonary disorders
    Chronic infection
Psychosocial deprivation

(2) Calculate the mid-parental height in centimeters to estimate the target adult height:

$$\text{Girls} = \frac{\text{mother's height} + (\text{father's height} - 13)}{2}$$

$$\text{Boys} = \frac{\text{father's height} + (\text{mother's height} + 13)}{2}$$

b. Physical examination: *Complete physical examination* with emphasis on standing height and sitting height, preferably by stadiometer; weight (plot height, weight, and body mass index [BMI]); funduscopic and visual field examination (indicator of pituitary issue); tooth development (reflects skeletal age); thyroid; pubertal staging; neurologic (indicator of CNS issue); dysmorphism

Box 7-2   Endocrine Causes of Short Stature

Growth hormone deficiency
Hypothyroidism
Hypercortisolism (includes iatrogenic)
Hypogonadism
Pseudohypoparathyroidism
Poorly controlled diabetes mellitus
Rickets

4. Laboratory findings
  a. Skeletal age: Obtaining a left-hand and wrist film and comparing the epiphysial ossification sites with published standards for age allow assessment of the child's biologic age and therefore of his or her growth potential.
  b. Initial screening laboratory tests: done to rule out systemic disease and hypothyroidism (Box 7-3).
  c. GH insufficiency
    (1) Screening tests for GH insufficiency
      (a) Insulin-like growth factor-I (IGF-I): circulating peptide generated in response to GH, and mediating the effects of GH
      (b) Insulin-like growth factor binding protein-3 (IGFBP-3): circulating protein, generated in response to GH, which modulates IGF-I action

Note: A random GH is not a useful test in the evaluation of short stature because of the pulsatile (and largely nocturnal) pattern of GH secretion.

    (2) Provocative tests for GH insufficiency: In a short child with an abnormal growth velocity, adequate nutrition, no systemic illness, and low growth factors (IGF-I and IGFBP-3), provocative testing is recommended. Various pharmacologic and physiologic stimuli cause GH release (Table 7-1). GH is sampled at frequent intervals for 1 to several hours after provocation.
  d. Magnetic resonance imaging (MRI) of the brain with emphasis on the hypothalamus and pituitary using gadolinium contrast should be done in all children diagnosed with GH deficiency to rule out an anatomic CNS pathologic process.
5. Management
  a. Systemic disease: Treatment is directed at the underlying disorder (e.g., hypothyroidism, diabetes).
  b. Familial short stature: Reassurance (GH is not thought to augment final adult height)
  c. Constitutional delay of growth and maturation: Reassurance. Sex steroid therapy may be offer̶ed̶ ̶ ̶ ̶ ̶ ̶ ̶ ̶ ̶ ̶ ̶14 years of age who

Box 7-3   Shor̶

Electroly̶
Blood
Cr̶

Th̶
Urinaly̶
Chromosome̶
  rule out low-lev̶

Table 7-1 **Selected Stimuli That Cause Growth Hormone Release**

Stimulus	Preparation	Dose	GH Sample (min)*
Exercise	4-hr fast	20-min exercise	0, 20, 40
Insulin-induced hypoglycemia†	Overnight fast	0.1 U/kg intravenous push	0, 20, 30, 45, 60, 90
Clonidine	Overnight fast	5 µg/kg orally (250 µg max)	0, 30, 45, 60, 90
Levodopa	Overnight fast	125–500 mg orally	0, 20, 40, 60, 90
Glucagon	Overnight fast	0.1 mg/kg intramuscularly	0, 30, 60, 90, 120, 150, 180

*Obtain glucose with all GH samples
†Seizure precautions include having intravenous dextrose at bedside.
GH, growth hormone.
Although controversial, failure to produce a GH level above 10 µg/L on two provocative tests is considered diagnostic of GH deficiency.

are distressed by their late pubertal development. One regimen is 50 to 100 mg testosterone enanthate intramuscularly (IM) monthly for 6 months.

d. GH deficiency: Treatment is somatropin (recombinant human GH), 0.05 mg/kg/day subcutaneously. Reported rare side effects include hypothyroidism, intracranial hypertension, slipped capital femoral epiphysis, glucose intolerance, allergic reactions, GH antibody formation, and pancreatitis.

TALL STATURE

1. Definition: Tall stature is defined as height above the 97th percentile for age.
2. Etiology: The differential diagnosis of tall stature includes
   a. Genetic tall stature: This is the most common diagnosis in patients seen for tall stature.
   b. Obesity: Exogenous obesity is associated with a modest acceleration in growth and bone age.
   c. Precocious puberty: Sex steroids contribute to the normal acceleration of linear growth during puberty. In a prepubertal age child (girls younger than 8 years, boys younger than 9 years), excessive levels of androgens or estrogens will cause abnormal growth acceleration.
   d. Marfan's syndrome
   e. Homocystinuria
   f. Klinefelter's syndrome
   g. 47, XYY male
   h. Acromegaly (GH excess)
   i. Hyperthyroidism
3. Diagnosis
   a. History: Family heights and pubertal timing, complete review of systems, and growth velocity from previous records. Calculate the mid-parental height in centimeters to estimate target adult height (see Short Stature).
   b. Physical examination (see Short Stature)
   c. Diagnoses of clinical syndromes associated with tall stature are made on the basis of history and physical findings.
4. Laboratory findings
   a. Skeletal age (see Short Stature): May be useful to make a prediction of ultimate stature
   b. Laboratory evaluation is directed by history and physical examination.
      (1) Testosterone or estradiol, dehydroepiandrosterone-sulfate (DHEA-S), and 17-hydroxyprogesterone should be obtained in suspected precocious puberty.
      (2) Serum and urine amino acids are indicated to confirm elevated homocystine concentrations in suspected homocystinuria.
      (3) Elevated GH and IGF-1 concentrations, followed by abnormal suppression of GH to a glucose challenge, confirm suspected GH excess. An MRI of the brain with emphasis on the hypothalamus and pituitary using gadolinium contrast should be done in all children diagnosed with GH excess, looking for a pituitary adenoma.

5. Management
   a. The treatment of precocious puberty is directed at the cause (see also Precocious Puberty).
   b. Genetic tall stature: Estrogens can be used to promote rapid epiphyseal fusion and therefore limit ultimate adult height. Therapy is indicated for psychological distress. An effective oral estrogen dose has been shown to be 0.15 to 0.5 mg/day of ethinyl estradiol.
   c. The treatment of GH-secreting pituitary tumors is transsphenoidal surgery. Somatostatin analogs may be of some use in decreasing GH secretion and shrinking tumor size.
   d. The treatment of hyperthyroidism is discussed in the section 7.2, Thyroid Disorders.

7.2 Thyroid Disorders

NORMAL PHYSIOLOGY

1. Normal thyroid function is essential for normal growth and development in childhood and is regulated by thyroid-stimulating hormone (TSH) and circulating iodide level. TSH is synthesized and released in the pituitary gland in response to hypothalamic thyrotropin-releasing hormone (TRH). TSH is inhibited by somatostatin and dopamine. TRH is modulated by temperature.
2. The thyroid gland concentrates iodine and returns it to the circulation as the hormones thyroxine (T_4) and triiodothyronine (T_3). Most circulating T_3 is synthesized (monodeiodinated) from T_4 in the periphery. Thyroid hormones modulate the synthesis and secretion of TSH and TRH.
3. Thyroid hormones circulate largely bound to thyroid-binding globulin (TBG), thyroid-binding prealbumin (TBPA), and albumin.
4. The effects of thyroid hormones, including thermogenesis, growth and development, and acceleration of metabolic pathways, are mediated by nuclear T_3 receptors in various cell types.

CONGENITAL HYPOTHYROIDISM

Congenital hypothyroidism is one of the most common treatable causes of mental retardation.

1. Fetal and neonatal thyroid physiology
   a. The hypothalamic-pituitary-thyroid axis begins to function in the second trimester.
   b. Free and total T_4 rise steadily beginning at 18 to 20 weeks' gestation until term. T_3 remains low until 30 weeks' gestation, gradually increasing subsequently. Fetal TSH increases from mid-gestation to term. Although the majority of circulating fetal thyroid hormone is from the fetal thyroid, there is a maternal–fetal gradient of thyroid hormones during the second and third trimester that may be protective in the setting of congenital hypothyroidism.
   c. At birth there is a surge of TSH in response to cold stress, with subsequent increases in T_4 and T_3. During childhood there is a gradual decrease in free T_4, total T_4, and T_3 and TSH levels (Table 7-2).

Table 7-2 Normal Levels of T_4, Free T_4, T_3, and TSH in Childhood

Age	T_4 (μg/dL)	Free T_4 (ng/dL)	T_3 (ng/dL)	TSH* mIU/mL
1–3 days	11.0–21.5			
1–5 yr	7.2–15.6	0.7–1.7	100–380	<2.5–13.3
6–15 yr	6.4–13.3	0.7–1.7	102–264	0.6–6.3
16–20 yr	4.2–11.8	0.7–1.7	94–241	0.6–6.3
			80–210	0.2–7.6

*Peaks at 80–90 mIU/mL 30 min after birth in term newborns.
T_3, triiodothyronine; T_4, thyroxine; TSH, thyroid-stimulating hormone.
Adapted from Johnson KB: The Harriet Lane Handbook, 13th ed. St. Louis, Mosby, 1993, p 149.

2. Etiology and pathophysiology
   a. Thyroid dysgenesis, which comprises thyroid agenesis, hypogenesis, and ectopia, is the most common cause of permanent congenital hypothyroidism, with a prevalence of 1/4000 newborns. The cause is sporadic.
   b. Other, less common etiologies of permanent congenital hypothyroidism include
      (1) Defects in thyroid hormone biosynthesis (1/30,000), usually autosomal recessive
      (2) Hypothalamic-pituitary dysfunction (1/100,000)
      (3) Transient congenital hypothyroidism
3. Diagnosis
   a. There are no specific abnormalities at birth. By 6 to 12 weeks, infants may show lethargy, constipation, and hoarse cry. There may be bradycardia, large fontanelles, protuberant tongue, umbilical hernia, hypotonia, mottling, jaundice, and hypothermia.
   b. Lack of therapy by 2 to 3 months will result in delayed somatic and intellectual development and permanent developmental impairment.
4. Laboratory findings
   a. Newborn screening: Capillary blood on filter paper
      (1) Screen is best done at 3 to 5 days of age; with early discharge it is often done earlier.
      (2) Most North American programs screen for T_4, and then follow with a TSH for the lowest 10% of T_4 levels.
      (3) A low T_4 and a TSH above 20 to 25 mU/mL suggests primary congenital hypothyroidism.
      (4) Low T_4 and normal TSH may reflect prematurity, TBG deficiency, or hypothalamic-pituitary insufficiency.
   b. Diagnostic studies (initiated as soon as abnormal screen result is reported)
      (1) Repeat serum free T_4 and TSH to verify screen. Measuring free T_4 will avoid the need to adjust the total T_4 if there is a binding protein abnormality (Table 7-3).
      (2) Perform thyroid scan with technetium-99m or iodine-123 to distinguish thyroid dysgenesis from a thyroid hormone biosynthetic defect.
      (3) If no thyroid gland is detected by scan, thyroid ultrasonography may be useful to distinguish thyroid aplasia from a TSH receptor abnormality or TSH receptor-blocking antibodies.
5. Management
   a. As soon as the diagnosis is confirmed, begin L-thyroxine at 10 to 15 µg/kg/day (usually 25 to 50 µg/day) orally. Parents are instructed to crush the tablet, mix with a *small* amount of liquid, and administer. Check free T_4 and TSH 1 month after starting therapy.
   b. Children are followed in parallel with well-child visits to ensure appropriate therapy. Free T_4 and TSH are monitored frequently. Free T_4 should be in the upper range of normal for age and TSH in the normal range.

Table 7-3 Thyroid Function Tests: Interpretation

Condition	TSH	T_4	Free T_4
Primary hyperthyroidism	L	H	High N to H
Primary hypothyroidism	H	L	L
Hypothalamic-pituitary hypothyroidism	L, N, H*	L	L
Thyroid-binding globulin deficiency	N	L	N
Euthyroid sick syndrome	L, N, H*	L	L to low N
TSH adenoma or pituitary resistance	N to H	H	H
Compensated hypothyroidism†	H	N	N

*Can be normal, slightly low, or slightly high.
†Treatment may not be necessary.
L, low; N, normal; H, high; T_4, thyroxine; TSH, thyroid-stimulating hormone.
From Robertson J, Shilkofski N: The Harriet Lane Handbook, 17th ed. Philadelphia, Elsevier Mosby, 2005.

ACQUIRED HYPOTHYROIDISM

1. Etiology and pathophysiology
   a. The causes of acquired hypothyroidism in childhood are listed in Box 7-4. Autoimmune thyroid disease is the most common cause of acquired hypothyroidism in children.
   b. Autoimmune thyroid disease involves a genetic predisposition for alterations in the immune surveillance system, which leads to thyroid inflammation and injury.
      (1) Chronic lymphocytic thyroiditis (Hashimoto's thyroiditis) results in destruction of the thyroid gland by natural killer cell–mediated cytotoxicity; antibodies to certain thyroid proteins (antibody-dependent, cell-mediated cytotoxicity); and

Box 7-4 Causes of Acquired Hypothyroidism in Children

Autoimmune thyroid disease
Thyroid dysgenesis
Disorders of thyroid hormone biosynthesis
Iatrogenic
Exposure to goitrogens (drugs, foods)
Endemic iodine deficiency
Hypothalamic-pituitary hypothyroidism
Generalized resistance to thyroid hormone

complement-dependent, cell-mediated cytotoxicity. The thyroid gland may be goitrous or atrophic.

(2) Hashimoto's thyroiditis may be associated with multiple endocrine deficiencies, most commonly type 1 diabetes mellitus with or without adrenal insufficiency.

(3) Hashimoto's thyroiditis occurs twice as frequently in girls as in boys, and more frequently in adolescence, but it has been reported in infancy.

2. Diagnosis
   a. History: There often is a family history of thyroid disease. Inquiry is made with respect to foods and medication that may interfere with thyroid function.
      (1) The most prominent feature of childhood-acquired hypothyroidism is linear growth failure. Weight is relatively spared.
      (2) Other manifestations include lethargy, somnolence, constipation, cold intolerance, and dry skin and hair.
   b. Physical examination may be significant for the following:
      (1) Short stature and decreased growth velocity
      (2) Moderately enlarged, firm thyroid gland
      (3) Bradycardia
      (4) Cool, dry extremities
      (5) Muscle hypertrophy and weakness
      (6) Delayed relaxation phase of deep tendon reflexes
      (7) Delayed or precocious sexual development
      (8) Myxedema

3. Laboratory findings
   a. Skeletal age: Delay equals or exceeds linear growth delay (see Short Stature).
   b. Initial laboratory evaluation includes a free T_4 and TSH. A low free T_4 and a high TSH are consistent with primary hypothyroidism; the addition of elevated antithyroglobulin or antithyroid peroxidase antibody titers suggests Hashimoto's thyroiditis.
      (1) If autoantibodies are absent, a thyroid scan is indicated to rule out thyroid dysgenesis or ectopia.
      (2) If a total T_4 is low and the TSH is normal, suspect either a TBG deficiency or a defect in the hypothalamus (TRH) or pituitary (TSH).
      (3) A T_3 is not very useful in the evaluation of hypothyroidism; T_3 is often normal in hypothyroidism because of increased conversion of T_4 to T_3.

4. Management
   a. L-Thyroxine: Dose (μg/kg/day) varies with age (Table 7-4).
   b. Treatment is recommended for children with an elevated TSH and a free T_4 in the low or normal range. Treatment is not recommended for a *euthyroid goiter* (i.e., if TSH and free T_4 are normal).
   c. Follow-up includes regular evaluation of growth, sexual maturation, thyroid function tests, and skeletal age. Behavioral changes are not uncommon as a result of thyroid hormone replacement.
   d. Most patients will require L-thytoxine indefinitely; 20% to 30% may undergo remission but continue to require follow-up.

Table 7-4   **Dosing of L-Thyroxine for Acquired Hypothyroidism**

Age	Dose (μg/kg)
0–3 mo	10–15
3–6 mo	8–10
6–12 mo	6–8
1–3 yr	4–6
3–10 yr	3–4
10–15 yr	2–4
>15 yr	2–3

ACQUIRED HYPERTHYROIDISM

1. Etiology and pathophysiology
   a. Hyperthyroidism in children is usually caused by Graves' disease, an autoimmune disorder developing in a genetically predisposed population. A defect in immune surveillance combined with an environmental stress results in the production of thyroid-stimulating immunoglobulin (TSI), also referred to as TSH receptor-stimulating antibody (TRS-Ab). The TSI stimulates the production of thyroid hormone through the TSH receptor. Graves' disease is more common in adolescence than in early childhood and is six to eight times more common in girls than in boys. There is often a family history of autoimmune thyroid disease.
   b. A hyperthyroid phase may be seen in the clinical course of chronic lymphocytic thyroiditis, which eventually results in clinical hypothyroidism. This entity has been termed *hashitoxicosis*. The hyperthyroid phase may result from inflammatory destruction of thyroid follicles and the release of T_4 and T_3 or stimulation from TSI.
   c. Subacute thyroiditis is a self-limited inflammation of the thyroid gland associated with an upper respiratory infection. Hyperthyroidism results from the release of T_4 and T_3 with destruction of thyroid follicles. The thyroid is usually tender.
2. Diagnosis
   a. History: Common complaints of hyperthyroid children are listed in Box 7-5.
   b. Physical examination: An examination is remarkable for goiter (unless autonomous nodule or factitious), restlessness, tremulousness, staring appearance and lid lag, tachycardia, wide pulse pressure, shortened relaxation phase of deep tendon reflexes, and growth acceleration. Exophthalmos due to ophthalmopathy may be seen in Graves' disease; dermopathy is rare in children.
3. Laboratory findings
   a. Initial laboratory studies include T_4, T_3, and TSH.
      (1) If T_4 and T_3 are high and TSH is low, primary hyperthyroidism is present. T_3 may be elevated in excess of T_4.

Box 7-5   Symptoms of Hyperthyroidism

Nervousness
Behavior deterioration and declining school performance
Heat intolerance
Sweating
Increased appetite
Weight loss
Palpitations
Weakness
Sleeplessness
Diarrhea

  (2) If T_4 and T_3 are high and TSH is normal, consider thyroid hormone binding abnormality.
  (3) If T_4 and T_3 are high and TSH is normal or high, consider pituitary resistance to thyroid hormone or TSH adenoma.
 b. Further laboratory studies
  (1) TSI (to confirm suspicion of Graves' disease) and also antithyroglobulin and antithyroid peroxidase antibodies.
  (2) Normal free T_4 and free T_3 (and normal TSH) suggest an abnormality of thyroid hormone binding.
  (3) An MRI is indicated if a pituitary adenoma is suspected.
  (4) Thyroid iodine-123 scan will show uptake in an autonomous functioning nodule.
  (5) Thyroid ultrasonography may be useful to evaluate thyroid gland anatomy as an adjunct to thyroid scan.
  (6) Fine-needle aspiration and cytology of a functioning nodule may be considered.
  (7) Skeletal age in young children with increased growth velocity (see Growth Disorders)
4. Management: Therapeutic options for Graves' disease include antithyroid drugs, radioactive iodine ablation, and near-total thyroidectomy. In addition, propranolol 0.5 to 2.0 mg/kg/day divided every 6 to 8 hours may be used to block the sympathetic hyperactivity characteristic of untreated hyperthyroidism.
 a. Inhibition of thyroid hormone synthesis using thioureylene antithyroid drugs is the first line of treatment for autoimmune hyperthyroidism in children.
  (1) Propylthiouracil (PTU): Also inhibits T_4-to-T_3 conversion; 5 to 10 mg/kg/day up to 450 mg divided every 8 hours
  (2) Methimazole (MMI): 0.5 to 1.0 mg/kg/day up to 30 mg divided every 12 hours. Toxic reactions to thioureylene drugs include agranulocytosis (1/1000), drug fever, hepatitis, nephritis, arthritis, rash, and lupus-like syndrome. Approximately 25% of children on medical therapy are expected to achieve remission every 2 years.

b. Ablation with iodine-131 has been proved safe in adolescents and adults. Remission may require several weeks to months after iodine-131 ablation, and thus interval treatment with antithyroid drugs may be necessary. Hypothyroidism occurs in 10% to 20% in the first year, 3% to 5% a year thereafter.

c. Surgery remains the treatment of choice for an autonomous hyperfunctioning nodule. It is also an option for Graves' disease if antithyroid drugs and radioactive iodine are not acceptable alternatives.

d. Iodides (Lugol's and saturated solution potassium iodide [SSKI]) quickly inhibit thyroid hormone synthesis and release and are useful in addition to thioureylene drugs in acute *thyroid storm* or before surgery.

7.3 Disorders of Sexual Maturation

AMBIGUOUS GENITALIA

The birth of an infant with ambiguous genitalia is psychologically stressful for the family. A prompt evaluation must be initiated by an experienced multidisciplinary team to identify a possible life-threatening medical condition and assign appropriate gender.

1. Etiology: The differential diagnosis of ambiguous genitalia in the newborn may be divided into three broad categories (Box 7-6).
2. Clinical features
   a. History: The history may reveal maternal androgen exposure or virilization during pregnancy, siblings with genital ambiguity, or neonatal demise.
   b. Physical examination: An examination should determine the presence of gonads, the degree of labioscrotal fusion, and the stretched phallus length.
3. Laboratory findings
   a. Initial studies to determine broad category
      (1) Chromosome analysis on peripheral blood leukocytes
      (2) Pelvic ultrasonogram and genitogram through the urogenital sinus to assess degree of müllerian duct development
   b. Directed studies to determine the specific diagnosis
      (1) 17-Hydroxyprogesterone, testosterone, steroid precursors
      (2) Electrolytes
      (3) Adrenocorticotropic hormone (ACTH) or human chorionic gonadotropin (hCG) stimulation tests
      (4) Gonadal biopsy
      (5) Genital skin biopsy for 5-α reductase or androgen receptor activity
4. Management
   a. Sex assignment is made by a multidisciplinary team including staff from pediatrics, endocrinology, surgery, genetics, and social services. Potential for normal physical appearance, sexual function, and fertility is considered.
   b. Medical
      (1) Glucocorticoids and mineralocorticoids in forms of congenital adrenal hyperplasia (CAH)
      (2) Sex steroid replacement at puberty and in adulthood

> Box 7-6   Features in Disorders Presenting with Hypocalcemia
>
> *Female Pseudohermaphroditism*
>
> Externally virilized individuals with 46, XX chromosomes, ovaries, and a normal uterus, cervix, and fallopian tubes.
>   Congenital adrenal hyperplasia
>   21-Hydroxylase deficiency
>   11-Hydroxylase deficiency
>   3-β-Hydroxysteroid dehydrogenase deficiency
>   Maternally derived androgens
>
> *Male Pseudohermaphroditism*
>
> Undervirilized individuals with 46, XY chromosomes with testes and variable development of epididymides, vas deferentia, and seminal vesicles.
>   Inadequate production of androgen
>   Testosterone biosynthetic defects
>   Leydig cell hypoplasia
>   5-α-Reductase deficiency
>   Peripheral unresponsiveness to androgen (partial androgen insensitivity)
>
> *Gonadal Differentiation Disorders*
>
> Gonadal dysgenesis—phenotype varies with amount of müllerian inhibiting substance and testosterone in utero produced by abnormal gonads.
>   46, XY partial gonadal dysgenesis (symmetric dysgenetic gonads)
>   45, X/46, XY gonadal dysgenesis (mixed gonadal dysgenesis)
>   True hermaphroditism

  c. Surgical
      (1) External genitalia reconstruction concordant with sex assignment
      (2) Removal of internal structure discordant with sex assignment
  d. Psychological: intervention required at birth and at later developmental stages

DISORDERS OF PUBERTY

Puberty or adolescence is the time period between the onset of secondary sex characteristics and completion of physical maturation.

Normal Pubertal Development

1. The fetal hypothalamic-pituitary-gonadal axis is functional by midgestation. By early childhood, however, CNS inhibition of gonadotropin-releasing hormone (GnRH), in combination with highly sensitive steroid negative feedback at the pituitary and hypothalamus, render this system quiescent.

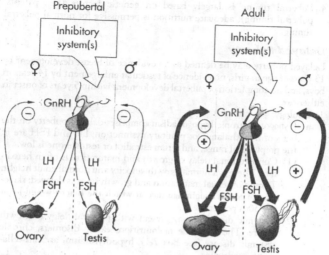

Figure 7-1 Hypothalamic-pituitary-gonadal axis showing the differences between children and adults. FSH, follicle-stimulating hormone; GnRH, gonadotropin-releasing hormone; LH, luteinizing hormone. (Redrawn from Bacon GE, Spencer ML, Hopwood NJ, Kelch RP: Practical Approach to Pediatric Endocrinology, 3rd ed. St. Louis, Mosby, 1990.)

2. At puberty, an unknown trigger diminishes the central inhibition, and the hypothalamus begins secreting GnRH, which stimulates the pituitary to secrete the gonadotropins luteinizing hormone (LH) and follicle-stimulating hormone (FSH). The gonads make sex steroids and mature germ cells in response to gonadotropins (Fig. 7-1).
3. Physical changes of puberty (see Appendix V)
   a. In girls, breast development begins first in puberty in response to rising ovarian estradiol (E$_2$) levels. The average age of menarche is 12.5 years. The growth spurt is early, peaking at approximately Tanner stage III.
   b. In boys, the first sign of puberty is testicular enlargement in response to gonadotropins and testosterone. The penis, prostate, and sexual hair develop in response to rising levels of testosterone, dihydrotestosterone (DHT), and adrenal androgens (see later). The average age of sperm production is 13.5 years. The growth spurt is late, at approximately Tanner stage IV to V.
   c. Adrenarche, that is, adrenal androgen secretion, is initiated in parallel with hypothalamic-pituitary-gonadal activation. Adrenal androgens, particularly DHEA-S, together with ovarian androgens are responsible for pubic and axillary hair in girls.
   d. The adolescent growth spurt requires adequate thyroid hormone, GH, and sex steroids.

4. Pubertal timing is largely based on genetic factors (i.e., parents' pubertal timing); adequate nutrition is permissive for normal pubertal timing.

Delayed Puberty

Delayed puberty may be defined as no evidence of breast development by 13 years of age in girls, no evidence of testicular enlargement by 14 years in boys, and no completion of pubertal development within 5 years of onset in either sex.

1. Etiology
   a. *Hypo*gonadotropic hypogonadism comprises delayed puberty on the basis of hypothalamic or pituitary dysfunction; LH and FSH are in the prepubertal range, and serum estradiol or testosterone is low.
      (1) Constitutional delay of growth and maturation is often hereditary. There is a normal growth velocity and normal adult height. Timing of sexual maturation and growth spurt is delayed; skeletal age equals height age (age at which the height would be at the 50th percentile).
      (2) Systemic disorders may present with pubertal delay or growth failure. These include malnutrition, eating disorders, chronic systemic disease (see Box 7-1), hypothyroidism, and miscellaneous syndromes.
      (3) Congenital hypothalamic or pituitary malformation may be associated with
         (a) Kallmann's syndrome (GnRH deficiency and anosmia)
         (b) Cleft lip or palate
         (c) Septo-optic dysplasia (other pituitary insufficiencies may coexist)
      (4) Acquired hypothalamic or pituitary disease may be associated with
         (a) Tumors, including craniopharyngioma, dysgerminoma, pituitary adenoma (particularly prolactinoma), and glioma
         (b) Infiltrative processes, particularly Langerhans cell histiocytosis
         (c) Infection
         (d) Inflammation, including autoimmune
         (e) Trauma, including radiation
         (f) Drugs
   b. *Hyper*gonadotropic hypogonadism comprises delayed puberty on the basis of primary gonadal disorders. LH and FSH are abnormally elevated, and estradiol or testosterone is normal or low.
      (1) Female
         (a) Turner's syndrome is the most common form of gonadal failure in girls, with a 1/2000 incidence. External and internal genitalia are female; ovaries are replaced by fibrous streaks of connective tissue. Karyotype is 45, XO in 50% of individuals, with mosaic forms and partial X-chromosome deletions in the remainder.
         (b) Gonadal radiation therapy or systemic chemotherapy
         (c) Autoimmune oophoritis (may or may not be associated with other autoimmune disorders)
         (d) Resistance to gonadotropins

(2) Male
  (a) Klinefelter's syndrome is the most common form of primary gonadal failure in boys, with a 1/500 incidence. There are normal prepubertal external genitalia. In adolescence boys are noted to have small testes, gynecomastia, eunuchoid body proportions, and decreased body hair. Karyotype is usually 47, XXY.
  (b) Gonadal radiation therapy or systemic chemotherapy
  (c) Cryptorchidism
  (d) Resistance to gonadotropins
2. Clinical features
  a. History: Complete history includes previous illness, family heights and pubertal timing, complete review of systems, and growth velocity from previous records.
  b. Physical examination: A *complete physical examination* should be done, with emphasis on height, weight, body mass index, funduscopic and visual field examination, sense of smell, thyroid, galactorrhea, pubertal staging, neurologic, dysmorphology, (consider gynecologic examination for primary or secondary amenorrhea)
3. Laboratory findings
  a. Skeletal age (see Short Stature)
  b. Initial laboratory tests, including LH, FSH, estradiol, or testosterone
    (1) If LH and FSH are elevated (no history of radiation therapy or chemotherapy), obtain karyotype.
    (2) If LH and FSH are low/normal, obtain
      (a) Screening laboratory tests to rule out systemic disease and hypothyroidism (see Box 7-3)
      (b) Prolactin, IGF-1, and IGFBP-3; *then,*
      (c) If evidence of systemic disease exists, evaluate and treat illness.
      (d) If prolactin is increased, proceed with MRI of the brain, with emphasis on the hypothalamus and pituitary, using gadolinium contrast.
      (e) If low IGF-1 and IGFBP-3, and no systemic disease, proceed with provocative pituitary hormone testing (see Short Stature).
      (f) If no systemic disease and no other pituitary abnormality suspected, consider MRI of the brain as previously, especially in girls.
4. Management
  a. Hypogonadotropic hypogonadism
    (1) Constitutional delay of growth and maturation
      (a) Reassurance
      (b) Low-dose sex steroids to initiate puberty
        (i) Girls (>13 years; rarely needed): conjugated estrogens (Premarin) 0.3 mg orally every other day for 6 months
        (ii) Boys (>14 years): testosterone enanthate 50 to 100 mg IM every 4 weeks for four to six doses
      (c) Counseling if indicated
    (2) Systemic disease: Treatment is directed at the underlying disorder.

(3) Congenital hypothalamic or pituitary malformation
 (a) Sex steroid replacement
  (i) Girls: (1) Conjugated estrogens (Premarin) 0.3 mg orally every day for 6 months; increase to 0.625 mg orally every day for subsequent 6 months; once spotting begins, begin cycling with conjugated estrogens 0.625 mg orally every day, days 1 to 25 of each month. (2) Medroxyprogesterone acetate 10 mg every day, days 16 to 25 of each month. (Menses occur after day 25.) (3) Oral contraceptives containing low-dose estrogen are an option when growth is complete.
  (ii) Boys: Testosterone enanthate 50 to 100 mg IM every 4 weeks, increasing the dose by 50 mg every 6 months to a dose of 200 to 300 mg every 3 weeks. Transdermal testosterone may be an option in fully virilized boys.
 (b) Other pituitary hormone replacement if indicated
(4) Acquired hypothalamic or pituitary disease: Treatment is directed at the underlying disorder. Hormone replacement as in congenital hypothalamic or pituitary malformation.
 b. Hypergonadotropic hypogonadism: sex steroid replacement

Precocious Puberty

Precocious puberty may be defined as breast development or pubic hair before 8 years of age in girls or testicular enlargement or pubic hair before 9 years of age in boys. *Isosexual* precocious puberty refers to early development that is appropriate for the sex of the individual, whereas *contrasexual* precocious puberty refers to virilization in girls and feminization in boys. Precocious puberty is much more common in girls than in boys, but is much more likely to be associated with a significant pathologic process in boys.

1. Etiology and pathophysiology
 a. Isosexual precocious puberty
  (1) *Central precocious puberty* refers to premature activation of the hypothalamic-pituitary-gonadal axis.
   (a) Idiopathic: 90% of girls, 20% of boys
   (b) Hypothalamic hamartoma: Nonenhancing heterotopic, hyperplastic neuronal tissue
   (c) Intracranial pathology, including tumor, head trauma, hydrocephalus, and postinfection
   (d) Profound hypothyroidism
   (e) Normal variant: Premature thelarche
  (2) *Peripheral precocious puberty* refers to development resulting from elevated sex steroids independent of the hypothalamic-pituitary-gonadal axis.
   (a) CAH
   (b) McCune-Albright syndrome (MAS)
   (c) Familial male precocious puberty (boys only)
   (d) Tumor
    (i) Steroid producing: Adrenal, ovary, testis
    (ii) hCG producing: Retroperitoneal, retropleural, intracranial, or hepatoblastoma (boys only)

(e) Exogenous sex steroids

(f) Normal variant: premature adrenarche

b. Contrasexual precocious puberty

    (1) Virilization in girls

       (a) CAH: 21-hydroxylase, 11-hydroxylase, and 3-β-hydroxy-steroid dehydrogenase deficiencies

       (b) Polycystic ovary disease

       (c) Ovarian or adrenal tumor

       (d) Exogenous androgens

    (2) Feminization in boys

       (a) Testicular or adrenal tumor

       (b) Exogenous estrogens

       (c) Normal variant: Adolescent gynecomastia

       (d) Liver dysfunction

2. Clinical features of isosexual precocious puberty

a. History is significant for rapid linear growth. There may be concern about pubic or axillary hair. There may be breast development or menstrual bleeding in girls, genital or testicular enlargement in boys. There may be a long-standing neurologic disorder or a more recent onset of neurologic complaints such as headache or vision change. There may be abdominal pain. Café au lait spots and bone pain may suggest MAS.

b. Physical examination is complete with emphasis on height, growth velocity, funduscopic examination, visual fields, thyroid, abdomen, pelvis, neurologic, skin, and Tanner stage of pubic hair in girls and boys and of breasts in girls. Testes should be carefully measured with either a 15-cm ruler or an orchidometer. Stretched penile length is obtained.

c. Laboratory findings

    (1) Initial tests

       (a) Boys: LH, FSH, testosterone, DHEA-S, 17-hydroxyprogesterone, free T_4, TSH, hCG

       (b) Girls: LH, FSH, estradiol, free T_4, TSH, as well as DHEA-S, 17-hydroxyprogesterone, and testosterone if there is adrenarche in addition to breast development

       (c) Both: Skeletal age (see Growth Disorders)

    (2) Adrenal computed tomography (CT) scan/gonadal ultrasonography

    (3) GnRH stimulation testing: 100 μg GnRH (Factrel) given intravenously (IV). LH and FSH are obtained by immunochemiluminescent assay at times 0, 30 minutes, and 60 minutes. Compare patient results with laboratory standards.

    (4) Boys

       (a) Testes are enlarged on physical examination: If hCG is then elevated, look for hCG-secreting tumor. If result of GnRH stimulation test is pubertal level (diagnosis is central precocious puberty), proceed with MRI of the brain. However, if GnRH stimulation test result is prepubertal or suppressed, consider MAS or familial male precocious puberty. Also, check free T_4 and TSH; if free T_4 is low and TSH is high, the diagnosis is hypothyroidism.

(b) Testes are not enlarged on physical examination: Look for adrenal or gonadal tumor on CT or ultrasonography, respectively, if screening androgens are high. Also, check for CAH if 17-hydroxyprogesterone, DHEA-S, and/or testosterone are high and imaging is negative: give 250 μg ACTH (Cortrosyn) IV; obtain 17-hydroxypregnenolone, 17-hydroxyprogesterone, DHEA, androstenedione, 11-deoxycortisol, and cortisol at 0 and 60 minutes. Compare patient results with laboratory standards. Finally, this could be secondary to premature adrenarche.

(5) Girls
    (a) Isolated breast development: Look for adrenal or gonadal tumor on CT or ultrasonography, respectively. If GnRH stimulation test result is pubertal level (diagnosis is central precocious puberty), proceed with MRI of the brain. If GnRH level is prepubertal or suppressed, consider MAS or premature thelarche. If free T_4 is low and TSH is high, the diagnosis is hypothyroidism.
    (b) Breast development and adrenarche: Look for adrenal or gonadal tumor CT or ultrasonography, respectively. Also check for CAH if 17-hydroxyprogesterone, DHEA-S, and/or testosterone are high and imaging is negative (see [4] [b], previously). If GnRH level is prepubertal or suppressed, consider MAS.
    (c) Isolated adrenarche Look for adrenal or gonadal tumor on CT or ultrasonography, respectively, if screening androgens are high. Look for CAH if 17-hydroxyprogesterone, DHEA-S, and/or testosterone are high and imaging is negative. The diagnosis is premature adrenarche if no evidence of tumor or CAH exists.

3. Management
   a. Adrenal or gonadal tumor: Primary therapy is surgical. Adrenalectomy requires glucocorticoid therapy during and after surgery for varying lengths of time.
   b. Intracranial pathologic process: Therapy (often surgical) is directed at the underlying disorder. The patient may also need therapy for central precocious puberty.
   c. Central precocious puberty: GnRH agonist therapy desensitizes the pituitary gonadotrophs to endogenous GnRH, blocking LH, FSH, and gonadal sex steroid production.
      (1) Leuprolide: 50 μg/kg/day subcutaneously
      (2) Depot leuprolide: 7.5 to 15 mg (start 0.3 mg/kg) IM every 4 weeks
      (3) Note: Children on GnRH agonist therapy usually are followed with GnRH stimulation testing to document suppression.
   d. CAH (see Adrenal Disorders)
   e. MAS and familial male precocious puberty
      (1) Girls (MAS only)
          (a) Letrozole, an aromatase inhibitor, blocks estrogen biosynthesis.

(2) Boys
    (a) Ketoconazole, a cytochrome P450 inhibitor, blocks testosterone biosynthesis.
    (b) Alternatively, letrozole, an aromatase inhibitor, in combination with spironolactone, an androgen receptor blocker, may be prescribed.

7.4 Disorders of Mineral Metabolism

CALCIUM DISORDERS

Calcium Homeostasis

1 Normal calcium and ionized calcium levels in childhood are 8.9 to 9.8 mg/dL and 4.2 to 5.2 mg/dL, respectively. Calcium level may drop as low as 7.6 mg/dL in term and 6.2 mg/dL in preterm infants 1 to 2 days after birth.

2. Calcium is present largely in the structural tissues of the skeleton and in solution in extracellular fluid.

3. The biologically active component of extracellular calcium is the ionized calcium. Approximately 40% of circulating calcium is bound to albumin.

4. Calcium is essential for signal transduction in nerve, muscle, endocrine, and other tissues.

5. Ionized calcium is tightly regulated by the parathyroid glands and the vitamin D endocrine system. Parathyroid hormone (PTH) raises calcium by increasing bone resorption, decreasing urinary calcium excretion, and enhancing synthesis of 1,25-dihydroxyvitamin D_3 (1,25[OH]$_2$D$_3$).

6. Calcitonin, produced in the C cells of the thyroid gland, decreases serum calcium and phosphate concentration by effects at bone and kidney.

Hypocalcemia

1. Etiology and pathophysiology
    a. Early neonatal hypocalcemia by definition occurs in the first 3 days of life, and it is an exaggeration of the physiologic fall in calcium at birth. The precise mechanisms are unclear, although there are associations with prematurity, diabetes in pregnancy, and cardiorespiratory distress.
    b. Late neonatal hypocalcemia typically presents in healthy term infants at 5 to 10 days of age. Etiologies include the following:
        (1) Neonatal hypoparathyroidism may be transient, due to maternal hypercalcemia, or permanent, due to parathyroid gland hypoplasia or a PTH biosynthetic defect (e.g., calcium-sensing receptor gain-of-function mutation, DiGeorge's syndrome).
        (2) Hyperphosphatemia shifts extracellular calcium into bone and reduces 1,25(OH)$_2$D$_3$ synthesis, leading to hypocalcemia.

Causes include cow's milk formula feeding because of the high phosphate content of cow's milk formulas, and renal failure because it results in decreased phosphate excretion and hyperphosphatemia.

   (3) Hypomagnesemia

   (4) Vitamin D deficiency (maternal deficiency or inherited disorder)

  c. Hypocalcemia may present beyond the newborn period.

   (1) Hypoparathyroidism due to abnormally low PTH secretion may develop from congenital or acquired lesions (e.g., congenital hypoparathyroidism, DiGeorge's syndrome, autoimmune, postsurgical, infiltrative).

   (2) Pseudohypoparathyroidism, that is, end-organ resistance to PTH, results in hypocalcemia, hyperphosphatemia, and *increased* PTH. Hypothyroidism and hypogonadism may be associated.

   (3) Vitamin D–deficiency rickets is most commonly caused by poor sunlight exposure and inadequate vitamin D intake. Precipitating factors include prolonged breast-feeding, gastrointestinal disease, and anticonvulsant therapy.

2. Clinical features

  a. History: Hypocalcemia may precipitate paresthesias, carpopedal spasm, muscle cramps, muscle twitch, seizures, tetany, and laryngeal stridor.

  b. Physical examination: Examination may reveal acute signs of hypocalcemia such as Chvostek's or Trousseau's signs. Particular findings associated with selected causes of hypocalcemia are shown in Box 7-7.

3. Laboratory findings

  a. Obtain serum calcium, ionized calcium, phosphate, intact PTH, alkaline phosphatase, 25-hydroxyvitamin D_3 (25[OH]D_3), and 1,25(OH)$_2D_3$ (Table 7-5); also, serum electrolytes, blood urea nitrogen (BUN), creatinine, and magnesium and urine for calcium, phosphate, and creatinine.

  b. Findings on bone films are shown in Box 7-7.

4. Management

  a. For tetany or seizures, treat with 10% calcium gluconate IV at 2 mL/kg over 10 minutes to correct hypocalcemia. This may be followed by 5 to 8 mL/kg/day of 10% calcium gluconate by constant infusion or divided every 6 hours. Calcium levels must be monitored carefully.

   Note: Extravasation of IV calcium may cause tissue necrosis.

  b. For chronic hypocalcemia (usually due to hypoparathyroidism or pseudohypoparathyroidism), treatment is with 1,25(OH)$_2D_3$. Dosage is begun at 0.01 to 0.05 µg/kg/day and titrated gradually up to a maximum of 1 to 2 µg/day. Calcium supplementation at 50 mg/kg elemental calcium per day may be used in three or four divided doses. Calcium level should be maintained in the lower range of normal to avoid potential hypercalcemia, hypercalciuria, nephrocalcinosis, and CNS injury.

  c. For vitamin D deficiency, we recommend vitamin D 5000 to 10,000 IU orally once daily initially. Serum calcium, phosphorus, and alkaline

Box 7-7   Features in Disorders Presenting with Hypocalcemia

| | PHYSICAL FINDINGS | |
Hypoparathyroidism	Pseudohypoparathyroidism (Ia)	Vitamin D Deficiency
Papilledema Moniliasis	Mental retardation Round face Short stature Short metacarpals Ectopic calcifications Enlarged ribs (rachitic rosary)	Rickets Frontal bossing Bowed legs Bone pain Muscle weakness
	RADIOLOGIC FEATURES	
Hypoparathyroidism	Pseudohypoparathyroidism (Ia)	Vitamin D Deficiency
Widened medullary canals with coarse trabecular patterns	Widened medullary canals with coarse trabecular patterns	Metaphyseal cupping and fraying of long bones
± Osteomalacia	Subcutaneous bone formation	Osteopenia
± Bone resorption	Short metacarpals Thickened calvaria Basal ganglia calcifications	Cortical thinning

phosphatase are monitored weekly, and the dose is lowered as the parameters improve to avoid toxicity. The standard dose of vitamin D for prevention is 400 IU/day.

Hypercalcemia

1. Etiology and pathophysiology
   a. A childhood calcium level over 9.8 mg/dL is usually considered elevated, but check with your laboratory. Symptoms of hypercalcemia may occur with levels over 12 to 14 mg/dL (moderate hypercalcemia).
   b. Hyperparathyroidism allows increased bone and renal resorption of calcium and increased intestinal absorption of calcium through increased $1,25(OH)_2D_3$.
      (1) Primary hyperparathyroidism is uncommon in childhood and most frequently is familial or in association with multiple endocrine neoplasia (MEN) syndromes. The pathologic process may be parathyroid hyperplasia or adenoma.
      (2) Secondary or tertiary hyperparathyroidism may develop in response to hyperphosphatemia as in renal failure.

Diagnosis	Ca	PO₄	25(OH)D₃	1,25(OH)₂D₃	PTH	Alkaline Phosphatase
Hypoparathyroidism	L	H	N	L	L	N or H
Pseudohypoparathyroidism	L	H	N	L	H	H
Vitamin D deficiency	L	N or L	L	N or ±H	H	HHH

1,25(OH)₂D₃, 1,25-dihydroxyvitamin D₃; 25(OH)D₃, 25-hydroxyvitamin D₃; L, low; N, normal; H, high; PTH, parathyroid hormone.

   c. Idiopathic infantile hypercalcemia (Willia s' syndrome) is associated with dysmorphic facies, cardiovascu! . anomalies, and mental retardation.

   d. Immobilization, as with severe injury, results in bone resorption.

   e. Vitamin D intoxication results in increased intestinal absorption of calcium.

   f. Malignancy may result in rapid skeletal destruction by metastases or may induce bone resorption through synthesis and release of PTH-related peptide.

2. Clinical features: Conduct a thorough history and physical examination, including a careful family history looking for MEN syndromes. The symptoms of patients with moderate hypercalcemia may be related to gastrointestinal, CNS, neuromuscular, osseous, and renal systems, and they include vomiting, constipation, and abdominal discomfort; malaise, depression, or delusions; weakness and paresthesias; bone pain (with increased PTH); and polyuria, thirst, renal colic. Hypertension may be present on physical examination.

3. Laboratory findings

   a. Obtain serum calcium, phosphate, intact PTH, alkaline phosphatase, $25(OH)D_3$, and $1,25(OH)_2D_3$ (Table 7-6); also, electrolytes, BUN, creatinine.

   b. Obtain urine calcium, creatinine for calculation of calcium-to-creatinine ratio (Ca/Cr). Obtain urine PO_4 for calculation of the tubular reabsorption of phosphate (decreased in hyperparathyroidism; see later).

   c. Bone films (hyperparathyroidism) may show subperiosteal resorption in the phalanges and clavicles, lytic skull lesions, cysts in pelvic and long bones.

4. Management

   a. Immediate therapy to initiate calciuresis

     (1) Hydration with normal saline at two times maintenance over 24 to 48 hours

     (2) Furosemide 1 mg/kg every 6 hours

   b. Bisphosphonates, inhibitors of osteoclast function, may be used in the acute management of hypercalcemia; use pamidronate, 0.5 to 1.0 mg/kg/dose over 4 to 5 hours.

   c. Calcitonin 2 to 4 U/kg IV every 6 to 12 hours opposes bone resorption, but effects are transient.

   d. Hydrocortisone 1 mg/kg every 6 hours reduces intestinal absorption of calcium, and possibly bone resorption.

   e. Removal of the underlying cause of hypercalcemia is primary. Parathyroid adenomas and parathyroid hyperplasia are treated surgically.

   f. Avoid excess ingestion of vitamin D and calcium salts.

PHOSPHATE DISEASES

Phosphate Homeostasis

Serum phosphate level is regulated primarily by control of renal reabsorption of phosphate in the proximal tubule. Phosphate intake and PTH regulate this process. The normal adult serum phosphate level is 2.5 to 4.5 mg/dL. Plasma levels of phosphate are higher in children than in adults.

Diagnosis	Ca	PO₄	25(OH)D₃	1,25(OH)₂D₃	PTH
Hypoparathyroidism	H	L	N	H	H
Williams' syndrome	H	N	N	?L	?
Familial hypocalciuric hypercalcemia	H	N or L	N	N	N or H
Immobilization	H	N or H	H	L	L
Vitamin D intoxication	H	N or H	H	L	L
Malignancy	H	N	L	L	L

1,25(OH)₂D₃, 1,25-dihydroxyvitamin D₃; 25(OH)D₃, 25-hydroxyvitamin D₃; L, low; N, normal; H, high; PTH, parathyroid hormone.
From Gertner JM: Disorders of calcium and phosphorus homeostasis. Pediatr Clin North Am 37:1441-1465, 1990.

Hypophosphatemia

1. Etiology and pathophysiology: Chronic hypophosphatemia results in rickets (child) or osteomalacia (adult/adolescent). Phosphate level usually remains above 1.0 mg/dL in this setting and is not associated with other signs or symptoms.

   Note: Rickets may present without hypophosphatemia in individuals with vitamin D deficiency, or inherited and acquired defects in vitamin D metabolism or absorption (see Hypocalcemia). Common causes include

   a. Inadequate phosphate intake

   (1) Prematurity and breast-feeding: Phosphorus content of human milk is inadequate to meet the needs of a preterm infant, resulting in hypophosphatemia, elevated $1,25(OH)_2D_3$, increased bone resorption, and rickets.

   (2) Phosphate-binding antacid abuse results in poor intestinal absorption of phosphate.

   (3) Severe intestinal disease

   b. Renal tubular phosphate reabsorption defects (excess phosphate loss; e.g., renal hypoxic or toxic injury)

2. Laboratory findings

   a. Obtain serum calcium, phosphate, PTH, $25(OH)D_3$, $1,25(OH)_2D_3$, alkaline phosphatase, and creatinine, as well as urine calcium, phosphate, and creatinine (glucose and amino acids).

   b. Bone films may show osteopenia and nonspecific rachitic changes, including cupping and fraying of the metaphyses in long bones and widening of the anterior ribs.

3. Management: Fortification of human milk, with commercially available preparations rich in calcium and phosphorus, is provided for preterm infants and has decreased the development of rickets.

Hyperphosphatemia

1. Etiology: Excess intravascular phosphate results from

   a. The inability of the kidney to excrete adequate phosphate, as in

   (1) Renal failure

   (2) Hypoparathyroidism

   (3) Pseudohypoparathyroidism

   b. Excess intake, as in

   (1) Enemas

   (2) Cow's milk in infancy

   c. Transfer from the intracellular space, as in cell lysis after chemotherapy for hematogenous malignancies.

2. Clinical features

   a. The most important acute potential consequences of hyperphosphatemia are hypocalcemia and tetany (or seizures).

   b. In the setting of renal failure, hyperphosphatemia may result in soft tissue calcifications and secondary hyperparathyroidism.

3. Management

   a. Dietary phosphate restriction

   b. Phosphate binders to reduce intestinal absorption. Calcium salts (calcium acetate or calcium carbonate) with meals are recommended as first-line phosphate binders. Hypercalcemia should be avoided.

7.5 Disorders of Water Metabolism

WATER HOMEOSTASIS

1. Normal serum osmolality is between 280 and 290 mOsm/kg.
2. Sodium concentration is used to follow water gains and losses, as reflected in hyponatremic or hypernatremic laboratory findings. However, it is important to understand that sodium concentration is influenced not only by sodium transport but by water intake.
3. In the presence of circulating antidiuretic hormone (ADH), the renal collecting duct becomes permeable to water, which decreases urine volume.
4. The stimuli that initiate pituitary release of vasopressin include increasing osmolality, detected by an osmosensor anterior to the hypothalamus, as well as decreasing blood volume and pressure, detected by barosensors in the left atrium, carotid sinus, and aortic arch.
5. The osmosensor for thirst is thought to have a similar anatomic location and threshold as the osmosensor for ADH.

DIABETES INSIPIDUS

1. Definition: This condition refers to an inability to form concentrated urine.
2. Etiology: Diabetes insipidus (DI) results from the inability to synthesize, secrete, or respond to ADH normally. Causes include mutations in the gene(s) responsible for ADH synthesis and response, congenital malformations of the neurohypophysis such as septo-optic dysplasia; and destruction of the hypothalamus or neurohypophysis by tumor, histiocytosis, granulomatous disease, inflammation, infection, autoimmune neurohypophysitis, or trauma.
3. Clinical features
   a. History
      (1) History may include polyuria and polydipsia (often of abrupt onset), nocturia, enuresis, preference for iced water, clear urine on awakening.
      (2) May include declining linear growth velocity or precocious puberty, suggesting another hypothalamic-pituitary abnormality.
      (3) May include headache, vomiting, or vision changes, suggesting an intracranial process.
      (4) Rule out use of lithium, demeclocycline, or diuretics.
      (5) In infancy, nephrogenic DI may present with hypernatremia and failure to thrive.
   b. Physical examination may show signs of mild dehydration and confirm history suggestive of hypothalamic-pituitary or another intracranial disorder.
4. Laboratory findings
   a. Initial studies serve to rule out diabetes mellitus, hypercalcemia, primary polydipsia, or renal parenchymal disease as a cause of polyuria and screen for DI (Box 7-8).
      (1) Serum: Osmolality, sodium, potassium, glucose, calcium, BUN, creatinine
      (2) Urine: Urinalysis, osmolality, sodium, glucose

> **Box 7-8   Screening Studies for Diabetes Insipidus (DI)**
>
> 1. Serum osmolality >300 mOsm/kg and urine osmolality <300 mOsm/kg indicates DI is likely.
> 2. Serum osmolality <270 mOsm/kg or urine osmolality >600 mOsm/kg indicates DI is unlikely.
> 3. Serum osmolality >270 mOsm/kg but <300 mOsm/kg represents unclear results.
>
> If the first or third results occur, proceed with water deprivation testing.

b. Water deprivation test
   (1) Patient is stable and well hydrated for 24 hours.
   (2) Fluids are withheld for 6 hours. Urine specific gravity and volume, and body weight are measured hourly.
   (3) Serum electrolytes and osmolality, and urine osmolality are obtained at 0 and 6 hours.
   (4) In DI, specific gravity will remain under 1.005, urine osmolality will be under 150 mOsm/kg, and urine volume will not change. Weight loss is usually 3% to 5%. In primary polydipsia, specific gravity rises to more than 1.010, urine/plasma osmolality ratio is greater than 2, urine volume decreases, and there is no weight loss.
   (5) At the termination of water deprivation, 1-desamino-8-D-arginine vasopressin (DDAVP) is administered intranasally or IV and urine is monitored hourly for a response over 4 hours. A urine specific gravity of 1.014 or an increase of 100 mOsm/kg in urine osmolality confirms central DI.
   (6) *No response suggests nephrogenic DI.*
c. If the water deprivation and DDAVP responsiveness tests demonstrate central DI, brain MRI using gadolinium contrast is indicted to look for a CNS lesion.
d. If there is renal unresponsiveness to DDAVP (i.e., nephrogenic DI), renal ultrasonography is indicated to rule out obstructive uropathy.
5. Management
   a. Central DI
      (1) Treatment of any underlying CNS disorder is primary.
      (2) DDAVP is a synthetic analog of vasopressin with a duration of action between 8 and 24 hours. Dose is 5 to 30 µg (0.05 to 0.3 mL) per 24 hours intranasally divided one to two times a day, beginning with the lowest dose and working up to an effective dose. Dose by subcutaneous or IV injection is 10% of the intranasal dose. Patients should be instructed to allow for at least a 1-hour escape from antidiuresis before administering the next dose to avoid water intoxication.
      (3) During parenteral fluid therapy (i.e., postoperative)
         (a) Restrict fluids to 1 L/m²/day.

(b) Prescribe a constant infusion of 0.5 mU/kg/hr aqueous vasopressin. To start, double q 30 minutes to max of 10 mU/kg/hr.

(c) Follow urine and serum osmolality every 12 hours.

b. Nephrogenic DI

(1) Treat any underlying renal disease such as outflow obstruction, renal tubular acidosis, or pyelonephritis.

(2) Provide adequate water and adequate calories for growth. Nighttime feedings are usually required in infancy.

(3) Restrict sodium; breast milk is preferable to formula.

(4) Chlorothiazide, 30 mg/kg/day in three divided doses, increases urinary sodium losses, leading to volume contraction and increased proximal tubule reabsorption of water (sodium restriction is necessary for the desired effect). Potassium replacement may be necessary.

SYNDROME OF INAPPROPRIATE ANTIDIURETIC HORMONE SECRETION

1. Etiology and pathophysiology: This condition is *rare* in children.

   a. Excess secretion of ADH results in water retention, weight gain, and hyponatremia, with resulting aldosterone suppression and decreased proximal tubular resorption of sodium (high urine sodium losses).

   b. CNS disorders: Meningitis, encephalitis, trauma

   c. Pulmonary disorders: Pneumonia, tuberculosis, bronchopulmonary dysplasia

   d. Medications: Carbamazepine, chlorpropamide, cyclophosphamide, analgesics, barbiturates, vasopressin

   e. Paraneoplastic syndrome (*rare*)

2. Clinical features

   a. History

   (1) Symptoms may be referable to an underlying illness causing increased ADH: CNS changes, pulmonary complaints (cough, shortness of breath).

   (2) Symptoms may be referable specifically to hyponatremia: Weakness, weight gain, anorexia, lethargy, confusion, and seizures.

   b. Physical examination: A complete physical examination may reveal mental status changes, focal neurologic changes, or evidence of lung disease, supporting the suspicion of syndrome of inappropriate ADH secretion (SIADH).

3. Laboratory findings

   a. Diagnostic studies

   (1) Serum: Electrolytes ($\downarrow$Na), BUN, creatinine, osmolality ($\downarrow$)

   (2) Urine: Sodium ($\uparrow$), osmolality ($\uparrow$)

   b. In SIADH, hyponatremia is accompanied by normal serum potassium and high urine sodium losses.

4. Management

   a. Fluid restriction: Limit oral fluid to 1 L/m^2/day.

   b. Treat underlying cause of SIADH/hyponatremia.

   c. Avoid rapid correction of hyponatremia. If severe CNS symptoms develop and sodium is less than 120 mEq/L, 3% saline at 5 mL/kg, in combination with IV furosemide, may be administered slowly until an improvement in mental status occurs. Sodium should not rise faster than 2 mEq/L per hour.

7.6 Adrenal Disorders

ADRENAL CORTEX PHYSIOLOGY

1. The mature adrenal cortex synthesizes steroid hormones, including mineralocorticoids, glucocorticoids, and androgens, from cholesterol (Fig. 7-2).
2. Control of steroid hormone synthesis
   a. Mineralocorticoids, particularly aldosterone, are synthesized in the zona glomerulosa, controlled primarily by angiotensin II (renin-angiotensin system) and potassium concentration.
   b. Glucocorticoids, particularly cortisol, are synthesized in the zona fasciculata, primarily controlled by hypothalamic corticotropin-releasing hormone (CRH) and pituitary ACTH.
   c. Androgens, particularly DHEA, DHEA-S, and androstenedione, are synthesized in the zona reticularis, responsive to ACTH and other, unspecified factors.

ADRENAL INSUFFICIENCY

Inadequate mineralocorticoid effect results in salt and water loss and potassium retention (low sodium, high potassium, and dehydration). Inadequate glucocorticoid effect results in impaired glucose synthesis (hypoglycemia).

1. Etiology: Box 7-9
2. Clinical features
   a. History may include complaints of weakness, fatigue, anorexia, weight loss, abdominal pain, vomiting, and diarrhea. There may be salt craving. Young children may have symptoms of hypoglycemia. There may be a history of (nonadrenal) autoimmune disease such as

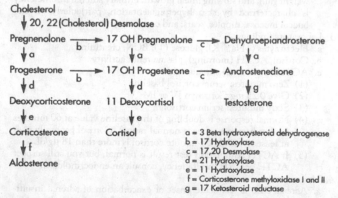

Figure 7-2 Steroid biosynthetic pathway.

Box 7-9   Causes of Adrenal Insufficiency

Primary Adrenal Insufficiency

Adrenal enzyme deficiencies (congenital adrenal hyperplasia)
    21-Hydroxylase
    3-β-Hydroxysteroid dehydrogenase
    17-α-Hydroxylase
    11-β-Hydroxylase
    20, 22 (cholesterol) Desmolase
Adrenal unresponsiveness to adrenocorticotropic hormone
Acquired adrenal insufficiency
    Adrenoleukodystrophy
    Autoimmune
    Infection (fungal, bacterial, viral, acquired immunodeficiency
        syndrome)
    Amyloidosis
    Metastases
    Hemorrhage

Secondary Adrenal Insufficiency

Associated with other pituitary insufficiencies
After prolonged glucocorticoid therapy

---

   diabetes mellitus, thyroiditis, pernicious anemia, vitiligo, alopecia, or
   chronic active hepatitis.
   b. Physical examination may be significant for low blood pressure, poor
      weight gain, and slowing linear growth. Primary adrenal insufficiency
      is characterized by skin hyperpigmentation, particularly on the
      buccal mucosa, nipples, scars, and creases.
3. Laboratory findings
   a. Electrolytes ($\downarrow$Na, $\uparrow$K), glucose ($\downarrow$), BUN, creatinine
   b. Cortisol, ACTH (morning), plasma renin activity
   c. ACTH (Cortrosyn) stimulation test
      (1) Zero minutes: serum cortisol baseline
      (2) Give 0.25 mg Cortrosyn IV or IM
      (3) Sixty minutes: serum cortisol
      (4) Normal response is doubling of the baseline value at 60 minutes
          (unless baseline exceeds normal range). Cortisol generally rises
          at least 10 μg/dL; 60-minute cortisol is more than 18 μg/dL.
      (5) If ACTH stimulation test result is normal, but you still suspect
          ACTH or CRH insufficiency, consult an endocrinologist.
4. Management
   a. *Adrenal crisis* is the acute onset or exacerbation of adrenal insuffi-
      ciency, often leading to electrolyte abnormalities, metabolic acido-
      sis, and shock. Immediately give

(1) Normal saline with 5% dextrose 20 mL/kg by IV bolus to treat hemodynamic instability and hypoglycemia, followed by constant infusion, *and*

(2) Hydrocortisone 50 mg/m^2 IV bolus, followed by 100 mg/m^2/day divided every 4 to 6 hours, *and*

(3) Treat any underlying disorder, such as infection.

b. Chronic adrenal insufficiency

(1) Hydrocortisone 8 to 15 mg/m^2/day orally in three divided doses. The dose is adjusted to avoid growth retardation. However, in virilizing forms of CAH, dose must be adequate to suppress excess adrenal androgens.

(2) Florinef (9-α-fluorocortisol) 0.05 to 0.1 mg/day (up to 0.2 mg/day in infants) orally for mineralocorticoid replacement in primary adrenal insufficiency

(3) Management of intercurrent illness or stress (fever or injury) includes the following:

(a) Three times the usual dose of hydrocortisone orally

(b) No change in mineralocorticoid dose

(c) If the patient is vomiting, parenteral hydrocortisone is indicated. Families are instructed in giving IM hydrocortisone in emergencies: 50 mg for young children, 100 mg for older children. The child should also be evaluated in the emergency department or office.

(d) For surgery, hydrocortisone, 100 mg/m^2/day IV divided every 6 hours, beginning on call to the operating room and for the following 24 to 48 hours

ADRENAL EXCESS

1. Cushing's syndrome

a. Etiology and pathophysiology: Excessive cortisol secretion may be due to an ACTH-secreting pituitary adenoma (Cushing's disease), a primary adrenal tumor, pigmented adrenocortical micronodular dysplasia (rare), or ectopic ACTH secretion (rare). A primary adrenal tumor is more likely in infancy and early childhood, whereas an ACTH-secreting pituitary adenoma is more likely after 7 years of age.

b. Diagnosis

(1) History is significant for weight gain and growth retardation.

(2) Physical examination often reveals obesity, slowed growth, delayed puberty, moon face, thinning of the skin, purple striae, hirsutism, muscle weakness, hypertension, and personality changes.

(3) Initial diagnostic studies may include a dexamethasone suppression test and 24-hour urinary free cortisol. Consult an endocrinologist.

c. Management

(1) Cushing's disease: Transsphenoidal adenomectomy is the current treatment of choice. Glucocorticoid coverage is indicated during surgery, and replacement therapy is required for varying lengths of time after surgery (see Adrenal Insufficiency).

(2) Adrenal disease
  (a) Adrenal adenoma: Adrenalectomy with glucocorticoid coverage during surgery followed by glucocorticoid replacement until contralateral gland is functioning (see Adrenal Insufficiency). Mineralocorticoid replacement is indicated after surgery in the case of bilateral adrenalectomy.
2. Sex steroid excess: Adrenal sex steroid excess occurs in certain forms of CAH and in androgen- or estrogen-secreting tumors (discussed in the sections on Ambiguous Genitalia and Precocious Puberty).

7.7 Diabetes Mellitus

1. Etiology, pathophysiology, and epidemiology: Clinically and genetically a heterogeneous group of diseases with the common characteristic of hyperglycemia, diabetes mellitus may be classified as type 1 (insulin-dependent, juvenile onset, ketosis prone), type 2 (non–insulin-dependent, adult onset), secondary (e.g., diabetes associated with cystic fibrosis), or other endocrine disorders (e.g., acromegaly or Cushing's syndrome).
2. Diabetes mellitus (all types) affects approximately 5% of the U.S. population.
   a. Type 1 diabetes accounts for 15% of all diabetes and occurs most commonly in children, adolescents, and young adults. It is characterized by the abrupt onset of polyuria, polydipsia, and weight loss that invariably progresses to ketoacidosis if untreated. The pathogenesis of type 1 diabetes is a result of an autoimmune process that causes loss of pancreatic beta cell mass and function. With the loss of insulin secretory capacity, hyperglycemia and a tendency toward ketosis develop.
   b. Type 2 diabetes is becoming increasingly more common in children and adolescents but still represents a minority of new cases of diabetes in this age group.

TYPE 1 DIABETES

1. Diagnosis: A definitive diagnosis of type 1 diabetes may be made in children and adolescents when the classic symptoms are present and unequivocal hyperglycemia (plasma glucose >200 mg/dL or 11.1 mmol/L) is detected. In rare cases in which symptoms are not yet present (e.g., if glycosuria is detected on a routine urinalysis), diagnosis may be based on fasting plasma glucose above 126 mg/dL (7.8 mmol/L) on two occasions, or plasma glucose over 200 mg/dL (11.1 mmol/L) that is sustained during an oral glucose tolerance test or random blood sugar.
2. Management of newly diagnosed type 1 diabetes (without ketoacidosis): At the onset of diabetes, priority should be given to correction of the metabolic perturbations while reassuring the patient and family. Hospitalization may be necessary to provide a period of metabolic stabilization, emotional adjustment, and family education. Seventy percent of new patients present without ketoacidosis (see Diabetic Ketoacidosis, later). The basic principles of management include the following:
   a. Initial insulin therapy: 0.15 to 0.3 U/kg subcutaneous regular insulin if significant ketonuria is present. As soon as possible, the timing

of insulin administration should be adjusted to coincide with meal-times. Children presenting with hyperglycemia but no ketonuria may be started on standard insulin therapy as described later.

b. When the patient's ketonuria has resolved, treatment may be modified to include longer-acting insulin. Multiple regimens are available, but the most commonly used are as follows:

(1) Two to three injections per day with a rapid-acting insulin analog (Lispro/Humalog or Aspart/NovoLog) before breakfast and supper, with an intermediate-acting insulin (N or NPH) also given at breakfast and dinner or bedtime. Total daily dose is usually in the range of 0.8 to 1.0 U/kg, depending on age and pubertal status, with approximately two thirds of the daily dose given before breakfast.

(2) A multiple daily injection regimen with a rapid-acting insulin given at meals and snacks in proportion to the carbohydrates ingested and a long-acting insulin analog (Glargine/Lantus) given once a day (morning or evening).

(3) Pumps are becoming increasingly more common in the pediatric age groups. However, insulin delivery by pump requires a multidisciplinary approach with a skilled diabetes nurse educator and nutritionist. Its use is often best reserved for those patients with longer duration of diabetes rather than the newly diagnosed.

c. Ongoing monitoring of blood glucose (by reagent strip meter) should be done before meals, before bed, and at or about 2:00 AM. Based on blood glucose readings, insulin can be adjusted to achieve an overall target range of 80 to 180 mg/dL (4.4 to 10 mmol/L). Ranges in infants and young children may be higher (100 to 200 mg/dL and 100 to 250 mg/dL, respectively) whereas adolescent ranges may be lower (90 to 150 mg/dL). Insulin adjustments may be made in 10% to 20% increments. In most cases, supplemental regular insulin need be used only for blood glucose above 300 mg/dL (16.7 mmol/L) or recurrence of ketonuria.

d. Because of the "dawn phenomenon" (an early-morning glucose rise), glucose nadirs usually occur at 4:00 to 5:00 AM. One approach to avoiding middle-of-the-night hypoglycemia is to set the target range for bedtime blood glucose higher than at other times of the day (100 to 180 mg/dL, or 5.6 to 10 mmol/L). In addition, regimens using N or NPH require a bedtime snack that includes protein and fat as well as carbohydrates.

e. Dietary education should be undertaken with several principles in mind: In children with diabetes younger than 3 years of age, timing and quality of meals may be difficult to control. In all children, dietary intake is profoundly affected by the patient's appetite, activity level, and preferences. In general, parents and patients will benefit the most from teaching sound dietary guidelines rather than providing a rigid diet. These guidelines should be aimed toward achieving a dietary composition of 50% to 55% of calories as carbohydrate, 15% to 20% as protein, and 30% to 35% as fat (polyunsaturated-to-saturated ratio of 1.2:1). In patients who are of normal weight for height, it is rarely necessary to designate a specific caloric intake. Carbohydrate counting is strongly encouraged in all families and is an essential part of dietary education.

3. Continuing care of type 1 diabetes: One approach to ongoing diabetes care, which is consistent with the current standards of care as outlined by the American Diabetes Association (ADA), is as follows:

a. Goals of therapy

(1) Normal growth and pubertal development should be an attainable goal in virtually all patients. This is achievable with "standard" care regimens.

(2) A primary treatment goal should be optimization of blood glucose control. Results of the Diabetes Control and Complications Trial (DCCT) indicated that at any level of glycemic control (as measured by glycated hemoglobin, such as HbA_{1c} or total glycohemoglobin), improvement may be associated with a decreased risk of long-term complications. Achieving "near-normal" levels of glycemia will, in most cases, require an intensive treatment regimen. Preferences of the patient, family, and health care team should be taken into account.

b. Practical aspects of ongoing care

(1) In newly diagnosed type 1 diabetes, it is often very easy to achieve tight control with standard regimens. This is due to a period that precedes total loss of endogenous insulin secretion (often referred to as the "honeymoon" period). During this phase, which may last from weeks to several years, insulin requirement may be minimal.

(2) Regardless of the treatment regimen used, ongoing monitoring of blood glucose at least several times per day is of benefit. Patients and families should be strongly encouraged to keep a diabetes log that includes insulin doses, blood glucose measurements, and documentation of other factors affecting diabetes care (e.g., intercurrent illnesses, changes in activity level).

(3) Some patients may achieve excellent glycemic control with a standard treatment regimen.

(4) Intensive treatment, in addition to multiple injections/insulin pump and frequent blood glucose monitoring (five times per day or more), requires frequent patient contact (weekly telephone contact and monthly visits) and the use of a multidisciplinary team (including physician, nurse educator, nutritionist, and psychiatrist/social worker). Without the latter component, the goal of tight glycemic control is often not achieved.

c. Long-term management

(1) Glycated hemoglobin measurements should be used to monitor glycemic control. These reflect the integrated serum glucose concentration over 6 to 10 weeks. Obtaining this test at each outpatient visit is warranted. Doing so provides the best long-term indicator of glycemic control.

(2) Ongoing monitoring for long-term complications

(a) Nephropathy: Occurs with a frequency similar to that seen with retinopathy. Once a child has had diabetes for 5 years and is at least 10 years of age, yearly screening for early nephropathy should be done. This can be accomplished by methods that detect microalbuminuria. Microalbuminuria, even in the absence of hypertension, is an indicator for treatment with angiotensin-converting enzyme inhibitors. Recent data indicate that this approach delays the development of diabetic nephropathy.

(b) Retinopathy: Background retinopathy occurs in over 40% of adolescents and almost 10% of children with type 1 diabetes after 15 years. It has been reported in patients with a diabetes duration of only 1 to 2 years; however, it is not usually recognized before 5 to 10 years of diabetes duration. Annual ophthalmologic screening with dilated funduscopic examination should commence is those children 10 years of age or older with a diabetes duration of 3 to 5 years. Early detection is imperative given the efficacy of laser photocoagulation in the treatment of the early stages of retinopathy.

(c) Dyslipidemia: A fasting lipid profile should be obtained in those patients older than 2 years of age with a strong family history of hypercholesterolemia or early atherosclerotic vascular disease. In those diabetic patients with reassuring family histories, the first fasting lipid profile should be obtained at puberty or at time of diagnosis in adolescents. If normal, the profile should be repeated every 5 years.

(d) Other long-term complications: Peripheral neuropathy, autonomic neuropathy, and macrovascular disease are unusual complications in childhood. Nonetheless, the approach to follow-up should take the risk of these complications into account.

(3) Associated autoimmune conditions

(a) Thyroid disease: Autoimmune thyroid disease is present in 17% of patients with type 1 diabetes. Thyroid function tests (TSH and total or free T_4) should be obtained in all newly diagnosed patients with diabetes once metabolic control has been established, or if clinically indicated. If normal TSH values are observed, a recheck is indicated every 1 to 2 years.

(b) Celiac disease: Celiac disease is now recognized to occur in association with type 1 diabetes with a prevalence of 1% to 16%, versus 0.3% to 1% of the general population. Many centers have initiated annual screens using tissue transglutaminase antibodies (immunoglobulin A [IgA] tTG). This assay is IgA based and thus IgA sufficiency must first be documented.

d. Other preventative measures

(1) Patients should wear medical alert identification.

(2) Cigarette smoking should be vigorously discouraged, given its compounding effect on development of macrovascular disease.

(3) Careful blood glucose monitoring aimed at avoiding hypoglycemia is particularly important in patients who drive an automobile.

(4) The risk of precipitating hypoglycemia by ingestion of alcohol should be stressed with adolescent patients.

e. Management of intercurrent illness

(1) At the onset of illness, around-the-clock monitoring every 4 hours of blood glucose and urinary ketones should begin.

(2) Antipyretics should be used as per routine indications.

(3) Use of antiemetics should be avoided.

(4) If the patient is unable to eat, intake of sugar-containing fluids, such as apple juice or regular soda, should be vigorously encouraged.

(5) If vomiting occurs or moderate to large ketones are detected in the urine, the use of regular insulin every 4 hours (0.15 to 0.3 U/kg, as required) should start (in place of the patient's usual insulin regimen). This insulin regimen should continue until the patient is able to resume normal or near-normal dietary intake and the ketones have cleared. In practice, administration of sufficient insulin to suppress ketosis may be limited by a tendency toward hypoglycemia, especially in young children and infants.

(6) Recurrent vomiting is an indication for immediate referral to the emergency department for clinical and laboratory evaluation.

f. Hypoglycemia in diabetes

(1) Early symptoms (referable, in part, to adrenergic effect): Pallor, diaphoresis, palpitations, tremors, hunger

(2) Progression of neuroglycopenia manifests as blurred vision, confusion, coma, or seizures.

(3) Insulin reactions in young children may present as irritability or drowsiness.

(4) Patients who succeed in obtaining tight glycemic control are prone to development of "hypoglycemia unawareness," in which the initial signs of an insulin reaction are lacking. These patients may have symptoms of neuroglycopenia before any other manifestations of hypoglycemia.

(5) Treatment of mild insulin reactions: 15 g of concentrated carbohydrate (juice or glucose tablets) by mouth followed by a repeat blood glucose measurement 15 minutes later ("Rule of 15s"). Repeated doses of carbohydrates may be needed. Depending on the insulin regimen, a snack may be required once normoglycemia has been achieved.

(6) Severe (defined as requiring assistance or unable to cooperate with administration of oral carbohydrate): oral glucose gel ("instant glucose" or cake frosting); glucagon 1 mg subcutaneously for patient older than 5 years of age, 0.5 mg subcutaneously if younger

(7) A severe reaction with a seizure or persistent altered level of consciousness is an indication for referral to the emergency department.

(8) Except for unusual instances in which other factors are present (e.g., fever, prodromal symptoms), severe reactions that manifest as seizures do not require evaluation or treatment for epilepsy. Patients may have signs of encephalopathy for several

hours after a severe reaction. This is also not an indication for a neurologic work-up.

(9) Repeated reactions of moderate or greater severity indicate that the patient's insulin regimen, diet, or both need modification.

DIABETIC KETOACIDOSIS

1. Clinical features: Persistent vomiting, whether occurring in newly diagnosed or established patients, nearly always heralds the onset of diabetic ketoacidosis. Abdominal pain and Kussmaul respirations are usually present, and the level of consciousness may be altered.

2. Laboratory findings
   a. Initial laboratory evaluation should include serum glucose, electrolytes, BUN, and urine ketones.
   b. Serum glucose greater than 700 mg/dL (39 mmol/L) is usually a reflection of severe dehydration. Under these circumstances, renal blood flow (and urinary glucose excretion) is impaired.
   c. The degree of ketoacidosis may be best interpreted by calculating the anion gap, which is accounted for largely by ketoacids. When serum total carbon dioxide is less than 6 to 8 mEq/L, determination of arterial blood gases is usually warranted. Severe acidosis (arterial pH <7.1) may produce central respiratory depression.
   d. The potassium deficit in ketoacidosis (usually 8 to 10 mEq/kg) may not be reflected in the serum potassium concentration. This lack of correlation is due to the inhibition of potassium transport from the extracellular to intracellular space that occurs with acidosis and diminished insulin effect. Examination of the electrocardiogram may reveal signs of hypokalemia, even in the presence of a normal serum potassium concentration.

3. Management: The goals of therapy are to (1) correct dehydration; (2) provide sufficient insulin to correct the hypoglycemia and, most important, to inhibit lipolysis and ketogenesis; and (3) correct metabolic acidosis and restore normal electrolyte balance.
   a. Fluid therapy
      (1) Because the dehydration in patients with diabetic ketoacidosis is hypertonic (thereby preserving extracellular fluid and plasma volumes), patients are not usually in shock. Initial restoration of intracellular dehydration volume can usually be achieved with the infusion of 10 mL/kg 0.9% saline over the first hour. Rapid administration of 0.9% saline in excess of 20 mL/kg should be undertaken with caution because some studies have correlated rapid fluid administration with development of cerebral edema in diabetic ketoacidosis.
      (2) Replacement and maintenance fluid should consist of 0.45% saline with 20 to 40 mmol/L potassium chloride. (Hypertonic fluid should be avoided because ketoacidosis is accompanied by a profound free-water deficit.) In most patients, initial deficits will approximate 100 mL/kg of water, 8 to 10 mmol/kg of sodium, and 8 to 10 mmol/kg of potassium. The rate of fluid administration should take into account ongoing insensible losses, ongoing renal losses (which may be excessive until hyperglycemia is

corrected), and repair of the deficit over 24 to 48 hours. When electrocardiographic signs of hypokalemia are present, higher concentrations of potassium chloride in the IV fluid may be required.

(3) Bolus administration of bicarbonate should be avoided except in "code" situations. However, the "physiologic" administration of bicarbonate in replacement fluids (a ratio of bicarbonate to chloride of 1:3 to 1:4) is safe and may prevent so-called dilutional acidosis. This practice is rarely undertaken unless serum pH is below 7.0, and if sodium bicarbonate is included in replacement IV fluids, it should be removed when serum bicarbonate exceeds approximately 14 mEq/L.

(4) Dextrose should be added to IV fluids when plasma glucose falls to approximately 250 mg/dL (14 mmol/L).

b. Insulin administration
   (1) "Low-dose" IV insulin is effective in treating ketoacidosis and should be started as early as possible. Dose is 0.1 U/kg as a priming bolus followed immediately by 0.1 U/kg/hr constant infusion.
   (2) In some patients, insulin resistance may require higher doses (up to 1 U/kg/hr).
   (3) The dose of IV insulin should not be routinely decreased based on falling plasma glucose. Such an approach risks exacerbation of ketosis and acidosis. Rather, the concentration of IV dextrose should be increased to permit continued administration of insulin at the effective dose of at least 0.1 U/kg/hr until acidosis is resolved.

c. Transition to subcutaneous insulin: Once the ketoacidosis has resolved, the patient may be transitioned to the standard subcutaneous insulin regimens.

TYPE 2 DIABETES IN CHILDREN AND ADOLESCENTS

1. Epidemiology, etiology, and pathophysiology
   a. The incidence of type 2 diabetes in the pediatric population has increased with the increasing prevalence of obesity. The exact incidence of type 2 diabetes in our youth is difficult to determine given the varied ages, races, degrees of obesity, and criteria used for diagnosis in patients studied. There are also no population-based studies, but among morbidly obese adolescents, 4% were found to have type 2 diabetes. In addition, some studies suggest up to 30% of new-onset diabetes mellitus in adolescents is type 2 diabetes.
   b. Type 2 diabetes is a result of both insulin resistance and insulin deficiency resulting from a failure of compensatory hyperinsulinemia.
   c. Initially, as beta cell function fails, basal insulin secretion is adequate but needs after carbohydrate load are not met. Clinically, this may result in a normal fasting glucose but hyperglycemia postprandially. As beta cell function fails, insulin deficiency becomes more profound and fasting hyperglycemia develops.
   d. Risk factors include obesity (particularly central or visceral adiposity), family history, abnormal birth weight (both intrauterine growth

retardation and large size for gestational age place infants at risk), and sedentary lifestyle.

2. Diagnosis and laboratory findings

   a. The diagnosis of type 2 diabetes in children and adolescents is identical to that in adults:

      (1) Symptoms of hyperglycemia (polyuria, polydipsia, weight loss) with a random blood glucose of at least 200 mg/dL (11.1 mmol/L).

      (2) Fasting blood glucose at least 126 mg/dL, *twice*.

      (3) Two-hour postload (1.75 g/kg to maximum of 75 g oral glucose load) blood glucose at least 200 mg/dL (11.1 mmol/L).

   b. Screening

      (1) In children and adolescents, screening should be restricted to those at risk:

         (a) Obese children (BMI >85th percentile), particularly if morbidly obese with the symptoms given in 2.a. (1) or 2.a. (2) above

         (b) Family history of type 2 diabetes in first- or second-degree relatives

         (c) Clinical or biochemical evidence of insulin resistance or the metabolic syndrome (acanthosis nigricans, hypertension, dyslipidemia, polycystic ovary syndrome)

      (2) The ADA suggests using a fasting plasma glucose as a screen, but many with impaired glucose intolerance or frank diabetes have preserved fasting glucose, with hyperglycemia occurring only after a carbohydrate challenge. The need for an oral glucose tolerance test should be individualized based on risk factors and clinical presentation.

   c. Measurement of autoantibodies should also be performed to avoid misdiagnosing patients with type 1 diabetes (who are at increased risk for ketoacidosis) as having type 2 diabetes.

3. Acute management

   a. Symptomatic and significant hyperglycemia may require insulin at diagnosis.

   b. Lifestyle modifications, including both exercise and dietary changes, are as efficacious as medical therapy in both preventing and initially treating type 2 diabetes. However, many patients are not compliant with this regimen and may also require oral agents or insulin.

   c. Oral agents include insulin sensitizers, insulin secretagogues, and α-glycosidase inhibitors.

      (1) Metformin is the only oral agent approved by the U.S. Food and Drug Administration for use in children. It acts by increasing hepatic insulin sensitivity and decreasing hepatic glucose production. It has lesser effects in the periphery, particularly muscle tissue. Metformin is the first-line agent for most children and adolescents with type 2 diabetes. Side effects are primarily gastrointestinal and can be minimized by slowly working up to a therapeutic dose.

      (2) Thiazolidinediones (TZDs; rosiglitazone, pioglitazone) decrease hepatic glucose production, increase glucose uptake in peripheral tissues, and inhibit lipolysis, thus improving glycemic control and dyslipidemia. Side effects include primarily weight gain

and fat redistribution. Edema occurs in those with background renal or cardiac disease. TZDs may be used alone or in combination with metformin, and are being studied in children and adolescents.

(3) Insulin secretagogues such as sulfonylureas (glyburide, glipizide) and meglitinides (repaglinide, nateglinide) act by stimulating insulin secretion. As a result, hypoglycemia and weight gain are reported side effects, and hence this class of oral agents is not used as routinely in children and adolescents.

d. Blood sugars should be monitored routinely and ideally be tested both preprandially and postprandially. The goals of management in this case should include maintaining blood sugars as close to the normal range as possible and HbA_{1c} levels at less than 6%. If insulin or insulin secretagogues are not used, this goal is achievable without concerns of hypoglycemia. Achieving this goal may require combination therapy or insulin therapy.

4. Long-term management
   a. Lifestyle modifications should be maintained lifelong—weight loss, exercise, dietary changes.
   b. Minimize other cardiac risk factors—smoking prevention/cessation, weight loss.
   c. Manage comorbidities—dyslipidemia, hypertension.
   d. Obtain routine HbA_{1c} to monitor true glycemic control.

5. Complications
   a. Microvascular complications are similar to those found in type 1 diabetes.
   b. Complications of insulin resistance or obesity may compound the care. These complications include dyslipidemia (low high-density lipoprotein, high triglycerides), hypertension, and, eventually, macrovascular disease.

7.8 Hypoglycemia

Hypoglycemia, although rare in infancy and childhood, can present with symptoms that are vague and nonspecific, thus requiring a high index of suspicion to make the diagnosis.

1. Definition: Beyond the newborn period, clinically significant hypoglycemia can be defined as blood glucose less than 2.2 mmol/L (40 mg/dL), if the patient is symptomatic.

2. Clinical features: In individuals of all ages, the signs and symptoms of hypoglycemia may be categorized into those associated with catecholamine release (tremors, diaphoresis, tachycardia, palpitations, pallor) and those due to neuroglycopenia (headache, lethargy or irritability, confusion, and progression to coma or seizures). In the newborn, symptoms are nonspecific and can include tremors, jitteriness, apnea, cyanosis, hypotonia, irritability, and feeding difficulties.

3. Diagnosis
   a. Although glucose meters are of great use in the setting of diabetes mellitus, they should *not* be used for the definitive diagnosis of

> ### Box 7-10   Diagnosis of Hypoglycemic Disorders: Analysis of Critical Samples
>
> **Blood (Serum or Plasma)**   **Urine**
>
> Glucose   Ketones
> Electrolytes   Organic acids
> Insulin   Amino acids
> Cortisol
> Growth hormone
> β-Hydroxybutyrate
> Quantitative amino acid
> Lactate and pyruvate
> Ammonia

hypoglycemia. Serum or plasma glucose concentration should be performed in a reliable clinical laboratory.

b. The specific diagnosis of a hypoglycemic disorder is best made when "critical blood and urine samples" are obtained. Such samples would be acquired at the time of symptomatic hypoglycemia, before treatment (Box 7-10).

c. If a patient's history is compatible with a hypoglycemic disorder but samples cannot be obtained during a hypoglycemic episode, two options are available:

   (1) Admit the patient to the hospital for a monitored, prolonged (≥24-hour) fast, or

   (2) Patients' parents can be given written instruction so that the appropriate tests can be obtained through an emergency department when the patient is symptomatic.

4. Laboratory findings: Once the critical tests are obtained, several decision-making branch points are possible, based on the following data interpretations:

a. Presence or absence of ketosis

   (1) The absence of ketonuria implies suppressed ketogenesis, due to either hyperinsulinemia or a primary defect in fatty acid oxidation.

   (2) Elevated plasma β-hydroxybutyrate may support a diagnosis of ketotic hypoglycemia.

If ketonemia is suppressed, hyperinsulinemia or fatty acid oxidation abnormalities should be considered.

b. Hormone concentrations

   (1) Insulin concentrations must be interpreted in light of plasma glucose level. A general guideline is that plasma insulin concentration, expressed as microunits per milliliter, should be less than one third of the glucose concentration in milligrams per deciliter.

    (2) At the time of hypoglycemia, circulating GH concentration should exceed 10 ng/mL.

    (3) Cortisol should exceed 10 μg/dL.

5. Specific hypoglycemic disorders: Clinical features, diagnosis, and management

  a. Hyperinsulinism

    (1) Etiology, clinical features, and diagnosis: This condition can result from a variety of pancreatic lesions, including diffuse functional abnormalities ("nesidioblastosis") and focal adenomas. Presentation occurs most often in infancy. Hyperinsulinism promotes peripheral glucose utilization while suppressing hepatic glucose production. The former leads to a hallmark of hyperinsulinism: increased requirement for IV dextrose (generally >10 mg/kg/min) to maintain euglycemia. As noted earlier, the diagnosis is supported by relative hyperinsulinemia and suppressed ketonemia.

    (2) Management should include suppressing insulin secretion using oral diazoxide 5 to 10 mg/kg/day (to a maximum of 25 mg/kg/day). Alternatively, glucocorticoids (e.g., prednisone 2 mg/kg/day) can be used to produce insulin resistance. Ultimately, surgical removal of part or all of the pancreas may need to be performed to control hypoglycemia.

  b. Hypopituitarism

    (1) Etiology and clinical features: Hypoglycemia is a potent stimulus for the release of GH and cortisol. Thus, the lack of an appropriate elevation in circulating GH or cortisol in response to hypoglycemia may indicate a hypothalamic-pituitary disorder or primary adrenal insufficiency. Clues as to the presence of hypopituitarism include microphallus in boys, prolonged hyperbilirubinemia (due to secondary or tertiary hypothyroidism), and linear growth failure.

    (2) Management: Hypoglycemia due to hypopituitarism may be prevented with daily administration of GH or glucocorticoids. As a manifestation of hypopituitarism, hypoglycemia does not usually persist past the age of 3 or 4 years.

  c. Ketotic hypoglycemia

    (1) Etiology and clinical features: This is a nonspecific designation applied, by exclusion of other disorders, to children in whom fasting leads to accelerated hypoglycemia accompanied by normal ketosis and, most important, by symptoms of hypoglycemia. Age of onset is typically before 18 months. Insulin, cortisol, and GH concentrations are normal (appropriate) at the time of hypoglycemia.

    (2) Management: Treatment consists of avoidance of prolonged fasts.

  d. Other disorders associated with hypoglycemia

    (1) Disorders of fatty acid metabolism: A defect in fatty acid beta-oxidation leads to hypoglycemia accompanied by hypoketonemia, with or without other characteristic findings, such as apnea ("near-miss sudden infant death syndrome"), encephalopathy,

  cardiomyopathy, skeletal myopathy, or hepatomegaly. Treatment tends to be palliative only, although oral carnitine and dietary avoidance of a particular class of fatty acid (e.g., long-chain) may be effective.

(2) Other mitochondrial disorders: These inheritable disorders in pyruvate dehydrogenase and the mitochondrial respiratory chain may present as lactic acidemia with hypoglycemia and encephalopathy or myopathy. At present, no effective therapy is available for these disorders.

(3) Glycogen storage disease: Type I glycogen storage disease is due to a defect in glucose-6-phosphatase activity and is associated with marked hepatomegaly. A subnormal glycemic response to glucagon is a hallmark of this disorder. The basis for therapy is avoidance of the fasted state, most often accomplished by feeding with raw (uncooked) cornstarch, which is slowly hydrolyzed in the gut, thereby providing a slow-release source of carbohydrate.

(4) Hereditary fructose intolerance: Characterized by severe hypoglycemia, lactic acidosis, and vomiting after fructose ingestion.

(5) Disorders of amino acid metabolism: Failure to thrive, vomiting, hepatomegaly, and fasting hypoglycemia may indicate the presence of any number of disorders of amino acid metabolism (e.g., branched-chain amino acids: leucine, isoleucine, valine).

(6) Other disorders: Hypoglycemia may result from severe hepatic dysfunction (neonatal hepatitis, galactosemia, and tyrosinemia). Hypoglycemia due to intoxication (e.g., with salicylates) should always be considered.

SUGGESTED READINGS

American Diabetes Association: Standards of medical care for patients with diabetes mellitus. Diabetes Care 28(Suppl 1), 2005.

Bloomgarden ZT: Type 2 diabetes in the young: The evolving epidemic. Diabetes Care 27:998-1010, 2004.

Bode HH: Disorders of the posterior pituitary. In Kaplan SA (ed): Clinical Pediatric Endocrinology. Philadelphia, WB Saunders, 1992, pp 63-86.

Diabetes Control and Complications Trial Research Group: The effect of intensive treatment of diabetes on the development and progression of long-term complications in insulin-dependent diabetes mellitus. N Engl J Med 329:977-986, 1993.

Drug and Therapeutics Committee, Lawson Wilkins Pediatric Endocrine Society: Guidelines for the use of growth hormone in children with short stature. J Pediatr 127:857-867, 1995.

Favus M (ed): Primer on the Metabolic Bone Diseases and Disorders of Mineral Metabolism, 5th ed. Philadelphia, Lippincott Williams & Wilkins, 2005.

Gertner JM: Disorders of calcium and phosphorus homeostasis. Pediatr Clin North Am 37:1441-1465, 1990.

Greulich WW, Pyle SI: Radiographic Atlas of Skeletal Development of the Hand and Wrist, 2nd ed. Palo Alto, Calif, Stanford University Press, 1959.

Halac I, Zimmerman D: Thyroid nodules and cancer in children. Endocrinol Metab Clin North Am 34:725-744, 2005.

Hannon TS, Rao G, Arslanian SA: Childhood obesity and type 2 diabetes mellitus. Pediatrics 116:473-480, 2005.

Kaplowitz K: Clinical characteristics of 104 children referred for evaluation of precocious puberty. J Clin Endocrinol Metab 89:3644-3650, 2004.

Lafranchi S: Congenital hypothyroidism: Etiologies, diagnosis and management. Thyroid 9:735-740, 1999.

Levine B, Carpenter TO: Rickets. In Radovick S, MacGillivray MH (eds): Pediatric Endocrinology: A Practical Clinical Guide. Totowa, NJ, Humana Press, 2003 pp 365-381.

Meyers-Seifer CH, Charest NJ: Diagnosis and management of patients with ambiguous genitalia. Semin Perinatol 16:332-339, 1992.

Miller, WL: The adrenal cortex. In Sperling MA (ed): Pediatric Endocrinology, 2nd ed. Philadelphia, WB Saunders, 2002, pp 385-438.

Nathan BM, Palmert MR: Regulation and disorders of pubertal timing. Endocrinol Metab Clin North Am 34:617-641, 2005

Ritszen EM: Early puberty: What is normal and when is treatment indicated? Horm Res 60(Suppl 3):31-34, 2003.

Root AW, Diamond FB: Disorders of calcium metabolism in the child and adolescent. In Sperling M (ed): Pediatric Endocrinology, 2nd ed. Philadelphia, WB Saunders, 2002, pp 629-670.

Wilson TA, Rose SR, Rogol AD et al: Update of guidelines for the use of growth hormone in children: The Lawson Wilkins Pediatric Endocrinology Society Drug and Therapeutics Committee. J Pediatr 143:415-421, 2003.

Zimmerman D: Fetal and neonatal hyperthyroidism. Thyroid 9:727-733, 1999

Renal Disorders

8

Natalia Golova, Anthony J. Alario, and
M. Khurram Faizan

8.1 HYPERTENSION

1. Definitions
   a. *Normal blood pressure* in children is defined as systolic or diastolic blood pressure below the 90th percentile for age, height, and sex. (See blood pressure charts in Appendix I.)
   b. *High normal blood pressure* in children is defined as systolic or diastolic blood pressure between the 90th and 95th percentile for age, height, and sex.
   c. *Hypertension* in children is defined as an average systolic or diastolic blood pressure equal to or greater than the 95th percentile for age, height, and sex, obtained on at least *three separate occasions*.
2. Measurement
   a. The blood pressure should be obtained with an appropriately sized cuff. The inflatable portion of the cuff must cover two thirds of the length and encompass at least 80% of the circumference of the upper arm. The first Korotkoff sound identifies the systolic blood pressure. The fifth Korotkoff sound (disappearance of pulsation sound on auscultation) identifies the diastolic blood pressure. When there is no total disappearance, as often occurs in infants and children younger than 13 years of age, the fourth Korotkoff sound (muffling of the sound's intensity) can be used to approximate the diastolic blood pressure.
   b. The American Academy of Pediatrics (AAP) recommends that the blood pressure be measured at least annually in children 3 years of age and older. However, the blood pressure should also be measured in *any child* with failure to thrive, seizures, recurrent headaches, cardiac disease, renal disease, or any illness of undetermined etiology.
3. Diagnosis/differential diagnosis
   a. Obtaining a thorough *history* and performing a *physical examination* are very important in focusing on a differential diagnosis for hypertension (shown in parentheses in the following). Items to inquire about include the following:
      (1) Neonatal course, prematurity, low birth weight, umbilical artery/ vein catheter, bronchopulmonary dysplasia, excess diuretics

(renal artery stenosis, renal vein thrombosis, pulmonary etiology, nephrocalcinosis)

(2) Family history of hypertension, preeclampsia, renal disease including renal cysts, tumors (essential hypertension, inherited renal disease, inherited endocrine disease)

(3) Drugs (oral contraceptives, corticosteroids, anabolic steroids, cocaine, phencyclidine, amphetamines, decongestants, nonsteroidal anti-inflammatory drugs [NSAIDs]) and tobacco use (drug-induced hypertension)

(4) Lead exposure, history of chronic toxicity (renal damage)

(5) Headaches, diplopia, changes in personality/memory, clumsiness, vomiting (increased intracranial pressure)

(6) Muscle cramps, weakness, constipation (hyperaldosteronism/mineralocorticoid excess)

(7) Arthritis, rashes, unexplained fevers (vasculitis, connective tissue disorder)

(8) Dysuria, frequency, nocturia, enuresis, abdominal/flank pain (urinary tract infections [UTIs], renal disease)

(9) Failure to gain weight, weight loss, sweating, flushing, palpitations, fevers (pheochromocytoma)

(10) Increased appetite with no weight gain or loss, nervousness, tremors, heat intolerance, resting tachycardia (hyperthyroidism)

b. Physical examination: Look for the following signs:

(1) Pallor, edema (renal disease)

(2) Moon faces, buffalo hump, striae, truncal obesity, hirsutism (Cushing's syndrome, glucocorticoid excess)

(3) Heart murmur, absent femoral pulses, blood pressure in lower extremities less than upper extremities, features of Turner's syndrome (coarctation of aorta)

(4) Tremors, tachycardia, sweating, enlarged thyroid (hyperthyroidism)

(5) Café au lait spots, hypopigmented lesions (neurofibromatosis, tuberous sclerosis)

(6) Abdominal masses (pheochromocytoma, neuroblastoma, Wilms' tumor, polycystic kidneys, hydronephrosis)

(7) Abdominal bruits (renal artery stenosis)

4. Laboratory evaluation

a. Initial laboratory evaluation should include

(1) Complete blood count (CBC; rule out anemia from chronic renal disease, hemolysis from hemolytic-uremic syndrome [HUS])

(2) Urinalysis (rule out nephrosis, nephritis, UTI)

(3) Electrolytes, blood urea nitrogen (BUN), and creatinine (assess renal function)

b. Optional

(1) Echocardiogram or electrocardiogram (ECG; rule out left ventricular hypertrophy from long-standing hypertension)

(2) Renal ultrasonography (rule out renal disease)

c. Based on history and physical, obtain the appropriate laboratory tests to confirm or exclude the secondary underlying etiology (e.g., cortisol levels in suspected Cushing's syndrome).

5. Management
    a. Mild hypertension (blood pressure between 95th and 99th percentile for age/sex)
        (1) Weight reduction if obese
        (2) Low-sodium diet
        (3) Exercise
        (4) Relaxation techniques
        (5) Follow-up every 6 months. If the patient is not responding to the previous measures over 6 to 12 months, experiences worsening hypertension, or shows evidence of end-organ damage (funduscopic, renal, or cardiac changes), pharmacologic treatment will be needed.
    b. Severe hypertension (blood pressure at or above the 99th percentile for age and sex)
        (1) Single-agent therapy is preferable, usually with a beta blocker, thiazide diuretic, angiotensin-converting enzyme (ACE) inhibitor, or a calcium channel blocker.
        (2) Consult a pediatric nephrologist or cardiologist.
    c. Hypertensive crisis (acute severe hypertension)
        (1) Antihypertensive agents (Table 8-1)
        (2) Mannitol, furosemide, hyperventilation if cerebral edema is present
        (3) Diuretics in patients with cardiovascular manifestations (congestive heart failure [CHF] with pulmonary edema)
        (4) Dialysis in patients with renal failure with fluid overload

8.2 Hematuria

1. Definitions
    a. *Hematuria* is the presence of blood in the urine.
    b. *Macroscopic* or *gross* hematuria is present when blood in the urine is evident to the naked eye (urine is usually tea or cola colored).
    c. *Microscopic hematuria* is present when the urine appears clear to the naked eye but has blood when examined under a microscope. The presence of more than five red blood cells (RBCs) per high-power field in a centrifuged specimen is considered significant.

    Note:
        (1) Not every red, pink, orange, or brown urine indicates hematuria. A number of drugs, foods, toxins, myoglobin, and hemoglobin can color the urine.
        (2) Not all positive dipsticks indicate hematuria. The urine dipsticks are very sensitive in detecting RBCs as well as minuscule amounts of myoglobin and hemoglobin. Therefore, a urinalysis is needed to diagnose hematuria in the presence of a positive dipstick.
        (3) "False-positive" dipsticks are caused by
            (a) Bacterial peroxidases from a UTI
            (b) Delay in reading the dipstick
            (c) Beets, aniline dyes, ascorbic acid
    d. *Hemoglobinuria* is the presence of hemoglobin in the urine; it is sometimes seen in conditions causing hemolysis.

8—Renal Disorders

Drug	Initial Daily Dose	Maximum Daily Dose	Frequency
Diuretics			
Hydrochlorothiazide	1–2 mg/kg (>6 mo)	100 mg	Twice daily
	3.0 mg/kg (<6 mo)	37.5 mg	Twice daily
Chlorothiazide	10–20 mg/kg (>6 mo)	1000 mg	Twice daily
	20–30 mg/kg (<6 mo)	375 mg	Twice daily
Furosemide	1–2 mg/kg	320 mg or 4 mg/kg	Twice daily, once daily
β-Adrenergic Blockers			
Selective			
Atenolol	0.5–1 mg/kg*	100 mg	Once daily
Metoprolol	1–2 mg/kg*	200 mg	Once daily, twice daily
Acebutolol	200–400 mg*	1200 mg	Once daily
Nonselective			
Propranolol	1–2 mg/kg	8 mg/kg	Twice daily
Nadolol	40 mg*	240–320 mg	Once daily
Direct Vasodilators			
Hydralazine	0.5–1.0 mg/kg (25 mg/m²)	4–8 mg/kg (200 mg)	Three to four times/day
Minoxidil	0.1 mg/kg	1 mg/kg (50 mg)	Twice daily, once daily
Calcium Channel Blockers°			
Nifedipine	0.25 mg/kg (10 mg)	1–2 mg/kg (180 mg)	Three to four times/day
Extended release		1–2 mg/kg (90 mg)	Once daily, twice daily
Diltiazem	1.5–2 mg/kg*	240 mg	Twice daily, once daily
Verapamil	3–4 mg/kg* (60 mg)	480 mg	Twice daily, once daily
Amlodipine	0.1 mg/kg (2.5–5 mg)	10 mg	Once daily

Peripheral α-Adrenergic Blockade			
Prazosin	2–2.5 µg/kg*	150 µg/kg (15 mg)	Two to three times/day
Angiotensin-Converting Enzyme Inhibitors			
Captopril	0.05–0.1 mg/kg	2 mg/kg	Two to three times/day
Enalapril (intravenous/oral)	0.08 mg/kg*	40 mg	Twice daily, once daily
Lisinopril	0.07 mg/kg*	40 mg	Twice daily, once daily
Central Sympatholytics			
Alpha methyldopa (intravenous/oral)	10 mg/kg (300 mg/m²)	65 mg/kg (2 g/m²)	Two to four times/day
Clonidine (patch vs. tablet)	0.05–0.1 mg tablet	2.4 mg by mouth	Two to three times/day
		0.6 mg by patch	Every week
Complex Adrenergic Antagonist			
Labetalol (intravenous/oral)	1–3 mg/kg	10–12 mg/kg (1200–2400 mg)	Twice daily

*Pediatric dosing not established.

Adapted from Jung FF, Ingelfinger JR: Hypertension in childhood and adolescence. Pediatr Rev 14:169–179, 1993.

    e. *Myoglobinuria* is the presence of myoglobin in the urine; it is some-
       times seen in conditions associated with muscular damage:
      (1) Trauma (crush injury)
      (2) Myocardial infarction
      (3) Strenuous exercise
      (4) Seizures
      (5) Heat stroke
      (6) Electric shock
      (7) Burns
2. Epidemiology: Approximately 5% of school-aged children have asymptomatic hematuria on routine screening. The incidence is higher in girls
   and increases with age.
3. Etiology: Most nontraumatic causes of hematuria in childhood are associated with *microscopic* hematuria, although some of these conditions
   can cause *gross* hematuria as well.
4. Diagnosis
    a. An algorithm for identifying the etiology of hematuria is shown in
      Figure 8-1.
    b. A stepwise work-up of a child with hematuria is indicated. Increase
      the level of evaluation depending on the child's condition and pre-
      sumed etiology (Box 8-1).
    c. Caveats
      (1) Gross *or* microscopic hematuria can be associated with
         hypercalciuria.
         (a) Age-specific urinary calcium/creatinine ratios*:
            (i) Younger than 7 months: <0.86
            (ii) 7 to 18 months: <0.60
            (iii) 19 months to 6 years: <0.42
            (iv) Older than 6 years: <0.22
         (b) Values are obtained from untimed random urine specimens.
         (c) Values indicate the 95th percentile for age. Values above
            the 95th percentile for age are considered abnormal.
      (2) Complements are often low in poststreptococcal glomerulone-
         phritis (GN) or systemic lupus erythematosus (SLE). They
         return to normal in 6 to 8 weeks in poststreptococcal GN.
         Persistently low complement levels indicate other forms of GN.
5. Localization of hematuria: Hematuria can usually be localized to either
   a glomerular or nonglomerular site (Table 8-2).
6. Indications for referral and possible renal biopsy in children with
   hematuria
    a. Persistent asymptomatic microscopic hematuria for more than 1 year
    b. Associated proteinuria
    c. Persistently low complement levels
    d. Family history of nephritis
    e. Sensorineural hearing loss
    f. Renal insufficiency
    g. Hypertension

---

*Data from Sargent JD, Stukel TA, Kresel J, Klein RZ: Normal values for random
urinary calcium/creatinine ratios in infancy. J Pediatr 123:393-397, 1993.

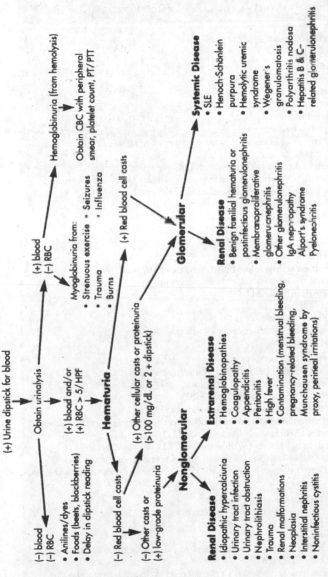

Figure 8-1 Algorithm for evaluation and diagnosis of hematuria. CBC, complete blood count; HPF, high-power field; PTT, partial thromboplastin time; RBC, red blood cell; SLE, systemic lupus erythematosus.

Box 8-1   Work-up of a Child with Hematuria

Initial Workup

HISTORY
Strenuous exercise
Fever and dehydration
Recent trauma
Recent bladder catheterization
Menstruation
Dysuria, frequency (UTI)
Intense back/flank pain, family history of renal stones (hypercalciuria, stone)
Recent throat or skin infection (group A streptococcal)
Recent or recurrent upper respiratory illness (adenovirus)
Rashes, arthralgia, or arthritis (SLE, HSP)
Bloody diarrhea (hemolytic-uremic syndrome)
Medications (antibiotics and cyclophosphamide)
Birth asphyxia or catheterization of umbilical vessels

FAMILY HISTORY
Hematuria or proteinuria
Deafness or hearing deficit (Alport's syndrome)
Renal failure, dialysis, or transplantation
Hypertension (PKD, GN)
Urolithiasis
Sickle cell disease or trait
Hemophilia or other coagulopathies
Hypercalciuria

PHYSICAL EXAMINATION
Blood pressure (acute renal failure, acute GN)
Weight and height (CRF, acidosis)
Fever, arthritis, or rash (SLE, HSP)
Edema (nephritis, nephrotic syndrome)
Eye grounds, lens abnormalities (Alport's syndrome, metabolic disease)
Costovertebral angle tenderness (UTI)
Abdominal masses (Wilms' tumor, PKD, hydronephrosis)
Genitalia—trauma, discharge, meatal stenosis, or foreign body
Pallor (anemia from CRF, HUS, hemoglobinopathy, leukemia, tumors)

INITIAL LABORATORY WORK-UP
Urinalysis—microscopy, proteinuria
Red blood cell morphology
Urine culture
Urinary calcium-to-creatinine ratio (see age-specific values later)
Sickle cell screen
Creatinine and blood urea nitrogen levels; complete blood count

---

Box 8-1 Workup of a Child with Hematuria—cont'd

Urine of first-degree relatives (rule out Alport's syndrome or benign familial hematuria)

Renal ultrasonography (rule out tumors, structural abnormalities, obstruction, stones)

Phase II Work-up (Guided by Initial Work-up)

Complement levels

Antistreptolysin-O and anti-DNAse B (poststreptococcal GN)

Antinuclear antibody (SLE)

Audiogram (Alport's syndrome)

Anti–glomerular basement membrane antibodies (Goodpasture's syndrome)

Antineutrophil cytoplasmic antibodies

Purified protein derivative

Advanced Work-up

Voiding cystourethrogram

Intravenous pyelography

Computed tomography scan

Magnetic resonance imaging

Renal scan

Renal biopsy

CRF, chronic renal failure; GN, glomerulonephritis; HSP, Henoch-Schönlein purpura; PKD, polycystic kidney disease; SLE, systemic lupus erythematosus; UTI, urinary tract infection.

Modified from Yadin O: Hematuria in children. Pediatr Ann 23:474–485, 1994.

h. Recurrent episodes of macroscopic hematuria not explained by a nonglomerular disease

i. Extreme parental anxiety with insistence on a specific diagnosis

7. When to stop the work-up

a. An etiology has been identified.

	Glomerular	Nonglomerular
Urine color	Brown, dark	Red, pink
RBC casts	+	−
Cellular casts	+	−
Proteinuria	+	−
Dysmorphic RBCs	+	−
Hypertension	+	−
Renal insufficiency	+	−
Blood clots	−	+

RBC, red blood cell.

    b. An etiology has not been identified (after a phase II work-up), but the patient has the following:

      (1) No proteinuria

      (2) No RBC casts

      (3) No hypertension

      (4) No renal insufficiency

      (5) No abnormalities on renal ultrasonography

      (6) These patients should be monitored periodically (every 3 to 6 months) with urinalysis, blood pressure, and kidney function tests (BUN and creatinine). If the hematuria resolves, then the work-up can be discontinued. If new findings appear, then an advanced work-up should proceed (see Box 8-1).

8. Management: The management of a child with hematuria depends on identification of the specific etiology and the clinical condition of the patient.

8.3 Proteinuria

1. Definition

    a. Protein of 1+ (30 mg/dL) in a urine dipstick (from a urine with a specific gravity below 1.015) can be classified as low-grade or minimal proteinuria and may not be associated with any genitourinary or renal disease.

    b. Protein of 2+ (100 mg/dL) in a urine dipstick (from a urine with a specific gravity above 1.015) usually is a more concerning degree of proteinuria.

    c. Protein above 4 mg/m²/hr in a timed 12- to 24-hour urine collection is considered significant proteinuria. Protein excretion above 40 mg/m²/hr is considered nephrotic-range proteinuria.

    d. Urinary protein-to-creatinine ratio (UPr/Cr): A ratio above 0.2 in children older than 2 years, or above 0.5 in children 6 months to 2 years of age, in a random urine specimen (do not use a postexercise specimen in children with severe nutritional deficiencies), indicates significant proteinuria. This is a simple, efficient way to detect significant proteinuria. If a repeat evaluation remains abnormal, a 24-hour specimen to measure total protein excretion should be obtained.

    e. Note: False-positive results to urinary protein by dipstick reactions can be due to the following factors:

      (1) Overlong immersion

      (2) Placing reagent strip directly in the urine stream

      (3) Alkaline urinary pH (pH >7.0)

      (4) Ammonium compounds and detergents

      (5) Pyuria

      (6) Bacteriuria

      (7) Mucoprotein

2. Epidemiology: Approximately 10% of school-aged children test positive for protein in urine dipstick at some time. When four specimens are obtained at different times, the prevalence falls to 1 in 1000. Only 10% of these children will have persistent proteinuria when followed for

6 to 12 months. The peak prevalence in girls is at 13 years of age and in boys at 16 years of age.
3. Etiology (Box 8-2)
4. Evaluation of the child with proteinuria
   a. A complete history should be taken and physical examination performed, looking specifically for the following conditions:
      (1) Hypertension
      (2) Edema
      (3) Short stature
      (4) Hearing deficits (Alport's syndrome)
      (5) Family history of renal disease
      (6) Café au lait spots, hypopigmented lesions (neurofibromatosis, tuberous sclerosis)
      (7) Rash, fever, arthralgias
   b. Perform an early-morning urinalysis for spot protein–creatinine (Pr/Cr) ratio.
   c. Do recumbent and ambulatory urinalyses. Obtain the first specimen right after patient wakes up and the second specimen several hours after normal ambulation. If abnormal, obtain a split 24-hour collection in both recumbent and ambulatory positions for quantitative protein measurement. For the diagnosis of orthostatic proteinuria to be made, the proteinuria in the recumbent specimen should be less than 4 $mg/m^2/hr$, or the spot Pr/Cr ratio should be less than 0.2. The protein in the ambulatory specimens may be elevated (two to four times the recumbent amount). The timed 24-hour protein excretion usually is below 1 g.
   d. Obtain CBC, electrolytes, BUN, creatinine, total protein, albumin, cholesterol, antistreptolysin-O titer (ASO), antinuclear antibody (ANA), and complement levels.
   e. Obtain renal ultrasonogram and voiding cystourethrogram if there is a history of recurrent UTI.
   f. If the preceding work-up does not reveal a particular diagnosis or the degree of proteinuria is significant, a renal biopsy may be indicated.
5. Management: Similar to hematuria, the management depends on the underlying etiology.

8.4 Nephrotic Syndrome

1. Definition: The four features that constitute nephrotic syndrome (NS) are as follows:
   a. Massive proteinuria (>40 $mg/m^2/hr$ or Pr/Cr >1.0)
   b. Hypoalbuminemia (albumin <2.5 g/dL)
   c. Edema
   d. Hyperlipidemia (hypercholesterolemia)
2. Epidemiology: The incidence is 1/100,000 among whites and 2.8/100,000 among nonwhites younger than 16 years of age. Two thirds of cases occur in children younger than 5 years of age, with a peak incidence between 2 and 3 years of age.
3. Etiology

Box 8-2   Classification and Etiologies of Proteinuria in Children and Adolescents

Functional/Transient (Usually below 2+ in Urine Dipstick)

Fever
Strenuous exercise
Cold exposure
Congestive heart failure
Seizures
Emotional stress

Isolated Proteinuria

Orthostatic proteinuria (very common cause)*
Persistent asymptomatic proteinuria (up to 80% of urine specimens
    may have protein)

Glomerular Disease

Minimal-change nephrotic syndrome
Focal segmental glomerulosclerosis
Glomerulonephritis
    Postinfectious
    Membranoproliferative
    Membranous
    Immunoglobulin A nephropathy
    Henoch-Schönlein purpura
    Systemic lupus erythematosus
    Hereditary nephritis

Tubulointerstitial Disease

Reflux nephropathy
Interstitial nephritis
Hypokalemic nephropathy
Cystinosis
Fanconi's syndrome
Tyrosinemia
Lowe's syndrome
Tubular toxins
    Drugs (e.g., aminoglycosides and penicillins)
    Heavy metals
Ischemic tubular injury

*Of all proteinuria seen in children, 60% is accounted for by orthostatic proteinuria.
Its incidence is higher in girls up to the age of 16 years, although usually proteinuria is
under 1 g/day, and the prognosis is excellent.
Adapted from Ettenger RB: The evaluation of the child with proteinuria. Pediatr Ann
23:486-494,1994.

  a. The most common association of NS in children is minimal-change disease (approximately 80% of cases), followed by focal segmental glomerulosclerosis (approximately 10%).

  b. The remaining 5% to 10% of cases are caused by the following conditions:

   (1) Membranous GN (most common cause in adults)

   (2) Mesangioproliferative GN

   (3) Membranoproliferative GN

   (4) Immunoglobulin A (IgA) nephropathy (Berger's disease)

   (5) Henoch-Schönlein purpura (HSP) nephritis (renal histology identical to IgA nephropathy)

   (6) SLE nephritis

   (7) Syphilis

   (8) Chronic hepatitis B, C infection

   (9) Human immunodeficiency virus (HIV) infection

   (10) Malaria

   (11) Drugs (mainly NSAIDs)

   (12) Heavy metal poisoning (e.g., lead, mercury)

4. Diagnosis: A thorough history and physical examination should focus on:

  a. History of periorbital edema on awakening (e.g., parents will complain that the child looks "puffy," pale, and clothes do not fit right)

  b. Recumbent, dependent, pitting edema (these children have marks left by socks, belts, tight clothing)

  c. History of recent drug ingestion

  d. History of travel to area endemic for malaria

  e. Rashes, arthralgia, fevers, pallor

  f. Purpura, abdominal pain

5. Laboratory findings

  a. Urine dipstick (usually above 3+)

  b. Urinalysis

  c. Quantitative protein in a 12- to 24-hour collection (>40 mg/m^2/hour) or a Pr/Cr above 1.0 in a random urine sample; CBC, electrolytes, BUN, creatinine, cholesterol, total protein, albumin

  d. ASO, ANA, C3 and C4 levels, and hepatitis serology for older children or those with a suggestive history

  e. Renal biopsy if the diagnosis of minimal-change NS (MCNS) is *not* suspected

   (1) Age-specific chances of having MCNS:

    (a) 1 to 7 years: 90%

    (b) 8 to 12 years: 50%

    (c) Older than 12 years: 20% to 30%

    (d) Adults: 25%

   (2) All of the following support the diagnosis of MCNS:

    (a) Age 1 to 7 years

    (b) Normal renal function (BUN, creatinine)

    (c) No gross hematuria or cellular casts (transient microscopic hematuria can be seen)

    (d) Complement levels (usually normal)

    (e) Negative ANA

    (f) No evidence of systemic disorders

       (g) Normal blood pressure

       (h) Elevated cholesterol

       (i) Positive response to steroids

6. Management

  a. Follow a low-sodium diet: 1 g/day for young children, 2 g/day for older children and adolescents.

  b. Fluid restriction is not necessary in most patients.

  c. Monitor strict intake and output and daily weights.

  d. In hospitalized patients with moderate to severe anasarca, treat with intravenous (IV) albumin infusion (25% albumin, 0.5 g/kg as initial dose), followed by a potent diuretic (usually furosemide, 1 to 2 mg/kg/dose IV). Repeated infusions might be needed.

  e. Steroid use in MCNS is outlined in Box 8-3.

    (1) Most patients (>90%) responding to steroids do so within the first month of treatment; 70% do so within 2 weeks.

Box 8-3 Prednisone Treatment in Minimal-Change Nephrotic Syndrome

Initial Episode

Prednisone/prednisolone 60 mg/m^2 (2 mg/kg) orally in two divided doses (maximum 80 mg/day) for 4 weeks

Followed by 40 mg/m^2 in a single morning dose on alternate days for 4–8 weeks. Taper gradually over the next 2–4 weeks. (Current evidence suggests that longer initial course of steroids is associated with diminished risk of subsequent relapse.)

Body surface area (BSA) may be calculated as follows:

$$BSA\ (m^2) = \sqrt{\frac{Height\ (cm) \times Weight\ (kg)}{3600}}$$

Relapse Episode

This is defined as 2+ or higher proteinuria for 3 consecutive days with acute weight gain.

Prednisone/prednisolone 60 mg/m^2 (2 mg/kg) orally in two divided doses (maximum 80 mg/day) until remission is achieved (absent or 1+ urine protein on 3 consecutive days)

Followed by 40 mg/m^2 in a single morning dose on alternate days for 2–4 weeks

Frequent Relapses

This is defined as three or more episodes per year.

Induce remission with previous regimen, followed by prednisone 0.25 to 1 mg/kg orally every other morning for 6–12 months.

Taper gradually over 1–2 months.

(2) Most patients (>90%) with MCNS respond to steroids, and most patients (>90%) who respond to steroids have MCNS.

f. Indications for renal biopsy
    (1) Patients who are not likely to have MCNS
    (2) Patients who fail to respond to daily steroids during the first month
    (3) Patients who relapse frequently
    (4) Patients who are experiencing steroid toxicity (refer all such patients to a pediatric nephrologist for a possible renal biopsy and alternative treatment)

g. Alternative treatment modalities: For patients who respond to steroids but experience significant toxicity, cyclosporine, chlorambucil, levamisole, mycophenolate mofetil, and cyclophosphamide have been used with varying success.

7. Prognosis
    a. Many patients (about 40%) may have a chronic relapsing course. Patients with MCNS respond to initial steroid therapy over 90% of the time, but relapse can occur in 70% to 80% of the cases.
    b. If a child remains relapse free for more than 1 year, there is a 95% chance that he or she will remain free of relapses thereafter.

8.5 Glomerulonephritis

1. Definition: The following features constitute the "nephritic syndrome":
    a. Proteinuria (usually not in the nephrotic range)
    b. Hematuria (gross or microscopic, with RBC casts in the urine)
    c. Hypertension (from fluid overload secondary to decreased glomerular filtration rate)
    d. Edema (from retention of salt and water or decreased oncotic pressure)

2. Etiology
    a. Acute postinfectious GN
    b. IgA nephropathy
    c. HSP nephritis
    d. SLE nephritis
    e. Rapidly progressive GN
    f. Wegener's granulomatosis/microscopic polyangiitis (associated with antineutrophil cytoplasmic antibodies [ANCA])
    g. Membranoproliferative GN (anti–glomerular basement membrane [GBM] antibodies are present)
    h. Hepatitis B- and hepatitis C-associated GN
    i. Goodpasture's syndrome
    j. Possible association of nephritis with chronic bacteremia (e.g., subacute bacterial endocarditis)

3. Clinical features and management of specific conditions
    a. Acute postinfectious GN
        (1) The most common form of postinfectious GN is acute poststreptococcal GN (APSGN), which in turn is the most common cause of GN in children. A number of other bacterial, viral, parasitic, rickettsial, and fungal agents cause infections that can be associated with an acute nephritic syndrome similar to the one that

follows an infection with a nephritogenic strain of group A beta-hemolytic streptococci (either pharyngitis or skin infection).

(2) Epidemiology: APSGN affects mainly school-aged children, with a mean age of 7 years, and is uncommon before the age of 3 years. The male-to-female ratio is 2:1. The interval between infection and the onset of GN is usually between 1 and 2 weeks, with a range of 5 days to 4 weeks.

(3) Clinical features
   (a) The most common presentation includes all the features of nephritic syndrome, plus nonspecific symptoms such as anorexia, vomiting, lethargy, abdominal pain, or headache.
   (b) The urine is usually dark (cola colored) and gross hematuria is present in up to 50% of the patients. Edema is present in at least 75% of patients and hypertension in 50% to 90%.

(4) Laboratory findings
   (a) Urinalysis
      (i) RBC casts are present in 60% to 85% of the patients.
      (ii) Hyaline, granular, and white blood cell (WBC) casts are often seen.
      (iii) Proteinuria is present in most patients.
   (b) Antistreptococcal antibodies (ASO, antihyaluronidase, and anti-DNase B) should be elevated to diagnose this entity with certainty. When all three antibodies are measured, proof of preceding infection is close to 100%.
   (c) Cultures should be taken if throat and skin lesions exist.
   (d) The C3 level is markedly decreased in at least 90% of patients. A follow-up level should be obtained 6 to 8 weeks after the onset of the illness. In APSGN, the C3 level returns to normal by this time. If the level is still decreased, other causes of GN should be sought, such as membranoproliferative GN or SLE nephritis.
   (e) ANA, ANCA, anti-GBM antibodies (to rule out other causes of nephritic syndrome)
   (f) Electrolytes, BUN, and creatinine: Hyponatremia or hypernatremia may be present. BUN is often elevated disproportionate to creatinine.

(5) Management entails mainly supportive measures:
   (a) Fluid and sodium restriction only if needed to control hypertension and fluid overload
   (b) Diuretics and antihypertensives
   (c) Throat or skin infections treated with antistreptococcal antibiotics

(6) Prognosis: More than 98% of patients recover completely over several months. The hypertension and gross hematuria usually resolve within 3 weeks, hypocomplementemia resolves in 6 to 8 weeks, the proteinuria over several months, and the microscopic hematuria can persist for years.

b. IgA nephropathy
   (1) Epidemiology and clinical features: The mean age of presentation is 9 years; 75% of the children affected are male. Hematuria occurs

within 24 hours of an intercurrent infection most commonly involving the upper respiratory tract (unlike with APSGN, there is no latent period—also called *synpharyngitic*). Microscopic hematuria is always present, and intermittent gross hematuria is present in 85% of the cases. Proteinuria is present in about 75% of the patients, but only 15% will have nephrotic-range proteinuria. Hypertension is present in 30% of patients. Fever, malaise, and abdominal or back pain are common presenting features, but most symptoms are secondary to the intercurrent infection.

(2) Diagnosis is confirmed by the demonstration of mesangial deposition of IgA on a renal biopsy.

(3) Management is mainly supportive. In patients with advanced kidney lesions, severe symptoms, or renal failure, prednisone and cytotoxic drugs have been tried, but, in general, there is no established treatment.

(4) Prognosis: Some children have a slowly progressive course, with up to 40% of patients developing chronic renal failure after 20 years of follow-up. Those at risk have persistent nephrotic-range proteinuria and hypertension.

c. HSP nephritis

(1) Etiology/epidemiology: HSP is a systemic (possibly autoimmune) vasculitis with a male predominance; most patients are younger than 5 years of age. The condition is often preceded by an upper respiratory infection 1 to 3 weeks earlier, with a peak incidence in the winter months.

(2) Clinical features

(a) Nonthrombocytopenic, palpable, purpuric rash, generally involving the lower extremities and buttocks. It may begin as a fine petechial rash. The petechiae eventually coalesce and form raised, swollen, generally nontender purpuric lesions. The rash primarily begins on the lower extremities, joints, and over the buttocks. It also can occur on the extensor surfaces of the upper extremities, sometimes accompanied by periorbital or labial edema.

(b) Arthritis/arthralgia is seen in almost 75% of patients.

(c) Crampy abdominal pain is seen in 50% of patients. The vasculitis can cause edema of the bowel wall and secondary intussusception or lower gastrointestinal bleeding. Symptoms may be severe and mimic appendicitis.

(d) Renal manifestations range from asymptomatic hematuria and proteinuria, to the complete nephritic/nephrotic syndrome. Most patients have microscopic hematuria and proteinuria, and gross hematuria and transient azotemia develop in up to 20% of patients. Acute renal failure is very rare. The renal lesion is identical to the one seen in IgA nephropathy.

(3) Management: Steroids (prednisone 1 to 2 mg/kg/day, twice daily for 5 to 7 days) have been proved to be beneficial in treating patients with severe abdominal pain and gastrointestinal bleeding, but there is no evidence to support their routine use for the

renal manifestations of the disease. NSAIDs (e.g., naproxen sodium) can be used for joint manifestations.

(4) Prognosis: The overall prognosis of HSP depends on the severity of the renal disease. Children with minor urinary abnormalities have an excellent prognosis, with complete recovery over several weeks, but those who present with acute nephritis or NS may develop chronic renal failure and end-stage renal disease (ESRD). After the acute manifestations, gastrointestinal and joint manifestations resolve over time. Recurrent or acute arthritis may recur but is usually mild.

d. SLE nephritis (see also Chapter 12)

(1) Epidemiology and clinical features: SLE usually presents in young adulthood, but up to 25% of the cases are diagnosed in the first two decades of life, with a male-to-female ratio of 1:8. Renal disease is present in 40% to 90% of patients, depending on the criteria used to diagnose SLE nephritis. Almost all patients have abnormalities on renal biopsy. Several histologic classes of SLE nephritis have been described (World Health Organization classes I-V).

(2) Diagnosis: At the time of diagnosis, complement levels are often low, and ANA and anti-dsDNA antibodies are elevated.

(3) Management: Many therapies have been used in SLE nephritis. Intermittent oral or IV cyclophosphamide, mycophenolate, and cyclosporine combined with steroids have all proved effective in reducing the risk of progression to ESRD disease.

8.6 Acute Renal Failure

1. Definitions: Acute renal failure (ARF) is the rapid cessation of renal function, with an inability of the kidney to control body homeostasis, resulting in azotemia and fluid and electrolyte imbalances. ARF can occur with or without diminished urine output. Children with ARF are usually oliguric.

a. *Oliguria* is defined as a urine output less than 0.5 mL/kg/hr in infants or less than 500 mL/1.73 m^2/day in older children.

b. *Anuria* is the total cessation of urinary output.

2. Etiology/classification

a. ARF can be classified into the following etiologic categories:

(1) Prerenal (the most common type, caused by hypoperfusion of the kidneys)

(2) Renal (intrinsic kidney disease)

(3) Postrenal (the least frequent type, caused by total or partial obstruction of the urinary tract)

b. Causes of ARF are shown in Box 8-4.

3. Diagnosis: In the evaluation of a child with ARF a thorough history and physical examination should be obtained, focusing on the following:

a. History of renal problems, poor growth and development, signs of renal osteodystrophy (to rule out ARF superimposed on chronic renal failure)

b. History of drug ingestion/administration

Box 8-4   Causes of Acute Renal Failure in Children

Prerenal Failure (Hypoperfusion)

DECREASED EFFECTIVE CIRCULATORY VOLUME

Hypovolemia

  Cutaneous losses (burns)

  Gastrointestinal losses (vomiting, diarrhea, ileostomy losses)

  Hemorrhage (trauma)

  Renal losses—polyuria (diabetes insipidus, diabetes mellitus, diuretics)

Maldistribution of blood

  Generalized vasodilation (anaphylaxis, antihypertensive drugs)

  Hypoperfusion secondary to occlusion of renal vessels (stenosis, thrombosis)

  Renal vasoconstriction (drugs—cyclosporine, α1-adrenergic agonist; hepatorenal syndrome)

  Shock (sepsis, toxins)

  Third space losses (abdominal surgery, peritonitis, pancreatitis, trauma, hypoalbuminemia–nephrotic syndrome, capillary leak syndrome)

DIMINISHED CARDIAC OUTPUT

Anatomic malformations (congenital heart diseases, acquired valvular diseases)

Arrhythmias

Cardiogenic shock

Cardiomyopathy (primary, secondary, or ischemic heart disease)

Renal: Intrinsic Acute Renal Failure

GLOMERULAR DISEASES (IMMUNE AND NONIMMUNE)

Acute postinfection glomerulonephritis

Anti–glomerular basement membrane glomerulonephritis (Goodpasture's syndrome)

Henoch-Schönlein purpura nephritis/immunoglobulin A nephritis

Membranoproliferative glomerulonephritis

Rapidly progressive glomerulonephritis

Systemic lupus erythematosus nephritis

VASCULAR LESIONS

Hemolytic-uremic syndrome

Hypersensitive vasculitis

Kawasaki's disease

Polyarteritis nodosa

Scleroderma

Wegener's granulomatosis

Continued

8—Renal Disorders

Box 8-4   Causes of Acute Renal Failure in Children—cont'd

TUBULAR LESIONS—ACUTE TUBULAR NECROSIS
Ischemia—all prerenal conditions
Nephrotoxins
    Drugs
        Antibiotics (aminoglycosides, tetracycline, cyclosporine, amphotericin B, and others)
        Anesthetics (methoxyflurane, halothane, enflurane)
        Chemotherapeutic agents (methotrexate, cisplatin)
        ACE inhibitors
        Ionic radiocontrast materials
    Toxins
        Ethylene glycol
        Heavy metals (lead, mercury)
        Hydrocarbons
        Organic solvents
    Pigments
        Hemoglobinuria (disseminated intravascular coagulation, transfusion reaction, glucose-6-phosphate dehydrogenase deficiency)
        Myoglobinuria (trauma, crush, injury, myositis, seizure)
Interstitial lesions
    Drug-induced (beta-lactam antibiotics, rifampin, acyclovir, nonsteroidal anti-inflammatory drugs, diuretics, ACE inhibitors)
    Infection (infectious mononucleosis, streptococcal infection)
    Infiltrative lesions (chronic pyelonephritis, tumor infiltration)
    Idiopathic interstitial nephritis with or without uveitis

Postrenal Failure

STRUCTURAL ABNORMALITIES (INTRINSIC/EXTRINSIC)
Bladder (fungus ball, stone)
Collecting duct (uric acid, oxalic acid)
Renal pelvis (acute papillary necrosis, ureteropelvic junction stenosis)
Ureter (stone, blood clots, postradiation stenosis, aberrant vessel, bowel impaction, retroperitoneal fibrosis, ureteral prolapse)
Urethral obstruction (posterior urethral valve, foreign body)

FUNCTIONAL ABNORMALITIES
Drugs (anticholinergic agents)
Neurogenic bladder (diabetes mellitus, meningomyelocele)

ACE, angiotensin-converting enzyme.
Adapted from Sehic A, Chesney RW: Acute renal failure: Diagnosis. Pediatr Rev 16:101, 1995.

   c. History of acute, recent fluid losses
   d. Assessment of fluid and cardiovascular/hemodynamic status
   e. Assessment of patency of urinary tract
   f. Signs of other organ involvement
4. Laboratory evaluation
   a. CBC with smear (anemia, low WBC count)
   b. Serum electrolytes (elevated K^+) and elevated uric acid, BUN, and creatinine
   c. Serum proteins (hypoalbuminemia)
   d. Urinalysis
   e. Urinary sodium, creatinine, osmolarity, and urea
   f. Urinary indices
      (1) UPr/Cr ratio
      (2) Urine/plasma osmolarity ratio
      (3) Fractional excretion of sodium (the most useful urinary index; see Chapter 9)
   g. C3 and C4 levels, antistreptococcal antibodies if APSGN is suspected
   h. ANA if SLE nephritis is suspected
   i. ANCA if vasculitis is suspected
   j. Renal ultrasonography with Doppler flow, including the lower urinary tract and bladder, should be considered in all patients with ARF.
   k. A renal biopsy might be indicated.
5. Management (Box 8-5): In most cases the treatment is conservative and mainly supportive.
   a. Treatment of underlying condition that led to ARF
   b. Maintenance of fluid and electrolyte balance
   c. Specific therapy for complications: hyperkalemia, hyponatremia or hypernatremia, hyperphosphatemia, hypocalcemia, fluid overload/CHF, hypertension, acidosis, uremia, and infection
   d. Dialysis is indicated in patients with the following conditions:
      (1) Volume overload with hypertension or CHF unresponsive to fluid therapy or antihypertensives
      (2) Hyperkalemia (potassium level >7.0 mEq/L, or <7.0 mEq/L accompanied by ECG changes)
      (3) Acidosis unresponsive to conservative measures
      (4) Uremic encephalopathy
      (5) Bleeding caused by uremia
      (6) Hypocalcemia and hyperphosphatemia severe enough to cause seizures
      (7) Severe hyponatremia or hypernatremia
      (8) Severe azotemia (BUN >150, specially if accompanied by mental status changes)
      (9) Need for removal of fluid to provide adequate nutrition, transfusions, or other therapies to the anuric or oliguric patient

8.7 Hemolytic-Uremic Syndrome

1. Epidemiology: The prevalence in the United States ranges from 0.3 to 10 cases per 100,000 children. HUS occurs more frequently in children 1 to 5 years of age, with whites being affected more often than blacks. There is no sex predilection. HUS is more common during the summer

Box 8-5 Conservative Management of Acute Renal Failure

Supportive Therapy

Stabilize

Monitor closely

Prevent sepsis (limit IV lines, remove indwelling urinary catheter, culture periodically, and administer antibiotics when indicated)

Administer ulcer prophylaxis

Adjust drugs according to renal function

Symptomatic Therapy

PRERENAL FAILURE AND EARLY CONVERSION TO OLIGURIC IN NONOLIGURIC FAILURE

Administer fluid challenge

  0.9% normal saline or 5% albumin 10–20 mL/kg/dose IV over 1 hr

  Response: urine output >1–3 mL/kg/hr within 2–3 hr

  Repeat fluid challenge and diuretics (loop) if no response and patient not in CHF

  Furosemide 2–5 mL/kg/dose IV

Give inotropic support for CHF

ESTABLISHED RENAL FAILURE

- **Restrict fluids**

Insensible loss: 400 mL/m^2/24 hr (25%–30% of maintenance fluid volume) as 5% or 10% glucose in water; *plus*

Urine output: 0.45% normal saline (mL for mL of output every 4–6 hr)

- **Treat hyponatremia**

Maintain serum sodium: 130–135 mEq/L, restricting free water

- **Treat metabolic acidosis**

Replace base deficit (BD) with sodium bicarbonate ($NaHCO_3$) if pH <7.2 or bicarbonate (HCO_3) <12 mEq/L and if cardiovascular status allows

$$BD = \frac{0.6 \times BW \ (body \ weight) \times (HCO_3 \ desired - HCO_3 \ observed)}{2}$$

½ over 2–3 hr, rest over next 24 hr

0.3 mol/L THAM (mL) dose = BD (mEq/L) × BW (kg)

- **Treat hyperphosphatemia**

Calcium carbonate: 300–400 mg/kg/day orally or by nasogastric tube

- **Treat tetany**

Calcium gluconate: 10% 0.5–1.0 mL/kg/dose IV

- **Treat hyperkalemia**

Serum potassium (K^+) >5.7 mEq/L

  Eliminate K^+ intake

  Cation exchange resin sodium polystyrene sulfonate: 1 g/kg/dose every 2–4 hr orally (in 70% sorbitol), rectally (in 25%–30% sorbitol or $D_{10}W$)

Box 8-5   Conservative Management of Acute
Renal Failure—cont'd

Serum K^+ >6.5 mEq/L with ECG changes:
  All of the above
  Calcium gluconate 10%: 0.5-1.0 mL/kg/dose IV slowly over
    10–15 min
  Glucose—$D_{25}W$ or $D_{50}W$ and regular insulin: dextrose and water,
    0.5–1.0 g/kg/dose IV; with insulin, 0.1 U/kg/dose IV or subcuta-
    neously
  Albuterol aerosol: 0.01–0.03 mL/kg/dose
  $NaHCO_3$ 7.5%: 1–2 mEq/kg/dose IV slow push or fast drip
• Treat hypertension
Nifedipine: 0.25–1 mg/kg/dose orally, SLQ (maximum 30 mg/dose)
Diazoxide: 3–10 mg/kg IV push (maximum 150 mg/dose)
Hydralazine: 1 mg/kg IV as first dose, then 0.1–0.3 mg/kg (maximum
  3.5 mg/kg/day)
Sodium nitroprusside: 0.5–10 μg/kg/min IV drip (maximum 800 μg/min)
Labetalol: 0.25–1.0 mg/kg IV bolus or 1–5 mg/kg/hr drip (maximum
  300 mg/day)
• Administer supplemental nutrition (400 kcal/m²/day)
Parenteral/enteral
  >70% carbohydrates, <20% lipids
  0.5–1.0 g/kg/day high–biological-value protein

CHF, congestive heart failure; IV, intravenous; SLQ, sublingual; THAM, tromethamine.
Adapted from Sehic A, Chesney RW: Acute renal failure: Therapy. Pediatr Rev
16:137, 1995.

and early fall. The most common form of HUS is associated with cyto-
toxin-producing organisms (verotoxin-producing *Escherichia coli* or
Shigatoxin-producing *Shigella dysenteriae*). The outcome is worse in the
non–diarrhea-associated HUS (Box 8-6). HUS is one of the most
common causes of ARF in children in developed countries.
2. Clinical features
  a. The syndrome consists of the following:
    (1) ARF
    (2) Microangiopathic hemolytic anemia
    (3) Thrombocytopenia
  b. The syndrome is often preceded by an acute gastroenteritis, consist-
    ing of bloody diarrhea, crampy abdominal pain, and vomiting, which
    usually lasts between 1 and 4 days. This prodrome precedes the onset
    of HUS by 3 to 12 days. The child becomes suddenly quite ill, mani-
    festing irritability, restlessness, and pallor. Oliguria then occurs, and
    signs and symptoms of fluid overload may develop.
  c. On diagnosis, hemolysis is present in all patients, and thrombocyto-
    penia (with platelet counts usually <40,000) in most of them. ARF
    occurs with the onset of hemolysis.

Box 8-6   Classification of Hemolytic-Uremic Syndromes

Diarrhea Associated

Typical, related to *Escherichia coli* O157:H7 (producing VT-1, VT-2)
Related to *Shigella dysenteriae* (type 1, producing Shigatoxin)
Related to other diarrhea-causing agents (*Campylobacter, Yersinia*)
Idiopathic

Non–Diarrhea Associated

Related to *Streptococcus pneumoniae* (neuraminidase associated)
Related to other infectious agents (Epstein-Barr virus, influenza virus, coxsackievirus)
Inherited
   Autosomal dominant
   Autosomal recessive
Pregnancy associated
Drug associated: cyclosporine, oral contraceptives, vaccines, chemotherapy
Radiation injury
Post-transplantation
Factor V Leiden deficiency (familial)
Malignancy associated
Idiopathic

Adapted from Stewart CL, Tina LU: Hemolytic uremic syndrome. Pediatr Rev 14:218-225, 1993.

    d. Central nervous system involvement in patients with HUS is manifested by irritability and lethargy. Some patients might even have seizures, ataxia, cerebral edema, hemiparesis, focal neurologic signs, and coma. These manifestations tend to be more severe in patients with non–diarrhea-associated HUS.
  3. Laboratory evaluation and findings (Box 8-7)
  4. Management
    a. Establish diagnosis and exclude alternative possibilities (i.e., post-infectious GN, SLE, sepsis/multisystem failure, vasculitis).
    b. Treat acute renal insufficiency.
      (1) Restrict fluids to insensible losses plus output.
      (2) Consider furosemide (1 to 2 mg/kg/day to maintain urine output, control edema), with replacement of urine output to avoid dehydration.
      (3) Consider early dialysis (manage as for ARF).
    c. Treat hematologic abnormalities.
      (1) Maintain hemoglobin above 8 g/dL.
      (2) Use platelet transfusion for symptomatic bleeding.
      (3) Consider plasma transfusion for hereditary HUS or prolonged or recurrent HUS.
      (4) Avoid plasma transfusion in pneumococcal-neuraminidase HUS.

> ### Box 8-7   Laboratory Evaluation and Findings in Hemolytic-Uremic Syndrome
>
> #### Hematology
>
> Platelet count ($\downarrow$)
> Platelet size ($\uparrow$)
> Hemolytic anemia (Coombs' test negative; helmet cells, schistocytes, and burr cells on smear); reticulocyte count ($\uparrow$)
> Haptoglobin ($\downarrow$)
> Prothrombin time/partial thromboplastin time (usually normal)
> Fibrin degradation products ($\uparrow$)
> Fibrinogen (normal or $\uparrow$)
> White blood cell count ($\uparrow$, left shift)
>
> #### Serum Chemistry
>
> Blood urea nitrogen ($\uparrow$)
> Potassium (variable)
> Serum protein ($\downarrow$)
> Bilirubin ($\uparrow$)
> Liver enzymes ($\uparrow$)
> Creatinine ($\uparrow$)
> Bicarbonate ($\downarrow$)
> Uric acid ($\uparrow$)
> Lipids ($\uparrow$)
>
> #### Urine
>
> Proteinuria
> Heme positive
> Leukocyte esterase positive
> Bilirubin $\pm$ positive
> Red blood cells (dysmorphic)
> White blood cells
> Casts (cellular, granular, pigmented, hyaline)

   d. Manage nutrition: Maintain caloric intake, enterally or parenterally.
   e. Antibiotics: There is currently no role for antibiotics in the treatment of E. coli O157:H7–positive HUS. In fact, recent studies suggest an increased risk of HUS after antibiotic treatment.
5. Prognosis
   a. HUS usually resolves in 1 to 3 months. Most patients recover completely, but approximately 15% of patients die or end up with significant renal dysfunction. In those who recover completely, the duration of oliguria or anuria averages 7 to 14 days. Poor prognostic factors are listed in Box 8-8.
   b. Renal transplantation can be performed in those children who progress to ESRD. However, recurrence of HUS has been noted in the transplanted kidney, for poorly understood reasons.

> **Box 8-8   Poor Prognostic Indicators of Hemolytic-Uremic Syndrome**
>
> Non–diarrhea-associated hemolytic-uremic syndrome (recurrent, hereditary): more progression to end-stage renal disease and increased mortality
> Very young or older age (under 1 year, over 5 years)
> Prolonged period of anuria (although patients have recovered even after 30 days of anuria)
> Severe hypertension
> Central nervous system findings (coma, seizure, hemiparesis/stroke)
> Elevated white blood cell count ($>20,000/mm^3$): on presentation and if remains elevated, in patients with diarrhea-associated hemolytic-uremic syndrome

    c. Approximately 10% of patients suffer some residual disease, with renal or neurologic involvement.

8.8 Chronic Renal Disease

1. Definitions
   a. *Impaired renal function*: The patient has a residual renal function less than 75% of normal and is asymptomatic.
   b. *Chronic renal insufficiency*: The patient has a residual renal function of 25% to 50% of normal. The patient is usually asymptomatic, but metabolic abnormalities may be present when the patient is stressed. Calcium and phosphorus levels are normal at the expense of an elevated parathyroid hormone, and growth is impaired. Dialysis is not needed at this stage.
   c. *Chronic renal failure*: The patient has a residual renal function less than 30% of normal. The patient shows metabolic abnormalities (osteodystrophy, anemia, acidosis, poor growth) even when not under stress. Hypertension might be present as well.
   d. *ESRD*: The patient has a residual renal function below 10% of normal. At this stage, renal replacement therapy is needed (dialysis or transplantation).
2. Etiology: The most common causes leading to chronic renal disease in children, in order of frequency, are as follows:
   a. Obstructive uropathy (reflux nephropathy or renal dysplasia secondary to obstruction)
   b. Renal hypoplasia/dysplasia
   c. Glomerulopathy/GN
   d. Polycystic kidney disease
3. Clinical features
   a. Growth failure

b. Hypertension
c. Nocturia, polyuria
d. Pruritus
e. Nausea, vomiting, anorexia
f. Peripheral neuropathy, lethargy, encephalopathy
g. Teeth and bone abnormalities
h. Anemia
4. Management
   a. Diet: At least 100% recommended daily caloric intake, but only 1 g/kg/day of protein and low sodium and low phosphorus
   b. Vitamin D and calcium supplements to prevent/treat renal osteodystrophy
   c. Iron supplements, erythropoietin if anemic
   d. Antihypertensive agent if hypertensive
   e. Sodium bicarbonate (or citrate) if acidosis is present
   f. Dialysis (see Section 8.10)

8.9 Indications for Renal Biopsy

1. In the presence of hematuria
   a. Persistent asymptomatic microscopic hematuria for more than 1 year
   b. Significant proteinuria (nephrotic range or >1 g/day)
   c. Persistently low C3 levels
   d. Family history of nephritis
   e. Hearing deficit
   f. Renal insufficiency
   g. Hypertension (after excluding anatomic and vascular anomalies)
   h. Recurrent episodes of macroscopic hematuria not explained by a nonglomerular disease
2. In the presence of proteinuria
   a. Persistent hematuria
   b. NS: Unresponsive to steroids, or with persistent hematuria, hypertension, or azotemia
   c. Azotemia or hypertension
   d. Persistently low C3 levels
   e. Systemic disease (SLE or HSP)
   f. Persistent (>80% of specimens), nonorthostatic, isolated proteinuria for more than 1 year
   g. Family history of chronic GN or unexplained renal failure
3. In the presence of GN
   a. Not likely to be acute postinfectious GN
   b. Systemic disease
   c. Renal insufficiency
4. In the presence of ARF
   a. No obvious cause
   b. Difficulty differentiating between acute tubular necrosis, glomerular or vascular lesions, and chronic renal failure
   c. Acute tubular necrosis is suspected, but anuria persists for more than 3 weeks

8.10 Indications for Dialysis

1. ESRD is a state of renal failure in which renal replacement therapy (dialysis or transplantation) is needed to sustain life. This usually occurs when the glomerular filtration rate is 5 to 10 mL/min/1.73 m^2. At this point the child can no longer function normally, is often tired, has decreased appetite, is constantly itching, cannot attend school, and has an overall poor quality of life.
2. Uremia (BUN >150 or rising rapidly)
3. Severe metabolic acidosis (pH <7.20)
4. Severe hyperkalemia unresponsive to conservative measures
5. Fluid overload with evidence of pulmonary edema or hypertension refractory to pharmacological therapy
6. Neurologic symptoms secondary to uremia or electrolyte imbalance
7. Severe hypocalcemia with tetany or seizures, in the presence of a very high serum phosphate
8. Need for fluid administration (nutrition, drugs) above insensible losses in anuric or oliguric patient
9. Acute intoxication with dialyzable substance/toxin that cannot be removed effectively or quickly enough in any other way. Molecules such as methanol, ethanol, ethylene glycol, and procainamide are some of the substances that can be removed by dialysis.
10. Types of dialysis (Table 8-3): The most common types of dialysis used in children are as follows:
    a. Hemodialysis
    b. Continuous ambulatory peritoneal dialysis
    c. Continuous cycling peritoneal dialysis
11. Complications
    a. Infection
    b. Hemorrhage
    c. Thrombosis
    d. Hypotension
    e. Cerebral edema (dysequilibrium syndrome)
    f. Peritonitis
    g. Peritoneal leak
    h. Outflow obstruction
    i. Hernias
    j. Protein loss

8.11 Renal Transplantation

1. Rationale: Renal transplantation provides the most humane and long-term solution for the child with ESRD.
2. Causes that lead to ESRD in children are listed in Box 8-9.
3. Outcome
    a. Approximately 40% of children who receive cadaveric transplants and 60% of those who receive a living related donor transplant are free of dialysis 10 years posttransplant. Some glomerulopathies can recur in the transplanted kidney. These include the following:
       (1) Focal segmental glomerulosclerosis

	Hemodialysis	Continuous Ambulatory Peritoneal Dialysis	Continuous Cycling Peritoneal Dialysis
Cost	Very expensive	Least expensive	Less expensive
Site	Hospital	Ambulatory (3 passes/day plus 1/night)	Ambulatory (no daytime pass)
Frequency	Several times per week (usually 3 times/wk for 3–4 hours)	Daily (bag change every 4–5 hours and once at night)	Daily (only connect to machine at night and disconnect in morning)
Access	Vascular access (arteriovenous fistula/subclavian catheter)	Peritoneal catheter	Peritoneal catheter

Box 8-9   Causes of End-Stage Renal Disease in Children

Congenital

Obstructive uropathy
Renal hypoplasia/dysplasia
Severe vesicoureteral reflux
Cystinosis
Polycystic kidney disease
Alport's syndrome

Acquired

Chronic glomerulonephritis
Renovascular disease
Bilateral Wilms' tumor
Hemolytic-uremic syndrome
Interstitial nephritis
Nephrotoxins

    (2) Goodpasture's syndrome
    (3) Membranoproliferative GN
    (4) Rapidly progressing GN
    (5) HSP/IgA nephropathy
    (6) SLE nephritis
    (7) Membranous GN
  b. The reader is referred to other sources for a more in-depth discussion
     of the management and complications encountered in patients who
     undergo renal transplantations.

SUGGESTED READING

Ettenger RB: The evaluation of the child with proteinuria. Pediatr Ann 23:486-494, 1994.

Grimm PC, Ogborn MR: Hemolytic uremic syndrome: The most common cause of acute renal failure in childhood. Pediatr Ann 23:505-511, 1994.

Jung FF, Ingelfinger JR: Hypertension in childhood and adolescence. Pediatr Rev 14:169-179, 1993.

National High Blood Pressure Education Program Working Group on Hypertension Control in Children and Adolescents: Update on the 1987 task force report on high blood pressure in children and adolescents: A working group report from the National High Blood Pressure Education Program. Pediatrics 98:649-658, 1996.

Sehic A, Chesney RW: Acute renal failure: Diagnosis. Pediatr Rev 16:101, 1995.

Sehic A, Chesney RW: Acute renal failure: Therapy. Pediatr Rev 16:137, 1995.

Stewart CL, Tina LU: Hemolytic uremic syndrome. Pediatr Rev 14:218-225, 1993.

Sargent JD, Stukel TA, Kresel J, Klein RZ: Normal values for random urinary calcium/creatinine ratios in infancy. J Pediatr 123:393-397, 1993.

Warshaw BL: Nephrotic syndrome in children. Pediatr Ann 23:495-504, 1994.

Wong CS, Jelacic S, Habeeb RL, et al: The risk of the hemolytic-uremic syndrome after antibiotic treatment of *Escherichia coli* O157:H7 infections. N Engl J Med 342:1930-1936, 2000.

Yadin O: Hematuria in children. Pediatr Ann 23:474-485, 1994.

Fluids and Electrolytes: Normal Requirements and Treatment of Dehydration and Electrolyte Disturbances

9

Anthony J. Alario

9.1 Physiologic Principles and Normal Requirements

1. Body water composition
   a. Much of an infant is water. Total body water (TBW) as a percentage of body weight is 75% to 80% of a newborn's birth weight, decreasing to 70% at 6 months and 55% to 60% at 1 year of age and beyond.
   b. Of the TBW, intracellular water plateaus at 40% to 45% of body weight during 1 to 3 years of age and extracellular water declines from 45% in the newborn to 25% by 1 year and 20% in adolescence.
2. Maintenance fluid requirements: The amount of fluid required to replace normal daily losses (from the respiratory system, skin, urinary and gastrointestinal tracts), whether the child is sick or well, determines the maintenance fluid requirement. Fluid losses are derived from the following sources:
   a. *Insensible (imperceptible) water loss:* Losses occur mainly from skin (two thirds) and respiratory (one third) losses.
      (1) Insensible losses are affected by humidity, clothing, body and ambient temperature, and the rate and depth of respiration.
      (2) There is a relationship between the volume of insensible losses (in milliliters) and energy expenditure (in calories), with 1 mL of water being lost for each calorie metabolized; calories expended are, in turn, related to body weight at any particular age.
      (3) Insensible losses through the skin under normal conditions account for about 30 mL/100 cal expended, and 15 mL/100 cal are expended through the pulmonary system. Therefore, a total of 45 mg/100 cal of fluid is expended through insensible loss.
      (4) If body temperature is elevated, insensible loss increases by 10% for each degree centigrade above normal or 7 mg/kg/24 hours for

each degree above 99° F. Note that excessive sweating (sensible water loss) may add another 5 to 20 mL (or more)/100 cal of water loss.

b. *Urinary loss:* The kidneys regulate and fine-tune fluid and electrolyte balance.

(1) Urine volume depends on renal solute load and urine osmolality. The usual endogenous solute load in children is 10 to 15 mOsm/100 cal expended.

(2) However, the amount of water that is obligately required for excretion increases as solute increases. Therefore, in calculations of fluid requirements the usual renal water allowance is 50 to 60 mL/100 cal metabolized.

c. *Stool losses:* Under normal conditions, in the absence of diarrhea, stool water losses are small, about 5 to 10 mL/100 cal expended.

d. A total of 85 to 100 mL of water/100 cal metabolized/day will provide adequate maintenance water replacement. In actuality, water can be *gained* by normal catabolism of carbohydrates and fats ("water of oxidation") to yield about 10 to 12 mL/100 cal metabolized (Table 9-1). Another 3 mL/100 cal can be gained in a state of tissue catabolism that exists during illness. The latter figures need to be considered when calculating fluid requirements only in situations in which *restriction* of maintenance fluid may be necessary (e.g., renal insufficiency or congestive heart failure).

3. Relationship of daily caloric expenditure, water requirement, and body weight

a. The maintenance water requirement is related to caloric expenditure and is based on the patient's weight in a relationship elucidated by Holiday and Segar (Fig. 9-1).

(1) In essence, based on requirements for insensible and urine losses already discussed, for the first 10 kg, 100 cal/kg or 100 mL/kg of water are expended (i.e., required).

Source	mL Water/100 cal/24 hr
Water Expended	
Insensible	45
Skin	30
Lungs	15
Sensible (sweat)	5-20
Urine	30-80
Stool	5-10
Total	85-155
Water Produced	
Water of oxidation (*total*):	10
Water needed to replace expenditures (total):	75-145

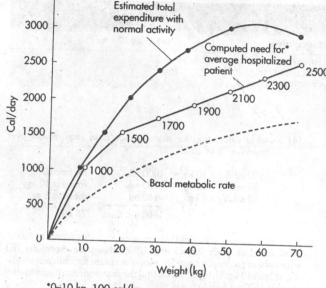

*0–10 kg, 100 cal/kg
10–20 kg, 1000 cal + 50 cal/kg for each kg over 10
20 kg and up, 1500 cal + 20 cal/kg for each kg over 20

Figure 9-1 Comparison of energy expenditure in basal and ideal state. (Redrawn from Segar WE: Parenteral fluid therapy. Curr Probl Pediatr 3[2]:4, 1972.)

    (2) The requirements change as body weight increases, as noted in the diagram. (Note that an inactive, recumbent hospitalized patient has less expenditure.)

    (3) A fasting, intubated, afebrile patient in the intensive care unit with normal renal function can be limited to basal expenditures (basal metabolic rate) alone. In such a patient, insensible loss may be limited to skin loss (30 to 40 mL/100 cal) with no or little loss from the lungs because of humidified air intake.

    (4) Urinary volume (expected to be 1 to 3 mL/hr/100 mL of maintenance fluid) would be replaced at 30 to 50 mL/100 cal, and gastrointestinal losses (e.g., from nasogastric drainage) also need to be replaced.

b. The basic calculation for 24-hour maintenance fluid requirements, based on patient weight, is easily determined as follows:

    (1) 100 mL/kg for *first* 10 kg

    (2) 50 mL/kg for *next* 10 kg

    (3) 20 mL/kg for *each kilogram* above 20

Electrolyte	mEq/kg/24 hr
Sodium	2-3
Potassium	1-2
Chloride	3-5

(4) Example calculation for maintenance fluid requirement over 24 hours for 28-kg child:

$$
\begin{array}{llll}
100 \text{ mL/kg} \times 10 \text{ kg} & = & 1000 \text{ mL} & \text{for first 10 kg} \\
50 \text{ mL/kg} \times 10 \text{ kg} & = & 500 \text{ mL} & \text{for next 10 kg} \\
20 \text{ mL/kg} \times 8 \text{ kg} & = & 160 \text{ mL} & \text{for next 8 kg} \\
\hline
& & 1660 \text{ mL fluid} & 28 \text{ kg}
\end{array}
$$

   c. Note that maintenance fluid requirements can also simply be calculated based on body surface area (BSA chart; see Appendix III) expressed as mL/m²/24 hours. It is most accurate for children weighing at least 10 kg. Using BSA, we find the maintenance fluid requirement is 1500 mL/m²/24 hours.

4. Maintenance electrolyte requirements
   a. In healthy children, the major source of electrolyte loss is the urine.
   b. Maintenance electrolyte requirements (based on urinary losses) are shown in Table 9-2.
   c. Electrolyte losses through skin and lungs under normal conditions are negligible unless excessive sweating occurs, and then considerable sodium and potassium may be lost.
   d. Stool electrolyte losses are minimal in the absence of significant diarrhea.
   e. Vomiting, burns, diuretics, and surgical drainage tubes may contribute to significant electrolyte losses (see later).
   f. In general, providing 2 to 3 mEq of sodium, potassium, and chloride per 100 mL of maintenance water will meet baseline electrolyte requirements.

9.2 Dehydration

PATHOPHYSIOLOGY

Despite their higher proportional water content compared with older children and adults, infants are much more susceptible to dehydration. The high proportional turnover of body fluid—especially extracellular water—predisposes infants to dehydration. The usual cause of dehydration is gastroenteritis with fluid loss from decreased intake or excessive stool output. When the cumulative effect of negative fluid balance exceeds 5% of body weight, symptoms and signs of dehydration may develop.

EVALUATION OF THE DEGREE OF DEHYDRATION

When concern arises over dehydration in an infant or child, a systemic evaluation should be undertaken, paying attention to four key elements of assessment using historical, examination, and laboratory information.

Assessment of Volume Deficit

A quantification should be made of whether a volume deficit exists and, if so, of what magnitude or severity. The severity of dehydration can be assessed in two major ways:

1. Actual weight loss (percentage). Using this formula:

$$\frac{\text{preillness wt} - \text{current wt (i.e., at time of visit)}}{\text{preillness wt}} \times 100 = \text{\% dehydration from weight loss}$$

   a. Comparison of preillness and postillness weights provides an accurate quantification of the percentage weight loss (and, indirectly, water loss and decreased lean body mass from tissue catabolism) due to the current illness. Unfortunately, in the usual clinical setting, a preillness weight that would have clinical utility is usually not available.

   b. Table 9-3 provides an estimate of the severity of dehydration based on the percentage of preillness weight lost through dehydration.

2. Historical and physical examination evidence: The following historical and examination findings provide additional clues with which to estimate the severity of dehydration. Although lacking the precision of comparative weight measurements, the history and physical examination are often the most expedient method.

   a. Historical factors

      (1) Output

         (a) Stools: Number, size, and consistency in previous 24 to 48 hours

         (b) Vomitus: Times and volume

         (c) Urine: Number of voids in previous 24 hours, time of last urination

If Estimated (or Actual) Weight Loss Is:	Dehydration Severity Is:
Infant	
5%	Mild
6%-10%	Moderate
>10%-15%	Severe
Older Child (≥15 kg)	
3%	Mild
4%-6%	Moderate
>7%-9%	Severe

(2) Intake
  (a) History of fluid intake in previous 24 to 48 hours; type of fluids (e.g., milk, skim milk, water, oral rehydrating solutions)
  b. Physical examination (Table 9-4): Assessment of key findings can assist in determining the degree of dehydration. However, many findings may be absent in severely dehydrated children or, conversely, present in children with milder forms of dehydration. The signs and symptoms are often affected by osmolality (see later). "Classic" signs such as sunken eyes, dry mouth, and absence of tears may not be as reliable as observation of decreased peripheral perfusion (e.g., capillary refill) and skin turgor changes.

Assessment of Osmolar Disturbance

1. The serum osmolality (number of osmotically active particles/1000 g water in a solution) is calculated by the following formula:

$$osmolality = 2(Na^+) + \frac{BUN(mg/dL)}{2.8} + \frac{glucose(mg/dL)}{1.8}$$

2. The normal range is 280 to 295 mOsm/L.
3. Except under conditions of extreme hyperglycemia, the body's osmolality (or tonicity) is reflected by the serum sodium concentration. Both intracellular fluid (ICF) and extracellular fluid (ECF) volumes are always in equilibrium regarding osmolality.
   a. The osmolal balance is carefully regulated by the kidney—by both its concentrating function and its response to changes in serum sodium concentration. In addition to the excretion or retention of water by the kidney, thirst, water intake, and iatrogenic sodium loss are important determinants of body fluid osmolality.
   b. Normally, osmolality varies between 280 and 295 mOsm/L; it is maintained within these limits by the precise control over water balance exerted by the kidneys.
   c. The clinical clues in Table 9-5 suggest that an osmolal disturbance may exist before laboratory evidence is available.
4. Although the serum sodium concentration by itself provides no useful information regarding the overall state of fluid balance, it is important to know the sodium concentration to determine whether an osmolar disturbance exists. Most cases of dehydration are associated with an isotonic (i.e., isonatremic) osmolal state. However, based on serum sodium concentration, the type of dehydration can be classified (and qualified) as in Table 9-6.
5. The typical fluid and electrolyte deficits that occur in the three most common types of dehydration are shown in Table 9-7.
6. The management of hypernatremic and hyponatremic dehydration is discussed in Section 9.3.

Assessment of an Acid-Base Disturbance

1. In the most common and pure state of dehydration associated with diarrhea, bicarbonate loss in the stool usually leads to a normal anion gap metabolic acidosis.

	Mild	Moderate	Severe
Urine output	Decreased	Markedly decreased	Anuria
Buccal mucosa	Slightly dry	Dry	Parched
Anterior fontanelle	Normal	Sunken	Markedly sunken
Eyes	Normal	Slightly sunken, dark circles	Markedly sunken
Skin turgor	Normal	Decreased	Tenting
Skin temperature	Normal	Cool	Cool, mottled, acrocyanosis
Pulse	Full, normal rate	Rapid	Rapid, weak/thready
Systolic blood pressure	Normal	Normal, low	Shock

Clinical Finding	Reason	Possible Osmolar Disturbance
Severe weight loss, yet no circulatory instability	Water loss occurs in greater amount than solute; fluid is redistributed between ICF and ECF to preserve the ECF compartment	Hypernatremia
Doughy skin, "tenting" of skin	Subcutaneous tissue hypertonicity alters skin retractability	Hypernatremia
Little or modest weight loss, yet clinical shock, impaired capillary refill (>3 sec)	Disproportionately greater solute loss relative to water occurs; fluid translocates into ICF to maintain osmotic equilibriums; intravascular volume is compromised	Hyponatremia

ECF, extracellular fluid; ICF, intracellular fluid.

	Sodium (mEq/L)	Serum Osmolality (mOsm/L)
Isotonic (isonatremic) dehydration	130-150	280-310
Hypertonic (hypernatremic) dehydration	>150	>310
Hypotonic (hyponatremic) dehydration	<130	<280

2. With severe dehydration, hypoperfusion, and renal underexcretion of acid, an accumulation of acid anions or lactic acid can further complicate the acidosis. Moreover, in infants with chronic pulmonary disease and underventilation, a "mixed metabolic–respiratory acidosis" (metabolic acidosis without appropriate ventilatory compensation) may occur.

3. The type of acid-base disturbance may be assessed by obtaining blood pH (normal, 7.35 to 7.45) and plotting the carbon dioxide tension (PCO_2; normal, 35 to 45 mm Hg) against the serum bicarbonate (normal, 24 to 29 mEq/L) using the diagram of the Henderson-Hasselbalch equation shown in Figure 10-1. The management of acid-base disturbances is discussed in Chapter 10.

Assessment of Potassium Disturbance

Potassium (K^+) is the principal cation of the ICF; its proportion to the ECF is controlled by multiple factors (e.g., body sodium and potassium). In addition, the serum potassium concentration is affected by acid-base balance; as acidemia develops (e.g., diabetic ketoacidosis), serum potassium may remain in the normal range (or increase) as potassium moves out of the ICF into the ECF, but *total body* potassium may be falling. Measurement of serum potassium concentration can thus be misleading, making it difficult to assess total body potassium stores. In states of dehydration, especially with significant losses in diarrheal stool, an estimated deficit of 8 to

		Deficits	
	Water (mL/kg)	Sodium (mEq/kg)	Potassium (mEq/kg)
Isonatremic	100-120	8-10	8-10
Hypernatremic	100-120	2-4	0-4
Hyponatremic	100-120	10-12	8-10

From Robson AM: Parenteral fluid therapy. In Behrman RE, Vaughan VC III, Nelson WE (eds): Textbook of Pediatrics, 13th ed. Philadelphia, WB Saunders, 1987, p 194.

10 mEq/kg or more of potassium can occur in isotonic or hypotonic dehydration, the deficit not being reflected in any abnormality of serum potassium. In hypertonic dehydration the potassium deficit is usually less, as little as 4 to 6 mEq/kg. If serum potassium is elevated in a state of dehydration, suspect acute renal failure (although rarely seen in dehydration), and proceed cautiously with potassium repletion.

1. The causes of *hypokalemia* (real or "measured" potassium deficiency) include
   a. Decreased total body content (associated with hypertension and increased urine potassium)
      (1) Renovascular disease
      (2) Excess renin
      (3) Excess mineralocorticoid
      (4) Cushing's syndrome
   b. Decreased total body content (associated with renal causes, normal blood pressure, and increased urine potassium)
      (1) Renal tubular acidosis (see Chapter 10)
      (2) Fanconi's syndrome (short stature, radial hypoplasia, hyperpigmentation, renal anomalies, pancytopenia)
      (3) Antibiotics
      (4) Diuretics
   c. Decreased total body content (associated with renal causes, normal blood pressure, and decreased urine potassium)
      (1) Skin loss (cystic fibrosis)
      (2) Gastrointestinal losses
      (3) Laxative or enema abuse
      (4) Anorexia nervosa
   d. Normal total body content (associated with increased urine potassium)
      (1) Alkalosis
      (2) Excessive insulin
      (3) Leukemia
2. The causes of *hyperkalemia* (real or "measured") include
   a. Increased total body content (increased urine potassium)
      (1) Cell breakdown
      (2) Transfusion with old, hemolyzed blood
      (3) Spitzer's syndrome
   b. Increased total body content (decreased urine potassium)
      (1) Congenital adrenal hyperplasia
      (2) Renal failure
      (3) Hypoaldosteronism
      (4) Aldosterone insensitivity
      (5) Low insulin
      (6) Potassium-sparing diuretics
   c. Normal total body content
      (1) Leukocytosis
      (2) Thrombocytosis
      (3) Metabolic acidosis (plasma potassium increases by 0.2 to 0.4 mEq/L for each 0.1 U decrease in arterial pH)
      (4) Hemolysis from blood drawing

3. Table 9-8 lists the symptoms and associated electrocardiographic (ECG) changes seen in conditions of hypokalemia and hyperkalemia.
4. Management
   a. Hypokalemia
      (1) If serum potassium is 2.5 mEq/kg or more and symptoms and ECG changes are absent:
         (a) Add 20 to 40 mEq potassium chloride/L to maintenance fluids
         (b) May supplement with 1 to 4 mEq/kg/day intravenous (IV) or oral potassium
      (2) If serum potassium is below 2.5 mEq/kg and symptoms or ECG abnormalities of hypokalemia are present:
         (a) Give potassium chloride 1 to 2 mEq/kg IV, slowly (0.5 to 1.0 mEq/kg/hr), to a maximum 20 mEq/hr
         (b) Follow serum potassium; repeat boluses as needed.
   b. Hyperkalemia: This is the most dangerous electrolyte disorder because it can lead to sudden death. Multiple treatment strategies may be required.
      (1) Alter the cardiotoxic effect of hyperkalemia by temporarily stabilizing cell membrane excitability with calcium infusion: Give calcium gluconate (10%) 0.2 to 0.5 mL/kg (minimum of 10 mL) IV over 2 to 5 minutes. This treatment is effective for up to 1 hour. Repeat if needed. Monitor ECG.
      (2) Decrease potassium in ECF by expanding ECF volume: Give sodium chloride 0.45%, 5% glucose, and 40 mEq/L sodium bicarbonate infused at a rate of 20 mL/kg/hr for 1 to 2 hours.
      (3) Decrease ECF potassium by transferring potassium into cells.
         (a) Give sodium bicarbonate 1 to 3 mEq/kg over 3 to 5 minutes (lasts several hours).

Note: Calcium gluconate solution is not compatible with sodium bicarbonate; flush line between infusions.

         (b) Give glucose 0.5 to 1.0 g/kg with 0.3 U insulin/g glucose over 1 to 2 hours.
         (c) Albuterol IV or by nebulizer has been shown to reduce hyperkalemia also.
      (4) Remove potassium from the body.
         (a) Give furosemide 1 mg/kg/dose IV over 1 to 2 minutes, or 2 to 3 mg/kg/day orally.
         (b) Give Kayexalate (sodium polystyrene resin) 1 to 2 g/kg with 3 mL sorbitol/g resin divided every 6 hours orally or with 5 mL sorbitol/g resin as retention enema over 4 to 6 hours; 1 g/kg of Kayexalate should lower potassium by 1 mEq/L.
         (c) Use peritoneal dialysis or hemodialysis if the preceding measures are unsuccessful.

Assessment of Renal Function

Although renal insufficiency/failure is extremely unusual in states of dehydration, it must be considered whenever there is a history of oliguria. Dehydrated children are often oliguric, failing to void for hours. However, obtaining only several milliliters of urine can be quite helpful in distinguishing prerenal

Serum Potassium (mEq/L)	Symptoms	Electrocardiogram Changes
Hypokalemia		
~2.5	Apathy, weakness, paresthesias	AV conduction defect, prominent U wave, ventricular arrhythmia, ST segment depression
Hyperkalemia		
~7.5	Weakness, paresthesias	T-wave elevation
~8		Loss of P wave, widening of QRS interval
~9	Tetany	ST segment depression, further widening of QRS interval
~10		Bradycardia, sine-wave QRS-T, primary AV block, ventricular arrhythmia, asystole

AV, atrioventricular.
From Feld LG, Kaskel FJ, Schoeneman MJ: The approach to fluid and electrolyte therapy in pediatrics. Adv Pediatr 35:497, 1988.

	Dehydration (Prerenal Azotemia)	Acute Renal Failure
Urine output	Decreased	Decreased
Urine specific gravity	>1.020	1.010-1.012
Urine osmolality (mOsm/kg water)	>500 (>350 newborn)	<350
Urine sodium (mEq/L)	<20	>40
Urine creatinine/ serum creatinine	>40	<20
FE(Na⁺) index*	<1%-2%	>2%-3%
Microscopic examination of sediment	No specific findings	Renal tubular cells (singly or casts)

*The following is the formula for calculating fractional excretion of sodium, FE(Na):

$$FE(Na) = \frac{U_{(Na)} / P_{(Na)}}{U_{(Cr)} / P_{(Cr)}} \times 100$$

$U_{(Na)}$ and $P_{(Na)}$ are the concentrations of sodium in urine and plasma, and $U_{(Cr)}$ and $P_{(Cr)}$ are the concentrations of creatinine in urine and plasma. Note that the blood urea nitrogen is *not* a reliable index of renal function (affected by dietary protein, tissue breakdown, and so forth); serum creatinine, although age dependent, is a better marker.

azotemia (secondary to dehydration) from acute renal failure. Table 9-9 outlines differences between dehydration and acute renal failure.

9.3 Management of Dehydration and Specific Fluid and Electrolyte Disturbances

1. The management of dehydration and electrolyte disturbances is dictated by
   a. The severity of the disturbance
   b. Associated clinical manifestations
   c. The underlying or comorbid conditions
2. In clinically apparent moderate to severe dehydration, obtaining serum electrolytes, glucose, calcium, blood urea nitrogen, creatinine, and a urinalysis are imperative to guide subsequent therapy. The following is a guide (with clinical examples) for fluid and electrolyte management.

EMERGENCY HYDRATING SOLUTIONS: INITIAL HYDRATION

1. Any child who is moderately to severely dehydrated should be weighed immediately and receive a hydrating dose of fluid to expand the intravascular compartment.

2. The most frequently used hydrating dose is 20 mL/kg of 0.9% sodium chloride given over 1 hour or faster by IV push, if needed.

3. Note: If signs of impending shock (decreased blood pressure, capillary refill >3 seconds) are present, continue to give an emergency hydrating solution (10 to 20 mL/kg) until blood pressure and the intravascular fluid compartment are stabilized. Reassess patient every 20 to 30 minutes.

4. Alternatively, 0.45% sodium chloride in 5% dextrose-water (D_5W) at a similar volume and rate has been advocated in the absence of hyperglycemia or shock. These solutions can be given safely to all children while awaiting the electrolyte results, and, in general, the volume given does *not* have to be figured into their other fluid requirements.

MAINTENANCE THERAPY

1. Fluid requirement: The maintenance fluid component, given after initial or emergency hydration, includes both insensible and urine losses. How many calories the patient needs is determined by the degree of his or her activity. This need will fall somewhere between the patient's basal metabolic rate and his or her energy expenditure at normal activity. As noted earlier, for every 100 calories metabolized, the patient requires 100 mL of fluid. The calories metabolized and the milliliters of fluid required are calculated for the typical state of isotonic (i.e., sodium between 130 and 150 mEq/L) dehydration using the guidelines in Table 9-10.

   a. Note that for patients with other forms of dehydration (such as hypertonic dehydration), maintenance and deficit therapies are different (see later).

   b. *Rate of administration* is calculated from the following formula:

$$\frac{\text{total fluid requirements per day}}{24\ \text{hours}} = \text{milliliters per hour intravenously (or nasogastric [NG]/orally)}$$

Body Weight	Fluid Maintenance/24 Hours
0-10 kg	100 mL/kg of weight per 24 hours (i.e., 8-kg infant will need 8 × 100 = 800 mL maintenance)
11-20 kg	100 mL/kg for the first 10 kg, *plus* 50 mL/kg of weight over the first 10 kg, per 24 hours (i.e., 14-kg child needs [10 × 100] + [4 × 50] = 1200 mL maintenance)
>20 kg	100 mL/kg for the first 10 kg, 50 mL/kg for the next 10 kg, *plus* 20 mL/kg of weight over 20 kg, per 24 hours (i.e., 25-kg child needs [10 × 100] + [10 × 50] + [5 × 20] = 1600 mL maintenance)

   c. Note: The final rate of fluid replacement, especially if deficit therapy is taken into consideration, will vary depending on the type of dehydration (see later).

   d. The role of glucose in IV solutions: Needed are 20 to 25 calories per 100 mL of fluids to prevent protein catabolism. This is accomplished by using 5% dextrose solutions (i.e., D_5W = 50 g/L of dextrose) rather than distilled water.

2. Electrolyte requirements

   a. Cations are to be added to the fluid maintenance according to

     (1) The weight of the child (sodium, 2 to 3 mEq/kg/24 hours; potassium 1 to 2 mEq/kg/24 hours) or

     (2) Per 100 mL of maintenance fluids per day (sodium, 3 mEq/100 mL; potassium, 2 mEq/100 mL).

   b. Potassium should always be withheld until the patient's renal function is known to be adequate.

   c. The safest way to administer potassium is to add it to the fluids after the patient voids. With few exceptions, the maximum concentration of potassium in the fluids should *not* exceed 40 mEq/L.

   d. Chloride is the usual accompanying anion with sodium, and therefore replacement/deficit calculations usually are not needed.

     (1) Excessive chloride losses can occur with significant vomiting in gastrointestinal conditions (e.g., pyloric stenosis), cystic fibrosis, or diuretic therapy. A metabolic alkalosis can occur as bicarbonate becomes the obligate anion (instead of chloride) to be reabsorbed with sodium in the kidney. In addition, the resultant secondary hyperaldosteronism leads to distal tubular secretion of hydrogen (and potassium), producing paradoxical aciduria.

     (2) Chloride disturbance is corrected by routine sodium chloride fluid replacement. Under certain conditions (e.g., severe diabetic ketoacidosis), the bicarbonate, acetate, or phosphate anion may be substituted for chloride to provide more buffering capacity.

   e. An example of 24-hour maintenance fluid electrolyte requirements for a 14-kg child may be written this way:

	Water (mL)	Sodium (mEq)	Potassium (mEq)
Maintenance	1200	36	24
Composition per liter	1000	30	20

     (1) Therefore, one would use a 0.2% sodium chloride (i.e., approximately 34 mEq/L sodium) solution in 5% dextrose, with 20 mEq potassium chloride per liter added after the patient has voided. The rate of administration is 50 mL/hr (i.e., 1200 mL ÷ 24 hours).

DEFICIT THERAPY

Once initial hydrating fluids have been given and maintenance requirements are calculated, the third component of fluid therapy is providing for deficit replacement. In this situation, it is important to know (1) the severity of dehydration, and (2) the serum osmolality (tonicity) as reflected by the sodium. The deficit requirements are then added to the calculated maintenance requirements. The following three sections illustrate deficit therapy (with case examples) using the serum sodium as a marker for the type of dehydration.

Isotonic Dehydration (Serum Sodium between 130 and 150 mEq/L)

1. The amount of fluid (water) to be given is determined based on the percentage of dehydration, calculated as follows:

If the child is:	The deficit fluid to be replaced is:
5% dehydrated	50 mL × wt (kg)
10% dehydrated	100 mL × wt (kg)
15% dehydrated	150 mL × wt (kg)

   a. Deficits are added in *addition* to calculated maintenance fluid requirement (as discussed earlier).
2. Electrolyte deficits may also be calculated based on the percentage of dehydration:

	Amount to be replaced of:	
% Dehydration	Sodium (mEq/kg/24 hr)	Potassium (mEq/kg/24 hr)
5	3-4	2-3
10	6-8	4-6
15	10-12	8-10

   a. Example: A 6-kg infant with 5% dehydration would require:

	Water (mL)	Sodium (mEq)	Potassium (mEq)
Maintenance	600	18	12
Deficit	300	24	18
Total fluids	900	42	30
Composition per liter	1000	46	33

   (1) Therefore, the child will get 0.33% sodium chloride (one-third saline has approximately 56 mEq/L sodium) in 5% dextrose (0.3 NS-D$_5$W); 33 mEq/L of potassium chloride should be added to 1000 mL after the patient has voided. The fluid correction can be accomplished by providing one half of the calculated fluid requirements over the first 8 hours and the other half over the next 16 hours (rate: first 8 hours, 56 mL/hr; next 16 hours, 30 mL/hr).

Hypertonic Dehydration/Hypernatremia (Serum Sodium over 150 mEq/L)

If shock is present (a late finding), treat as outlined earlier. In the absence of shock, the most important goal in treating hypertonic dehydration is not to drop the sodium too rapidly (i.e., no more than a 10- to 15-mEq/L drop in serum sodium in 24 hours). *Too rapid a correction can produce intracellular fluid overload, leading to cerebral and pulmonary edema.* Therefore, correction must take place over at least 48 to 72 hours instead of 24 hours. These children clinically appear less dehydrated than they really are; thus, it can be assumed that all have at least 8% to 10% dehydration.

1. Causes of hypernatremia (independent of hydration status) include
   a. Decreased free-water intake: Secondary to illness or iatrogenic causes (e.g., error in formula preparation with not enough free water added—a very common cause)
   b. Gastrointestinal losses of free water in excess of sodium: very common
   c. Skin losses
   d. Diuretic use
   e. Nephropathy
   f. Diabetes insipidus
   g. Excess sodium administered to dehydrated patients
   h. Mineralocorticoid excess
2. Correction of hypernatremia and hypertonic dehydration
   a. Deficit fluids can be calculated based on free water deficit or as in isotonic dehydration:
      (1) The *free-water deficit* can be calculated as follows: Free-water deficit = 4 mL/kg for every mEq that serum sodium exceeds 145 mEq/L *or*

      $$\text{Free-water deficit} = \frac{0.6(\text{wt in kg})(\text{sodium serum} - 140)}{140}$$

      (a) Example: Free-water deficit in a 12-kg child with serum sodium 165 =

      $$\frac{0.6 \times 12 \text{ kg} \times (165 - 140)}{140} = 1.3 \text{ L}$$

      (b) This patient should receive 1.3 L of free water to correct the hypernatremia. Note that water *cannot* be given without sodium chloride and glucose.
      (2) In actuality, calculating the fluid deficit based on 10% dehydration may quantitatively take into account the free-water deficit (see the example later for a 12-kg child).
   b. The typical solution used to treat hypernatremia would include a sodium concentration between 30 and 50 mEq/L: Either 0.2 or 0.33 sodium chloride, both in D_5W. There is no optimal solution, but the greater the tonicity of the solution, the longer the duration of correction (e.g., over 48 to 72 hours).
   c. Postacidotic tetany is a common complication of hypernatremia; therefore, obtain a serum calcium level. Tetany is prevented by adding 10 mL of 10% calcium gluconate to every 500 mL of solution used in treating hypertonic dehydration. Note that calcium cannot be added to any bicarbonate-containing solution.
   d. Obtain a blood glucose level because hyperglycemia may be seen in almost 50% of patients with hypernatremia. It is not usually necessary to correct the hyperglycemia rapidly because glucose provides buffering capacity, and, as a metabolic substance, it is a source of free water.
   e. It is extremely important to note that patients with hypertonic dehydration have excess antidiuretic hormone secretion and are

extremely oliguric. Therefore, maintenance fluid replacement should *not* be the same as isotonic dehydration. Maintenance replacement may be calculated at one half of what would be given for isotonic dehydration (see the following example).

f. Example: A 12-kg child with 10% dehydration (but no cardiovascular instability) and a serum sodium level of 165 mEq/L:

	Water (mL)	Sodium (mEq)	Potassium (mEq)
Maintenance (for 48 hr)	2200	72	48
Deficit (to be replaced in first 24 hr)	600	18	12
Deficit (replace in next 24 hr)	600	18	12
Total fluids for 48 hr	3400	108	72
Composition per liter	1000	32	21

(1) Note: Two days of maintenance fluids are added to the deficit, and the total is to be given over 48 hours. The deficit is corrected evenly over 48 hours to avoid central nervous system dysfunction. This child would get 0.2% sodium chloride (34 mEq/L Na) in D_5W with 20 mEq of potassium chloride per liter added after voiding. To correct the deficit slowly, run IV at 60 mL/hr for the first 12 hours, 70 mL/hr for the next 12 hours, and 80 mL/hr for the next 24 hours (see caveats, next). Add calcium as cited earlier. Follow electrolytes closely.

(2) Caveats on therapy for hypernatremic dehydration

(a) If serum bicarbonate is less than 12 mEq/L, add bicarbonate (see calculations later) until corrected—remember that bicarbonate and calcium do not mix in IV solution.

(b) Replace deficit slowly—try not to exceed 50 to 60 mL/kg/12 to 24 hours.

(c) Urine output will be low even in patients being rehydrated because of increased antidiuretic hormone secretion in hypernatremia.

(d) Giving a solution too high in sodium may lead to sodium overload and a natriuresis (increased urine output secondary to increase sodium).

(e) A serum sodium of 180 mEq/L or more may require peritoneal dialysis to correct the disturbance.

Hypotonic Dehydration/Hyponatremia (Serum Sodium below 130 mEq/L)

1. Causes of hyponatremia (independent of hydration status) include

a. Gastrointestinal losses of sodium (diarrhea is the most common cause), accompanied by low-solute fluid replacement (i.e., colas, fruit juice)

b. Third spacing

c. Skin losses

d. Nephrotic syndrome

e. Congestive heart failure

f. Syndrome of inappropriate antidiuretic hormone secretion (SIADH)
   (1) Causes a to e are associated with a decreased urine sodium level and a decreased urine volume.
   (2) SIADH can be associated with increased or decreased urine sodium and lowered urine volume.
   (3) Causes a to c are associated with weight loss.
   (4) Causes d to f are associated with weight gain (i.e., circulating volume is increased or normal; therefore, treatment is water restriction).
g. Factitious—that is, sodium is "falsely" decreased due to
   (1) Hyperlipidemia: Sodium "decreased" by 0.002 × lipid (mg/dL)
   (2) Hyperproteinemia: Sodium "decreased" by 0.25 × (protein [g/dL] − 8)
   (3) Hyperglycemia: Sodium "decreased" by 1.6 mEq/L for every 100-mg/dL rise in glucose
h. Renal losses (increased urine sodium, increased urine volume, decreased weight): Diuretics, adrenal insufficiency, hyperglycemia

2. Maintenance and deficit fluid and electrolyte needs in hyponatremia
   a. These patients are primarily losing fluid from intravascular (and ECF) compartments and are symptomatic early in course. Dehydration severity and fluid needs are calculated according to the isotonic dehydration guidelines described earlier. Because of excessive loss, sodium must be added to the maintenance and deficit fluids. The extra sodium required (i.e., sodium deficit) is calculated using the following formula:

$$(\text{Desired sodium} - \text{actual sodium}) \times 0.6 \times (\text{wt in kg})$$
$$= \text{extra sodium (mEq) needed}$$

   b. Note: If the patient's symptoms are alarming (i.e., change in consciousness, seizures), the sodium deficit can be replaced (in total or in part) in the first 1 to 2 hours using a hypertonic saline solution (3% sodium chloride)
   c. After calculation of the sodium needed from the preceding formula, the volume of 3% sodium chloride to give is calculated as follows:

$$\text{Vol in mL of 3\% sodium chloride} = \frac{\text{mEq sodium need}}{0.153 \text{ mEq sodium/mL}}$$

   (1) There is 0.513 mEq sodium per milliliter of 3% sodium chloride.
   d. If the patient is asymptomatic, correction can be made more gradually over 8 to 12 hours.
   e. Example: A 6-kg infant is 10% dehydrated and has a serum sodium level of 120 mEq/L, but is *not* symptomatic:

	Water (mL)	Sodium (mEq)	Potassium (mEq)
Maintenance	600	18	12
Deficit	600	48	36
Sodium deficit	—	54*	—
Total	1200	120	48

*(135 − 120) × 0.6 × 6 = 54 mEq

f. Patients with hyponatremia may be acidotic, so part of the sodium deficit may be corrected using sodium bicarbonate. Therefore, this child could receive 0.45% sodium chloride (approximately 77 mEq/L) in D$_5$W with 20 mEq sodium bicarbonate/L. Add 40 mEq of potassium chloride per liter after the patient voids. At a rate of administration of 60 mL/hr, in 24 hours almost all of the deficit will be corrected.

Correction of Metabolic Acidosis

See Chapter 10. When the metabolic acidosis is severe (serum bicarbonate 8 mEq/L or less), sodium bicarbonate can be given following either formula:

1. 2.5 mEq/L of sodium bicarbonate × (wt in kg) over half an hour will raise the serum bicarbonate by 5 mEq/L.
2. (Desired bicarbonate [i.e., 15 to 20 mEq/L] − actual bicarbonate) × 0.5 × (wt in kg) = mEq sodium bicarbonate to be given over 30 minutes.

CAVEATS TO ALL FLUID THERAPIES

1. All deficit calculations are based on the child's condition at the time fluid therapy is begun. Abnormal ongoing losses must be recognized and replaced accordingly.
2. Fluid orders for hospitalized patients must be written for exact 24-hour periods; otherwise, they become meaningless.
3. Do not hyperhydrate patients by overestimating their fluid deficits. The human body has many mechanisms to compensate for hypohydration, but very few for hyperhydration.
4. Always add potassium to the IV fluids if the patient is going to receive fluid for more than 24 hours.
5. Do not correct mild or moderate acidosis with sodium bicarbonate unless it is really necessary. Fluids, a bit of salt, and time will correct the problem, assuming normal renal function.
6. Remember that when you prescribe sodium bicarbonate, for every milliequivalent of bicarbonate that you give, the patient also receives 1 mEq of sodium.
7. In newborns and small infants, the most common cause of unexplained hyperkalemia is not Addison's disease but hemolysis of the blood sample.
8. Never give 5% glucose as the only IV solution.
9. Any infant with significant diarrhea who does not appear dehydrated but has a serum sodium above 150 mEq/L has *moderate* dehydration (the so-called "inapparent dehydration" of the hypernatremic state).
10. The most important end points in fluid therapy are clinical improvement, daily progress, and weight gain.
11. If possible, the rate of hydration is better accomplished slowly rather than too quickly. Table 9-11 shows the rate of deficit repletion over a 48-hour period. Percentages reflect the cumulative proportion of the total deficit that should be repleted by the designated time period.
12. Note that with certain clinical conditions, fluid losses can be substantially different than fluid losses from routine diarrheal illness, and replacement therapy needs to reflect those losses. Table 9-12 provides

Table 9-11 **Deficit Repletion over Time as a Cumulative Percentage**			
	0-12 Hours	**12-24 Hours**	**24-48 Hours**
Isonatremic	50%	100%*	
Hypernatremic	25%	50%	100%
Hyponatremic	75%	100%	

*By 24 hours the total deficit in isonatremic dehydration can be replaced.
Adapted from Kallen RJ: The management of diarrheal dehydration in infants using parenteral fluids. Pediatr Clin North Am 37:265-286, 1990.

guidelines for fluid composition based on the type of fluid lost. Note that the composition of the fluid for replacement is not necessarily identical to the actual fluid lost.

9.4 Oral Rehydration Therapy

1. Indications for use
   a. In the United States, in contrast to many other areas of the world, oral rehydration therapy (ORT) has not been used to its full potential. This is especially true for the early treatment of infants with mild to moderate dehydration who can maintain good oral intake.
   b. It would not be indicated for infants in shock or coma, or with severe dehydration, severe electrolyte/acid-base disturbances, intractable vomiting, or gastric distention. However, once these conditions are stabilized and neurologic and hemodynamic equilibrium returns to baseline, ORT can be safely instituted.
   c. ORT can be undertaken at home or in the office, emergency department, or hospital ward.
2. Techniques of administration
   a. ORT may be given by bottle, cup, spoon, syringe, or even by nasogastric tube with continuous infusion.
   b. The goal is to give small amounts frequently (e.g., 5 to 10 mL fluid every 5 to 10 minutes) to avoid vomiting secondary to ileus and abdominal distention.
   c. Increase the rate by 1 teaspoon (5 mL) every minute, as tolerated.
3. Replacement oral electrolyte solutions (OES)
   a. Similar to IV fluid rehydration, there are two basic goals of ORT:
      (1) Rehydration and deficit replacement
      (2) Maintenance therapy
   b. There are two types of OES:
      (1) *Rehydration/deficit replacement* OES has a higher sodium level (75 to 90 mEq/L), primarily to replace excessive sodium and chloride loss in severe diarrheal infections (e.g., cholera).
      (2) *Maintenance solution* has less sodium (45 to 60 mEq/L), which is more appropriate for the types of diarrheal conditions seen in developed countries. The types and composition of OES are shown in Table 9-13. The important formulation is having at least 45 to 50 mEq/L sodium *and* 2 to 3 g/dL of glucose in solution

9—Fluids and Electrolytes

Table 9-12 Composition of Replacement Fluid

Type of Fluid Loss	Sodium (mEq/L)	Potassium (mEq/L)	Chloride (mEq/L)	Bicarbonate (mEq/L)
Cystic fibrosis (sweat)	100-130	20-30	75-100	20-25
Gastric suctioning	75-100	30-40	100-140	0
Small intestinal drainage	100-140	20-30	75-110	20-40
Diarrheal	40-60	30-40	40-60	30-40

Table 9-13 Types and Composition of Oral Electrolyte Solutions

	Sodium (mEq/L)	Potassium (mEq/L)	Chloride (mEq/L)	Base (mEq/L)	Glucose (g/dL)
Rehydration Solutions					
Rehydralyte	75	20	65	30	2.5
World Health Organization formulation	90	20	80	30	2.0
Maintenance Solutions					
Pedialyte	45	20	35	30	2.5
Lytren	50	25	45	30	2.0
Resol	50	20	50	34	2.0

9—Fluids and Electrolytes

Table 9-14 **Composition of Clear Liquid Beverages**

Fluid	Sodium (mmol/L)	Potassium (mmol/L)	Carbohydrate (g/100 mL)	Osmolality (mmol/L)
Beef broths	110-248	2.5-17		300-390
Chicken broths	140-251	1.5-8.2		380-500
Apple juice	0.1-3.5	24-32	12	650-734
Grape juice	0.8-2.8	31-44	15	1170-1190
Colas	1.3-1.7	0.1	10.4-11.3	390-750
Ginger ale	0.8-5.5	0.1-1.5	5.3	520-560
7-Up	5.5-5.5	1.0-2.0	7.4	520-550
Kool-Aid	0.5-1.2	0.1-1.8	10.6	250-590
Popsicles	4.7-5.6	0.5-2.0	NA*	670-720
Jell-O	22-27	1.3-2.0	15.8	570-640
Tea (unsweetened)	0	5	0	
Gatorade	20	3	4.6	330

*Not available.
From Costeel HB, Fiedorek SC: Oral rehydration therapy. Pediatr Clin North Am 37:295-311, 1990.

to promote appropriate water, glucose, and electrolyte absorption from the intestines.

4. Rehydration/deficit replacement
    a. *For mild dehydration:* Replace at a rate of 50 to 60 mL/kg over 2 hours; use either rehydration or maintenance OES (see later).
    b. *For moderate dehydration:* Replace at a rate of 70 to 80 mL/kg over 2 hours. If there are significant stool losses, use at least 10 mL/kg of rehydration OES for each diarrheal stool seen in office/emergency department, or 20 to 50 mL/kg/day additional.
    c. Add deficit and maintenance fluids to be replaced over 8 to 12 hours.
    d. Continue breast-feeding during deficit replacement.
    e. Correct mild, asymptomatic hypernatremic dehydration (i.e., if sodium is 145 to 155 mEq/L) slowly over 12 to 24 hours.
    f. Provide ongoing monitoring of weight, urine output, stool losses, vomiting, and so forth.
        (1) If still clinically dehydrated, recalculate deficit, ongoing losses, and maintenance, and correct over 6 to 8 hours.
        (2) If rehydrated, proceed to maintenance phase.

5. Maintenance
    a. Use an OES with sodium of 40 to 60 mEq/L for this phase.
    b. Provide OES ad libitum (at least 100 mL/kg/day) for 24 hours. Continue breast-feeding, but monitor OES intake.
    c. Advance formula-fed infants after 24 hours of OES to one-half strength lactose-containing or lactose-free formula for next 12 to 24 hours; you may alternate with OES (at least 100 to 150 mL/kg/day total)
    d. Advance to full-strength formula in next 12 to 24 hours.
    e. Introduction of solid foods can occur after 24 to 48 hours of therapy. Avoid high-fat and high-carbohydrate food (fruit juices, ice cream, puddings high in sugar).
    f. Monitor for large stool volumes (can be seen as a consequence of OES). If carbohydrate malabsorption is present (evidenced by 0.5% or more on Clinitest/Test Tape) in more than two stools, ORT may need to be discontinued.
    g. An examination of the composition of clear liquid beverages (shown in Table 9-14) demonstrates that these solutions, although commonly used, may be inappropriate to treat acute dehydration in infants because, compared with OES, their concentration of sodium is either excessive (broths) or insufficient (sodas, Jell-O, Gatorade, tea); carbohydrate concentration is high (colas, juices); or potassium is low (colas).

SUGGESTED READING

Arnold WC, Kallen RJ (eds): Fluid and electrolyte therapy. Pediatr Clin North Am 37(2), 1990.

Acid-Base Disturbances

10

Fred F. Ferri and Anthony J. Alario

10.1 Basic Principles

1. The extracellular fluid pH in normal children is narrowly regulated between 7.38 and 7.45 pH units (Table 10-1 shows normal pH values). Regulating mechanisms include:
   a. Blood buffers (phosphate, bicarbonate)
   b. Changes in alveolar ventilation
   c. Renal regulation (recovery of filtered HCO_3 and acid excretion)
2. The identification of the type of disturbance is of great practical importance when deciding on a course of therapy.
   a. When the pH is altered by a single primary event (e.g., child with diarrhea losing excess HCO_3 in stool), then the disorder is characterized as a *simple* acid-base disorder.
   b. When a combination of simple disorders occurs (e.g., a child with cystic fibrosis is treated with diuretics), a *mixed* acid-base disorder can ensue (as in the case of the child with cystic fibrosis, mixed respiratory acidosis and metabolic alkalosis).
      (1) If the mixed disorders cause a pH deviation in the *same* direction, then the disorder can lead to a life-threatening acid-base disturbance (e.g., the child who develops secondary respiratory failure and acidosis from ingestion of ethylene glycol, a primary metabolic acidosis).
      (2) In addition, patients may develop an *acute* disturbance in face of a *chronic* one, as in the patient with cystic fibrosis.
3. The suffix *-osis* does not correspond to blood acidity but is used only to refer to the primary process generating OH^- or H^+.
   a. Acidosis: Process that generates H^+
   b. Alkalosis: Process that generates OH^-
4. The suffix *-emia* refers to blood acidity.
   a. Acidemia: pH <7.36
   b. Alkalemia: pH >7.44

Table 10-1 Age-dependent Normal Blood Values for pH

Blood Sample	pH	$Paco_2$ (mm Hg)	HCO_3 (mEq/L)	Total CO_2 (mEq/L)
Arterial: age <1 yr	7.33-7.40	35-45	23-27	20-24
Arterial: age >1 yr	7.38-7.45	35-45	23-27	24-28
Venous	7.35-7.40	45-50	24-29	25-30

10.2 Diagnosis and Approach to the Patient With Acid-Base Disturbances

DIAGNOSIS

An acid-base disturbance should be readily suspected given a history of predisposing risk factors (e.g., diabetes, ingestions, pernicious vomiting). Clinical features that would suggest an acid-base disturbance include the following:

1. History of pernicious vomiting (e.g., pyloric stenosis) or excessive diarrhea (e.g., more than 10 to 15 stools/day)
2. Cyanosis, ashen-gray appearance, mottling (acidosis)
3. Unusual breath odors (e.g., "fruity" smell from acetone, ethylene glycol ingestion)
4. Breathing pattern—rate, depth, rhythm (hyperpnea with salicylate ingestion, Kussmaul respirations with diabetic ketoacidosis)
5. Orthostatic changes in blood pressure (shock from acidosis)
6. Decreased capillary refill, poor peripheral perfusion, cold extremities (shock)
7. Grunting and flaring of alar nasi (respiratory acidosis in primary lung disease or metabolic acidosis from dehydration, shock)
8. Symptoms of acute anxiety, lightheadedness, tetany (acute respiratory alkalosis from psychogenic hyperventilation)

IDENTIFICATION OF AN ACID-BASE DISTURBANCE

Identifying the type of acid-base disturbance can be facilitated by the following steps:

1. Draw arterial blood gas (ABG) and electrolyte samples concomitantly; evaluate the following:
   a. Plasma HCO_3
      (1) Increased in metabolic alkalosis or respiratory acidosis (compensated)
      (2) Decreased in metabolic acidosis or respiratory alkalosis (compensated)
   b. Serum K^+ (ΔpH 0.1 units = ΔK^+ 0.6 mEq/L)
      (1) Increased in acidemia
      (2) Decreased in alkalemia
   c. Serum Cl^-: Compare with plasma sodium concentration; they should be proportionately increased or decreased if the change in Cl^- concentration is the result of a change in the hydration of the patient.
      (1) If the Cl^- is disproportionately increased, think of metabolic acidosis or respiratory alkalosis.
      (2) If the Cl^- is disproportionately decreased, think of metabolic alkalosis or respiratory acidosis.
2. Calculate the anion gap (AG):

$$AG = Na^+ - (Cl^- + HCO_3)$$

$$\text{Normal} = 9 \text{ to } 14 \text{ mEq/L}$$

   a. The anion gap represents unmeasured anions in the plasma (negative charges on plasma proteins and negative charges contributed by organic and inorganic anions normally present in the plasma but not routinely measured).

b. The normal reference range for the serum anion gap is 9 to 14 mEq/L. Some have proposed including the K^+ in the calculation (normal range then becomes 12 to 18 mEq/L). Others have proposed a downward shift of 3 to 11 mEq/L for normal range due primarily to an upward shift in laboratory measurements of serum chloride values.

c. The anion gap is used to divide the causes of metabolic acidosis into two main categories:

(1) Normal anion gap acidosis (hyperchloremic acidosis)

(2) Elevated anion gap acidosis (normochloremic acidosis)

d. An elevated anion gap is the result of the presence of acid ions (e.g., lactic acid) in the extracellular fluid.

e. The causes of an increased or decreased anion gap are shown in Box 10-1.

3. Evaluate ABGs to determine the type of disturbance present by examining pH, $PaCO_2$, and HCO_3.

a. Table 10-2 relates specific acid-base disorders to the primary physiologic abnormality, secondary (compensatory) responses, and the changes in body chemistry.

Box 10-1   Causes of Increased or Decreased Anion Gap

Increased Anion Gap

Decreased unmeasured cation: hypokalemia, hypocalcemia, hypomagnesemia

Increased unmeasured anion

  Organic anions, lactate, ketoacids

  Inorganic anions; phosphate, sulfate

  Proteins: hyperalbuminemia

  Exogenous anions: salicylate, nitrates, penicillins

  Incompletely identified anions: ethylene glycol, methanol and salicylate poisoning, uremia, hyperosmolar hyperglycemic non-ketotic coma

Decreased Anion Gap

Increased unmeasured cation

Increased normally present cation: hypermagnesemia

Decreased unmeasured anion: hypoalbuminemia

Laboratory error

  Systemic error: hyponatremia due to viscous serum, hyperchloremia in bromide intoxication

  Random error: falsely decreased serum sodium, falsely increased serum chloride or bicarbonate

---

Modified from Johnson KB: The Harriet Lane Handbook, 14th ed. St. Louis, Mosby, 1996.

Table 10-2	Primary Abnormality and Compensatory Responses in Simple Acid-Base Disorders				
Disorder	**Primary Abnormality**	**Secondary Response**	**pH**	**Paco$_2$**	**HCO$_3$**
Metabolic acidosis	Gain of H$^+$ or loss of HCO$_3$	↑ Ventilation (and chemical buffering)	→	→	→
Respiratory acidosis	Hypoventilation	HCO$_3$ generation	→	←	←
Metabolic alkalosis	Gain of HCO$_3$, or loss of H$^+$	↓ Ventilation (and chemical buffering)	←	←	←
Respiratory alkalosis	Hyperventilation	HCO$_3$ consumption	←	→	→

Adapted from Bia M, Thier S: Mixed acid base disturbances: A clinical approach. Med Clin North Am 65:347-361, 1981.

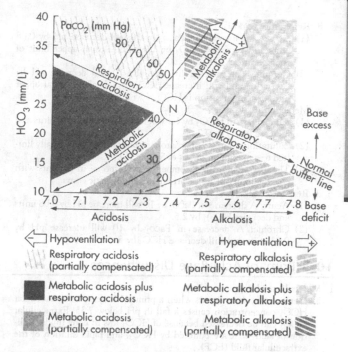

Figure 10-1 Graphic representation of the Henderson-Hasselbalch equation of acid-base relationships. (From Rosen P [chief ed]: Emergency Medicine: Concepts and Clinical Practice, 6th ed. St. Louis, Mosby, 2006.)

   b. Figure 10-1 is a graphic representation of the classic Henderson-Hasselbalch equation of acid-base relationships. This acid-base nomogram is constructed from arterial pH, $PaCO_2$, and HCO_3. The normal values are labeled N. This table is helpful in identifying specific acid-base disturbances, which can be determined by plotting the pH, $PaCO_2$, and HCO_3.
4. Calculate whether the degree of physiologic compensation is adequate. If the degree of compensation is inadequate, consider the simultaneous presence of two or more primary abnormalities (i.e., mixed acid-base disturbance—see later).
   a. Metabolic acidosis
      (1) If adequate compensation, $PaCO_2 = (1.5 \times HCO_3) + 8.4$; usually $PaCO_2$ = last two digits of the pH
      (2) If actual $PaCO_2$ greater than calculated, then metabolic acidosis and respiratory acidosis are present
      (3) If actual $PaCO_2$ less than calculated, then metabolic acidosis and respiratory alkalosis are present

b. Respiratory acidosis
  (1) Acute: An increase in $PaCO_2$ by 10 will decrease pH by 0.08 units and increase HCO_3 by 1.0 mEq/L; usual upper limit of compensation is $HCO_3 = 30$ mEq/L.
  (2) Chronic: An increase in $PaCO_2$ by 10 will decrease pH by 0.03 units and will increase HCO_3 by 3.5 mEq/L; usual upper limit of compensation is $HCO_3 = 55$ mEq/L.
c. Metabolic alkalosis
  (1) An increase in HCO_3 by 1.0 will increase pH by 0.015 units and increase $PaCO_2$ by 0.7.
  (2) Limitations: The compensatory response ($PaCO_2$) is usually limited to a maximum $PaCO_2$ of 55 mm Hg.
  (3) There is an impaired compensatory response in patients with chronic lung disease, heart failure, and hepatic coma.
d. Respiratory alkalosis
  (1) Acute: A decrease in $PaCO_2$ by 10 will increase pH by 0.08 units and decrease HCO_3 by 2.5.
  (2) Chronic: A decrease in $PaCO_2$ by 10 will increase pH by 0.03 units and will decrease HCO_3 by 5.

10.3 Primary Acid-Base Disturbances

1. Metabolic acidosis
   a. Metabolic acidosis occurs when a primary decrease in extracellular HCO_3 concentration causes a fall in pH below 7.35. Extracellular HCO_3 can be decreased because of HCO_3 loss in body fluids, addition of acids that are buffered by HCO_3, and rapid dilution of the extracellular fluid (ECF).
   b. Metabolic acidosis with increased anion gap (normochloremic acidosis)
      (1) Lactic acidosis (most common cause of acidosis in ill children); secondary to tissue hypoxia (shock, hypovolemia, dehydration, respiratory failure [asphyxia], severe congestive heart failure, sepsis, inborn errors of carbohydrate or pyruvate metabolism)
      (2) Ketoacidosis (diabetes mellitus, ethanol intoxication, starvation, inborn errors of amino acid or organic acid metabolism)
      (3) Uremia (chronic renal failure)
      (4) Ingestion of toxins (paraldehyde, methanol, salicylate, ethylene glycol)
   c. Metabolic acidosis with normal anion gap (hyperchloremic acidosis; Box 10-2)
      (1) Intestinal loss of bicarbonate (diarrhea—most common cause of normal anion gap acidosis; pancreatic fistula)
      (2) Renal tubular acidosis (RTA)
         (a) RTA-associated hyperchloremic metabolic acidosis occurs secondary to excess renal tubular loss of bicarbonate, or a failure to excrete dietary acid, or both.
         (b) There are multiple causes of RTA: Idiopathic (inherited) or secondary to renal disease (obstructive nephropathy, nephrocalcinosis), systemic diseases (diabetes, syndromes, systemic

> ### Box 10-2   Urinary Anion Gap and Urinary pH in Hyperchloremic Metabolic Acidosis
>
> The measurement of the urinary anion gap ($U_{Na} + U_K - U_{Cl}$) and urinary pH is useful in the differential diagnosis of hyperchloremic metabolic acidosis:
>
> 1. Negative urinary anion gap suggests gastrointestinal loss of bicarbonate.
> 2. Positive urinary anion gap suggests altered distal urinary acidification.
> 3. Low urinary pH and elevated plasma K^+ in patients with positive urinary anion gap suggest selective aldosterone deficiency.
> 4. Urinary pH greater than 5.5 and elevated plasma K^+ suggest hyperkalemic distal renal tubular acidosis.
> 5. Urinary pH greater than 5.5 and normal or decreased plasma K^+ indicate classic renal tubular acidosis.

       lupus erythematosus), or medications (amphotericin, lithium, aminoglycosides).

       (c) See Table 10-3 for characteristics of the three major types.

    (3) Ureteral diversion with bowel (ureterosigmoidostomy)

    (4) Exogenous Cl -containing compounds ($CaCl_2$, $MgCl_2$)

    (5) Carbonic anhydrase inhibitors (acetazolamide)

    (6) Dilutional (rapid expansion of ECF with bicarbonate-free isotonic saline)

    (7) Mineralocorticoid deficiency

2. Respiratory acidosis

  a. A primary increase in $Paco_2$ (usually secondary to alveolar hypoventilation) will create a respiratory acidosis with a blood gas pH under 7.35.

  b. Associated causes

    (1) Pulmonary disease (severe pneumonia, pulmonary edema, interstitial fibrosis)

    (2) Acute airway obstruction (foreign body, aspiration, severe bronchospasm, croup, epiglottitis)

    (3) Thoracic cage disorders (pneumothorax, flail chest, kyphoscoliosis)

    (4) Defects in muscles of respiration (myasthenia gravis, hypokalemia, muscular dystrophy)

    (5) Defects in peripheral nervous system (poliomyelitis, Guillain-Barré syndrome, botulism, tetanus, organophosphate poisoning, spinal cord injury)

    (6) Depression of respiratory center (anesthesia, narcotics, sedatives, vertebral artery embolism or thrombosis, increased intracranial pressure)

    (7) Chronic lung disease: Cystic fibrosis, bronchopulmonary dysplasia

    (8) Failure of mechanical ventilator

Table 10-3 Renal Tubular Acidosis Characteristics

	Type		
	1 (Distal)	2 (Proximal)	3 (Hyperkalemic)
Failure to thrive	Yes	Yes	Yes
Polyuria/polydipsia	Yes	Yes	No
Renal function	WNL	WNL	WNL or ↓
HCO_3 loss	Often	Significant	Less
Urine maximally acidic	No (pH >6)	Yes	Yes
Nephrocalcinosis/nephrolithiasis	Yes	No	No

WNL, within normal limits.

3. Metabolic alkalosis
   a. A primary increase in ECF concentration of HCO_3 sufficient to raise pH above 7.45 will create a metabolic alkalosis. Conditions that result in loss of H^+, gain of HCO_3, or loss of ECF Cl^- in excess of HCO_3 all contribute to the alkalosis. In addition, to maintain the alkalosis, factors that prevent the kidneys from excreting HCO_3 must also be present, as outlined in Box 10-3.
   b. Metabolic alkalosis can be divided into *chloride-responsive* (urinary chloride concentration <15 mEq/L) and *chloride-unresponsive* forms (urinary chloride >15 mEq/L).
      (1) Chloride-responsive
         (a) Vomiting
         (b) Nasogastric suction
         (c) Diuretics
         (d) Posthypercapnic alkalosis
         (e) Stool losses (laxative abuse, cystic fibrosis, villous adenoma)
         (f) Massive blood transfusion
         (g) Exogenous alkali administration
      (2) Chloride-unresponsive
         (a) Hyperadrenocorticoid states (Cushing's syndrome, primary hyperaldosteronism, secondary mineralocorticoidism [licorice, chewing tobacco])

Box 10-3   Etiology of Metabolic Alkalosis

Contributors to Metabolic Alkalosis

1. Loss of H^+
   a. Gastrointestinal (vomiting, nasogastric aspiration, congential Cl^--wasting diarrhea, laxative abuse)
   b. Renal
      Diuretics (thiazides, furosemide, ethacrynic acid)
      Excess mineralocorticoid
         Endogenous (hyperaldosteronism, Cushing's disease, adrenogenital syndrome)
         Exogenous (steroid therapy, licorice, chewing tobacco)
         Bartter's syndrome
         Cl^--deficient infant formula
      Posthypercapnia
2. Gain of HCO_3: Exogenous alkali (HCO_3, citrate, acetate, lactate)
3. Contraction of extracellular volume: Cystic fibrosis (infants)

Maintenance of Metabolic Alkalosis

1. Renal failure
2. Extracellular volume depletion
3. Increased mineralocorticoid
4. Potassium depletion
5. Cl^- depletion

      (b) Hypokalemia
      (c) Bartter's syndrome

4. Respiratory alkalosis
  a. Respiratory alkalosis results from a primary decrease in $Paco_2$ sufficient to increase blood gas pH above 7.45.
  b. This is probably the most common primary acid-base disturbance in childhood, resulting from hyperventilation from a variety of causes:
    (1) Fever
    (2) Sepsis
    (3) Hypoxemia (pneumonia, pulmonary embolism, atelectasis, high-altitude living)
    (4) Drugs (salicylates, xanthines, progesterone, epinephrine, thyroxine)
    (5) Central nervous system disorders (tumor, cerebrovascular accident, trauma, infections)
    (6) Psychogenic hyperventilation (anxiety, hysteria)
    (7) Hepatic encephalopathy
    (8) Sudden recovery from metabolic acidosis
    (9) Mechanical ventilation

10.4 Common Causes of Mixed Disturbances

A *mixed* acid-base disturbance arises when two or more primary disorders occur simultaneously. One disorder is usually metabolic acidosis. Common associations include the following:

1. Mixed anion gap acidosis
  a. Ketoacidosis and lactic acidosis
  b. Methanol or ethylene glycol intoxication and lactic acidosis
  c. Uremic acidosis and ketoacidosis
  d. Sepsis (late; lactic and respiratory acidosis)
2. Mixed anion gap and hyperchloremic acidosis
  a. Diarrhea and lactic acidosis or ketoacidosis
  b. Progressive renal failure
  c. Type IV RTA and diabetic ketoacidosis
  d. Diabetic ketoacidosis during treatment
3. Mixed hyperchloremic acidosis
  a. Diarrhea and RTA
  b. Diarrhea and hyperalimentation
  c. Diarrhea and acetazolamide or mafenide
4. Anion gap acidosis or hyperchloremic acidosis and metabolic alkalosis
  a. Ketoacidosis and protracted vomiting or nasogastric suction
  b. Chronic renal failure and vomiting or nasogastric suction
  c. Diarrhea and vomiting or nasogastric suction
  d. RTA and vomiting
  e. Lactic or ketoacidosis plus $NaHCO_3$ therapy
5. Anion gap acidosis or hyperchloremic acidosis and respiratory alkalosis
  a. Salicylate poisoning
  b. Hepatic disease
  c. Sepsis (early)
  d. Pulmonary edema

6. Anion gap acidosis or hyperchloremic acidosis and respiratory acidosis
   a. Cardiopulmonary arrest
   b. Pulmonary edema
   c. Respiratory failure in chronic lung disease
   d. Phosphate depletion
   e. Drug overdose and poisoning

10.5 Management

In general, once an acid-base disturbance is detected, treatment is directed primarily toward ameliorating the underlying cause of the acid-base disorder (e.g., restoration of ECF volume, correction of K^+ or Cl^- deficiency, removal of toxic substance, and improvement in alveolar ventilation). Prompt and appropriate treatment of the underlying cause in most instances, given normal respiratory and renal compensation, will lead to eventual correction of the acid-base disturbance. Note that secondary respiratory compensation for a metabolic disorder begins within minutes and within 12 to 24 hours is complete, whereas secondary metabolic compensation for a respiratory disorder occurs slowly, beginning within hours and taking 2 to 5 days for completion. The management of specific simple acid-base disorders follows.

1. Metabolic acidosis
   a. Correct underlying cause (e.g., diabetic ketoacidosis, diarrhea, uremia).
   b. Give $NaHCO_3$ therapy for cases of life-threatening metabolic acidosis. However, routine use for simple disorders that respond to correcting the underlying condition has become controversial.
   c. When the metabolic acidosis is severe (pH <7.2, HCO_3 ≤8 mEq/L), the amount of $NaHCO_3$ to be given can be calculated following either formula given in Box 10-4.
   d. Overaggressive $NaHCO_3$ therapy can lead to "overshoot alkalosis"; therefore, aim for a pH of 7.25 and correct the bicarbonate blood level to approximately 15 mEq/L. In non–life-threatening situations, only half the bicarbonate deficit should be corrected over a 12-hour period.
   e. Hypernatremia and fluid overload after $NaHCO_3$ therapy is of concern, particularly in patients with renal failure or congestive heart failure.

Box 10-4   Amount of $NaHCO_3$ To Be Given in Severe Metabolic Acidosis

1. 2.5 mEq/L of $NaHCO_3$ × (wt in kg) over half an hour will raise the serum bicarbonate by 5 mEq/L.
2. (Desired bicarbonate [i.e., 15 mEq/L] – actual bicarbonate) × 0.5 × (wt in kg) = mEq $NaHCO_3$ to be given over 30 minutes or longer.

   f. Patients on beta blockers do not have the protective effects on the circulatory system that endogenous catecholamines provide in acidosis. Therefore, begin $NaHCO_3$ therapy at a higher pH (7.25 to 7.30, rather than 7.20).

   g. Patients who are already hypernatremic (hyperosmolar) and acidotic may not tolerate $NaHCO_3$ therapy. Hemodialysis or peritoneal dialysis with HCO_3 in the dialysate should be considered.

   h. Before $NaHCO_3$ is given, the patient's K^+ should be determined (i.e., in acidosis, K^+ moves from the intracellular fluid compartment to the ECF). If K^+ in blood is low or low normal, the patient is total-body K^+ depleted. As K^+ moves back into cells with $NaHCO_3$ therapy, and the total-body K^+ pool is *not* replenished, life-threatening respiratory muscle paralysis can occur from severe hypokalemia.

   i. Rapid correction of metabolic acidosis can lead to a respiratory alkalosis (i.e., the cerebrospinal fluid pH change lags behind that of the ECF, and the respiratory drive continues to be accelerated *despite* a normalizing pH). Conversely, if impending respiratory failure is superimposed on metabolic acidosis, $NaHCO_3$ therapy may lead to central nervous system–mediated hypoventilation and a mixed acidosis.

2. Respiratory acidosis

   a. The goal of management in this situation is to compensate for alveolar hypoventilation with mechanical ventilatory support to lower a rising $Paco_2$.

   b. Renal compensatory mechanisms (acid excretion as NH_4^+ and tubular reabsorption of HCO_3) will also help if there is normal renal function.

3. Metabolic alkalosis

   a. Correct underlying cause (e.g., surgery for pyloric obstruction).

   b. Further therapy will vary with the underlying cause:

     (1) Chloride-responsive forms are treated with saline administration and correction of accompanying hypokalemia.

     (2) Chloride-resistant forms require correction of underlying cause and associated potassium depletion.

   c. Severe metabolic alkalosis (pH >7.55) rarely requires treatment with an exogenous acidifying solution such as dilute HCl, NH_4Cl, or arginine HCl. The administration of these agents is problematic: dilute HCl at 150 mEq/L must be delivered slowly into a large (i.e., central) vein to avoid hemolysis. NH_4Cl cannot be given to patients with hepatic failure (i.e., it raises blood ammonia); arginine HCl has been associated with severe hyperkalemia. Hemodialysis or peritoneal dialysis high in Cl^- and low in HCO_3 may be the best therapeutic option.

4. Respiratory alkalosis

   a. Therapy of respiratory alkalosis is aimed at its underlying cause.

   b. Symptomatic patients with psychogenic hyperventilation often require some form of rebreathing apparatus (e.g., paper bag, breathing 5% CO_2 by mask); rarely is sedation needed.

   c. Patients should be educated on avoiding triggers of anxiety and using techniques of relaxation to avoid recurrences.

SUGGESTED READING

Batlle DC, Hizon M, Cohen E, et al: The use of urinary anion gap in the diagnosis of hyperchloremic metabolic acidosis. N Engl J Med 318:594-599, 1988.

Bia M, Thier S: Mixed acid base disturbances: A clinical approach. Med Clin North Am 65:347-361, 1981.

Brewer ED: Disorders of acid-base balance. Pediatr Clin North Am 37:429-447, 1990.

Chattha G, Arieff AI, Cummings C, Tierney LM Jr: Lactic acidosis complicating the acquired immunodeficiency syndrome. Ann Intern Med 118:37-39, 1993.

Dubose TD Jr: Clinical approach to patients with acid-base disorders. Med Clin North Am 67:799-813, 1983.

Salem MM, Mujais SK: Gaps in the anion gap. Arch Intern Med 152:1625-1629, 1992.

Orthopedic Conditions

Craig P. Eberson, Christopher DiGiovanni,
Manuel F. DaSilva, and Michael G. Ehrlich

11.1 Orthopedic Problems Present in Infants and Toddlers

DEVELOPMENTAL DISLOCATION OF THE HIP

1. Epidemiology: Two percent of infants will have one or more *postural* deformities (e.g., developmental dislocation of the hip [DDH], facial deformities, scoliosis, metatarsus adductus).
2. Pathogenesis: Lax ligaments or immature capsule leads to acetabular dysplasia, which in turn leads to a dislocatable/subluxable hip.
3. Clinical features. DDH more likely:
   a. If other postural deformities are present (or neuromuscular disorders) in infancy
   b. With first pregnancies
   c. In female infants (susceptibility to maternal estrogen leads to ligamentous laxity)
   d. With previous positive family history for DDH
   e. With breech presentation
   f. With prolonged gestation and increased body weight
   g. With amniotic fluid abnormalities
4. Diagnosis
   a. Screening examination: Ortolani and Barlow maneuver (most useful in first month; Fig. 11-1)
      (1) The examiner adducts the hip, then pushes down to try to dislocate it (Barlow), and then, lifting with the fingers behind the trochanter while keeping some gentle pressure on the limb, abducts the hip (Ortolani). A dislocatable hip responds with a "clunk."
      (2) After the first month, findings are limited to abduction, shortening, and asymmetric gluteal folds. By 6 months, ligaments are too tight to make the examination useful.
   b. Other clues in older infants
      (1) Incomplete or asymmetric abduction of the hip appears on the involved side.

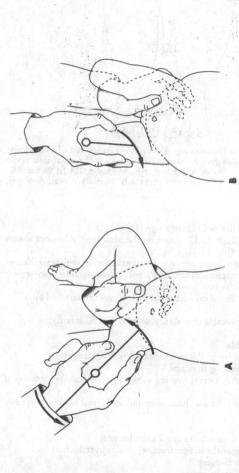

Figure 11-1 **A,** Ortolani maneuver. Hold opposite pelvis steady with one hand while the limb to be examined is grasped with the other. Flex hip and knee. Gently pulling the femur forward, abduct the limb using the greater trochanter as a fulcrum. A palpable or audible "click" manifested by a sudden shift in position of the proximal femur signifies reduction of dislocation. **B,** Barlow test. This provocation test for dislocatability uses the same initial positioning as for the Ortolani maneuver. Place your thumb over the lesser trochanter and the tip of your middle finger over the greater trochanter. With the thumb over the lesser trochanter and the hip and knee in flexion, exert gentle pressure. A sudden shift of the proximal femur, often with a "clunk," suggests dislocatability. Reverse any dislocation with the Ortolani maneuver. (Adapted from Scoles PV: Pediatric Orthopedics in Clinical Practice, 2nd ed. Chicago, Year Book, 1988.)

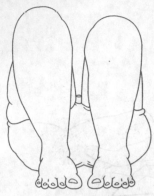

Figure 11-2 Allis' or Galeazzi's sign. Knee is lower on affected side when knees and hips are flexed because the femoral head lies posterior to the acetabulum in this position. (Redrawn after Shelov MD, Mezey AP, Edelmann CM Jr, Barnett HL: Primary Care Pediatrics: A Symptomatic Approach. Norwalk, Conn, Appleton-Century-Crofts, 1984.)

      (2) Positive Allis' or Galeazzi's sign (Fig. 11-2).
      (3) An extra thigh fold is noted on the abnormal side—*not* always diagnostic (Fig. 11-3).
      (4) A leg length discrepancy can be appreciated in unilateral disease.
      (5) Routine anteroposterior (AP) pelvic radiographs can appear normal in the first 3 months of life.
   c. Classification. Based on examination, hip can be classified as:
      (1) Normal
      (2) Lax or subluxable (instability; seen in 1 of 60 infants)
      (3) Clicking
      (4) Dislocatable
      (5) Dislocated (reducible/irreducible; 1 of 1000 infants)
5. Laboratory and imaging findings:
   a. Radiographs: AP, lateral frog-leg view of pelvis (can be negative if hip relocates)
   b. Ultrasonography: Stress ultrasonography is the test of choice in newborns/infants.
6. Management
   a. Younger than 6 months in age: Pavlik harness
   b. Older than 6 months in age: traction to obtain reduction
   c. Older patients: Surgery
      (1) Open reduction *and/or*
      (2) Pelvic osteotomy to remodel acetabulum

CLUB FOOT (TALIPES EQUINOVARUS)

1. Introduction: This diagnosis is made at the time of birth. The foot faces inward with severe metatarsus adductus; the heel is in the equinus and varus position and the foot is twisted inward (Fig. 11-4).

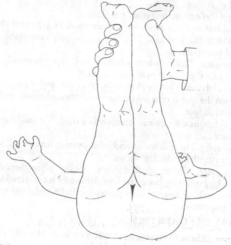

Figure 11-3 Asymmetry of gluteal fold. (Redrawn after Shelov MD, Mezey AP, Edelmann CM Jr, Barnett HL: Primary Care Pediatrics: A Symptomatic Approach. Norwalk, Conn, Appleton-Century-Crofts, 1984.)

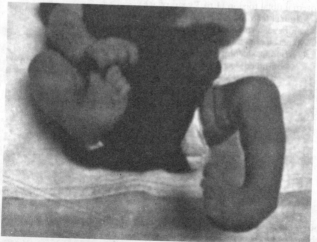

Figure 11-4 Infant with bilateral club feet.

2. Positional club foot
   a. Etiology: Reflects intrauterine positioning
   b. Clinical features: In a newborn examination, fold the child back into the intrauterine position. The foot is passively correctable without forceful manipulation.
   c. Management: This problem usually corrects spontaneously within a few weeks, otherwise it may need casting.
3. Neurologic club foot: This condition corrects easily with casting but recurs rapidly when the cast is removed if there is continued muscle imbalance.
4. Anatomic club foot
   a. Clinical features: Examination reveals a rigid, not easily correctable deformity.
   b. Radiographs: The calcaneus and talus overlap on the AP view, and they are parallel on lateral views.
   c. Management: Either casting with weekly adjustments/recasting followed by splinting once the foot deformity is corrected (may take 2 to 3 years); or surgery with posteromedial and lateral releases for recalcitrant cases

TORSIONAL DEFORMITIES

There are three common "toeing in" conditions in childhood.
1. Metatarsus adductus (in-toeing; Fig. 11-5)
   a. Etiology: Likely caused by intrauterine positioning
   b. Clinical features: When the bottom of the forefoot is pressed, instead of the heel lining up with the second metatarsal, the forefoot faces in with a curved or "bean" shape (the curve is in the midfoot; the heel cord is flexible).
   c. Management: Stretching exercises and out-flare shoes (if corrected easily by stretching). If rigid, treatment is casting by an orthopedist.
2. Internal tibial torsion (1 to 3 years of age)
   a. Clinical features: When the child's patella points forward, the tibia can be seen to be rotated and the position of the foot is inward.
   b. Management
      (1) Supine sleeping position to allow gravity to rotate foot outward; continued sleeping on the back to avoid recurrence of symptoms

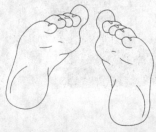

Figure 11-5 Metatarsus adductus. (Redrawn after Shelov MD, Mezey AP, Edelmann CM Jr, Barnett HL: Primary Care Pediatrics: A Symptomatic Approach. Norwalk, Conn, Appleton-Century-Crofts, 1984.)

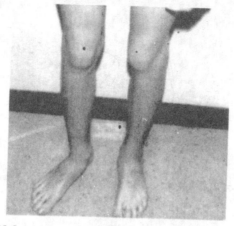

Figure 11-6 Child demonstrating increased femoral anteversion—kneecaps facing one another.

    (2) Denis Browne splint or Fillauer bar attached to shoes with 30- to 45-degree outward rotation during sleep for about 4 months

3. Internal femoral torsion (3 to 6 years of age; Fig. 11-6)
   a. Clinical features: The amount of internal rotation of the hip is much greater than the amount of external rotation (normally the other way around).
   b. Management
     (1) Normally expected to resolve spontaneously by about 10 years of age, as the femur becomes less anteverted
     (2) Night bar to hold feet in external rotation
     (3) Knee immobilizer to transmit force up to the hip
     (4) Supine position when sleeping

"TURNING OUT"

This condition is often called *external rotation contracture of infancy* (when caused by intrauterine positioning).

1. Clinical features: Most commonly occurs from the hips. In this case, when rotation of the hip is tested, the hip will turn out about 90 degrees but does not turn in at all past midline.
2. Management: The condition is self-correcting when the child starts walking. (Be sure to check for hip dislocation in infants and slipped capital femoral epiphysis [SCFE] in adolescents.)

BOWING OR GENU VARUS

1. Clinical features (Fig. 11-7)
   a. Normal in children 18 months to 2 years of age

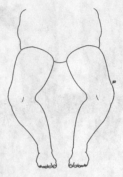

Figure 11-7 Genu varus.

b. Severe bowing accompanied by internal tibial torsion can be associated with
   (1) Blount's disease (growth disturbance of medial portion of proximal tibial physis), especially if the patient is an early walker or overweight
   (2) Phosphate diabetes (inherited)
   (3) Renal tubular acidosis
   (4) Renal failure
2. Diagnosis
   a. Serum phosphate: Low levels for vitamin D resistance or dietary rickets; high in renal failure
   b. Radiographs: Rule out metabolic disease or Blount's disease (metaphyseal beaking and sloped epiphysis).
3. Management
   a. No treatment is required for young children with physiologic bowing.
   b. For young children with severe physiologic bowing or early Blount's disease: Night bar with feet turned out 45 degrees
   c. For older children: Formal single, upright bowleg brace
   d. For older children with bowing deformity: Osteotomy or asymmetric stapling of physis. Teenagers with Blount's may require leg lengthening.
   e. If phosphate diabetes exists, replace phosphate, including doses at night, and usually add vitamin D supplements.

KNOCK KNEES OR GENU VALGUM

1. Clinical features: Family history is often positive. Usually seen after 2 years of age, severity may peak at 3 years, and normalize by 5 years of age (see Chapter 2).
2. Management
   a. Older child: Nighttime knock-knee brace
   b. Arch supports: Scaphoid pads with a UCB heel to hold the foot in slight varus, thus shifting weight-bearing line

c. The teenager or child with severe deformity may require osteotomy of leg or thigh, or asymmetric stapling of physis.

11.2 Upper Extremity Orthopedic Conditions

CLAVICLE FRACTURE

1. Clinical features: Pain and deformity (an elevation or step-off has a "ping-pong" feel in infants, in which there is a sudden release when depressing the clavicle)
2. Management
   a. Evaluate for neurovascular injury.
   b. Wear figure-of-eight splint for 3 to 4 weeks.
   c. Return to sports at 6 weeks.
   d. Usually heals with permanent lump—tell parents beforehand!
   e. Surgery is indicated for nonunion or open fracture.

NURSEMAID'S ELBOW OR TRAUMATIC SUBLUXATION OF THE RADIAL HEAD

1. Etiology and pathophysiology
   a. Generally occurs in younger children with underdeveloped annular ligaments
   b. The child is lifted by the hand, "yanked," cries, and stops using arm.
2. Clinical features: The arm is held in flexion, pronated, and close to the chest (radiographs are negative and not needed).
3. Management: Supinate the forearm while gently pulling into extension. The child should reuse the arm within 15 to 20 minutes (if not moving, the arm may go into a cast in supination for a few weeks).

BRACHIAL PLEXUS PALSY

1. Etiology and pathophysiology: This palsy usually occurs with large infants (the mothers frequently have diabetes).
2. Clinical features
   a. Klumpke's or lower brachial plexus palsy: Hand function is involved and prognosis is poor. A particularly bad prognostic sign is Horner's syndrome, which suggests root avulsion.
   b. Erb's palsy or upper brachial plexus palsy: The upper plexus is affected, with shoulder and elbow weakness; treated with passive range-of-motion exercises, it has a better prognosis, with most patients making at least a partial recovery. Avoid abduction splints, which lead to contractures.

11.3 Lower Extremity Orthopedic Conditions

HIP (ALL PRESENT WITH A LIMP)

1. Legg-Calvé-Perthes disease (avascular necrosis of femoral head; 4 to 8 years of age)

a. Clinical features
   (1) Painless limp or hip pain
   (2) Loss of abduction and internal rotation
   (3) Referred hip pain may lead to mild ache in groin or knee.
b. Diagnosis
   (1) Bone scan or magnetic resonance image (MRI) will show early changes, before radiographic changes.
   (2) Radiographs: AP and frog-leg lateral (Fig. 11-8)
       (a) Early: Radiographs may show only widening of the teardrop head distance or subchondral crack on the frog-leg lateral projection.
       (b) Later: A phase of bony sclerosis is followed by the disappearance of all or part of femoral head.
       (c) Ultimately: Reconstitution occurs.
c. Management
   (1) Traction or exercises to regain motion
   (2) Surgery to improve containment and remodeling of hip

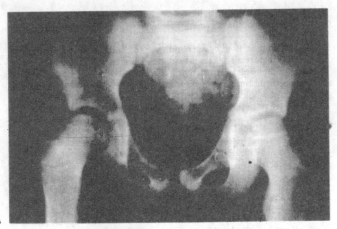

A

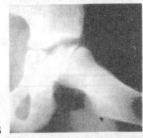

B

Figure 11-8 Radiographs showing widening teardrop head distance (A) and subchondral crack (B).

2. Toxic synovitis
   a. Clinical features
      (1) Refusal to walk—usually, no walking in the morning, but running by midday
      (2) Occasional groin or thigh pain
      (3) Limited abduction and internal rotation
      (4) Slight fever (<102° F) with mild rise (≤30) in erythrocyte sedimentation rate (ESR)
   b. Diagnosis
      (1) Blood tests are usually normal.
      (2) Symptoms may occasionally persist over several weeks.
      (3) Be sure to distinguish between toxic synovitis and septic hip (which has very limited range of motion). For example, with a septic hip:
         (a) The hip is held rigidly flexed and externally rotated.
         (b) Radiographs may show widening of the joint space.
         (c) Ultrasonography can demonstrate the presence of a large effusion.
         (d) Loss of motion will worsen (hip motion will improve with toxic synovitis).
      (4) Hip aspiration should be performed to rule out joint sepsis if any concern exists, with debridement to follow if positive (e.g., pus aspirated from the joint). The physician should have a very low threshold for performing this procedure (i.e., low risk, high yield).
      (5) Symptoms may last several weeks with gradual improvement. If symptoms of toxic synovitis remain for more than a month, suspect Legg-Calvé-Perthes disease.
   c. Management
      (1) Reassurance and bed rest for a few days
      (2) Nonsteroidal anti-inflammatory drugs (NSAIDs) occasionally useful
3. Slipped Capital Femoral Epiphysis (10 to 16 years of age; Fig. 11-9): SCFE (pronounced 'skiffee').
   a. Clinical features
      (1) Walking: The foot on the involved side is externally rotated while walking. There usually is a limp or even an inability to bear weight.
      (2) Examination: Limited abduction and internal rotation; external rotation on flexion of hip
      (3) Pain: Low-grade ache in groin or thigh or knee
      (4) Body habitus: Children tend to be obese/large; if seen in a thin child or one younger than 10 or older than 16 years of age, consider endocrinopathy (i.e., hypothyroidism) or renal failure.
   b. Diagnosis: Obtain AP and frog-leg lateral radiographs of pelvis (the condition is often misdiagnosed as a groin pull).
   c. Management
      (1) The patient should be taken immediately to the hospital or an orthopedist to prevent acute slip.
      (2) Minor slips can be pinned by a surgeon, with a single pin; more severe ones may require an osteotomy.

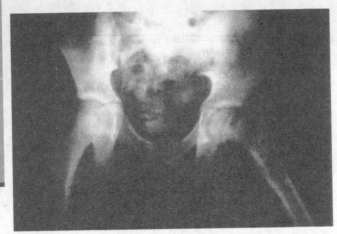

Figure 11-9 Radiograph of slipped epiphysis.

(3) Acute slips with severe complications can occur after minor injury in a patient preweakened by a chronic slip.

KNEE INJURY

Figure 11-10 shows the decision tree for diagnosis of subacute knee injury.
1. Diagnosis
   a. History of injury: Acute versus chronic or gradual onset
   b. Pain or instability (giving way); often associated with a limp in severe cases
   c. Palpate tender areas: Joint effusion means there is an intra-articular injury, such as patellar dislocation, ligament rupture (usually anterior cruciate ligament [ACL]), osteochondral fracture, or meniscal tear.
   d. Test ligaments for resistance to stress: Excessive movement/laxity suggests rupture or tear.
   e. Obtain radiographs as indicated by the degree of injury on examination (knee pain is often referred from the hip, so rule out primary hip process).
2. Osgood-Schlatter disease
   a. Introduction: Osgood-Schlatter disease represents the most common location of apophysitis (inflammation of growth plates) in children (other types of apophysitis and their respective growth plate involvement are listed in Table 11-1).
   b. Clinical features
      (1) Pain arises in the tibial tubercle, usually after exercise or while kneeling on it.
      (2) May present with a warm, tender lump over the anterior tibial tuberosity.

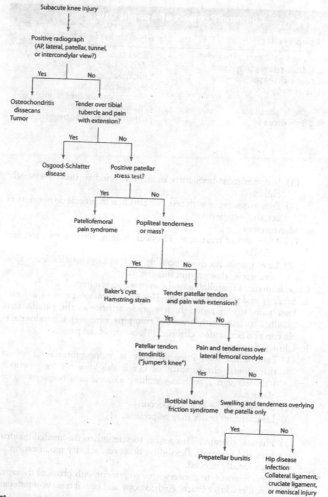

Figure 11-10 Decision tree for diagnosis of subacute knee injury. (From Gunn V, Nechyba C [eds]: The Harriet Lane Handbook, 16th ed. Philadelphia, Mosby, 2002.)

Table 11-1 **Common Regions of Apophysitis**	
Apophysitis	**Growth Plate Involved**
Osgood-Schlatter disease	Tibial tubercle
Sindig-Larsen-Johansson disease	Inferior pole of patella
Sever's disease	Calcaneal apophysis
Little-leaguer's elbow	Medial epicondyle (occasionally olecranon)
Pitcher's shoulder	Proximal humerus
Iselin's disease	Fifth metatarsal tuberosity

  (3) It occurs most frequently in athletic children (also overweight children).

  (4) Pain may subside with rest, but children in general do not restrict activity sufficiently.

 c. Management

  (1) Mainstays of treatment: Physical therapy, relative rest, ice, and NSAIDs

  (2) Late complications are possible, such as loose ossicles or avulsion of tubercle, that require surgery.

3. Chondromalacia (patellofemoral compression syndrome)

 a. Etiology and pathophysiology: The most common cause of anterior knee pain, it may represent low-grade arthritis of the patella. It is usually associated with "overuse" (jumping, running). Chondromalacia can also occur after chronic dislocation of the patella.

 b. Clinical features

  (1) Pain under the kneecap that is more pronounced when the patient climbs stairs or bends the knee for long periods ("theater sign"), such as watching a movie or sitting in a car or classroom.

  (2) Buckling of the knee can occur.

  (3) Ligamentous laxity may be present.

 c. Management

  (1) Physical therapy: The goal is to strengthen the medial quadriceps and maintain flexibility; however, activity modification is occasionally needed.

  (2) If no response to conservative treatment with physical therapy, consider a knee brace. Arthroscopy and lateral release of patellar ligament is required in some cases.

4. Meniscal tear

 a. Etiology and pathophysiology: History of twisting injury

 b. Clinical features: Knee effusion, unable fully to flex knee, tenderness over the joint line, clicking or pain with *McMurray's test*

 c. Diagnosis: MRI is helpful only if the diagnosis is in doubt. Meniscal vascularity in children often is mistaken for a tear on MRI.

 d. Management: Treat with rest, physical therapy, or surgery for recalcitrant cases.

5. ACL tear
   a. Etiology and pathophysiology: May be caused by valgus-force directed blow or by twisting injury
   b. Clinical features
      (1) History of hearing "pop"
      (2) Knee rapidly fills with blood, leading to large effusion
      (3) Instability detected with anterior drawer or Lachman test (look for excessive anterior motion of the tibia on the femur)
      (4) Associated injury to the medial collateral ligament or medial meniscus (O'Donohugh's triad) may be present.
   c. Management: Initial treatment is physical therapy, but surgery is an option for persistent symptoms, preferably in skeletally mature patients.
6. Osteochondritis desiccans (see Fig. 11-14)
   a. Etiology and pathophysiology: Subchondral fracture of joint surface, ranging from a small crack with an intact joint surface to a detached fragment
   b. Clinical features
      (1) History of pain and swelling with activity
      (2) Most commonly seen in lateral part of medial femoral condyle
      (3) Imaging
         (a) Radiographs should include a "tunnel view," which shows sclerosis or focal fragmentation. This may be a normal variant, so films of the opposite knee are helpful for comparison.
         (b) MRI can be helpful to confirm the diagnosis and guide treatment.
   c. Management: Skeletally immature patients often heal with rest, immobilization, or casting; mature patients often require surgery.
7. Patellar dislocation
   a. Etiology and pathophysiology: May be due to direct blow or twisting injury
   b. Clinical features
      (1) The patella is seen as a "lump" laterally.
      (2) Very painful: The examination reveals tenderness over medial patellar retinaculum, effusion, and apprehension when the patella is pushed gently laterally.
   c. Diagnosis: Radiographs and occasionally MRI are helpful to rule out associated fracture.
   d. Management: Reduction by slow extension of flexed knee and then treat with rest, braces, rehabilitation; surgery if acute fracture present or if recurrent dislocation occurs

FOOT AND ANKLE INJURIES

1. Ankle sprain
   a. Skeletally immature patients: Usually a Salter-Harris type I fracture of the distal fibula. Radiographs show only soft tissue swelling, and treatment is 3 weeks in a weight-bearing cast.
   b. Skeletally mature patients: Usually injure lateral ankle ligaments, particularly anterior talofibular and calcaneofibular. Treatment is primarily physical therapy.

2. Sever's disease (calcaneal apophysitis)
   a. Etiology and pathophysiology: Insertion of tendon into growth plate causes pain with overuse because of inflammation of the growth plate. Probably represents a low-grade stress fracture (8 to 12 years of age).
   b. Clinical features: Pain in heel, generally after activity (e.g., soccer), that lasts for a few days before it goes away
   c. Management: Stretching exercises and NSAIDs or heel lift are helpful; if resistant, then 6 weeks in a walking cast. Note that the child will outgrow the condition, but pain can be intermittent for several years, although there are no serious complications

DIFFERENTIATION OF COMMON GAIT ABNORMALITIES

Figure 11-11 outlines the common gait abnormalities.

11.4 Spinal Deformities

SCOLIOSIS

1. Introduction: *Scoliosis* is defined as a spinal curve in the coronal plane, usually with associated rotation of vertebral bodies.
2. Etiology and pathophysiology
   a. Idiopathic (most common diagnosis): Familial with girls, usually in teen or preteen years
   b. Congenital malformation: In infants (especially heart disease), early surgery required to prevent progression
   c. Other: Scoliosis can also be seen secondary to neurofibromatosis, radiation of the spine, chest surgery, and neurologic problems (e.g., cerebral palsy, epidural lipoma, spinal cord tethering, nerve and bone tumors, polio, and leg length discrepancies).
3. Clinical features: Signs of scoliosis include apparent elevation of the pelvis on one side (pelvic tilt) or prominence of a scapula or shoulder blade. The hump becomes more noticeable when the child bends forward (forward bending test; Fig. 11-12). A scoliometer may be helpful in screening as well.
4. Diagnosis
   a. Radiography: Evaluate the severity of the curve.
      (1) Obtain standing AP radiographs of the thoracolumbar spine.
      (2) If there is a leg length discrepancy, get a sitting AP spine radiograph.
      (3) Calculate the Cobb angle (Fig. 11-13): Draw lines parallel to the two most angled vertebrae and drop a perpendicular line from each. The angle at which these two perpendicular lines intersect is the Cobb angle.
5. Management
   a. Curves less than 20 degrees do not require treatment, only careful follow-up (a curve of 10 degrees occurs in 2% to 3% of the population).
   b. Patients with curves greater than 20 or 30 degrees may require night, or day and night, bracing.
   c. Progressive curves greater than 45 or 50 degrees may require surgery.

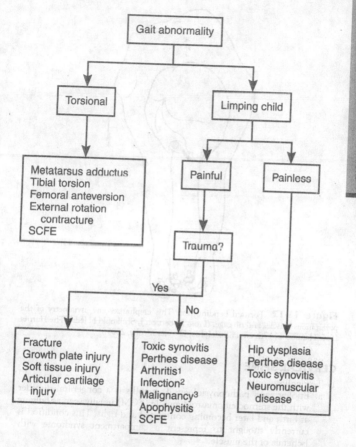

¹Arthritis includes: JRA, Lyme arthritis, reactive arthritis, other (SLE, ARF, spondyloarthritis)
²Infection includes: septic arthritis, osteomyelitis, diskitis, bursitis
³Malignancy includes: bone tumors, leukemia (severe bone pain out of proportion to exam findings)

Figure 11-11 Differentiation of common gait abnormalities. ARF, acute rheumatic fever; JRA, juvenile rheumatoid arthritis; SCFE, slipped capital femoral epiphysis; SLE, systemic lupus erythematosus.

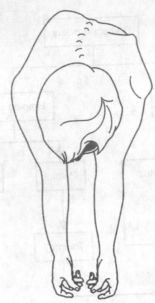

Figure 11-12 Forward bending test. This emphasizes any asymmetry of the paraspinous muscles and rib cage. (From Robertson J, Shilkofski N [eds]: The Harriet Lane Handbook, 17th ed. Philadelphia, Elsevier Mosby, 2005.)

CERVICAL SPINE

1. Torticollis
   a. Etiology and pathophysiology: Torticollis is a congenital disorder with the sternocleidomastoid muscle (SCM) usually seen as bulging at birth and later becoming contracted and tight. This condition is currently thought to represent a compartment syndrome with ischemia of the muscle.
   b. Clinical features
      (1) The neck is tipped to one side and usually rotated (e.g., if the right SCM is involved, the right ear tilts to the right shoulder, but the chin faces to the left).
      (2) Movement may or may not be painful.
      (3) Radiographs are often difficult to obtain if the deformity is marked.
   c. Management
      (1) Infants: Passive stretching, and positioning so the child faces the opposite way. For example, for a tight right SCM, tip the left ear to the left shoulder, and rotate the head to the right. Also position in the crib so the child has to turn to the right.
      (2) Older children: Surgical releases are required.

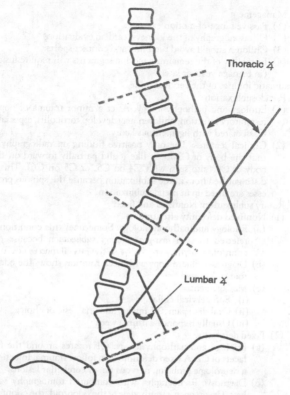

Figure 11-13 The Cobb measurement. The vertebrae with the greatest amount of tilt are selected as the end vertebrae. The angle formed at the intersection of these lines is the Cobb angle. If a second curve is present below the primary curve, the original curve's lower vertebra becomes the top vertebra for measuring the second curve, and the same line along its surface is used. (From Herring JA [ed]: Tachdjian's Pediatric Orthopaedics, 3rd ed. Philadelphia, WB Saunders, 2002.)

2. Congenital torticollis secondary to Klippel-Feil syndrome
   a. Etiology and pathophysiology: This condition is characterized by fusion of two or more vertebral bodies and often is associated with Sprengel's deformity, cardiac abnormalities, high congenital scoliosis, and about 30% of the time with major renal anomalies.
   b. Clinical features: Children often present with a twisted neck, but most characteristically with a short neck. It should be distinguished from bilateral Sprengel's deformity (short neck).
   c. Diagnosis: Best made on AP and lateral radiographs of the cervical spine

d. Management
   (1) Passive range-of-motion exercises
   (2) Ultrasonography of the kidneys, cardiac evaluation
   (3) Children should avoid tumbling and contact sports.
   (4) Instability of the remaining motion segments will require fusion (in teenage years or later).
3. Traumatic injuries of the cervical spine
   a. Pseudosubluxation
      (1) Etiology and pathophysiology: After a minor trauma or upper respiratory infection, children may develop torticollis, especially if associated with ligamentous laxity.
      (2) Clinical features: The only positive finding on radiography is that the body of C3 looks like it slid partially forward on the body of C4 (also seen with C4 on C5, or C5 on C6). This is distinguished from a true subluxation because the spinous processes are lined up in pseudosubluxation.
   b. Rotary subluxation: Nonfixed and fixed
      (1) Nonfixed deformity after trauma
         (a) Etiology and pathophysiology: Sometimes this condition is referred to as a *first-grade rotary subluxation* because the odontoid is asymmetric between the lateral masses of C1.
         (b) Diagnosis: Fluoroscopy with neck rotation shows the odontoid is centered.
         (c) Management
            (i) Soft cervical collar
            (ii) Oral diazepam, 0.1 mg/kg, and analgesic of choice
            (iii) Usually responds within a week
      (2) Fixed deformity
         (a) Etiology and pathophysiology: C1 rotates around the flat facets of C2. A fixed deformity can follow trauma, infection, a neurologic problem, nervous tic, or cerebellar lesions.
         (b) Diagnosis: Radiographs, with computed tomography scan best. On an open-mouth view of the odontoid, the odontoid is asymmetric between the lateral masses of C1.
         (c) Management: When fixed, the deformity needs reduction in traction, and possibly fusion or a halo jacket.
   c. Fractures and dislocations
      (1) Clinical features: Children with cervical fractures and dislocations/subluxations may present only with torticollis.
      (2) Diagnosis
         (a) Measurement of C1-C2 motion is different than that in adults. C1 may be 5 mm forward on the odontoid and still be normal in a child. However, the difference between flexion and extension should not be greater than 3 mm.
         (b) A clue to serious injury can be gauged by measuring the prevertebral soft tissue (i.e., behind the trachea) on an inspiratory plain film.
            (i) Above C4: Under 7 mm indicates serious injury.
            (ii) Below C4: The prevertebral soft tissue should be two-thirds the AP width of a vertebral body.

(3) Management: Conservative management includes rest, bracing, and NSAIDs; however, surgery occasionally is required.

11.5 Injuries to Extremities: Fractures, Sprains, and Strains

1. Fractures
   a. Clinical features: Most common cause of pain, point tenderness over involved area is an important diagnostic finding.
   b. Diagnosis
      (1) In addition to radiographs of site, additional radiographs of uninvolved side for comparison may be needed.
      (2) Secondary centers of ossification may be misinterpreted as avulsion injuries or fractures.
      (3) In the elbow, the medial epicondyle is occasionally superimposed on the lateral epicondyle or trapped in the joint. Radiographs of the opposite side would reveal that it is missing.
2. Salter-Harris fractures: Growth plate fractures
   a. Clinical features: These fractures present with point tenderness over the growth plate (or physis) and can follow even trivial trauma.
   b. Diagnosis: Plain radiographs are obtained to determine the Salter-Harris classification (I through V; Fig. 11-14). Note that an undisplaced growth plate fracture is classified as Salter I and has no abnormal radiologic features.
   c. Management
      (1) Nondisplaced growth plate fractures (Salter-Harris I, II, or V): Cast for 3 to 4 weeks
      (2) Displaced growth plate fractures: May need surgery, especially if they involve the joint surface (Salter-Harris III or IV)
3. Sprains or strains
   a. Etiology and pathophysiology
      (1) Rare in children with open physes (the growth plate is generally open in girls younger than 14 and boys younger than 15 to 16 years of age) because the physis is actually weaker than the ligaments.

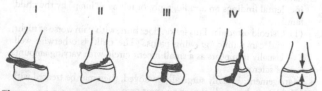

Figure 11-14   Salter-Harris classification of growth plate injury. Class I, fracture along growth plate; class II, fracture along growth plate with metaphyseal extension; class III, fracture along growth plate with epiphyseal extension; class IV, fracture across growth plate, including metaphysis and epiphysis; class V, crush injury to growth plate without obvious fracture. (From Robertson J, Shilkofski N [eds]: The Harriet Lane Handbook, 17th ed. Philadelphia, Elsevier Mosby, 2005.)

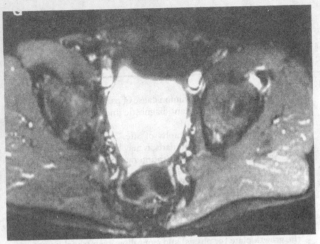

Figure 11-15   Avulsion of the iliac spine. (Courtesy of Michael G. Ehrlich, MD, Brown University School of Medicine, Providence, RI.)

    (2) Children do not get muscle pulls. They are more likely to avulse the apophysis to which the muscle is attached—that is, to rip off the ischial tuberosity or iliac spine, rather than tear the hamstring or have a rectus tear (Fig. 11-15).
  b. Diagnosis: Radiographs may show a small flake of bone pulled off the pelvis.
  c. Management: Supportive with rest and NSAIDs

11.6 Bone Tumors

1. Benign neoplasms
  a. Clinical features: Most benign neoplasms are not painful and are incidental findings on a radiograph, or felt as a "lump" by the child/family.
    (1) Osteoid osteoma: This lesion does hurt, with pain worse at night, and can mimic "growing pains." The child is otherwise well. Usually it appears as a small lucent circle with varying amounts of sclerosis.
  b. Management: Usually surgically removed, they may be treated with NSAIDs and even disappear on their own.
2. Pathologic fracture
  a. Etiology and pathophysiology
    (1) Pathologic fractures may develop because of weakening of bone due to a growth. (If such a lesion is discovered, it is advisable to seek orthopedic consultation.)

(2) Another consideration is child abuse characterized by
    (a) Multiple fractures at different stages of healing
    (b) Spiral fractures, suggesting twisting
    (c) Avulsion fractures from the end of the bone

3. Malignant neoplasms (osteogenic sarcoma [56%], Ewing's sarcoma [34%])
  a. Clinical features
    (1) These may present with pain, rapidly spreading mass, or pathologic fracture.
    (2) Often presentation is similar to infection, especially Ewing's sarcoma (i.e., presenting with fever, elevated ESR and destructive changes).
    (3) Laboratory findings: Elevated serum alkaline phosphatase and lactate dehydrogenase
    (4) Radiologic findings: Osteogenic sarcoma: "sunburst" pattern of ossification; Ewing's sarcoma: periosteal "onion-skin" appearance
  b. Management: Surgery, multiagent chemotherapy, radiation
  c. Prognosis: The 5-year survival rate for both tumors is approximately 60%; it is somewhat lower for Ewing's sarcoma.

SUGGESTED READING

Aboulafia AJ, Kennon RE, Jelinek JS: Benign bone tumors of childhood. J Am Acad Orthop Surg 7:377-388, 1999.

Bradford DS, Lonstein JE, Moe JH, et al: Moe's Textbook of Scoliosis and Other Spinal Deformities. Philadelphia, WB Saunders, 1987.

Ginsburg GM, Bassett GS: Back pain in children and adolescents: Evaluation and differential diagnosis. J Am Acad Orthop Surg 5(2):67-78, 1997.

Kujala UM, Kvist M, Heinonen O: Osgood-Schlatter's disease in adolescent athletes: Retrospective study of incidence and duration. Am J Sports Med 13:236-241, 1985.

Noonan KJ, Richards BS: Nonsurgical management of idiopathic clubfoot. J Am Acad Orthop Surg 11:392-402, 2003.

O'Connor MI, Pritchard DJ: Ewing's sarcoma: Prognostic factors, disease control, and re-emerging role of surgical treatment. Clin Orthop Relat Res 262:78-87, 1991.

Staheli LT: Rotational problems in children. Instr Course Lect 43:199-209, 1994.

Staheli LT, Corbett M, Wyss C, King H: Lower extremity rotational problems in children: Normal values to guide management. J Bone Joint Surg Am 67:39-47, 1985.

Tada K, Tsuyuguchi Y, Kawai H: Birth palsy: Natural recovery course and combined root avulsion. J Pediatr Orthop 4:279-284, 1984.

Terjesen T, Osthus P: Ultrasound in the diagnosis and follow-up of transient synovitis of the hip. J Pediatr Orthop 11:608-613, 1991.

WEBSITES

American Academy of Orthopaedic Surgeons: www.aaos.org
Open Directory Project (dmoz): http://dmoz.org/Health/Medicine/Surgery/Orthopedics
thoseek: www.orthoseek.com/topics.html

Ali Yalcindag, Bradley J. Bloom, and
Anthony J. Alario

12.1 Approach to the Patient with Painful or Swollen Joints

Extremity pain or joint swelling are common problems encountered during childhood. The etiology of these problems ranges from relatively benign conditions like joint hypermobility to more severe and sometimes chronic conditions like inflammatory or infectious arthritis or even neoplasms. Often the etiology of the problem is obvious (e.g., trauma, soft tissue swelling from an insect bite); at other times a thoughtful work-up is necessary. Salient features in the evaluation of a joint condition are outlined here.

1. History: Elements of history are important in differentiating between conditions characterized by synovial inflammation and mechanical conditions. In general, inflammatory pain is more prominent after prolonged rest and in the morning hours (morning stiffness), whereas mechanical conditions are exacerbated by activity and relieved by rest. Severe pain localizing to the bones that wakes a child up from sleep suggests malignancy. The following features of history are important in evaluating children with extremity pain.

   a. Duration of joint involvement: Is it transient (minutes, hours) or chronic (days, weeks, or months)?

   b. Pattern of joint involvement: Is it fixed or migratory? How many joints are involved (Fig. 12-1)?

   c. Fever: Height, duration, pattern. Fever can be a sign of septic arthritis. Quotidian fever of systemic-onset juvenile idiopathic arthritis is characterized by daily spikes of late evening to early morning. Leukemias and lymphomas can present with fevers.

   d. Rash: Generalized versus localized

   e. Morning stiffness (a reliable marker for chronic arthritis; joint fluid "gels" from inflammation)

   f. Activities of daily living: Can the patient put on socks and turn knobs?

   g. Ancillary complaints: Abdominal pain, diarrhea, weight loss, bloody stools raise suspicion for inflammatory bowel disease

(IBD)–associated arthritis. Recurrent painless oral ulcers are seen in systemic lupus erythematosus (SLE).
  h. Residence in or travel to Lyme disease endemic areas
  i. Family history: Important features include identifying family members with the following conditions, which may accompany rheumatic diseases:
     (1) Inflammatory low back pain (spondyloarthropathy)
     (2) Heel pain (spondyloarthropathy)
     (3) Knee problems
     (4) Arthritis or other rheumatic disease
     (5) IBD (colitis/ileitis)
     (6) Prostatitis/urethritis/cervicitis (Reiter's syndrome)
     (7) Uveitis/iritis/conjunctivitis/blepharitis (Reiter's syndrome, juvenile idiopathic arthritis [JIA])
     (8) Psoriasis (psoriatic arthritis)
2. Physical examination
  a. The examination should include an assessment of the following:
     (1) Overall appearance and stigmata of chronic disease
     (2) Growth data (plot height and weight)
     (3) General examination: Skin, nails, mucous membranes
     (4) Soft tissue examination
     (5) Muscle examination: Inspection, palpation, strength (measure circumference of greatest muscle mass proximal to involved joint because chronic arthritis leads to muscle atrophy)
  b. The examination specific to the joints includes the following:
     (1) Inspection
        (a) Loss of normal contour and landmarks
        (b) Distention and fullness
        (c) Angulation and deformity
     (2) Palpation
        (a) Pain, tenderness, warmth
        (b) Effusion and distention
        (c) Induration ("boggy" swelling)
        (d) Nodules
     (3) Movement
        (a) Range of motion
        (b) Stability
        (c) Gait
     (4) Strength: Muscle strength grading
3. Laboratory and radiographic studies
  a. Complete blood cell count (CBC) with differential count: Leukocytosis suggests infection or inflammation; thrombocytosis can be seen in the setting of chronic inflammation. Cytopenias should raise a suspicion for hematologic malignancies.
  b. Erythrocyte sedimentation rate (ESR): ESR is an indirect way of measuring elevated concentrations of acute-phase–response plasma proteins (see later). Normal level is reassuring, but should not be used in isolation. Normal ranges widely vary by age, sex, red blood cell morphology, and anemia/polycythemia. It may remain elevated for a while even if the inflammatory stimulus (infection) has resolved.

c. Acute-phase–response (APR) proteins: APR refers to the alteration of plasma protein synthesis by hepatocytes in response to systemic inflammation. C-reactive protein, complement proteins, haptoglobin, fibrinogen levels are elevated, whereas albumin and transferrin levels drop. These markers are more useful in following systemic inflammatory response than ESR.

d. Rheumatoid factor* (RF): RFs are autoantibodies directed against immunoglobulin G (IgG) molecules. Although RF measurement can be useful in evaluating adult rheumatoid arthritis, it has a very limited role in the diagnostic work-up of children with extremity pain or joint swelling.

e. Antinuclear antibody* (ANA): ANAs are antibodies directed against nuclear antigens. They can be found in the setting of several autoimmune conditions like arthritis and SLE. However, ANAs can be transiently elevated after viral infections and can be elevated in otherwise healthy individuals. Therefore, an elevated ANA should not be used to diagnose an autoimmune condition in isolation.

f. Serum chemistry panel (blood urea nitrogen/creatinine, liver function tests, muscle enzymes—as a screen for metabolic disease, hepatitis)

g. Urinalysis (rule out infection versus nephritis or vasculitis)

h. Quantitative IgG, IgM, IgA.* Arthritis can be seen in the setting of antibody deficiency.

i. Complement components:* Elevated levels can be seen with systemic inflammation. Depressed levels are seen in active consumption states like active SLE. Congenital absence of early complement components predisposes to SLE.

j. Streptococcal titers (rule out acute rheumatic fever)

k. Tuberculin skin test

l. Lyme titers. Positive enzyme-linked immunosorbent assays (ELISA) should be confirmed with Western blot.

m. Radiography. Plain radiographs can show bony tumors, cysts, lytic lesions, joint effusions, soft tissue swelling. Chronic arthritic changes in the form of periarticular osteopenia, narrowing of joint spaces, erosions in the cartilage can also be seen by plain radiography, but these findings lag behind the clinical disease. Magnetic resonance imaging (MRI) with gadolinium enhancement is useful for demonstrating synovial inflammation. Ultrasonography can be used to detect subclinical joint effusions.

n. Joint fluid analysis/culture indications: Single joint with severe pain or total disuse ± severe inflammatory signs, fever, or other evidence of systemic infection (pauciarticular/monoarticular versus infection)

o. Blood culture (if febrile)†

p. Slit-lamp examination of the eye* (rule out uveitis)

q. Technetium bone scan† (infection versus tumor or arthritis)

r. Bone marrow examination (malignancy)†

---

*Identifies some populations especially susceptible to rheumatic disease.
†In selected cases when signs and symptoms suggest a particular diagnosis.

    s. Intestinal series for IBD[†]
    t. Stool analysis/culture (rule out parasites, *Clostridium difficile, Yersinia*)[†]
    u. Echocardiogram (Kawasaki's disease, acute rheumatic fever)[†]
    v. Human leukocyte antigen (HLA) B27[*]
    w. Parvovirus titer[†]
    x. Work-up for sexually transmitted diseases[†]
4. Conditions in the pediatric age group associated with joint effusions or arthritis
    a. Rheumatic diseases
        (1) JRA/JIA
        (2) SLE
        (3) Rheumatic fever
        (4) Juvenile ankylosing spondylitis
        (5) Dermatomyositis/polymyositis
        (6) Scleroderma
        (7) Sjögren's syndrome
        (8) Psoriatic arthritis
        (9) Reiter's syndrome
        (10) Sarcoidosis
    b. Infectious diseases
        (1) Septic arthritis
        (2) Osteomyelitis
        (3) Reactive or postinfectious arthritis
        (4) Lyme disease
    c. Heritable disorders
        (1) Hemophilia
        (2) Sickle cell disease
        (3) Mucopolysaccharidosis
        (4) Immune deficiency syndromes
    d. Neoplastic diseases
        (1) Leukemia
        (2) Lymphoma
        (3) Neuroblastoma
    e. Miscellaneous
        (1) Trauma and orthopedic conditions (e.g., fracture, sprain, chondromalacia, patella-femoral syndrome)
        (2) Toxic synovitis
        (3) Hypermobility syndrome
        (4) Kawasaki disease
        (5) Anaphylactoid purpura
        (6) IBD
        (7) Vasculitis syndromes (Henoch-Schönlein purpura)
        (8) Child abuse
5. Differential diagnosis
    a. Figure 12-1 outlines possible etiologies based on number of joints involved and whether there is associated *fever*.

---

[*]Identifies some populations especially susceptible to rheumatic disease.
[†]In selected cases when signs and symptoms suggest a particular diagnosis.

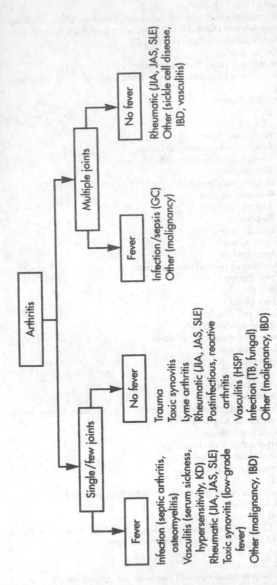

Figure 12-1 Differential diagnosis of acute arthritis. GC, gonococcal; HSP, Henoch-Schönlein purpura; IBD, inflammatory bowel disease; JIA, juvenile idiopathic (rheumatoid) arthritis; JAS, juvenile ankylosing spondylitis; KD, Kawasaki's disease; TB, tuberculosis; SLE, systemic lupus erythematosus.

> Box 12-1   Differential Diagnosis of Arthritis
>
> **Single Joint**
>
> ACUTE
> Septic arthritis
> Oligoarticular JIA
> Spondyloarthropathy/enthesitis-associated arthritis
> Lyme disease
> Reactive arthritis
> Malignancy (leukemia, neuroblastoma)
> Hemophilia
> Trauma
>
> CHRONIC
> Oligoarticular JIA
> Chronic infection (tuberculosis)
> Sarcoidosis
> Pigmented villonodular synovitis
> Hemangioma
> Discoid meniscus
> Psoriatic arthritis
> Spondyloarthropathy/enthesitis-associated arthritis
>
> **Multiple Joints**
>
> Polyarticular JIA
> Systemic lupus erythematosus
> Sarcoidosis
> Lyme disease
> Reactive arthritis
> Viral arthritis
> Psoriatic arthritis
> Spondyloarthropathy/enthesitis-associated arthritis
> Mucopolysaccharidoses

JIA, juvenile idiopathic arthritis

   b. Box 12-1 also outlines possible etiologies based on the number of joints involved and whether the onset is *acute* or *chronic*.

12.2 Juvenile Idiopathic Arthritis (Juvenile Rheumatoid Arthritis)

1. Definition: Onset of arthritis occurs in a child before 16 years of age, lasts for at least 6 weeks. *Arthritis* is defined as joint swelling or limited range of motion accompanied by pain. Arthralgia alone is *not* sufficient for diagnosis.
2. Clinical features and diagnosis: Three major subtypes exist: Oligoarticular (60% of JIA/JRA cases), polyarticular (30%), and systemic (10%).

Subtype classification is determined by assessing the patient's involvement at 6 months from onset of symptoms.

a. Oligoarticular
   (1) This type is defined by involvement of four joints or fewer (small joints, e.g., metacarpophalangeals, count as one joint). This subtype is further divided into persistent and extended oligoarticular categories based on the number of joints involved within the first 6 months. Up to 50% of patients with oligoarticular JIA may have inflammation in more than four joints (i.e., extended oligoarticular phenotype).
   (2) There is strong female predominance.
   (3) The average age at onset is 2 years.
   (4) Monoarticular onset appears in 75% of cases; most of these involve the knee. Ankles and elbows may also be involved. Hip involvement is rare.
   (5) Eye involvement: Anterior uveitis (iridocyclitis) develops in 20% of patients. Eye involvement is usually asymptomatic, and its course does not necessarily correlate with arthritis activity. Patients with positive ANA are at higher risk for uveitis. Routine screening is needed every 3 months until the disease is inactive for 5 years. Total blindness occurred in up to 24% before routine screening and aggressive therapy; now it is rare.
   (6) Forty percent of patients are ANA positive; 70% of patients with iridocyclitis are ANA positive.
   (7) Major conditions in the differential diagnosis of oligoarticular JIA include the following:
      (a) Septic arthritis (bacterial, tubercular)
      (b) Lyme arthritis
      (c) Trauma
      (d) Postinfectious (viruses)
      (e) Malignancy
      (f) Spondyloarthropathy

b. Polyarticular
   (1) This subtype involves five or more joints with arthritis (cervical spine, both temporomandibular joints, carpus, and tarsus are counted as one joint each). Differential diagnosis includes
      (a) Psoriasis
      (b) SLE
      (c) Spondyloarthropathies
      (d) Infectious or postinfectious
   (2) Two subtypes, seronegative and seropositive, are defined by absence or presence of RF.
      (a) Seronegative polyarthritis: The more common subtype, it represents 85% of patients with polyarthritis. The median age at onset is 3 years, with female predominance. Uveitis is uncommon except in those who had pauciarticular onset or are ANA positive (25%).
      (b) Seropositive polyarthritis: This subtype is defined by the presence of RF (native IgM antibodies to native IgG) in serum. Nodules (mobile, nontender) may develop over

extensor surfaces. Female predominance exists, and this form usually presents in adolescence—essentially it is an early presentation of adult-type rheumatoid arthritis. It comprises only 6% of all JIA. Therefore RF is not generally a useful test in juvenile arthritis unless the patient has polyarthritis and fits the already cited demographics.

c. Systemic-onset arthritis (Still's disease) is defined by the presence of arthritis plus the following:

(1) Daily high-spiking fevers (>38.5° C), with a return to normal or below normal, especially during therapy

(2) Salmon-pink, evanescent rash, macular, occasionally papular, rarely urticarial, typically on the trunk and proximal extremities; it may be elicited by scratching or pressure (Köbner's phenomenon).

(3) The median onset is at 5 years of age, but it can arise at any age, including adulthood; its incidence is equal in boys and girls. Systemic onset represents 10% of all JIA.

(4) Other features include anemia (of chronic disease, or occasionally hemolytic), hypoalbuminemia, leukocytosis, thrombocytosis, lymphadenopathy, hepatosplenomegaly, and pericarditis. Systemic features may precede arthritis. Some patients may develop macrophage activation syndrome characterized by hepatic failure, hemophagocytosis, disseminated intravascular coagulation, and sometimes renal failure.

(5) Differential diagnosis of systemic-onset JIA includes all causes of fever of undetermined origin: Infection, malignancy, IBD, other

3. Management

a. Oligoarticular arthritis

(1) A large majority of patients have a good response to nonsteroidal anti-inflammatory drugs (NSAIDs). Naproxen,*† ibuprofen,*† tolmetin,* aspirin* and its derivatives (such as magnesium choline salicylate*†), indomethacin,† and others have all been used with similar efficacy.

(2) Physical therapy is crucial for maintaining function and normal strength and range of motion.

(3) Night splinting may be needed for large contractures; shoe lifts may be needed for leg-length discrepancy.

(4) Intra-articular steroids are the best alternative to NSAIDs; effects may last for several months. Disease-modifying antirheumatic drugs (DMARDs; see [b], Polyarticular arthritis, for examples) are needed if NSAIDs or intra-articular steroid injections fail.

b. Polyarticular arthritis

(1) Treatment initially is similar to that for pauciarticular disease.

(2) DMARDs may be effective; early use of methotrexate is now proven to be very effective and safe.

---

*Medication approved by the U.S. Food and Drug Administration for children younger than 12 years of age for the indication of arthritis.
†Available in a liquid suspension.

(3) Indications for methotrexate:
   (a) Radiographic evidence of bony erosion or cartilage loss
   (b) Severe dysfunction (unremitting pain, average of about 1 hour or more, or morning stiffness or disuse of an extremity [e.g., inability to ambulate]) despite adequate trial of at least one NSAID over about 3 months
   (c) Most patients with seropositive disease
(4) There is an increasing trend toward early use of DMARDs in severe cases.
(5) Tumor necrosis factor antagonists: Etanercept is used in rapidly progressing moderate to severe polyarticular JIA unresponsive to therapies mentioned previously.
(6) Other potential therapies include the following:
   (a) Intramuscular gold
   (b) Sulfasalazine
   (c) Hydroxychloroquine, penicillamine, oral gold (all, however, have been shown to be no more effective than a placebo in controlled trials)
   (d) Immunoglobulin, azathioprine, cyclosporine, or cyclophosphamide may help in refractory cases (only anecdotal evidence exists).
(7) Low-dose oral prednisone or intermittent intravenous pulses of methylprednisolone may be useful adjuncts in maintaining normal function, but they probably do not alter the disease's course and should not be used as primary therapy or on a prolonged basis because of side effects.
(8) Physical and occupational therapy, orthotics, and corrective surgeries (including total joint replacements) can be crucial to maintaining function.
(9) Treatment of seropositive disease is similar to that of seronegative; however, there is an increasing tendency to start these patients on DMARDs earlier because of the aggressive nature of the disease.

c. Systemic arthritis is treated as in polyarticular disease. Systemic features are often controlled with high doses of NSAIDs. Steroid therapy is indicated for the following:
(1) Symptomatic anemia, fever, and malaise leading to an inability to attend school or perform activities of daily living
(2) Pericarditis
(3) Patients who fail to come under adequate control with a short course of steroid therapy or who become steroid dependent can respond to methotrexate, cyclosporine, tumor necrosis factor antagonists, cyclophosphamide. Recent studies support a role for thalidomide in the management of treatment-resistant systemic JIA. Early studies with interleukin (IL)-1 receptor antagonist and anti-IL-6 antibody have also revealed promising results for such patients.

4. Prognosis
a. Oligoarticular arthritis is usually controlled easily; periodic flares over several years may occur. About 10% of patients progress to

polyarticular disease. Usually no significant residual joint destruction or deformity occurs. Uveitis can be chronic or severe, despite therapy, in 10% of patients with eye involvement.

b. Polyarticular arthritis

(1) *Seronegative* disease generally "burns out" after several years' activity, usually by adolescence. However, joint-related disabilities may remain in up to 25%, and 10% may have some active disease into adulthood.

(2) *Seropositive* polyarthritis persists into adulthood. Early joint destruction is common. Many patients have severe disability, but prognosis for normal function is good with aggressive treatment. The prognosis is poorer in late adulthood; therefore, life expectancy is slightly shorter than normal.

c. Systemic arthritis symptoms usually resolve within several months, but arthritis continues in 25% and is chronic and severely destructive in 10%. Growth impairment and developmental delay can occur with all forms of JIA.

12.3 Juvenile Spondyloarthropathy

1. Definition: Spondyloarthropathy refers to disorders that share several common features, including arthritis (primarily axial, although children tend to get more peripheral involvement), enthesitis (inflammation of tendon insertion sites), and association with HLA B27. There is a strong familial occurrence and male predominance. Juvenile ankylosing spondylitis (JAS), juvenile psoriatic arthritis, IBD-associated arthritis, and Reiter's syndrome are included in this category.

2. Clinical features and diagnosis

a. The median age of onset of JAS is approximately 12 years, and there is a strong male predominance. JAS most frequently affects large joints in a lower extremity, including hips. Sacroiliac and toe joints (especially the first metatarsophalangeal) are commonly involved. Enthesitis (pain/inflammation at soft tissue insertions into bone) is frequent, most commonly at the Achilles tendon or plantar fascia insertions. Back involvement is less common in childhood.

b. Patients may have an onset as Reiter's syndrome (triad: arthritis, urethritis, and conjunctivitis or uveitis) with or without preceding infections such as chlamydial urethritis/cervicitis or *Yersinia/Salmonella/Shigella* enteritis.

c. Juvenile psoriatic arthritis presents with asymmetric large and small joint arthritis. Involvement of joints of fingers and toes with tenosynovitis is common (sausage digits). Skin disease may be absent at the time of diagnosis. Unlike other spondyloarthropathies, girls tend to be more commonly affected, and ANA can be positive.

d. IBD-associated arthritis involves axial and large peripheral joints in an asymmetric distribution. The axial disease does not correlate with the activity of IBD.

e. Up to 25% of patients with spondyloarthropathies will develop uveitis (anterior or posterior), although possibly not until adulthood; it is often symptomatic.

f. Other rare systemic manifestations include aortic insufficiency, cutaneous balanitis, and keratoderma blenorrhagicum.

g. Seventy percent of patients are positive for HLA B27, but patients have this condition without HLA B27 positivity (7% of the general population are HLA B27 positive). It is estimated that spondyloarthropathy will develop in 7% of HLA B27–positive patients over their lifetimes.

3. Management: NSAIDs, especially indomethacin, may be efficacious (first line). Sulfasalazine and methotrexate have been proven effective in adult studies and are also helpful in children (second line). Tumor necrosis factor antagonists are used for disease resistant to first- and second-line agents.

4. Prognosis
   a. Twenty-five percent have a single attack of disease, 50% have a relapsing/remitting course, and 25% have disease that is always active to some degree. Disease in the latter groups may persist into adulthood, but only a minority have any joint destruction. Only 2% progress to full-blown ankylosing spondylitis.
   b. Children often have a mild disease presentation and a course limited to intermittent enthesopathy and large joint arthritis, referred to as seronegative enthesopathy/arthropathy syndrome.

12.4 Dermatomyositis/Polymyositis

1. Definition: Presumably, dermatomyositis is an immune-mediated inflammatory myopathy resulting in muscle weakness, accompanied by skin vasculitis (in dermatomyositis), leading to typical rashes. The underlying pathologic process is vasculitis in striated muscles, skin, and gastrointestinal tract.

2. Clinical features and diagnosis
   a. Diagnosis is based on the four criteria of Bohan and Peter, listed here. Three of four criteria are needed to diagnose polymyositis. Dermatomyositis is confirmed by three of four criteria plus typical rashes (see later).
      (1) Proximal muscle weakness. This can begin acutely but usually follows a subacute indolent course and mostly involves shoulder and pelvic girdle.
      (2) Elevation of muscle-derived enzymes: creatine phosphokinase, aldolase (very helpful), alanine aminotransferase, aspartate aminotransferase, lactate dehydrogenase
      (3) Typical electromyographic findings of inflammatory myopathy (small-amplitude/short-duration motor unit potentials, fibrillations, spontaneous high-frequency discharges)
      (4) Typical pathologic findings on muscle biopsy (perifascicular atrophy, perivascular lymphocytic infiltrates)
      (5) Note: Although these diagnostic criteria are still in use, muscle biopsy and electromyography are rarely used today because of their invasive nature and their tendency to miss the diagnosis if an uninvolved muscle site is chosen for sampling. Instead, MRI (fat-suppressed, T2-weighted) images of proximal muscle groups

(e.g., proximal thighs) readily demonstrates the muscle inflammation required by the diagnostic criteria.

b. Rashes consistent with dermatomyositis
   (1) Periorbital heliotrope (purplish, erythematous, flat rash, often with cutaneous edema)
   (2) Gottron's papules (erythematous, raised, sometimes scaly rash over extensor surfaces of joints, especially knuckles and elbows)

c. Other cutaneous features include a malar rash similar to a periorbital rash, usually extending into nasolabial folds (unlike lupus); and a photosensitive rash, often in a "shawl" distribution over the shoulders, upper back, and chest. A vasculopathy of nailbeds shows dilated or infarcted capillary loops, often visible when active with minimal magnification (e.g., otoscope), and cutaneous calcinosis (usually late).

d. Systemic features: Palatopharyngeal muscle weakness may lead to dysphagia and aspiration. Respiratory failure may occur with severe involvement of chest wall muscles. Ten percent have cardiac muscle involvement, usually mild, but suggesting the potential for congestive heart failure. Gastrointestinal vasculitis may cause intestinal cramping, malabsorption, or catastrophic perforations. Reflexes are preserved.

e. Laboratory findings: Elevated enzymes are as described earlier. Forty percent are ANA positive. Von Willebrand's factor antigen elevation correlates with active disease in some patients, but sensitivity and specificity are not ideal. Other markers of vasculitis may be better, but are not widely available in commercial or hospital laboratories (e.g., neopterin).

f. Differential diagnosis includes rhabdomyolysis, muscular dystrophy, toxins, myasthenia gravis, Guillain-Barré syndrome, and postviral myositis.

3. Management
   a. Initial treatment with corticosteroids: 1 to 2 mg/kg/day of prednisone or equivalent orally; often treatment is more effective in split doses (i.e., twice a day) in initial phases. Early treatment with high-dose intravenous methylprednisolone therapy (30 mg/kg/day, up to 1 g daily for 3 days) may suppress disease activity more quickly. Long-term treatment with intravenous pulse therapy intermittently (e.g., every 2 to 8 weeks) may lead to fewer steroid- and disease-related complications.

   b. Adjunctive therapies
      (1) Methotrexate may be effective as a steroid-sparing agent and as treatment of refractory disease.
      (2) Intravenous immunoglobulin is very effective for muscle and skin disease, but frequent and chronic dosing is needed to maintain remissions.
      (3) Cyclosporine may also be effective.
      (4) Hydroxychloroquine is used as an adjunct by some; it may lead to quicker resolution of muscle disease and refractory skin disease, but ocular toxicity and idiosyncratic worsening of rash may occur.

4. Prognosis/course
    a. Different disease courses are described.
        (1) Monocyclic: Typically, presentation is acute; after 1 to 2 years of treatment, disease generally resolves without recurrence.
        (2) Polycyclic: The disease is usually well controlled but will recur after period of quiescence off therapy.
        (3) Chronic/continuous: Patients have some degree of disease activity at most times over years despite aggressive therapies. May continue into adulthood.
    b. There is increasing evidence that early aggressive treatment with the aforementioned agents tends to reduce the risk of a polycyclic or chronic course and later sequelae like calcinosis cutis.
    c. Long-term sequelae
        (1) Calcinosis cutis: Subcutaneous deposits of calcium can occur anywhere, but their predilection is for pressure points (extensor joint surfaces, ischial tuberosities). They can be diffuse and debilitating. They may extrude calcium, and superinfection is common. There is a strong association with uncontrolled disease, but they can occur in any patient.
        (2) Acquired lipodystrophy: Insulin resistance, loss of subcutaneous fat, and hyperlipidemia characterize this condition. Secondary features are amenorrhea and acanthosis nigrans. The prognosis is unknown, but patients with the congenital form of this disease die prematurely of diabetic and hyperlipidemic complications.

12.5 Systemic Lupus Erythematosus

1. Definition, clinical features, and diagnosis: SLE is a multisystem disease defined by the presence of 4 of 11 clinical criteria (Box 12-2).
    a. Other features include fatigue, alopecia, Raynaud's phenomenon, myocarditis/endocarditis, pulmonary infiltrates/hemorrhage, hepatitis, and colitis. Isolated discoid lupus is rare in childhood. Systemic disease develops in fewer than 20% of such patients.
    b. The peak onset is in adolescence. The female-to-male ratio is at least 8:1, but is 1:1 in children younger than 5 years of age. A higher incidence occurs in Asians and African Americans and in the XXY karyotype (Klinefelter's syndrome).
    c. Laboratory findings include autoantibodies as described earlier. *Caution should be taken in interpreting positive ANA alone.* ANA positivity can be seen in 5% to 7% of normal children, healthy relatives of people with autoimmune disease, other rheumatic diseases (juvenile rheumatoid arthritis, dermatomyositis, scleroderma), and nonrheumatic conditions, including trivial viral infections and anticonvulsant therapy.
        (1) Double-stranded DNA (dsDNA) antibodies are very specific to SLE, especially in high titer. Other antibodies and their relative frequency of occurrence in patients with SLE include the following:
            (a) Anti-Sm antibodies (25% to 60%)
            (b) Anti SS-A (10% to 30%)
            (c) Anti SS-B (10%)

Box 12-2   Clinical Criteria for Systemic Lupus Erythematosus*

Positive antinuclear antibody testing

Immunologic abnormality (one of the following): False-positive serologic test for syphilis (or antiphospholipid antibodies), antibodies to native (double-stranded) DNA, anti-Smith antibody, positive LE cell preparation [antibodies to RNP, RO(SS-A), La(SS-B)]

Photosensitivity (usually blistering rash to minimal ultraviolet light exposure)

Mucosal ulcerations (oral or nasal, usually painless)

Malar rash (sparing nasolabial folds, crossing bridge of nose) [leukocytoclastic vasculitis, purpuric rash]

Discoid lupus

Arthritis (typically symmetric, large joints, nonerosive) [arthralgia]

Serositis–pleuritis, pericarditis, peritonitis (frequently accompanied by effusions)

Hematologic abnormalities (any one of the following): Coombs-positive hemolytic anemia, leukopenia (total lymphocyte count <4000) or lymphopenia (total lymphocyte count <1500), thrombocytopenia [anemia of chronic disease]

Neurologic abnormalities (one of the following): Seizures, psychosis [organic brain syndrome, mononeuritis multiplex, chorea, myasthenia]

Renal abnormalities (one of the following): Proteinuria (3+ by dipstick, over 0.5 g/24 hours), cellular casts

*Related features not meeting diagnostic criteria are in brackets.

(2) Complement levels decrease (as measured by C3, C4, total hemolytic complement [CH_{50}]) owing to consumption in immune complexes, decreased synthesis, and possibly increased clearance by the reticuloendothelial system. Increases in dsDNA titer with decreasing levels of complement often correlate with disease flares.

2. Management

   a. For mild disease (less common in children than adults), including constitutional symptoms, arthritis, cutaneous/mucosal manifestations without internal systems involvement:

      (1) NSAIDs for arthritis as in JIA are recommended.

      (2) Hydroxychloroquine is well tolerated and effective for arthritis, cutaneous disease, and fatigue. It is necessary to monitor for retinal toxicity.

      (3) Prednisone: Low doses may be helpful to restore the patient to a normal lifestyle.

   b. For moderate to severe disease, including involvement of internal organ systems:

      (1) Oral corticosteroids (prednisone) are the mainstay of therapy (initial doses of 1 to 2 mg/kg/day).

(2) Hydroxychloroquine is helpful and may also help stabilize immune abnormalities.

c. Agents used in refractory cases or as steroid-sparing agents:
   (1) High doses of intravenous corticosteroids (30 mg/kg/day to a maximum of 1 g for 1 to 3 days every 2 to 12 weeks)
   (2) Azathioprine: daily oral therapy
   (3) Cyclophosphamide: Intravenous pulses are commonly used for diffuse proliferative glomerulonephritis.
   (4) Methotrexate: Weekly oral or intramuscular therapy, similar to antiarthritic doses. No controlled trials have been done, but it is anecdotally effective and probably less toxic than other immunosuppressive agents.
   (5) Immunoglobulin: Intravenous therapy is helpful for autoimmune thrombocytopenia.
   (6) Plasmapheresis is unproven in trials but is anecdotally helpful in severe cases.
   (7) There are anecdotal reports of success with B-cell–targeted therapies like rituximab.

3. Prognosis: Now, at least 80% have a 20-year survival. The most common cause of death is from infections (especially encapsulated bacteria, but also other bacteria, fungi, *Pneumocystis*, and disseminated varicella), probably as a result of the more aggressive use of immunosuppressives. However, improved surveillance for infections, antibiotics, and supportive/intensive care modalities continues to decrease deaths from infection. Severe nephritis and central nervous system involvement worsen the prognosis.

12.6 Scleroderma

LOCALIZED DISEASE

1. Definition, clinical features, and diagnosis
   a. Localized scleroderma is a self-limited condition affecting local areas of skin only.
   b. Two types
      (1) *Morphea*: This type has well-circumscribed patches of shiny, indurated skin; it is usually limited to one or a few areas but may involve many areas. Usually it occurs in self-limited patches, but lesions may expand over time.
      (2) *Linear*: This type is similar to morphea but has a linear distribution, frequently overlying extensor joint surfaces. It may lead to joint limitation or atrophy of affected extremity. It may overlie the midface/forehead ("en coup de sabre" pattern), leading to cosmetic deformity. Rarely, underlying brain abnormalities/seizures exist (possibly related to Perry-Romberg syndrome, which is facial hemiatrophy with underlying central nervous system abnormalities).
   c. Progression to systemic disease is almost never seen (isolated case reports).
   d. Laboratory findings: 40% to 50% of patients with each type are positive for ANA or RF.

2. Management is usually limited to adjunctive therapies, such as physical therapy and plastic surgery in rare cases. D-Penicillamine and methotrexate may lead to improvement, but trials are lacking, and potential toxicity makes these therapies justified only in severe cases. Oral, topical, or intralesional steroids may lead to some transient skin softening, but they do not improve long-term outcome.

SYSTEMIC SCLEROSIS

1. Definition, clinical features, and diagnosis
   a. The classic form involves *diffuse cutaneous* involvement and internal organ involvement, including esophageal dysmotility, restrictive lung disease, myocarditis or pericarditis, and renal vascular disease. Severe Raynaud's phenomenon is almost universal. Another subtype, called *limited cutaneous*, involves less skin involvement and more indolent internal organ disease. One form of this is called CREST syndrome, an acronym for calcinosis, Raynaud's phenomenon, esophageal dysmotility, sclerodactyly, and telangiectases. It is associated with anticentromere antibodies.
   b. Laboratory findings: Most patients are ANA positive, often in a nucleolar pattern. Anti–Scl-70 (topoisomerase III) antibodies are highly specific but not sensitive. An upper gastrointestinal series shows a dilated distal esophagus with poor motility and reflux. Pulmonary function testing often shows a restrictive deficit. Cardiac testing may reveal myocardial dysfunction, pericardial effusions, and dysrhythmias (especially ventricular ectopy). Skin biopsy usually is not necessary for diagnosis, but if done shows dense collagen deposition in the dermis with a loss of adnexal structures; lymphocytic or eosinophilic infiltrates are also common in early disease.

2. Management
   a. Many medications have been used for scleroderma. Unfortunately, no proven curative or remittive agents exist. The following agents continue to be used frequently, although therapeutic trials have been equivocal and not well controlled.
      (1) D-Penicillamine: Some studies have shown modest improvements on this medication, including skin softening and improvements in visceral disease and long-term survival.
      (2) Corticosteroids: These do not alter the long-term prognosis. However, they may help specific manifestations, such as pericardial effusions and myositis. They also decrease pain and swelling in the initial edematous phase of skin disease.
      (3) Immunosuppressives, especially methotrexate, have been tried with some anecdotal success.
   b. *Survival and quality of life have been increased, mostly because of improved supportive care.*
      (1) Aggressive treatment or prevention of skin breakdown is helpful.
      (2) Gastrointestinal management includes antisecretory and promotility agents, the prevention of bacterial overgrowth, nutritional supplementation, and the prevention/treatment of severe constipation.

(3) Physical and occupational therapy help maintain activities of daily living.

(4) Vasoactive medications: Calcium channel blockers are helpful for Raynaud's phenomenon; angiotensin-converting enzyme inhibitors may prevent or slow the progression of renal and pulmonary vascular disease.

(5) Monitoring of cardiac status, with treatment of myocardial dysfunction/dysrhythmias if necessary.

3. The prognosis for adults in 60% to 70% of patients is 10-year survival, and is somewhat better in limited cutaneous disease. Most common causes of death are related to acute renal vascular crisis and cardiac (congestive heart failure from myocardial dysfunction, sudden death from arrhythmias) and pulmonary (especially pulmonary hypertension) complications.

12.7 Vasculitis

Vasculitis is characterized by inflammatory infiltrates in or around vascular structures, ultimately leading to damage of the tissues fed by these vessels. The most common vasculitis syndromes of childhood (by far) are Kawasaki's disease and Henoch-Schönlein purpura. Rare types of vasculitis are generally conceptualized by the size of blood vessel predominantly affected (i.e., small, medium, or large). The rarer types include polyarteritis nodosa (medium vessels), Takayasu's arteritis (large vessels), Wegener's granulomatosis, and Churg-Strauss syndrome (necrotizing vasculitis), and should be considered in children with unexplained systemic illness.

12.8 Benign Rheumatologic Conditions

In contrast to most of the previous conditions, *chronic* but benign musculoskeletal complaints in childhood are very common. Box 12-3 provides distinguishing features that can help differentiate benign from serious musculoskeletal pain.

Box 12-3 Benign versus Serious Limb Pains	
Benign	**Serious**
Nonarticular, diffuse	Articular or deep bone pain
Intermittent	Regular intervals or unremitting
No or minimal inflammation	Inflammation
Systemically well	Systemically ill
Not debilitating; no limp or disuse	Debilitating; limp or disuse (especially reliable in patient younger than 5 years of age)
Evening pain, pain after activity	Morning pain or stiffness

GROWING PAINS

1. Clinical features and diagnosis
   a. Growing pains present as crampy pain late in the day (often at bedtime). Usually it is in the legs (calves, shins, or thighs) and bilateral, but it may occasionally present in the arms. Rarely, pain may awaken the child from sleep; however, this must raise suspicion of other conditions, such as malignancies, or benign tumors, such as osteoid osteoma.
   b. Symptoms commonly occur at irregular intervals.
   c. The peak onset is at 3 to 5 and 8 to 12 years of age, and it is slightly more common in girls. Such pains occur in at least 5% of all children, perhaps up to 15%.
   d. Diagnostic criteria have been developed to serve as a general guideline for diagnosis.
      (1) Three-month history of pain
      (2) Symptom-free intervals of days to months
      (3) Pain late in day or on awakening
      (4) Pain not specifically related to joints
      (5) Pain of sufficient severity to interrupt normal activity
      (6) Normal physical examination results. Note: Normal laboratory (e.g., CBC, ESR) and radiologic data reinforce this diagnosis but are usually not necessary when children have classic symptoms.
2. Pathophysiology is unknown. However, pain is probably not related to growing. These children have normal growth, and peak onset is during years of relatively less growth. Most children with growing pains do not have orthopedic abnormalities or psychological dysfunction.
3. Management and prognosis: Massaging affected areas and providing reassurance is usually the best course of management. Maintaining the bedtime atmosphere and rituals is also helpful. In more severe cases, intermittent dosing of acetaminophen or ibuprofen may be useful. The prognosis is good; the vast majority of cases resolve some time in adolescence, if not before.

BENIGN HYPERMOBILITY SYNDROME

1. Definition, clinical features, and diagnosis
   a. This condition is defined as musculoskeletal complaints related to increased joint mobility. It may present with a wide variety of intermittent articular and nonarticular limb pains. Although usually mild, symptoms may include episodic arthritis with mild effusions.
   b. Mild hypermobility in a few joints is so common that specific criteria have been devised to qualify for this diagnosis. Although this approach may exclude a few patients with pain due to mild hypermobility, it decreases the tendency to blame all musculoskeletal problems on hypermobility when there may truly be another underlying diagnosis. Criteria are as follows:
      (1) Passive apposition of the thumbs to the flexor aspect of the forearms
      (2) Hyperextension of the fingers so that they lie parallel to the extensor aspect of the forearms
      (3) Hyperextension of the elbows above 10 degrees

      (4) Flexion of the trunk with the knees extended so that the palms rest on the floor

  c. Approximately 18% of girls and 9% of boys meet these criteria. There is often a family history of hypermobility, sometimes with similar pain. These children tend to be athletic and are often participants in sports requiring extreme mobility such as gymnastics and ballet.

2. Management is generally supportive: Stretching and strengthening exercises, intermittent doses of acetaminophen or NSAIDs. Withdrawal from activities is usually more disappointing to the patient than the pain, and thus not recommended. Maintain suspicion for disorders of collagen synthesis, such as Marfan's syndrome or Ehlers-Danlos syndrome.

FIBROMYALGIA

1. Definition, clinical features, and diagnosis
  a. Fibromyalgia is a syndrome of fatigue and diffuse musculoskeletal pains. It is usually idiopathic but may be preceded by trauma or a specific infection; it may coincide with other rheumatic conditions. There is also a strong association with sleep disturbances and affective disorders. Therefore fibromyalgia is best thought of as a syndrome with many causes, not as a specific disease.
  b. Diagnostic criteria have been devised by the American College of Rheumatology.
    (1) Widespread musculoskeletal pain is defined as follows:
      (a) Pain in axial distribution
      (b) Pain on the left and right sides of the body
      (c) Pain above and below the waist
    (2) Tenderness at 11 of 18 (9 pairs) specified tender points on moderate palpation with thumb or forefinger:
      (a) Insertion of nuchal muscles into the occiput
      (b) Mid-portion of the upper border of the trapezius
      (c) Muscle attachments to the upper medial border of the scapula
      (d) Anterior aspects of the C5 and C7 intertransverse spaces
      (e) Second rib space about 3 cm lateral to the sternal border
      (f) Muscle attachments to lateral epicondyle about 2 cm below bony prominence
      (g) Upper outer quadrant of gluteal muscles
      (h) Muscle attachments just posterior to greater trochanter
      (i) Medial fat pad of knee proximal to joint space
  c. Associated symptoms are fatigue, nonrestorative sleep, headache, irritable bowel, heat–cold intolerance and depression.

2. Management: General conditioning and strengthening will decrease pain and lead to a greater sense of well-being. Acetaminophen or NSAIDs may help intermittently but not over time. Low doses of tricyclic antidepressants (10% to 40% of doses used for depression) often restore the normal sleep pattern and lead to decreased pain.

3. Prognosis: Adult studies have suggested that fibromyalgia is a chronic condition. One pediatric study showed a more favorable outcome (75% remission after 30 months); this is likely to be the case in most children.

PATELLOFEMORAL SYNDROME (CHONDROMALACIA PATELLAE)

1. Definition, clinical features, and diagnosis
   a. This is a syndrome of anterior knee pain, with onset usually in adolescence and female predominance. Pain typically worsens with prolonged activity, stair descent, or prolonged knee flexion (e.g., sitting in a theater or class for long periods). Sometimes it is accompanied by small knee or suprapatellar effusions and associated with obesity or hypermobility.
   b. Diagnosis is based on history combined with physical findings:
      (1) Tenderness on patellar compression
      (2) Patellar grinding
      (3) Quadriceps wasting or asymmetry
      (4) Patellar inhibition sign: When relaxed, have patient flex the knee 5 to 10 degrees. Push downward and caudally on patella with your thumb and forefinger each bracing one side of the patella. As you are completing this maneuver, have the patient fully contract quadriceps muscles. If this maneuver elicits pain, the sign is positive.
   c. Radiographs, MRI, and arthroscopy are frequently used to diagnose this condition but are usually unnecessary.
2. Management: Isometric exercises of quadriceps femoris muscles are usually sufficient. Have the patient lie supine, lift the whole leg 10 to 12 inches off ground, hold up for about 10 seconds, and repeat. Start with 10 repetitions once a day and increase toward 20, twice daily. Then the patient can use 2- to 5-lb leg weights. NSAIDs or acetaminophen are sometimes helpful. Arthroscopic shaving and patellectomy are radical procedures for this condition and rarely, if ever, needed. Bracing of the knee is usually not helpful unless there is patellar instability.

REFLEX SYMPATHETIC DYSTROPHY

1. Definition, clinical features, and diagnosis
   a. This is a syndrome of pain and disuse of a limb accompanied by evidence of increased activity of the sympathetic nervous system.
   b. Classic findings are cutaneous hypersensitivity (e.g., extreme pain elicited even with very light touch), cool temperature, nonpitting edema, and mottled coloration. After weeks to months, trophic changes such as limb atrophy, fixed joint contractures, and increased hair growth may occur.
   c. There is often a history of minor trauma (out of proportion to the degree of pain and physical findings) or prolonged immobilization for another purpose (e.g., casting for fracture). Patients frequently have psychological stressors, most commonly depression, chaotic home situation, or an aversion to sports or physical education (remember, even if the child excels at a sport, she or he may hate it or feel an excessive pressure from parents or coaches to excel).
2. Management: Aggressive physical therapy over many months seems most helpful. The key to therapy is starting with an initial gentle desensitization phase (the affected extremity is exposed to various different

textures and temperatures), which will gradually lead to a decrease in the cutaneous hypersensitivity. Mobilization, then strengthening exercises follow. NSAIDs and tricyclic antidepressants in low doses may be helpful adjuncts.

SUGGESTED READING

Cassidy JT, Petty RE (eds): Textbook of Pediatric Rheumatology, 4th ed. Philadelphia, WB Saunders, 2001.

Jacobs JC: Pediatric Rheumatology for the Practitioner, 2nd ed. New York, Springer, 1992.

Laxer RM (ed): Pediatric rheumatology. Pediatr Clin North Am 52(2), 2005.

Pediatric Dermatology

13

Monika Upadhye Curlin, Priya Swamy Zeikus,
and Jennie J. Muglia

13.1 Introduction/Terminology

1. Lesions types: The terminology defined in the following not only is useful for making a diagnosis, it promotes accurate and effective communication between physicians.
   a. Macules: A circumscribed change in skin color without elevation or depression
   b. Papule: A solid elevated lesion 0.5 cm or less in diameter
   c. Plaque: A raised lesion that has a greater area compared with its elevation above the skin surface
   d. Wheal (hive): A rounded or flat-topped elevated lesion formed by local dermal edema
   e. Nodule: A palpable solid lesion of varying size, greater than 0.5 cm and less than 2 cm in diameter, that may be present in the epidermis, dermis, or subcutis
   f. Vesicle: A circumscribed elevated lesion 0.5 cm or less in diameter that contains free fluid. Bullae/blisters are fluid-filled vesicles.
   g. Pustule (abscess): A circumscribed elevated lesion that contains pus. An abscess is usually in the dermis or subcutis.
   h. Purpura: Nonblanching erythema or violaceous color due to extravasation of blood into the tissue
   i. Lichenification: Epidermis thickened and rough surfaced—almost like tree bark
2. Topical preparations
   a. Commonly used preparations are described. Ointments, gels, creams, and lotions contain varying amounts of water and oil.
      (1) Ointments: Essentially pure petroleum and thus ideal emollients with good skin penetration and adherence to surfaces
      (2) Gels: Semisolid systems consisting of a suspension interpenetrated by a liquid. Gels are compatible with many substances and may contain penetration enhancers for anti-inflammatory medications.
      (3) Creams: Consist of medicaments dissolved or suspended in water removable or emollient bases

(4) Lotions: Fluid suspensions or emulsions (mostly water) ideal for lubricating intertriginous areas between the fingers, thighs, and arms

b. Uses
(1) Ointment and gels for areas where skin is thick (palms, soles), lichenified, or severely involved
(2) Lotions and solutions for hairy areas or sensitive skin

13.2 Acne

1. Epidemiology
   a. Affects neonates and adolescents
   b. Neonatal acne is a self-limited condition during the first few months of life (Fig. 13-1, color insert).
   c. More than 80% of adolescents and young adults are affected by acne.
2. Pathophysiology and etiology
   a. Abnormal keratinization at the lower infundibulum of the hair follicle leads to plugging of the follicular duct. Impaction and distention of the duct give rise to open and closed comedones.
   b. Androgenic stimulation of the sebaceous glands at puberty increases sebum production.
   c. *Propionibacterium acnes* hydrolyzes sebum and secretes proinflammatory and chemotactic factors to attract neutrophils.
   d. The neutrophils release lysosomal enzymes, which lead to rupture of the follicle, causing inflammatory papules and pustules.
3. Clinical features
   a. The primary lesion of acne is the comedone, which can be open (blackhead) or closed (whitehead). Other lesions may include papules, pustules, and cysts.
   b. Distribution includes the face, chest, back, and shoulders, areas that have the largest numbers of sebaceous glands.
   c. Resolution of lesions can occur with dyspigmentation and indented or hypertrophic scarring.
4. Differential diagnosis includes folliculitis, keratosis pilaris, and miliaria.
5. Management (Table 13-1)
   a. Mild acne
      (1) Topical antibiotics
         (a) Clindamycin (solution, lotion, gel, foam)
         (b) Erythromycin (gel)
         (c) Sodium sulfacetamide (Sulfacet R)
      (2) Benzoyl peroxide agents—bactericidal and comedolytic
         (a) Gels, lotions, creams, and washes are available in concentrations of 2.5% to 10%.
         (b) Side effects: Irritation and pigmentary changes
         (c) Combinations of benzoyl peroxide and topical antibiotics: BenzaClin, Benzamycin
      (3) Topical retinoids—prevents follicular hyperkeratosis
         (a) Mainstay for the treatment of comedonal acne

Table 13-1	Therapeutic Modalities for Acne Vulgaris	
	Dose/Application	**Strengths**
Topical Agents		
Tretinoin	Once nightly	0.025%, 0.05%, 0.1% cream; 0.01%, 0.025% gel/ 0.05% liquid
Benzoyl peroxide	Once or twice daily	2.5%, 5%, 10% gel or wash
Erythromycin	Once daily	2% gel, liquid
Clindamycin	Once or twice daily	1% gel, liquid, lotion
Azelaic acid	Twice daily	20% cream
Adapalene	Once nightly	0.1% gel
Systemic Agents		
Tetracycline	250–500 mg PO twice daily	
Erythromycin	250–500 mg PO twice daily	
Minocycline	50–100 mg PO twice daily	
Doxycycline	100 mg PO once or twice daily	

PO, orally.

(b) Topical tretinoin (Retin A, Avita) available in cream, gel, in strengths of 0.025%, 0.05%, 0.1%; or Retin A Micro (0.04% or 0.1%)

(c) Adapalene (Differin) 0.1% gel or cream

(d) Tazarotene (Tazorac) 0.05%, 0.1% cream or gel

(e) Gels are useful for oily skin, but can be an irritant because of alcohol base.

(f) Use lowest strength initially, increasing to higher strength if comedones persist.

(g) Apply to very dry skin to avoid erythema and irritation. An amount the size of a pea is sufficient to cover the entire face.

(h) Combination of benzoyl peroxide plus a topical antibiotic and tretinoin is beneficial as a synergistic approach (e.g., BenzaClin + Retin A). Each agent should be applied separately at different times of the day because benzoyl peroxide agents can deactivate tretinoin.

(4) Other topical agents

(a) Salicylic acid: Comedolytic, found in many over-the-counter creams, washes, solutions

(b) Azelaic acid (Finacea, Azelex): Comedolytic, anti-inflammatory, and used for postinflammatory hyperpigmentation

b. Moderate acne—inflammatory or nodular acne (Fig. 13-2, color insert)

(1) Oral antibiotics—decrease inflammation and suppress P. acnes organisms

(a) Tetracycline, erythromycin, doxycycline, and minocycline
    (i) Tetracycline, doxycycline, and minocycline carry a risk of photosensitivity.
    (ii) Minocycline may cause blue-gray hyperpigmentation of the skin.
    (iii) Antibiotic therapy should be used for a minimum of 6 to 8 weeks before progress is evaluated.
(b) All antibiotics carry a risk of vulvovaginal candidiasis in female patients, and risk of decreased efficacy of the birth control pill. Gram-negative folliculitis, a sudden exacerbation of acne distributed around the nose, is a risk with oral therapy. Treatment of gram-negative folliculitis is with ampicillin or isotretinoin.
(2) Oral contraceptives: Ortho Tri-Cyclen
c. Severe nodulocystic acne (Fig. 13-3, color insert): isotretinoin
    (1) Most effective dose is 1 mg/kg/day, given as a 4- to 5-month course.
    (2) Most important side effect involves teratogenicity, seen in approximately 25% of women exposed to the drug during pregnancy. Extensive counseling and administration of contraceptives should be done in conjunction with a gynecologist.
    (3) Medication must be given only in 30-day supplies, with monthly serum β-human chorionic gonadotropin, complete blood cell count, liver function tests, and lipid profile before refills.
    (4) Side effects include elevation of triglycerides and cholesterol, hepatotoxicity, cheilitis and xerosis, night blindness, pseudotumor cerebri, alopecia, myalgias, and arthralgias.

13.3 Alopecia

1. Epidemiology
   a. Incidence of alopecia areata is 17.2 per 100,000 persons.
   b. The first attack usually occurs in patients younger than 25 years of age.
2. Pathophysiology and etiology
   a. There are two phases of hair growth: anagen (active growth) and telogen (resting phase).
   b. Disruption of either phase can result in alopecia.
   c. Alopecia can be described as nonscarring and scarring. In the pediatric population, nonscarring alopecia is more common.
   d. Causes of nonscarring alopecia include telogen effluvium, anagen effluvium, alopecia areata, and hair shaft abnormalities such as monilethrix, pill torti, and pili annulati.
   e. The more common causes of scarring alopecia include resolution of kerion and acne keloidalis.
3. Clinical features
   a. Telogen effluvium
      (1) Nonscarring alopecia associated with diffuse generalized hair loss with acute onset
      (2) Shift of hairs into telogen phase or the resting phase
      (3) Reactive process caused by severe illness, surgery, emotional stress, crash diets, pregnancy, or endocrine disease

(4) Time course between the stressful event and the loss of hair is approximately 3 months.
  b. Anagen effluvium
    (1) Sudden loss of anagen hair after a systemic insult such as chemotherapy or radiation therapy to the scalp
    (2) Examination of hair shafts reveals a preponderance of anagen hairs, or hairs in the active growth phase.
  c. Alopecia areata (Fig. 13-4, color insert)
    (1) Discrete, circumscribed, round patches of noninflammatory, nonscarring alopecia up to several centimeters in diameter
    (2) Common sites are the scalp, beard, eyebrows, and eyelashes. Valuable diagnostic clue is the presence of "exclamation-point hairs" (hair shafts tapered at the base) found at the periphery of the patches
  d. Hair shaft abnormalities such as pill torti, trichorrhexis nodosa, and monilethrix. Fragile hair shafts break easily because of abnormal hair structure.
4. Diagnosis and differential diagnosis
  a. Primary method of distinguishing between scarring and nonscarring alopecia is with skin biopsy.
  b. Diagnosis of alopecia in the pediatric population is often based on historical features.
  c. Diseases of the hair shaft often present as hair that does not grow to a desired length.
  d. Diagnosis is aided by light microscopy of plucked hair.
  e. Alopecia areata can be diagnosed by the presence of exclamation-point hairs at the periphery of the alopecia.
  f. Telogen effluvium and anagen effluvium are suggested if there is an underlying systemic insult.
  g. Differential diagnosis: Black-dot tinea should also be included in the differential diagnosis of alopecia areata, as well as trichotillomania (compulsion to pull one's hair out) and traction alopecia.
5. Management
  a. Telogen effluvium: Treatment (or removal, remediation) of underlying cause results in spontaneous regrowth.
  b. Alopecia areata: Options include topical minoxidil, tar preparations, anthralin, ultraviolet light therapy, and high-potency topical steroids or intralesional steroids once monthly.
    (1) Steroid use should be monitored closely because continued usage may produce scalp atrophy.
    (2) Many cases resolve spontaneously within 1 to 2 years.
  c. Hair shaft abnormalities: Treatment options are limited owing to the inherent defect in the hair structure. Avoidance of chemical processing, curling irons, and excessive brushing and combing may help minimize breakage.

13.4 Tinea Capitis

1. Epidemiology: Dermatophytic infection of the scalp with peak incidence in children aged 3 to 9 years

2. Pathophysiology and etiology
   a. Most common cause in children is a fungal infection with *Trichophyton tonsurans*.
   b. Person-to-person transmission and from fomites (combs, clothing, bedding, vinyl chairs, couches, toy bears, dolls, phone receivers)
3. Clinical features
   a. Red or skin-colored, scaly papules on the scalp associated with brittle hairs (Fig. 13-5, color insert)
   b. Pruritus may be present with alopecia in the affected areas.
   c. May progress to a kerion, which is a large, boggy inflammatory mass (possibly autoimmune) associated with scarring alopecia.
   d. Cervical lymphadenopathy may be present.
4. Diagnosis and differential diagnosis
   a. Potassium hydroxide preparations of plucked hair under the microscope show hyphae.
   b. Fungal culture of plucked hairs
   c. Woods lamp examination of scalp (certain fungal infections [*Microsporum* species] will cause infected hairs to fluoresce)
5. Management
   a. Ultramicrosize griseofulvin tablets 10 to 12 mg/kg/day or micronized griseofulvin suspension 15 mg/kg/day for 6 to 8 weeks
      (1) Administration with a fat-containing meal aids in absorption.
      (2) If child is healthy and therapy lasts less than 3 months, blood work is not needed.
   b. Terbinafine (Lamisil) tablets 3 to 6 mg/kg/day for 2 to 4 weeks
   c. Ketoconazole and itraconazole are second-line treatments.
   d. Selenium sulfide 2.5% shampoo can be used topically as an adjunct to systemic therapy.
   e. All household contacts should be treated with twice-weekly selenium sulfide shampoo to eradicate the carrier state (forming spores) and prevent reinfection.
   f. For kerion infection, prednisone 1 mg/kg/day is used in conjunction with griseofulvin until lesions clear.
   g. Antibiotics should be considered if regional lymphadenopathy persists.

13.5 Atopic Dermatitis

1. Epidemiology: Most common dermatologic disorder in childhood, affecting 10% to 20% of the pediatric population. Papulosquamous eruption seen in all pediatric age groups (Fig. 13-6, color insert).
2. Pathophysiology and etiology
   a. May be associated with atopic diatheses such as hay fever, allergies, asthma, or family history of atopy. Also associated with elevated immunoglobulin E (IgE) levels in response to triggering agents.
   b. Unknown etiology. Immunologic, genetic, physiologic, pharmacologic, and psychological factors may all contribute to the cause.
3. Clinical features
   a. Papulosquamous eruption: Scaling papules and plaques on the extensor surfaces of the extremities, face, and trunk (Fig. 13-7, color insert). Clinical presentation differs depending on age.

(1) *Infantile form*: Extensor surfaces are more affected than flexors. Truncal, facial, and scalp involvement is common, with sparing of the diaper area.

(2) *Early to middle childhood*: Flexural surfaces are more severely involved.

(3) *Late childhood and adolescence*: Lesions tend to be restricted to skin creases and hand dermatitis.

b. Markedly pruritic, often aggravated by bathing in hot water, contact with wool, or use of drying soaps.

c. Associated xerosis, with "atopic shiners" and hyperlinearity of the palms.

d. Complications include impetiginization due to *Staphylococcus aureus*, or eczema herpeticum due to superinfection with herpes simplex virus. Adjunct treatment is with antibiotics or oral acyclovir.

4. Diagnosis and differential diagnosis
   a. Contact dermatitis or irritant dermatitis
   b. If eczema is unremitting or associated with systemic illnesses such as infections and failure to thrive, consider immunologic disorders such as Bruton's agammaglobulinemia, Job's syndrome, Wiskott-Aldrich syndrome, and chronic granulomatous disease.
   c. Umbilicated vesicles should suggest the diagnosis of eczema herpeticum.

5. Management
   a. Removal of exacerbating agents, avoidance of hot water baths, use of mild soaps (Dove, Lever 2000), emollients, and cotton clothing
   b. Steroids: 1- to 2-week courses of low- to medium-potency topical steroids (Table 13-2)
      (1) Topical steroid preparations are grouped according to relative anti-inflammatory activity, but activity may vary considerably depending on the vehicle, the site of application, disease, the individual patient, and whether an occlusive dressing is used.
      (2) Side effects to prolonged use include atrophy of skin, telangiectases, and striae.
      (3) Application of even low-potency topical steroids to large areas of inflamed skin may result in systemic absorption.
      (4) Systemic or high-potency steroids should be used in consultation with a dermatologist.
   c. Lubrication is essential; parents should be instructed to apply creams or petrolatum-based products two to three times daily and to wet skin after bathing.
   d. Impetiginization (honey-colored crusting) is a sign of superinfection and should be treated with oral antibiotics such as dicloxacillin or cephalexin (Box 13-1).
   e. Antihistamines such as hydroxyzine 2 mg/kg/day or diphenhydramine 5 mg/kg/day in divided doses should be used around the clock to prevent scratching.
   f. Topical immunomodulators: tacrolimus (Protopic), pimecrolimus (Elidel)
      (1) Second-line agent to topical steroids

Table 13-2 Topical Steroid Potency

Generic Name	Brand Name	Strength
Low Potency		
Hydrocortisone	Cortate, Unicort, Cortisporin	0.5%, 1%, 2.5% cream, ointment, and lotion
Alclometasone dipropionate	Aclovate	0.05% cream and ointment
Betamethasone valerate	Betnovate, Celestoderm	0.05%, 0.1% cream
Betamethasone dipropionate	Diprosone	0.05% cream and ointment
Desoximetasone	Topicort	0.05% cream
Medium Potency		
Fluocinonide	Lidex, Lidemol	0.01%, 0.05% cream, ointment, and gel
Fluocinolone acetonide	Synalar, Synemol, Derma-Smooth	0.01%, 0.025%, 0.01% cream, solution, and ointment
Triamcinolone acetonide	Aristocort D, Aristocort R, Kenalog, Vicoderm-KC	0.025%, 0.1% cream, ointment
Betamethasone dipropionate	Propaderm, Diprosone, Diprolene Glycol	0.025%, 0.05% cream, ointment
Betamethasone dipropionate, augmented	Diprolene	0.05% cream
High Potency		
Desoximetasone	Topicort	0.25% cream and ointment; 0.05% gel
Fluocinolone acetonide	Synalar HP	0.2% cream
Halcinonide	Halog	0.1% cream, ointment
Triamcinolone acetonide	Aristocort A	0.5% cream and ointment
Betamethasone dipropionate, augmented	Diprolene	0.05% ointment and gel
Very High Potency		
Clobetasol propionate	Temovate	0.05% cream and ointment
Diflorasone diacetate	Psorcon	0.05% ointment
Halobetasol propionate	Ultravate	0.05% cream and ointment

> ### Box 13-1   Skin Care Products for Patients with Eczema
>
> *Cleansers:* Dove, Oil of Olay, Aveeno, Cetaphil bars, Aquanil liquids
> *Ointments:* Aquaphor, Vaseline
> *Creams:* Eucerin, Moisturel, Cetaphil
> *Lotions:* Eucerin, Moisturel, Cetaphil, Lubriderm

    (2) Short-term or intermittent therapy for moderate to severe atopic dermatitis in children older than 2 years who are unresponsive to conventional therapies
    (3) Potential concern for secondary malignancies

13.6 Allergic Contact Dermatitis/Rhus Dermatitis

1. Pathophysiology and etiology
   a. Allergic contact dermatitis is an example of a type IV hypersensitivity reaction. Development of lesions occurs within 48 to 72 hours after exposure to the antigen. Uncommon in children younger than 1 year of age. Should be considered in any linear or bizarrely shaped eczematous or vesicular eruption.
   b. Common contact allergens: nickel sulfate (belts, jewelry), Neomycin, balsam of Peru, fragrance mix, thimerosal, Bacitracin
   c. Rhus dermatitis is due to contact with poison ivy, oak, or sumac. It occurs after contact with the roots, leaves, or twigs of plants.
2. Clinical features
   a. Vesicular or eczematous eruption with sharply demarcated or linear borders (Figs. 13-8 and 13-9, color insert)
   b. Rhus dermatitis is characterized by linear pruritic vesicles, papules, or bullae.
3. Diagnosis and differential diagnosis
   a. The diagnosis is based on history and distribution of skin lesions.
   b. Skin biopsy can be nonspecific, and patch testing often is not done on the pediatric population.
4. Management
   a. Avoidance of the allergen
   b. Short course (2 weeks) of medium- to high-potency topical steroids
   c. Systemic steroids are reserved for cases involving the face or genitals or if large areas of the body are affected. Steroid course should cover 3 weeks to avoid a rebound phenomenon. A depot preparation of steroids (e.g., triamcinolone 60 to 120 mg intramuscular) can provide up to 3 weeks of effect but should be reserved only for the most severe cases.

13.7 Pigmented Birthmarks

CAFÉ AU LAIT MACULES

1. Epidemiology: Light brown macules found in 10% to 20% of the population
2. Clinical features: Lesions can occur at any site and may be up to 20 cm in diameter, with an even, light brown macular discoloration and presentation at birth (Fig. 13-10, color insert).
3. Diagnosis and differential diagnosis
   a. The diagnosis is usually by visual inspection.
   b. Differential diagnosis: Congenital nevus
      (1) Congenital nevus is usually darker and more raised, with terminal hairs.
      (2) Skin biopsy may be helpful in distinguishing these two entities.
   c. Associated diseases to exclude include neurofibromatosis (NF), tuberous sclerosis, and McCune-Albright syndrome.
      (1) NF type 1 (NF1): Major criterion for diagnosis is the presence of six or more café au lait macules greater than 0.5 cm diameter before puberty or greater than 1.5 cm diameter after puberty (Fig. 13-11, color insert).
4. Management
   a. There is no risk of malignant transformation in café au lait macules, and treatment is unnecessary.
   b. For known NF1 diagnosis, see Chapters 4 (Dysmorphology, Common Syndromes, and Genetic Counseling) and 20 (Neurologic Disorders).

MELANOCYTIC NEVI

1. Epidemiology: Most common neoplasm found in humans; occurs in 1% of neonates.
2. Pathophysiology and etiology
   a. Histologically, melanocytic nevi are composed of nests of melanocytes, referred to as *nevus cells*. There is a general transformation of nevus cell morphology, from epithelioid and rounded in the higher dermis, to spindle-shaped and elongated in the lower dermis.
   b. In general, junctional nevi are found more commonly in the pediatric population. In this subtype, nevus cells in nests are located at the dermoepidermal junction on biopsy.
3. Clinical features: Three categories of melanocytic nevi, based on the location of nevus cells in the skin
   a. *Junctional nevi* have nevus cells confined to the epidermis; they are macular and generally found in children (Fig. 13-12, color insert).
   b. *Compound nevi* can be found at birth but are more commonly seen in older children and adults. The nevus cells in this category are located at the dermoepidermal junction (Fig. 13-13, color insert).
   c. *Intradermal nevi* are seen in adults and are characterized by nevus cells entirely in the dermis (Fig. 13-14, color insert).
4. Diagnosis and differential diagnosis
   a. Melanocytic nevi can be confused with café au lait macules, lentigines, and mongolian spots.
   b. Diagnosis is most often by physical examination.

> ### Box 13-2   ABCDs of Melanoma
>
> Asymmetry
> Border irregularities
> Color variegation
> Diameter greater than 6 mm

5. Management
   a. Changes in lesions should be taken seriously and corresponding lesions excised.
   b. Lesions should be observed for ABCDs of melanoma (Box 13-2).
   c. Strict use of sunscreens (SPF 30) in children older than 6 months of age
   d. Management of congenital melanocytic nevi depends on the size of the lesion.
      (1) Small congenital nevi (<1.5 cm in diameter; Fig. 13-15, color insert)
          (a) Low (4.5%) risk of malignant transformation
          (b) Most cases of malignancy have occurred after puberty, so lesions can be observed clinically and excised after puberty.
      (2) Medium congenital nevi (lesions 1.5 to 20 cm in diameter)
          (a) No studies have demonstrated a definitive risk for progression to melanoma.
          (b) Larger lesions may be followed for changes, with prompt excision if changes arise.
      (3) Large or giant congenital melanocytic nevi (>20 cm in diameter; Fig. 13-16, color insert)
          (a) Approximately 10% lifetime risk for melanoma
          (b) These should be removed, but excisions require large-scale grafts.

VASCULAR BIRTHMARKS

1. Clinical features and pathophysiology
   a. Salmon patch (Fig. 13-17, color insert)
      (1) Flat, dull pink macule on the nape of the neck, glabella, forehead, upper eyelids, and nasolabial region. It is the most common vascular lesion of infancy ("stork bite").
      (2) Ninety-five percent of salmon patches (except those on the nuchal region) fade within the first year of life.
   b. Port-wine stain (Fig. 13-18, color insert)
      (1) Present at birth and persists throughout life, often with darkening or thickening over the years
      (2) The port-wine stain or nevus flammeus is a congenital malformation composed of dilated capillaries.
   c. Hemangioma (strawberry hemangioma; Fig. 13-19, color insert)
      (1) Hemangiomas are benign neoplasms composed of proliferating vascular endothelium. They are commonly seen on the head and neck as red to purple papules or nodules.

    (2) May present at birth but usually develop during the first few months of life.

    (3) Rapid growth during the first 6 months of life, most reaching their maximum growth by the first year

    (4) In 50% of cases, the hemangiomas disappear by 5 years of age; by 7 years, 70% of hemangiomas are resolved; and 90% of hemangiomas disappear by 9 years of age.

2. Diagnosis and differential diagnosis

  a. Sturge-Weber syndrome

    (1) Port-wine stains in the trigeminal (cranial nerve V-1) distribution or extending into the maxillary and mandibular regions

    (2) Clinical features include seizures, mental retardation, hemiplegia, and glaucoma.

  b. Klippel-Trenaunay-Weber syndrome

    (1) Extensive nevus flammeus of a limb with underlying venous varicosities

    (2) Bone and soft tissue hypertrophy of the affected limb

3. Management

  a. Salmon patch: Treatment is not necessary because most fade spontaneously.

  b. Hemangiomas

    (1) Ninety percent of hemangiomas disappear by 9 years of age.

    (2) Treatment is usually not necessary but often sought for cosmetic reasons.

    (3) Criteria for aggressive treatment include location (periorbital, auditory canal, pharynx, and larynx), rapid growth rate, ulceration, hemorrhage, infection, or Kasabach-Merritt syndrome (consumptive coagulopathy most often seen with larger and deeper lesions).

      (a) Intralesional corticosteroid therapy for discrete, smaller lesions, or oral prednisone in a dosage of 1 to 2 mg/kg/day for 7 weeks, with gradual taper.

      (b) Other modalities include surgery, laser treatment, and sclerosing, but conservative therapy is most often recommended.

13.8 Diaper Dermatitis

1. Pathophysiology and etiology: Multifactorial in etiology

  a. Friction (Fig. 13-20, color insert)

  b. Irritant or allergic dermatitis due to contact with harsh soaps, detergents, or topical medications

  c. Moisture or urinary wetness increases skin pH, leading to increased permeability to irritants.

2. Clinical features

  a. Localized to the convex areas exposed to the wet diaper ("napkin dermatitis").

  b. Sparing of intertriginous areas

  c. Skin is erythematous with shiny or glazed appearance.

  d. Erosions or ulcerations are present in severe cases.

3. Differential diagnosis

  a. Seborrheic dermatitis .

        (1) Salmon-colored greasy plaques with yellow scale

        (2) Examining for other sites of involvement (scalp, face, neck, flexural folds, and postauricular region) may help make diagnosis.

    b. Cutaneous candidiasis (Fig. 13-21, color insert)

        (1) Beefy red plaques on the lower abdomen, inner aspects of the thighs, and buttocks

        (2) Pinpoint satellite pustules and papules aid in diagnosis.

        (3) *Candida* can superinfect all intertriginous rashes.

    c. Other differential diagnoses: Dermatophyte infection, psoriasis, congenital syphilis, Letterer-Siwe disease, and acrodermatitis enteropathica

4. Management

    a. Areas must be kept dry and clean.

    b. Limit use of occlusive plastic diapers or macerating agents such as talc.

    c. Frequent diaper changes with thorough cleansing and drying of skin

    d. Topical steroids should be minimized in the intertriginous region to avoid cutaneous atrophy and striae.

    e. Low-potency agent such as hydrocortisone 1% should be used for 5 to 7 days only.

    f. Associated candidiasis should be treated with clotrimazole or ketoconazole cream.

    g. If candidiasis is resistant to topical therapy, a course of oral nystatin (200,000 U four times a day) for 1 week may be helpful.

13.9 Lice (Pediculosis)

1. Pathophysiology and etiology

    a. Acquired by person-to-person contact

    b. Three varieties of lice attack humans: *Pediculus humanus* var. *capitis* (the head louse), *Pediculus humanus* var. *corporis* (the body louse), and *Pthirus pubis* (the crab louse).

2. Clinical features: The hallmark for all types is pruritus.

    a. Pediculosis capitis (head lice) is the most common form of louse infestation.

        (1) Can occur on the scalp or eyelids, with transmission by the sharing of combs, brushes, and headgear.

        (2) Nits or eggs are visible along the hair shaft (a Woods lamp aids in visualization).

    b. In pediculosis corporis (body lice), the parasite lives in clothing or bedding, and is rarely observed on the skin. The primary lesion is a pinpoint red papule with central hemorrhagic punctum.

    c. Pediculosis pubis (crab or pubic lice) can occur on the pubic area, as well as the eyebrows and eyelashes of children.

3. Diagnosis and differential diagnosis

    a. Microscopy or visualization of the lice is usually diagnostic.

    b. Differential includes scabies, eczema, and contact dermatitis.

4. Management

    a. Pediculosis capitis (head lice)

        (1) Pyrethrins such as RID or 1% permethrin (Nix) cream rinse. Both available on an over-the-counter basis. Head should be

shampooed and pyrethrins or permethrin rinse should be applied for 10 minutes. Use fine-toothed comb to remove the nits. Repeat in 7 days.
(2) Lindane (Kwell) is a second-line agent used only if there is no response to permethrin or pyrethrins. Treatment has been associated with seizures.
(3) Alternative treatment is suffocation of lice by application of petroleum jelly to cover scalp for 24 hours.
(4) Bed sheets and clothing are cleaned, with particular attention to the seams of clothing. Combs and brushes should be soaked in the pediculicide for 15 minutes.
b. Pediculosis corporis (body lice): Eradication occurs with washing clothing in hot water or storing clothes for at least 2 weeks (starving louse). Lindane may be used to eradicate any lice on body hair.
c. Pediculosis pubis (crab or pubic lice)
(1) Permethrin or pyrethrins for 10 minutes, with concomitant treatment of sexual partners
(2) Involvement of the eyelids may be treated with petrolatum jelly twice daily for 1 week, followed by mechanical removal of the nits.
(3) Screen patient for common sexually transmitted diseases or signs of sexual abuse.

13.10 Scabies

1. Epidemiology
   a. Occurs in any age group, race, or socioeconomic class
   b. Epidemics can occur in institutions such as group homes or colleges.
2. Pathophysiology and etiology: Caused by the eight-legged mite *Sarcoptes scabiei* var. *hominis*
3. Clinical features
   a. Intensely pruritic exanthem, with linear burrows, and pink-encrusted papules on the wrists, trunk, extremities, and finger webs (Fig. 13-22, color insert)
   b. Small children and infants often have extensive involvement of the face, palms, and soles, with blisters in some cases. Older children and adolescents rarely have facial involvement.
   c. Lesions can become impetiginized (superinfected secondary excoriations).
   d. Secondary "Id" (hypersensitivity to mite components) reaction can occur, characterized by extensive erythematous papules.
4. Diagnosis and differential diagnosis
   a. Physical examination and identification of the female mite under mineral oil microscopy
   b. Burrow should be scraped and evaluated for the characteristic eggs, mite, or feces. Negative scrapings in children are common, and should not dissuade from treating.
5. Management
   a. 5% permethrin cream (Elimite)
   (1) Treatment should include an 8- to 12-hour application to the neck and body for young children, adding the head and scalp

for infants. Palms, soles, umbilicus, and subungual regions must also be treated.

(2) Applications may be repeated in 1 to 2 weeks.

(3) Precipitated sulfur (6%) in a petrolatum base can be applied twice a day for 5 days for infants younger than 2 months of age.

(4) Pruritus and rash may take several weeks to resolve, and should not be treated again with antiscabietics unless advised by a physician.

b. Close personal contacts should be treated, and clothing and linen should be washed in warm water. Because the incubation time for scabies infection is up to 1 month, all family members and sexual partners, regardless of symptoms, should be treated.

13.11 Molluscum Contagiosum

1. Pathophysiology and etiology
   a. Common disorder caused by a poxvirus
   b. Spread with the simple skin-to-skin contact of children, but sexual transmission can also occur
   c. Autoinoculation due to scratching can lead to extensive lesions in children with atopic dermatitis.
2. Clinical features: Discrete or multiple, flesh-toned or pink, umbilicated, dome-shaped, waxy papules on the face, trunk, and extremities (Fig. 13-23, color insert). The papules may range from 1 mm to 1 cm in size.
3. Diagnosis is based on clinical appearance.
4. Management
   a. Medication: 35% trichloroacetic acid. Tretinoin 0.025% cream or adapalene (Differin) cream or gel every day may be better tolerated for lesions on the groin or the face.
   b. Other: Cryotherapy or curettage
   c. Some lesions spontaneously resolve.

13.12 Warts (Verrucae)

1. Epidemiology: Common in children and adolescents, with a peak incidence at 10 to 19 years of age.
2. Pathophysiology and etiology
   a. Caused by viral infection with the human papillomavirus of the papova group
   b. Inoculation occurs from direct or indirect contact. Small breaks in the skin can lead to inoculation.
3. Clinical features
   a. Verrucae vulgaris (common warts) affect dorsal digits or periungual regions (Fig. 13-24, color insert).
   b. Verrucae plantaris (plantar warts) affect the plantar surfaces of the feet and are very uncomfortable to walk on.
   c. Verrucae plana or flat warts occur on the face, neck, arms, and legs. Irritation from shaving can lead to spread on the legs of women or the beard area of men.
   d. Linear lesions can occur because of autoinoculation from picking or scratching.

4. The diagnosis of warts is based on physical examination.
5. Management
   a. Medical
      (1) Cantharidin (blister beetle extract)
      (2) Salicylic acid/lactic acid preparations
         (a) Over-the-counter preparations include Wart-Off, Duofilm, Compound W.
         (b) Forty percent salicylic acid plasters (Mediplast) may be used for larger plantar warts.
      (3) Cryotherapy
      (4) Cimetidine: For extensive or resistant cases; increases T-cell response to verrucae in children (35 to 40 mg/kg for 1 to 2 months).
   b. Surgical: Laser ablation or surgical excision, along with topical application of bichloracetic acid
   c. Other: Warm-water soaks followed by paring down warts with a pumice stone or emery board; duct tape completely covering the wart for several weeks is safe and inexpensive. The power of suggestion, "charming the wart," can be very effective in susceptible individuals.

13.13 Erythema Multiforme

1. Epidemiology: The true incidence of erythema multiforme (EM) is unknown. EM minor accounts for 80% of all cases of EM; however, only 20% of EM minor cases occur in childhood. EM major (i.e., Stevens-Johnson syndrome), although much less common overall, is more likely to occur in children.
2. Pathophysiology and etiology: Hypersensitivity disorder to a number of entities, most commonly herpes simplex virus or medications
3. Clinical features
   a. EM minor
      (1) Annular or targetoid lesions occurring acrally, with palms and soles most often involved (Fig. 13-25, color insert). Lesions may extend to the trunk, face, and neck. Lesions in various stages of change can be seen (i.e., papules, vesicles, target erythema). Lesions may also become vesiculobullous with time.
      (2) One mucous membrane area may be involved, with ulcerations predominant.
      (3) Eruptions last about 1 week, although recurrences are common with the herpes simplex–induced cases.
      (4) Systemic manifestations are rare.
   b. EM major (Stevens-Johnson syndrome)
      (1) Systemic manifestations include high fever, constitutional symptoms, and bullae.
      (2) Two or more mucous membrane areas are involved with bullae and overlying hemorrhagic crust.
      (3) Causative agents more likely to be drugs or *Mycoplasma* infection.

4. Differential diagnosis
    a. Toxic epidermal necrolysis (TEN): Tenderness limited to the erythematous area
    b. Staphylococcal scalded skin syndrome: Fever, malaise, and generalized macular erythema that quickly progresses to diffuse exfoliation; diffusely tender skin (contrast to limited tenderness in TEN); radial fissures around the mouth; watch for in children younger than 5 years of age.
5. Management
    a. Supportive treatment in uncomplicated EM minor cases
    b. Patients with extensive mucosal and skin lesions require management of fluid-electrolyte balance to replace insensible water loss from denuded areas of skin.
    c. Systemic corticosteroids (prednisone 1 to 2 mg/kg/day in two doses) are controversial because no adequate studies show a positive effect on outcome. Advocates of steroid therapy agree that they must be administered very early in the course of the disease to be of benefit.
    d. EM major (Stevens-Johnson syndrome) is a life-threatening illness that usually requires treatment in a burn unit facility.

13.14 Pityriasis Rosea

1. Epidemiology: Peak incidence in adolescents and young adults
2. Pathophysiology and etiology: Acute, benign, self-limiting eruption. A viral etiology has been proposed (human herpes virus types 6 and 7), but not proved.
3. Clinical features
    a. Starts with the herald patch, an annular scaling plaque, located on the upper arms, trunks, or neck
    b. Prodromal symptoms of fever and malaise nay appear before development of herald patch.
    c. After 5 to 10 days, an exanthem appears consisting of groups of round or oval, salmon-colored to pink, scaling papules and plaques distributed in a "Christmas tree" pattern on the trunk (Fig. 13-26, color insert).
    d. Many lesions have a cigarette-paper–like collarette of scale in the central aspect.
    e. Papular variant or inverse pityriasis rosea, with lesions distributed on the face, wrists, and extremities, can also be seen in children.
    f. Pruritus can be an associated symptom.
    g. Lesion can be intensified by heat (bathing, sun exposure).
4. Diagnosis and differential diagnosis: Diagnosis is based on clinical examination, and a history of herald patch is helpful to confirm.
5. Management
    a. Treatment not required
    b. Spontaneous resolution usually in 8 weeks
    c. Treatment of pruritus can be provided with Sarna lotion, pramoxine lotions, antihistamines, or ultraviolet B phototherapy.
    d. Low- to medium-potency topical steroids may be used for pruritus for 2 weeks.

WEBSITES

American Academy of Dermatology: www.aad.org
DermNet NZ: www.dermnetnz.org
Dermatology Image Atlas: www.dermatlas.com
eMedicine: www.emedicine.com

Hematologic/ Oncologic Disorders 14

Christopher Paul Keuker and Edwin N. Forman

14.1 Red Blood Cell Disorders

HEMOGLOBINOPATHY

1. Etiology and pathophysiology: Hemoglobinopathies are red blood cell (RBC) disorders caused by variations in the molecular structure of hemoglobin. The predominant hemoglobin after infancy is hemoglobin A, composed of two α-globin chains and two β-globin chains. More than 500 hemoglobin variants have been described. Depending on the location of the structural alteration in the hemoglobin molecule, hemoglobinopathies can result in polymerization or crystallization of hemoglobin molecules, gross molecular instability with hemoglobin precipitation (Heinz bodies), or changes in oxygen affinity.

2. Clinical features: Most hemoglobin variants, with the exception of Hb S (see Sickle Cell Syndromes), have no physical or functional abnormalities. Other common hemoglobin variants, including C, E, and D-Los Angeles, are all stable structural variants of the β-globin chains.

THALASSEMIA

1. Etiology and pathophysiology: Thalassemia ("the sea in the blood") is a disorder caused by abnormal hemoglobin production. Specifically, the α- or β-globin chains of hemoglobin molecules are not produced because of a mutation in the gene encoding the globin chains. This mutation in the α- or β-globin gene cluster inhibits gene expression. The basic RBC defect is imbalanced globin chain synthesis, resulting in ineffective erythropoiesis and intracellular precipitation of excess α- or β-globin chains.

   a. Molecular pathology: Deletions in one or more of the four α-globin genes on chromosome 16 result in α-thalassemia; point mutations in one or both β-globin genes on chromosome 11 result in β-thalassemia.

   b. Prevalence: α-Thalassemia 1 is the most common in Southeast Asia and Mediterranean. α-Thalassemia 2 is the most common in Africa, the Mediterranean region, the Middle East, throughout Southeast Asia, and parts of the Indian subcontinent. $\beta^{0/+}$-Thalassemia mutations are distributed predominantly in the Mediterranean region and parts

of Africa, the Middle East, the Indian subcontinent, and Southeast Asia.
2. Clinical features: The clinical and laboratory expression or phenotype varies among the different thalassemia syndromes (Table 14-1). Microcytic anemia is the common finding in thalassemia. Peripheral blood smear may show target cells, polychromasia, nucleated RBCs, and basophilic stippling.
3. Management (thalassemia intermedia and major)
   a. Hypertransfusion therapy to keep hemoglobin (Hb) above 11.0 g/dL and reduce hematopoiesis
   b. Chelation therapy when indicated for iron overload
   c. Splenectomy after 5 years of age (or sooner, after the age of 2 years, if sequelae are severe) to reduce transfusion requirements after splenic removal and breakdown of the abnormal thalassemia RBCs
   d. Antibiotics: prevention and treatment of postsplenectomy sepsis and infections

RED BLOOD CELL MEMBRANE DEFECT: HEREDITARY SPHEROCYTOSIS

1. Etiology and pathophysiology: Hereditary spherocytosis (HS) is a corpuscular hemolytic anemia caused by a primary defect or deficiency of a specific red cell skeletal protein (ankyrin, Band 3, α- or β-spectrin, or pallidin), resulting in RBC membrane loss and decreased cell surface-to-volume ratio. HS usually shows autosomal dominant inheritance, although autosomal recessive inheritance and spontaneous mutations

Syndrome	Major (Onset in Infancy)	Intermedia (Later Onset)	Minor (Asymptomatic)
Clinical			
Splenomegaly	++++	+++ – ++++	0–+
Jaundice	+++	+–+++	0–+
Skeletal changes	++++	++–++++	0
Transfusion	+–+++	0–+	0
Hematologic			
Anemia (Hb)	<7	7–10	>10
RBC count	↓	↓	N–↑
Microcytosis	+	+	+
Nucleated RBC	++–++++	+–+++	0
RBC morphology	++++	++	+
Biochemical			
HbF	10%–95%+	10%–95%+	N or <10%
HbA$_2$	N or ↑	N or ↑	N or ↑ (>3.5%)

Hb, hemoglobin; RBC, red blood cell.
Modified from Pearson HA, Berman LC, Crocker AC (eds): Thalassemia intermedia: A region I conference. Arlington, Va, National Center for Education in Maternal and Child Health, 1997.

exist; it is most common in people of northern European descent, with a frequency of 1 in 5000 in this population. The pathophysiology of HS is sequestration and destruction, in splenic sinusoids, of poorly deformable "spherocytic red cells."

2. Clinical features: HS is usually diagnosed before puberty from a family history or as part of a work-up for secondary anemia or jaundice (most cases have a history of neonatal hyperbilirubinemia). It may rarely present as symptomatic gallstones in childhood.

3. Laboratory findings
   a. The presence of hyperchromatic spherostomatocytes ("microspherocytes") on peripheral blood smear
   b. Increased RBC osmotic fragility secondary to decreased RBC surface area and an inherent increased membrane permeability to sodium and potassium

4. Management
   a. Splenectomy is universally "curative" of HS. In severe HS cases, splenectomy after the age of 3 years (preferably after 5 years of age) is recommended to reduce the morbidity associated with chronic severe anemia.
   b. Vaccinations: Splenectomized patients should receive *Haemophilus influenzae* type B and pneumococcal vaccinations 2 weeks before splenectomy procedure.
   c. Chemoprophylaxis: Splenectomized patients with HS should receive chemoprophylaxis for pneumococcal sepsis with penicillin (125 mg two times a day for children younger than 3 years of age; 250 mg two times a day for children 3 years of age and older), given until 17 years of age or at least 1 year after splenectomy. Folate supplementation (1 mg every day) is also recommended.

5. Clinical complications
   a. Aplastic crisis: Dramatic and sudden fall in hemoglobin concentration associated with arrest of marrow red cell production; most important clinical complication of HS; frequently associated with parvovirus B19 infection
   b. Hemolytic crisis: Transient increase in hemolysis and jaundice; usually precipitated by infection
   c. Pigment gallstone: Increased incidence with age
   d. Folate deficiency: Increased marrow utilization secondary to increased RBC turnover

RED BLOOD CELL ENZYME DEFECTS

Glucose-6-phosphate dehydrogenase (G6PD) deficiency and pyruvate kinase (PK) deficiency account for over 97% of all cases of RBC enzyme defects in childhood.

1. G6PD deficiency: G6PD is an enzyme of the pentose phosphate pathway of glucose metabolism. Deficiency decreases the reductive energy (decreased nicotinamide adenosine dinucleotide phosphate [NADPH] and glutathione) of RBCs, resulting in hemolysis, which is exacerbated by exposure to oxidative agents. Inherited in a sex-linked recessive mode, it is found most frequently in blacks, populations of Mediterranean ancestry, and certain Chinese and Southeast Asian populations.

Box 14-1   Major Drugs Known to Induce Hemolysis
in G6PD Deficiency

Antimalarial drugs: pamaquine, pentaquine, primaquine
Sulfonamides and sulfones: Azulfidine, Bactrim, Dapsone, Gantrisin,
   Pediazole, Septra, sulfacetamide
Other antibacterial drugs: chloramphenicol, Macrodantin
Analgesics/antipyretics: aspirin, probenecid, Pyridium
Miscellaneous: dimercaprol (BAL), hydralazine, methylene blue,
   naphthalene (moth balls), synthetic substitutes for vitamin K

G6PD deficiency commonly presents as episodes of acute hemolytic anemia ("crisis") produced by drugs (Box 14-1), fava beans, or infection; it may uncommonly present as a chronic nonspherocytic hemolytic anemia. Acute drug-induced hemolytic anemia is a normocytic, normochromic anemia with degmacytes ("bite cells") and Heinz bodies on peripheral smear; reticulocytosis and hemoglobinuria are prominent. Diagnosis is made by measuring G6PD activities in blood. Management includes removal of the oxidizing agent or infection; hemolytic crisis in patients with G6PD deficiency is usually self-limited.

2. PK deficiency: Deficiency of PK in RBCs causes reduced adenosine triphosphate (ATP) levels, resulting in increased cation permeability of the RBC and osmotic loss of intracellular water with resulting autohemolysis. PK deficiency is inherited in an autosomal recessive mode; it is less common than G6PD deficiency. Severity is variable. Affected patients present with anemia and jaundice; peripheral blood smear shows contracted, crenated RBCs (echinocytes), polychromasia, and occasionally macrocytosis; reticulocytosis is prominent; splenomegaly may be present. Diagnosis is made by measuring PK activity in blood. Management includes supportive transfusion therapy and folic acid supplementation; splenectomy may be indicated in patients with increased transfusion requirement.

IMMUNE HEMOLYTIC ANEMIA: AUTOIMMUNE HEMOLYTIC ANEMIA

1. Etiology and pathophysiology: Autoimmune hemolytic anemia (AIHA) is a rare extracorpuscular hemolytic anemia caused by the action of autoimmunoglobulins on the RBC membrane antibodies, usually of the immunoglobulin G (IgG) class or IgM associated with cold agglutinins. Most cases of AIHA in childhood are secondary to an acute infection, usually mild and involving the upper respiratory tract (e.g., Mycoplasma pneumoniae or Epstein-Barr virus [EBV] infection). Other cases are idiopathic or related to drugs and chemicals (penicillins, sulfonamides, cephalosporins, acetaminophen, ibuprofen, insecticides), immunizations, neoplasia, hematologic disorders, collagen-vascular disorders, and immune-based disorders (Evan's syndrome).

2. Clinical features: Onset is sudden with pallor, malaise, and jaundice with dark urine; splenomegaly with or without hepatomegaly may be seen.
3. Laboratory findings: These include normocytic, normochromic anemia (Hb may be under 6 g/dL), with reticulocytosis; positive direct Coombs' test; hyperbilirubinemia; decreased haptoglobin. The peripheral blood smear is noted for prominent microspherocytosis and polychromatophilia. Hemoglobinuria (and increased urobilinogen), neutropenia, and thrombocytopenia may occasionally be found.
4. Management: Although many cases of AIHA require no treatment, some may be severe and life-threatening (platelet count <5000), requiring immediate medical treatment with high-dose corticosteroids (2 to 10 mg/kg/day of prednisone with taper). Splenectomy may be indicated in patients with persistent hemolysis not controlled by other therapies.

14.2 White Blood Cell Disorders

SEVERE CHRONIC NEUTROPENIA

1. Definition: Severe chronic neutropenia (SCN) comprises a heterogeneous group of diseases characterized by an absolute neutrophil count (ANC) under 500/mm³. SCN may be congenital (present in the first 4 weeks of life) or acquired, and may be a primary disorder or associated with an underlying disorder or syndrome. SCN should be suspected in a child with documented severe neutropenia and history of recurrent infections.
2. Clinical features: Symptoms depend on the severity and duration of neutropenia; patients may complain of fever and malaise; findings include aphthous stomatitis, pharyngitis, otitis media, respiratory infections, cellulitis, and perianal abscesses; bacterial infections (staphylococcal, streptococcal) are most common; opportunistic (fungal, yeast, parasites) and viral infections occur infrequently; leukemic transformation is reported.
3. Types of SCN
   a. Severe congenital neutropenia (Kostmann's syndrome), present at birth
   b. Cyclic neutropenia: ANC oscillates from normal (>2000/mm³) to near zero, with a typical cycle length of 21 days.
   c. Autoimmune neutropenia: Neutropenia in the first 2 years of life, with recovery usually by age 4 years; serum neutrophil-specific antibody assays may be positive.
   d. Glycogen storage disease type 1b: A metabolic disorder cause by a defect in glucose-6-phosphate transport; with short stature, hepatosplenomegaly, and hypoglycemia. Neutropenia severity is variable.
4. Diagnosis
   a. SCN as a clinical entity may be defined as an ANC <500/mm³ on at least three occasions in a 3-month period that is not drug-induced.
   b. Serial complete blood counts (CBCs) with differentials; CBCs should be taken three times per week for at least 6 weeks if cyclic neutropenia is suspected.
   c. Serum antineutrophil antibody testing, if available

    d. Bone marrow aspiration/trephine biopsy with cytogenetic and molecular testing

5. Management
   a. Identification and treatment with broad-spectrum antibiotics of infection and fever
   b. Granulocyte colony-stimulating factor (G-CSF) titrated to maintain ANC at 1500 to 10,000/mm^3; median dose range 3 to 12 µg/kg/day
   c. Bone marrow transplantation

TRANSIENT NEUTROPENIA

1. Drug-induced neutropenia: Many drugs and chemicals (Box 14-2) may cause severe neutropenia (ANC <200/mm^3) as a result of dose-dependent suppression of granulocytosis or an idiosyncratic reaction; onset of neutropenia is usually 7 to 14 days after exposure and duration is variable. Treatment is removal of the offending drug or chemical; G-CSF may be used to shorten duration of neutropenia.

2. Infection-associated neutropenia: Neutropenia with or without low total white blood cell (WBC) count may develop during the first 2 days of an infection (Box 14-3) and may last for 1 to 2 weeks (median, 8 days; range, 7 to 44 days). The cause of neutropenia is not clear, but an alteration in the distribution of neutrophils (margination), aggregation, or microbial destruction are suspected. The clinical course of neutropenia is generally benign; the development of secondary bacterial infection or fungal infection is uncommon. Empirical treatment with broad-spectrum antibiotics is not indicated.

Box 14-2   Drugs and Chemicals Causing Neutropenia

Analgesics and nonsteroidal anti-inflammatory drugs (aminopyrine,* ibuprofen, indomethacin, acetaminophen)

Antibiotics (penicillins, cephalosporins, gentamicin, clindamycin, antimalarials)

Anticonvulsant drugs (phenytoin, carbamazepine)

Antihistamines (cimetidine, ranitidine)

Antimetabolites* (6-mercaptopurine, methotrexate)

Antipsychotic, sedative, antidepressant drugs (chlorpromazine,* imipramine)

Cardiovascular drugs (nifedipine, propranolol, thiazides)

Cytotoxic drugs* (cyclophosphamide)

Hair dyes

Heavy metals (gold, arsenic)

Metoclopramide

Penicillamine

Sulfonamides* (sulfamethoxazole, sulfasalazine)

---

*Most frequently associated with agranulocytosis

> ### Box 14-3 Infections Associated with Secondary Neutropenia
>
> Viral infection—adenovirus, coxsackievirus, Epstein-Barr virus, hepatitis (A and B), influenza, measles, mumps, respiratory syncytial virus, retrovirus (human immunodeficiency virus), rubella
> Bacterial infection—brucellosis, malaria, rickettsiosis, tuberculosis, typhoid, overwhelming bacterial sepsis

CHRONIC GRANULOMATOUS DISEASE

1. Etiology and pathophysiology: Chronic granulomatous disease is caused by gene mutations resulting in a defect in one of the components of NADPH oxidase. This results in the inability of neutrophils, eosinophils, and monocytes to produce a respiratory burst. There are both X-linked (60%) and autosomal recessive (40%) variants.
2. Epidemiology: Incidence in the United States is 1/200,000 to 250,000 people.
3. Clinical features: See Box 14-4.
4. Diagnosis: Laboratory tests include nitroblue tetrazolium slide test, direct genetic testing of patient and family members, and dihydrorhodamine flow cytometry
5. Management includes early and aggressive treatment of infections, antimicrobial prophylaxis (Bactrim and itraconazole 5 to 10 mg/kg/day), interferon gamma, and possible bone marrow transplantation.

> ### Box 14-4 Clinical Findings Associated with Chronic Granulomatous Disease
>
> Unusual catalase-positive infections (*Staphylococcus*, gram-negative enteric bacteria, *Pseudomonas*, yeast, fungi)
> Recurrent suppurative lymphadenitis
> Recurrent fungal or bacterial pneumonia
> Abscesses of liver, spleen, lung, brain
> Perianal or perirectal abscesses
> Multifocal osteomyelitis
> Purulent skin and scalp infections
> Granulomas of skin, gastrointestinal and genitourinary tracts
> Diarrhea secondary to enteritis
> Ulcerative stomatitis
> Rash of ears and nares
> Family history of recurrent infections

EOSINOPHILIA

Reactive eosinophilia is a benign reaction to a disease process. In pediatrics, allergy is the most common cause of reactive eosinophilia. An acronym for conditions in which eosinophilia is common is **NAACP**.

> **N**eoplasm: Hodgkin's lymphoma, non-Hodgkin's lymphoma, myeloproliferative disorders
>
> **A**llergy: Asthma, hay fever, urticaria, drug hypersensitivity, atopic dermatitis, eczema, irritable bowel disease, milk precipitin disease
>
> **A**spergillosis: Bronchopulmonary *Aspergillus* infection, rarely other fungal infections
>
> **C**ollagen-vascular disease: Rheumatoid arthritis, Goodpasture's syndrome, sarcoidosis, periarteritis nodosa
>
> **P**arasitic disease: Helminths (*Ascaris, Trichinella spiralis, Toxocara canis* with levels >50,000/mm^3), protozoa (*Plasmodium, Toxoplasma, Pneumocystis*)

14.3 Platelet Disorders

THROMBOCYTOPENIA

1. Definition: *Thrombocytopenia* is defined as a platelet count under 150,000/mm^3.
2. Etiology and pathophysiology: Thrombocytopenia is a result of a disorder causing increased platelet destruction (thrombolytic thrombocytopenia), decreased platelet production, or platelet trapping/sequestration. The risk of bleeding usually correlates with the degree of thrombocytopenia (Box 14-5).
3. Types of thrombocytopenia
   a. Immune thrombocytopenic purpura (ITP)
      (1) Etiology and pathophysiology
         (a) Thrombocytopenia mediated by autoantibodies that specifically bind to epitopes on the platelet membrane, resulting in their rapid destruction or removal from circulation by the reticuloendothelial system (spleen, liver). This is the most frequent cause of thrombolytic thrombocytopenia.
         (b) The majority of cases of ITP are associated with an antecedent viral illness (upper respiratory infection, varicella,

---

> **Box 14-5 Degree of Thrombocytopenia and Bleeding Risk**
>
> <90,000/mm^3: Bleeding increased with contact sports and surgical procedures
> 50,000 to 90,000/mm^3: Increased bruising with known trauma
> 20,000 to 50,000/mm^3: Spontaneous bruising, bleeding from mucous membranes
> <20,000/mm^3: Petechiae, very rare occurrence of serious bleeding
> <12,000/mm^3: Rare occurrence of serious bleeding, including intracranial hemorrhages

cytomegalovirus [CMV], EBV, hepatitis, measles, mumps, rubella, rubeola); rare cases are associated with recent measles vaccination, bacterial infection, and drug use (valproic acid and other antiseizure medications, antibiotics, analgesics, sedatives, hypnotics); some cases are secondary to human immunodeficiency virus (HIV) infection, systemic lupus erythematosus (SLE), and other connective tissue diseases.

   (c) Childhood ITP (<10 years of age) affects both sexes equally, with an incidence of about 6 cases per 100,000 children per year; the peak age for the diagnosis of ITP is 2 to 6 years.

(2) Clinical features: ITP is typically characterized by rapid onset of bleeding symptoms in a generally healthy child; in 50% to 80% of cases, there is a history of a recent viral illness (usually upper respiratory infection) within 3 weeks before the onset of thrombocytopenia.

   (a) Purpura of the skin (ecchymoses and petechiae) and mucous membranes ("oozing" and petechiae) are common at onset.

   (b) Bleeding from the nose, gums, gastrointestinal (GI) tract, and kidneys (hematuria), and conjunctival hemorrhages can be present. Menorrhagia may occur in adolescent girls.

   (c) Splenomegaly is not present.

(3) Laboratory findings

   (a) A CBC shows thrombocytopenia (platelet count usually <20,000/mm³ at onset) without any other abnormalities (anemia may be present if there has been prolonged bleeding).

   (b) Platelets in patients with ITP have a greatly decreased life span and are larger (younger platelets are larger), usually resulting in an increase of mean platelet volume.

(4) Diagnosis: A diagnosis of exclusion (occasionally bone marrow aspiration is indicated to rule out leukemia, aplastic anemia). Normal or increased numbers of megakaryocytes in the bone marrow confirms the diagnosis of ITP.

(5) Management: Goal of treatment is prevention of serious bleeding during periods of thrombocytopenia; decision to treat is individualized. Intravenous immune globulin (IVIG) or WinRho (see later) will not mask a diagnosis of leukemia. *Therapy for ITP does not affect the course of the disease.*

   (a) Prednisone (2 to 4 mg/kg/day orally tapered over 2 to 4 weeks)

   (b) IVIG (800 mg/kg/day IV for 1 to 2 days)

   (c) Prednisone and IVIG therapy may be used in combination

   (d) Anti-Rh(D) immunoglobulin (WinRho; 50-75 µg/kg given as a short 3- to 5-minute IV infusion) in patients who are Rh(D) positive.

   (e) Platelet transfusion in ITP is not effective in raising platelet counts because of very rapid consumption of antibody-coated platelets. Serious, life-threatening bleeding episodes secondary to ITP are managed with platelet transfusion combined with IVIG therapy or corticosteroids.

(f) Splenectomy may be indicated in cases of chronic ITP and cases of acute ITP refractory to medical management.

(g) Expectant or watchful observation is appropriate in cases without serious bleeding. Restriction from contact sports and dangerous activities is required.

(6) Prognosis and complications: On average, ITP in children resolves in 4 to 6 weeks. Most cases have a spontaneous remission by 6 months (acute ITP); 20% of cases have persistent, fluctuating thrombocytopenia lasting longer than 6 months (chronic ITP). The risk for chronicity is increased in infants (<2 years of age) and older children (>10 years of age). Rare complications of ITP are intracranial hemorrhage, gross hematuria, and severe GI bleeding.

b. Thrombotic microangiopathies: severe microvascular occlusions characterized by aggregation of platelets in small blood vessels, resulting in thrombocytopenia and microangiopathic hemolytic anemia

(1) Etiology and pathophysiology: Two types of thrombotic microangiopathies

(a) Thrombotic thrombocytopenic purpura (TTP): Caused by absent or low levels of von Willebrand factor (VWF)–cleaving protease, resulting in accumulation of unusually large multimers of VWF. Microangiopathy is usually systemic. Acquired TTP occurs in older children and adults (median age at onset is 35 years).

(b) Hemolytic-uremic syndrome (HUS) is usually caused by exposure to Shiga toxin, most commonly from GI infection with *Escherichia coli* O157:H7. It occurs mostly in children and can be sporadic or epidemic.

(2) Clinical features: Classic signs and symptoms of thrombotic microangiopathies are fever with neurologic (progressive lethargy, confusion) and renal dysfunction (decreased urine output, increased blood urea nitrogen/creatinine).

(3) Laboratory findings: Hematologic abnormalities are moderate to severe thrombocytopenia (<50,000/mm^3) and hemolysis with RBC fragmentation (schistocytes) and polychromasia. The serum lactate dehydrogenase (LDH) is elevated. It is distinguished from disseminated intravascular coagulation by the absence of consumptive coagulopathy (i.e., normal prothrombin time [PT], partial thromboplastin time [PTT], and fibrinogen levels; D-dimers may be slightly elevated).

(4) Diagnosis

(a) TTP: Pentad of thrombocytopenia, microangiopathic hemolytic anemia, neurologic abnormalities, renal failure, and fever. Pretreatment plasma may be tested for ADAMTS-13 activity and VWF multimeric analyses.

(b) HUS: Microangiopathic hemolytic anemia and renal insufficiency 1 week after an episode of bloody diarrhea. Stool may be cultured for *E. coli* O157:H7.

(5) Management: TTP is considered a hematologic emergency; a majority of patients respond to plasma exchange or fresh frozen

plasma infusion. Supportive management of renal disease, if present, is indicated in both HUS and TTP. Bleeding in TTP and HUS from thrombocytopenia is usually not severe; platelet transfusion is not indicated, except for life-threatening bleeding, because it may exacerbate microvascular thrombosis. Children and infants with HUS have a mortality rate of 5% and a 10% chance of development of end-stage renal disease.

THROMBOCYTOSIS

Etiology and pathophysiology: Elevated platelet count above 500,000/mm^3 in children is usually a benign reaction to a disease process (reactive thrombocytosis). In reactive thrombocytosis, the elevation in platelet count is transitory, with thrombotic and hemorrhagic events extremely rare. See Box 14-6 for conditions associated with reactive thrombocytopenia.

14.4 Bone Marrow Failure

ACQUIRED APLASTIC ANEMIA

1. Definition: Acquired aplastic anemia is characterized by pancytopenia (hemoglobin = 10 g/dL, platelet count = 50,000/mm^3, WBC count = 3500/mm^3) and reduced hematopoietic activity in the bone marrow without evidence of malignancy or an inherited syndrome.
2. Etiology and pathophysiology: Acquired aplastic anemia is believed to be due to immune-mediated destruction of hematopoietic cells, apparently by cytotoxic T lymphocytes. In most cases (70% to 80%) of acquired aplastic anemia the cause is unknown (idiopathic); many drugs, chemicals, toxins, and infections, however, have been associated with acquired aplastic anemia (Box 14-7).
3. Clinical features: Patients with acquired aplastic anemia have the insidious onset of fatigue, pallor, bruising, and increased susceptibility to infections; hepatosplenomegaly and lymphadenopathy are not found.
4. Laboratory findings: In severe aplastic anemia, marked hypocellular (<25% cellular) bone marrow with peripheral neutropenia

---

Box 14-6   Conditions Associated with Reactive Thrombocytosis

Infection (bacterial, viral)
Anemia (iron-deficiency anemia, hemolytic anemia)
Trauma (surgery, fracture, acute blood loss)
Stress, exercise
Asplenia (splenectomy)
Inflammatory disease (Kawasaki's disease, connective tissue disorders, inflammatory bowel disease)
Medication/drug use (vincristine, corticosteroids, epinephrine)
Malignancy

> **Box 14-7   Factors Associated with Acquired Aplastic Anemia**
>
> Drugs: cytotoxic chemotherapy; antibiotics (tetracyclines, chloramphenicol, sulfonamides); anticonvulsants (carbamazepine, phenytoin); antimalarial (chloroquine)
> Chemicals: insecticides, benzene, carbon tetrachloride, glue, toluene
> Infections: viruses (hepatitis, Epstein-Barr virus, cytomegalovirus, human immunodeficiency virus, measles, mumps, rubella, parvovirus, influenza); Rocky Mountain spotted fever
> Autoimmune disorders: juvenile rheumatoid arthritis, systemic lupus erythematosus
> Radiation exposure
> Graft-versus-host disease
> Malnutrition

(ANC <500/mm^3), platelet count below 20,000/mm^3, and reticulocyte count less than 1% (corrected for anemia)

5. Diagnosis: Work-up for acquired aplastic anemia involves documenting pancytopenia and marrow aplasia, exploring for possible causes, and excluding other disorders (e.g., myelodysplasia, acute leukemia).
   a. Hematologic: CBC with differential, reticulocyte count, bone marrow aspiration/biopsy with cytogenetic analysis
   b. Genetic: Chromosome fragility testing to rule out Fanconi's anemia (see later)
   c. Infectious: Viral serology (EBV, CMV, HIV, hepatitis, parvovirus)
   d. Immune studies: Quantitative immunoglobulins, antinuclear factor
   e. Other: Sugar water test or Ham acid serum test to rule out paroxysmal nocturnal hemoglobinuria
6. Management: Generally supportive to treat any infections, bleeding, or anemia. Febrile neutropenic patients should be worked up for infection and started on broad-spectrum antibiotics. Blood products should be single-donor irradiated platelets, used judiciously to prevent donor sensitization. Exposure to a causative agent, if identified, should be removed. Definitive therapy includes the following:
   a. Bone marrow transplantation; allogeneic transplantation from a human leukocyte antigen (HLA)–matched sibling is considered front-line therapy.
   b. Immunosuppressive therapy: Antithymocyte globulin (40 mg/kg/day for 4 days) ± cyclosporine A (2 mg/kg/dose twice daily) ± methylprednisolone ± colony-stimulating factors (granulocyte-macrophage [GM]-CSF, G-CSF).
7. Prognosis: Up to 90% of patients treated with bone marrow transplantation have long-term survival; immunosuppressive therapy is curative only in approximately 50% of patients.

FANCONI'S ANEMIA

1. Etiology: Fanconi's anemia (FA) is an autosomal recessive disorder with familial aplastic anemia and congenital physical abnormalities.
2. Clinical features: Gradual onset of bone marrow failure, usually with the development of thrombocytopenia first; aplastic anemia usually is diagnosed at a mean age of 6 to 8 years. Some may present with varied physical abnormalities (Box 14-8).
3. Diagnosis: Demonstration of increased chromosome breakage to clastogenic agents; classic chromosome fragility testing is performed with diepoxybutane (DEB).
4. Management: Androgen therapy (oxymetholone 2 to 5 mg/kg/day) in conjunction with corticosteroid (prednisone 5 to 10 mg every other day), cytokine therapy (G-CSF, erythropoietin), and transfusion (platelet, RBC), as indicated. For long-term management, allogeneic bone marrow transplant from a matched related sibling who has been screened for FA.
5. Prognosis for patients with FA is poor, with most patients dying within 2 years of the onset of aplastic anemia with only supportive treatment.

PURE RED BLOOD CELL APLASIA

1. Transient erythroblastopenia of childhood (TEC): This acquired clinical entity results from the transient cessation of marrow erythropoiesis and is usually preceded by a viral illness 1 to 2 months before the onset of anemia and is characterized by transient anemia with reticulocytopenia and a normal platelet count and WBC count. TEC is distinguished

---

Box 14-8   Frequent Sites of Congenital Malformations and Abnormalities Associated with Fanconi's Anemia

Skin pigmentation (64%)*
Growth retardation/short stature (60%)
Radial ray defects—thumb, radii (49%)
Eye (41%)
Renal and urinary tract (34%)
Neurodevelopment (26%)
Other skeletal—congenital hip, vertebral, scoliosis, rib, clubfoot (22%)
Male genitalia (20%)
Ear (15%)
Gastrointestinal—anorectal, duodenal atresia, tracheoesophageal fistula, esophageal atresia (14%)
Heart (13%)
Hearing loss (11%)
Central nervous system—hydrocephalus, absent corpus callosum (7%)
Oral cavity (4%)

*Percentage frequency.

from hemolytic anemia with an acute aplastic crisis by the absence of a history of anemia, normal RBC morphology, absence of jaundice, negative Coombs' test, and normal serum haptoglobin. TEC is a self-limited disorder, with spontaneous recovery within 4 to 8 weeks.

2. Diamond-Blackfan anemia: This rare congenital anemia presents in the first year of life because of an intrinsic abnormality of erythroid progenitor cells. Inheritance is unclear; both autosomal dominant and autosomal recessive modes of inheritance occur. Physical abnormalities (25% of cases) include musculoskeletal abnormalities of the head, face, and upper limbs, short stature, and renal and cardiac anomalies. Laboratory features include macrocytic anemia and increased RBC fetal hemoglobin and i antigen. Bone marrow examination shows selective deficiency of RBC precursors in an otherwise normocellular bone marrow. Management includes long-term RBC transfusions, prednisone or prednisolone therapy (2 mg/kg/day), and bone marrow transplantation from HLA-matched sibling donors for those patients who do not respond to steroid therapy.

3. Pure red cell aplasia: Acquired pure red cell aplasia (PRCA) is a disorder of RBC proliferation associated with several causal factors such as medications (antiepileptics, sulfonamides, INH), viral infection (parvovirus B19, EBV, HIV), malignancy, collagen-vascular disease (SLE), pregnancy, and vitamin deficiency (folate, B_{12}). Laboratory findings include normocytic (macrocytosis is seen in some conditions) and normochromic anemia with reticulocytopenia. PRCA may precipitate severe anemia (aplastic crisis) in patients with congenital hemolytic anemias. Bone marrow examination shows deficiency of erythroid precursors. Treatment of PRCA includes removal of the causative agent, immunosuppressive therapy, and supportive RBC transfusion if indicated.

14.5 Sickle Cell Syndromes

1. Etiology: Sickle cell disease is a hemoglobinopathy resulting from the substitution of glutamic acid by valine at the sixth amino acid from the N-terminus of the β-globin chain. The sickle cell gene (Hb S) may be heterozygous, usually producing no clinical symptoms (sickle cell trait), or homozygous (sickle cell disease-SS). Sickle cell trait, or the carrier state of Hb S, is inherited as an autosomal dominant disorder, and the homozygous state sickle cell disease as autosomal recessive; 8% of African Americans carry Hb S and about 1 of 600 newborn African Americans are homozygous for Hb S.

2. Pathophysiology: The sickle mutation induces abnormal polymerization of deoxygenated hemoglobin in the RBC, which causes membrane changes and loss of normal deformability, resulting in the characteristic sickle shape (drepanocyte). The deformed RBCs occlude capillary beds, causing hemolysis and vaso-occlusion. Sickling is usually reversible with oxygenation.

3. Clinical features: Clinical complications of sickle cell disease are a consequence of hemolytic anemia, sickling causing vaso-occlusion, and functional asplenia resulting in susceptibility to infection. The onset, frequency, and clinical severity of symptoms related to sickle cell anemia

and its variants are quite variable for each patient. The clinical syndromes that occur in patients with sickle cell disease include the following:

a. *Acute pain crisis:* Vaso-occlusion causing infarction and pain occurring in long bones, joints, spine, chest, skin, and abdomen (liver, spleen, and lymph nodes); may be precipitated by dehydration, fever, exposure to cold, and infection (acidosis).

b. *Dactylitis (hand-foot syndrome):* Infarction of metacarpals and metatarsals in infants causing painful swelling of hands and feet

c. *Acute chest syndrome (pulmonary infarction versus pneumonitis):* Defined as a new infiltrate on chest radiograph plus tachypnea, chest pain, fever greater than 38.5° C, hypoxia (oxygen saturation [SaO_2] on room air 3% to 5% points less than baseline), and leukocytosis

d. *Splenic sequestration crisis:* Infants and young children (5 months to 2 years of age) with splenomegaly who have not yet undergone fibrosis may have an acute increase in spleen size together with a decrease in hemoglobin, with or without thrombocytopenia.

e. *Stroke:* Vaso-occlusion of small or medium-sized arteries in the central nervous system (CNS) can cause ischemia and infarction. Ten percent of patients with sickle cell disease have clinically evident stroke by 20 years of age; risk is increased in sickle cell disease-SS, in patients 2 to 10 years of age, and in patients with silent stroke (magnetic resonance imaging [MRI] evidence of cerebral ischemia without focal deficits).

f. *Priapism:* Vaso-occlusion of corpora cavernosa can result in painful erection persisting more than 1 hour. Onset in early childhood or adolescence and can result in impotence.

g. *Aplastic crisis:* Infection, usually viral, may diminish RBC production, resulting in rapid decrease of hemoglobin.

h. *Cholelithiasis:* Chronically increased serum bilirubin levels from hemolysis produce gallstones. Complications include acute cholecystitis, bile duct obstruction, and chronic right upper quadrant pain.

i. *Infection:* Overwhelming sepsis and meningitis with *Streptococcus pneumoniae, Neisseria meningitides,* and *H. influenzae* type b are serious consequences of loss of normal splenic function; the period of greatest risk for death from these severe infections is during the first 5 years of life. Patients with sickle cell disease are also at increased risk for *Salmonella* osteomyelitis.

4. Diagnosis: Hb S is identified and quantified using hemoglobin electrophoresis. Hb S is a mandatory part of newborn screening in most states.

5. Management

a. Routine health care maintenance for children with sickle cell disease

(1) Comprehensive pediatric hematology visits every 2 to 4 months until 2 years of age, every 6 months until 12 years of age, and every 6 to 12 months after 12 years of age.

(2) Avoidance of dehydration and cold

(3) Penicillin prophylaxis until 5 years of age (125 mg orally [PO] twice daily, birth to 36 months of age; 250 mg PO twice daily, 3 to 5 years of age).

(4) Folic acid supplementation (prescription—1 mg PO once a day; OTC—400 μg once a day from multivitamin) for patients with

elevated hemolysis (reticulocyte count >10%) helps prevent acute pain crisis.

(5) Hydroxyurea for patients with severe sickle cell disease

(6) Simple transfusion to increase hemoglobin to 10 g/dL in surgical settings

(7) Pneumococcal vaccination (PCV7 and PPV23)

(8) Influenza, inactivated vaccination given annually after 6 months of age

(9) Transcranial Doppler ultrasonography every 6 to 12 months from 3 to 16 years of age to screen for increase risk of stroke

(10) Dental care annually after 2 years of age

(11) Ophthalmology examination annually after 10 years of age

b. Specific therapy of sickle cell syndromes

(1) Pain crisis: Children older than 12 months of age and adolescents with moderate to severe acute pain crisis should be offered symptomatic and supportive treatment.

(a) IV fluid bolus if dehydration present and IV fluids at 11/4 maintenance rate

(b) Opiate pain medication administered regularly

(i) Morphine sulfate IV (0.1 mg/kg to a maximum 5-mg bolus, then 0.05 mg/kg every 20 minutes)

(ii) Hydromorphone (Dilaudid) IV (0.015 mg/kg to a maximum 2-mg bolus, then 0.008 mg/kg every 20 minutes)

(iii) Methadone IV (0.1 mg/kg to a maximum 10-mg bolus every 4 to 6 hours)

(c) Anti-inflammatory medication adjunct

(i) Ketorolac IV (0.5 mg/kg to a maximum of 30 mg every 6 hours)

(ii) Ibuprofen PO (10 mg/kg to a maximum of 800 mg every 6 hours)

(iii) Methylprednisolone IV (15 mg/kg to a maximum of 1000 mg)

(iv) Choline magnesium trisalicylate PO (25 mg/kg/day divided in two daily doses)

(2) Acute chest syndrome: Treat with broad-spectrum parenteral antibiotics (e.g., ceftriaxone) plus macrolide (e.g., azithromycin) if clinically indicated, IV fluid bolus, oxygen, bronchodilators and corticosteroids, and simple or exchange transfusion.

(3) Splenic sequestration crisis: Evaluate and treat hypovolemia with volume expanders (IV fluids, normal saline, or blood) if present. Also perform simple transfusion with or without exchange transfusion. Long-term management with splenectomy should be considered in patients with severe or recurrent sequestration.

(4) Stroke: Perform exchange transfusion as soon as possible in the event of a suspected or likely acute infarct stroke. Perform MRI/magnetic resonance angiography for diagnostic purposes. Long-term management consists of chronic transfusion therapy to reduce Hb S to less than 30% to prevent strokes in children with abnormal results on transcranial Doppler ultrasonography and silent stroke.

(5) Priapism: Obtain urologic consultation for penile aspiration with epinephrine irrigation, hydrate, and give analgesia (IV or oral), pseudoephedrine (4 mg/kg/day to a maximum of 240 mg), and exchange transfusion if persistent.

(6) Aplastic crisis: close monitoring with or without slow simple transfusion as indicated

(7) Cholelithiasis: elective cholecystectomy for symptomatic stones

(8) Infection: Patients with fever greater than 101° F younger than 36 months of age or 102° F older than 3 years of age should have blood cultures drawn and empirical parenteral antibiotic (ceftriaxone 50 mg/kg to a maximum of 1 g) given as soon as blood cultures are obtained.

6. Prognosis: Mortality from complications of sickle cell disease in children is highest in the first 3 years of life, although this rate is reduced in developed countries. The average life span of patients with sickle cell disease-SS is 50 years in developed countries.

14.6 Approach to the Child with Anemia

BACKGROUND

1. Anemia is defined as a reduction in the quantity of Hb or RBC mass below age-specific normal values. Normal values of Hb and hematocrit (Hct) vary with age and sex; the World Health Organization defines anemia in children 6 months to 6 years of age as Hb less than 11 g/dL (Table 14-2).

2. Spurious Hb (false-positive values or laboratory errors), statistical anemia ("normal" outliers), and nonphysiologic anemia (dehydration or volume overload) must be considered.

3. Historical information: Age, sex, race, ethnic extraction, neonatal history of jaundice, diet, drug use, infection, diarrhea, and family history of anemia, jaundice, gallstones, or splenectomy are important in determining the etiology of anemia.

4. Initial laboratory assessment includes a CBC, reticulocyte count, and examination of the peripheral blood smear.

CLASSIFICATION OF ANEMIA

Anemia in children is most easily classified on the basis of RBC size or mean corpuscular volume (MCV). MCV is equivalent to the ratio of Hct to RBC count.

1. *Microcytic anemia* (MCV <70 fL all ages; MCV <75 fL 2 to 18 years of age): Reflects a quantitative defect in hemoglobin synthesis. Causes of hypochromatic microcytic anemia are listed in Table 14-3.

2. *Normocytic anemia* (MCV 75 to 95 fL 2 to 6 years of age; MCV 78 to 100 fL 12 to 18 years of age): Causes of normocytic anemia in children may be differentiated by using the reticulocyte count to assess RBC production.

   a. *Normocytic anemia with reticulocytosis* (reticulocyte index [percentage reticulocytes corrected for degree of anemia] >3; elevated absolute number of reticulocytes).

      (1) Bleeding/acute blood loss

Table 14-2 Normal Hematologic Values in Children[a]

Age	Hemoglobin (g/dL)		Hematocrit (%)		Red Cell Count (10¹²/L)		MCV (fL)		MCH (pg)		MCHC (g/dL)	
	Mean	±2 SD	Mean	±2 SD	Mean	±2 SD	Mean	±2 SD	Mean	±2 SD	Mean	±2 SD
Birth (cord blood)	16.5	13.5	51	42	4.7	3.9	108	98	34	31	33	30
1-3 days (capillary)	18.5	14.5	56	45	5.3	4.0	108	95	34	31	33	29
1 wk	17.5	13.5	54	42	5.1	3.9	107	88	34	28	33	28
2 wk	16.5	12.5	51	39	4.9	3.6	105	86	34	28	33	28
1 mo	14.0	10.0	43	31	4.2	3.0	104	85	34	28	33	29
2 mo	11.5	9.0	35	28	3.8	2.7	96	77	30	26	33	29
3-6 mo	11.5	9.5	35	29	3.8	3.1	91	74	30	25	33	30
0.5-2 yr	12.0	10.5	36	33	4.5	3.7	78	70	27	23	33	30
2-6 yr	12.5	11.5	37	34	4.6	3.9	81	75	27	24	34	31
6-12 yr	13.5	11.5	40	35	4.6	4.0	86	77	29	25	34	31
12-18 yr												
Female	14.0	12.0	41	36	4.6	4.1	90	78	30	25	34	31
Male	14.5	13.0	43	37	4.9	4.5	88	78	30	25	34	31
18-49 yr												
Female	14.0	12.0	41	36	4.6	4.0	90	80	30	26	34	31
Male	15.5	13.5	47	41	5.2	4.5	90	80	30	26	34	31

[a]These data have been compiled from several sources. Emphasis is given to studies using electronic counters and to the selection of populations that are likely to exclude individuals with iron deficiency. The mean ±2 SD can be expected to include 95% of the observations in a normal population. MCH, mean corpuscular hemoglobin; MCHC, mean corpuscular hemoglobin concentration; MCV, mean corpuscular volume.
From Dallman PR: In Rudolph A (ed): Pediatrics, 16th ed. New York, Appleton-Century-Crofts, p 1111, 1977.

Table 14-3 Differentiating among Causes of Microcytic Anemia

Differential Diagnosis	Diagnostic Red Cell Features	Other Laboratory Tests
Iron deficiency	Marked variation in size of red cells (anisocytosis); marked hypochromasia; target cells	Ferritin low FEP elevated Serum iron low
Thalassemia/HbE	RBC count high; mean corpuscular hemoglobin concentration normal; target cells; RBC basophilic stippling (ribosome aggregates) may be present	Hb electrophoresis
Lead poisoning/ sideroblastic anemia	Marked RBC basophilic stippling	FEP elevated Lead levels high
Anemia of inflammation	Microcytosis and hypochromia usually mild	Ferritin high Serum iron low Sedimentation rate high

	Serum Ferritin	FEP	Serum Iron	Lead Level	HbA$_2$
Iron deficiency	D	I	D	N	N/D
β-Thalassemia trait	N	N	N	N	I
Anemia of inflammation	I	I	D	N	N
Lead poisoning	I	I	N/I	I	N

FEP, free erythrocyte porphyrin; Hb, hemoglobin; RBC, red blood cell; N, normal; D, decreased; I, increased.

    (2) Hemolytic anemia: Characterized by shortened RBC life span usually secondary to a hemolytic process; may be demonstrated by the presence of low serum levels of free haptoglobin or, occasionally, elevated serum LDH with hyperbilirubinemia or hemoglobinuria (see Red Blood Cell Disorders).
        (a) Extracorpuscular (extrinsic) hemolytic anemia (Table 14-4)
        (b) Corpuscular (intrinsic) hemolytic anemia
  b. *Normocytic anemia with reticulocytopenia* (inappropriate reticulocytosis for degree of anemia; reticulocyte index <3): Usually the result of some process of bone marrow aplasia or depression.
    (1) Aplastic anemia (see Marrow Failure)
    (2) Transient erythroblastopenia of childhood (see Marrow Failure)
    (3) Malignancy involving bone marrow
    (4) Renal failure

Table 14-4   **Extracorpuscular versus Corpuscular Hemolytic Anemia**

Differential Diagnosis	Diagnostic Red Cell Features	Other Laboratory Tests
Extracorpuscular Hemolytic Anemia		
Autoimmune hemolytic anemia	Microspherocytosis; marked polychromasia	Direct Coombs' test positive
ABO isoimmune hemolytic disease of newborn	Spherocytosis; nucleated red blood cells; marked polychromasia	Direct/indirect Coombs' test positive; immunoglobulin G in maternal serum
MAHA/"Waring blender" syndrome*	Fragmented red cells (schistocytes)	Platelet count usually decreased; Coombs' test negative
Hypersplenism	RBC morphology usually normal	Leukopenia and thrombocytopenia usually present
Nonimmune hemolytic anemia†	Nonspecific	Coombs' test negative
Corpuscular Hemolytic Anemia		
Sickle cell anemia (Hb SS)/other hemoglobinopathies	Sickle cells, target cells, occasional nucleated red blood cell	Hb electrophoresis
Enzymopathies	Poikilocytosis (burr cells)	Glucose 6-phosphate dehydrogenase/pyruvate kinase screen
HS/HE‡	Spherocytosis, elliptocytosis	Osmotic fragility increased

*Microangiopathic hemolytic anemia ("Waring blender" syndrome) causes include disseminated intravascular coagulation, hemangiomas, hemolytic-uremic syndrome, thrombotic thrombocytopenic purpura, severe valvular heart disease, and surgical correction of endocardial cushion defects.
†Nonimmune, secondary causes of red blood cell hemolysis: infection—malaria, babesiosis, *Clostridium*, *Escherichia coli*, *Salmonella*, *Streptococcus*, Epstein-Barr virus, hepatitis, cytomegalovirus; drugs/toxins—vitamin K, sulfones, lead, snake and spider bites.
‡Hereditary spherocytosis/hereditary elliptocytosis.

3. *Macrocytic anemia* (MCV >95 fL 6 months to 12 years of age; MCV >100 fL 12 to 18 years of age)
   a. Megaloblastic anemia: Characterized by ineffective erythropoiesis secondary to defects in DNA replication; MCV usually greater than 110 fL; megaloblastic erythroid maturation in marrow is seen; hypersegmented neutrophils (nuclei with more than five lobes) may be seen. Causes include
      (1) Folate deficiency secondary to goat's milk–fed infants, tropical sprue, celiac disease
      (2) Vitamin B_{12} deficiency: Intrinsic factor deficiency (pernicious anemia)
      (3) Drug induced: Sources include antimetabolite chemotherapy agents, anticonvulsants.
      (4) Congenital dyserythropoietic anemia
   b. Congenital bone marrow failure: Etiology may include Diamond-Blackfan anemia or FA (see Marrow Failure).
   c. Trisomy 21
   d. Hypothyroidism
   e. Active hemolysis with marked reticulocytosis

IRON-DEFICIENCY ANEMIA

1. Etiology and pathophysiology: Iron-deficiency anemia is a decrease in RBC Hb production secondary to inadequate body iron stores. Poor dietary intake of iron is the primary cause of iron deficiency in children younger than 2 years of age; the National Health and Nutrition Examination Survey reported that 13% of 1-year-olds were iron deficient. GI blood loss should be considered as a cause of iron deficiency in all children older than 2 years of age. Common causes of iron deficiency in childhood include
   a. Poor dietary intake of iron (bioavailability of food iron is greatest in meat and animal products because iron is in the heme form; vegetable sources of iron are in the nonheme form, which is poorly absorbed)
   b. Fetal/neonatal blood loss
   c. Early transition from iron-fortified formula to cow's milk
   d. Cow's milk intolerance with resulting blood loss secondary to exudative enteropathy
   e. Increased physiologic requirements during rapid growth in infancy and adolescence (especially girls)
   f. Excess menstrual blood loss
   g. Decreased vitamin C intake (vitamin C plays an important role in absorption of nonheme iron)
   h. Chronic GI blood loss from inflammatory bowel disease
   i. Tea ingestion (tannates in tea chelate iron)
2. Diagnosis
   a. CBC for Hb, MCV, and RBC distribution width (RDW), reticulocyte count, and examination of peripheral blood smear (see Table 14-2 and 14-3)
   b. Stool for occult blood and serum albumin (severe iron deficiency can itself cause an exudative enteropathy, resulting in occult blood and protein loss)

3. Management
   a. Oral iron salts (ferrous sulfate) at 3 to 6 mg of elemental iron/kg/day (to a maximum of 60 to 120 mg) to correct anemia, and an additional 2 months to replace iron stores
   b. Vitamin C to increase absorption, optional
   c. Increase in reticulocytes should be noted in 5 to 10 days after starting iron therapy, followed by a rise in hemoglobin by 0.2 to 0.4 g/dL/day.
   d. No improvement in Hb (<1 g/dL increase) after 1 month of iron therapy requires further evaluation to confirm iron deficiency and search for possible sources of blood loss.

14.7 Coagulation Disorders

Normal hemostasis, or the arrest of bleeding, depends on blood vessels (vascular phase), platelets (platelet phase), and the plasma coagulation cascade (plasma phase). The plasma phase of coagulation includes not only processes leading to the formation of a fibrin clot, but those that regulate clotting (Fig. 14-1).

PHYSIOLOGIC COAGULATION

1. Definition: Coagulation is the process of clot formation and is composed of primary and secondary mechanisms.
   a. Primary coagulation: Formation of a temporary platelet plug (vascular and platelet phases)
   b. Secondary coagulation: Conversion of factor II (prothrombin) to thrombin, which catalyzes the production of fibrin from factor I (fibrinogen) and the formation of a clot or stable platelet plug (plasma phase)
      (1) Intrinsic pathway: Factor VIII (antihemophilic factor), factor IX (Christmas factor), factor XI (plasma thromboplastin), and factor XII (Hageman factor); activated by subendothelial collagen, endotoxin, complement, and others; requires phospholipid contributed by the platelet membrane (see Fig. 14-1)
      (2) Extrinsic pathway: Factor VII (stable factor) activated by factor III (tissue thromboplastin) and other tissue factors (see Fig. 14-1)
      (3) Common pathway: Prothrombin is converted to thrombin and involves factor X and factor V; requires phospholipid contributed by the platelet membrane (platelet factor 3). Fibrin clots are stabilized by activated factor XIII (fibrin-stabilizing factor).

COAGULOPATHY

1. Etiology and pathophysiology: Deficient quantity or function of the components of the platelet phase or plasma phase is inherited or acquired and results in excessive bleeding after trauma or surgery or predisposes to excessive or spontaneous bleeding. Coagulation is modulated by antithrombin III, protein C, protein S, and plasminogen, the latter of which is converted to plasmin and catalyzes fibrinolysis or clot lysis. Inhibitors of plasmin are α_2-antiplasmin, α_1-antitrypsin, α_2-macroglobulin, and antithrombin III.
2. Problems with the formation of a platelet plug (vascular and platelet phases) result in "small" vessel or capillary bleeding—petechiae/ecchymosis of

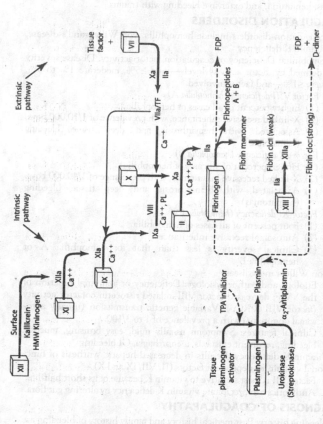

Figure 14-1 Coagulation cascade. FDP, fibrin/fibrinogen degradation products; HMW, high molecular weight; PL, platelet membrane phospholipid; TF, tissue factor; TPA, tissue plasminogen activator. (From Noble J: Textbook of Primary Care Medicine, 3rd ed. Philadelphia, Mosby, 2001.)

the skin, mucous membrane bleeding or "wet purpura" (epistaxis, oozing from gums, oral petechiae), and GI bleeding. These include disorders of von Willebrand protein, which is necessary for normal platelet–endothelial cell and platelet–platelet interaction, quantitative and qualitative platelet disorders (see Platelet Disorders), and vasculitis.

3. Problems with secondary coagulation (plasma phase) are related to "large" vessel bleeding and produce hemarthrosis, soft tissue hematomas, hematuria, and extensive bleeding with trauma.

COAGULATION DISORDERS

The coagulation disorders include hemophilia, von Willebrand's disease, and vitamin K deficiency.

1. Hemophilia: Deficiency of coagulation factor activity. Disease severity is defined by factor activity levels—mild ≥5%, moderate 1% to 5%, severe ≤1%—and factor involved.

   a. *Factor VIII deficiency (hemophilia A)*
      (1) Eighty percent of all cases of hemophilia
      (2) X-linked recessive inheritance, with prevalence of 1/10,000 boys
      (3) Associated with hemarthrosis and deep tissue bleeding (hematomas)

   b. *Factor IX deficiency (hemophilia B)*
      (1) Fifteen percent of all cases of hemophilia
      (2) X-linked recessive inheritance, with prevalence of 1/40,000 boys
      (3) Associated with hemarthrosis and deep tissue bleeding (hematomas)

   c. *Factor XI deficiency (hemophilia C)*
      (1) Four percent of all cases of hemophilia
      (2) Autosomal recessive inheritance
      (3) Clinical severity is less than that for hemophilia A or hemophilia B

2. Von Willebrand's disease

   a. Etiology and pathophysiology: Deficiency or abnormal function of the VWF; decreased factor VIII–related ristocetin cofactor activity (factor VIII R:RCo). Variable genetic transmission (usually autosomal dominant) with a prevalence of 1 to 3/100.

   b. Clinical features: Symptoms usually mild, easy bruising, mucosal bleeding, recurrent epistaxis, menorrhagia, GI bleeding

3. Vitamin K deficiency: Results in decreased hepatic synthesis of functional vitamin K–dependent factors (II, VII, IX and X)

   a. Factor VII is most sensitive to vitamin K because of its short half-life.

   b. Antibiotics can precipitate vitamin K deficiency by altering gut flora.

DIAGNOSIS OF COAGULAPATHY

1. Bleeding history: Past medical history and family history of bleeding are very important in the evaluation of a child with a suspected coagulation disorder. Questions to be asked include

   a. Is the bleeding lifelong or recent onset?

   b. Is the bleeding from more than one site (i.e., is epistaxis bilateral or unilateral)?

   c. Was there excessive bleeding with tonsillectomy, dental extractions, or other minor surgery?

d. Was there bleeding requiring hospitalization or transfusions?
e. Is bruising with trauma early and large?
2. Laboratory findings: PT, activated PTT, and platelet count (Fig. 14-2)
   a. *Bleeding time* measures platelet function and vascular integrity and is prolonged in von Willebrand's disease and qualitative platelet disorders. However, abnormal values are not reliable because the method is poorly standardized and the results altered by many variables. A *platelet function* analyzer has greater specificity.
   b. Screening for von Willebrand's disease includes factor VIII R:Ag (VWF antigen) level, factor VIII R:RCo activity level, factor VIII activity level, and VWF multimeric analysis.

MANAGEMENT OF COAGULATION DISORDERS

1. Hemophilia: Typical bleeds are treated with purified factor concentrates with dosing recommendations based on the type of hemorrhage (Table 14-5).
   a. Hemophilia A: One unit of factor VIII concentrate is equivalent to the amount of factor in 1 mL of normal pooled plasma; 1 U/kg of factor VIII yields an increase of 2% of plasma factor activity. Half-life 12 to 15 hours.
      (1) Recombinant-prepared (Recombinate, Kogenate, ReFacto, Advate)
      (2) Monoclonal, plasma derived (Monarc-M)
   b. Hemophilia B: One unit of factor IX concentrate is equivalent to the amount of factor in 1 mL of normal pooled plasma; 1 U/kg of factor IX yields an increase of 1% of plasma factor activity. Half-life 18 to 30 hours.
      (1) Monoclonal, plasma derived (Alphanine SD)
      (2) Recombinant-prepared (Benefix)
   c. Patients with high inhibitor titer (>10 Bethesda units) or for those patients with low inhibitor levels who do not respond to factor concentrates:
      (1) Activated prothrombin complex concentrate (anti-inhibitor coagulation complex)
         (a) Feiba VH intravenous (plasma derived) 50 to 100 U/kg every 6 hours; monitor for thrombosis.
      (2) Activated factor VII concentrate
         (a) NovoSeven intravenous (recombinant) 90 to 120 μg/kg every 2 hours; monitor for thrombosis.
   d. Desmopressin acetate (DDAVP), 0.3 μg/kg IV, can be used in patients with mild to moderate hemophilia A with minor bleeding episodes.
   e. Epsilon aminocaproic acid (Amicar-Immunex Co.) 100 mg/kg every 6 hours orally for 3 to 5 days as an adjuvant to factor replacement in the control of oral mucosal bleeding and dental extractions
   f. Ice therapy for 20 minutes and immobilization for 48 hours in hemarthrosis and soft tissue hematoma
2. Von Willebrand's disease
   a. DDAVP
      (1) Stimate intranasal (DDAVP 1.5 mg/mL), one spray in each nostril (300 μg) in patients 50 kg or more; single spray in patients less than 50 kg

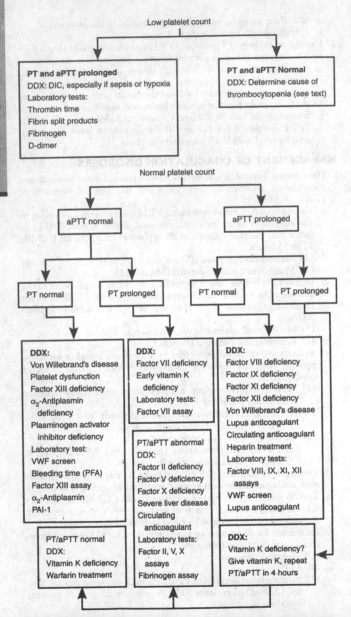

Low platelet count

PT and aPTT prolonged
DDX: DIC, especially if sepsis or hypoxia
Laboratory tests:
Thrombin time
Fibrin split products
Fibrinogen
D-dimer

PT and aPTT Normal
DDX: Determine cause of
thrombocytopenia (see text)

Normal platelet count

aPTT normal

aPTT prolonged

PT normal

PT prolonged

PT normal

PT prolonged

DDX:
Von Willebrand's disease
Platelet dysfunction
Factor XIII deficiency
α_2-Antiplasmin
deficiency
Plasminogen activator
inhibitor deficiency
Laboratory test:
VWF screen
Bleeding time (PFA)
Factor XIII assay
α_2-Antiplasmin
PAI-1

DDX:
Factor VII deficiency
Early vitamin K
deficiency
Laboratory tests:
Factor VII assay

PT/aPTT abnormal
DDX:
Factor II deficiency
Factor V deficiency
Factor X deficiency
Severe liver disease
Circulating
anticoagulant
Laboratory tests:
Factor II, V, X
assays
Fibrinogen assay

DDX:
Factor VIII deficiency
Factor IX deficiency
Factor XI deficiency
Factor XII deficiency
Von Willebrand's disease
Lupus anticoagulant
Circulating anticoagulant
Heparin treatment
Laboratory tests:
Factor VIII, IX, XI, XII
assays
VWF screen
Lupus anticoagulant

PT/aPTT normal
DDX:
Vitamin K deficiency
Warfarin treatment

DDX:
Vitamin K deficiency?
Give vitamin K, repeat
PT/aPTT in 4 hours

Figure 14-2 Differential diagnosis of bleeding disorders. aPTT, activated partial thromboplastin time; DIC, disseminated intravascular coagulation; PAI, plasminogen activator inhibitor; PT, prothrombin time; VWF, von Willebrand factor. (Adapted from Robertson J, Shilkofski N: The Harriet Lane Handbook, 17th ed. Philadelphia, Elsevier Mosby, 2005.)

      (2) Humate-P IV for patients with moderate or severe von Willebrand's disease or who do not respond to DDAVP:
        (a) Minor hemorrhage: 40 to 50 U/kg (one or two doses)
        (b) Major hemorrhage: Loading dose 50 to 75 U/kg, then 40 to 60 U/kg every 8 to 12 hours for 3 days
3. Vitamin K deficiency
  a. Vitamin K_1 1 mg as a subcutaneous injection
  b. Fresh frozen plasma (to replace vitamin K–dependent coagulation factors) in patients with hemorrhagic events
  c. Factor IX concentrates (to bypass vitamin K–dependent factor steps in the clotting cascade)

THROMBOPHILIA

1. Definition: Thrombophilia is a disorder in which there is a tendency for recurrent thrombosis.
2. Etiology and pathophysiology: The etiology of thrombophilia is either acquired (lupus anticoagulant, hyperlipidemia, paroxysmal nocturnal hemoglobinuria, or hypohomocysteinemia) or inherited (deficiency of antithrombin III or protein C or S, factor V Leiden mutation, prothrombin mutation, or hyperhomocysteinemia). Deficiencies of antithrombin III or protein C or S cause a 20-fold increase in venous thrombotic risk. Venous thrombosis in children with a heterozygous (single gene defect) inherited thrombophilia usually results from an additional procoagulation factor (e.g., prematurity, central venous line, congenital heart disease, oral contraception, malignancy/myeloproliferative disorder, prolonged immobilization, trauma).
3. Diagnosis
  a. Acquired thrombophilia: Work-up depends on suspected etiology (e.g., ANA, C3, C4, total hemolytic complement [CH_{50}], antiphospholipid and anticardiolipin antibodies for SLE).

Table 14-5 **Desired Factor Replacement in Hemophilia (First Dose)**	
Bleeding Site	**Desired Level (%)**
Joint	8–100
Soft tissue/hematoma	50–70
Dental extraction	50–100
Gastrointestinal	70–100
Oral mucosa	70–100
Head injury	100
Major surgery (dental, orthopedic, other)	100

b. Evaluation for an inherited thrombophilia should be done in children with a high probability of congenital thrombophilia (e.g., unexplained neonatal thrombosis, sinovenous thrombosis, recurrent spontaneous venous thrombosis, family history of thromboembolic disease, relatives of patients with inherited thrombophilia):

(1) Activated protein C resistance (APCR) functional assay; followed by factor V Leiden genetic assay if APCR is low

(2) Functional assay of protein C and S, and antithrombin III

c. Homocysteine ultraquantitative serum analysis

4. Management: Children with identified thrombophilia should avoid external factors associated with thrombosis and consider indefinite oral anticoagulation with first venous thromboembolic event (secondary prophylaxis).

14.8 Hematologic Malignancies: Acute Leukemias

INTRODUCTION

From 1996 through 2002, leukemia represented 40% of all cancer cases occurring among children and adolescents 0 to 19 years of age; 23% were lymphomas. Classification as follows:

1. Lymphoproliferative disorders
   a. Acute lymphocytic leukemia (see Acute Leukemias).
   b. Lymphoma (see Neoplastic Tumors in Pediatrics).
2. Myeloproliferative disorders
   a. Acute myelogenous leukemia (see Acute Leukemias).
   b. Chronic myeloproliferative syndromes: These are unusual in childhood and include chronic myelogenous leukemia, with excess production of mature granulocytes (Philadelphia chromosome positive), chronic myelomonocytic leukemia, and myelodysplastic syndrome.

ACUTE LYMPHOBLASTIC LEUKEMIA

1. Classification
   a. *Precursor B-cell acute lymphoblastic leukemia (pre B-ALL; 80% to 85%)*: Leukemic transformation of B-cell lymphoid precursors
   b. *T-cell ALL (13% to 15%)*: Leukemic transformation of T-cell lymphoid precursors
   c. *B-cell ALL (<3%)*: Leukemic transformation of mature B cells; indistinguishable from the malignant B cells of small, noncleaved non-Hodgkin's lymphoma
2. Epidemiology: ALL represents 78% of the total cases of leukemia in children younger than 15 years of age and has an annual incidence of 34/1,000,000, with a peak incidence among 2- to 3-year-olds (>80/1,000,000). There is a twofold higher incidence for white children compared with black children. Incidence of ALL in children has shown a moderate increase in the past 20 years.
3. Clinical features
   a. Symptoms: Anorexia/weight loss, fatigue, very severe bone and joint pain causing limp or refusal to walk (may be present 2 to 6 weeks or longer before the diagnosis of acute leukemia is made)

b. Signs: Fever with or without documented infections, pallor, bleeding/ bruising, petechiae or purpura, hepatosplenomegaly, lymphadenopathy, and rarely neurologic signs or cranial nerve palsies

c. Laboratory findings: The CBC shows a WBC count that may be low, normal, or elevated (>50,000/mm³ in approximately 20% of cases) at diagnosis; neutropenia (absolute neutrophil count <1000/mm³), thrombocytopenia (platelet count <100,000/mm³ in 75%), and normocytic anemia (Hb <10 g/dL in 80%) are usually present; identifiable blast cells on peripheral blood smear may be present.

d. Radiologic findings

(1) Pulmonary hilar lymphadenopathy and mediastinal mass (seen in 5% to 10% of cases; frequent in T-cell ALL)

(2) Skeletal abnormalities (diffuse or localized) on plain radiographs (50%): Metaphyseal lucent bands, osteoporosis (occasionally with associated compression fractures), localized areas of bone destruction/absorption (osteolytic lesions), areas of increased bone density or sclerosis, and periosteal elevation with new bone formation

(3) Radionuclide bone scans may show many areas of increased uptake.

4. Diagnosis. Examination of peripheral blood and bone marrow aspiration with immunophenotyping and cytogenetic analysis will classify the type of leukemia and direct treatment.

5. Management: Successful treatment of ALL requires induction of remission as well as treatment or prophylaxis of extramedullary disease (CNS, testes). Children with acute leukemia have a better outcome when treated on national cooperative group treatment protocols (e.g., Children's Oncology Group [COG]).

a. Induction: Standard induction chemotherapy regimens for pre-B ALL uses three or four drugs (prednisone/dexamethasone, vincristine, and asparaginase, ± daunomycin for children with high-risk features) with intrathecal therapy (methotrexate, cytarabine) given for CNS prophylaxis. Cranial irradiation is reserved for those patients with excessive CNS disease at diagnosis. Induction therapy lasts 28 days.

b. Consolidation: After induction, consolidation therapy to treat residual disease and maintenance or continuation therapy to treat "dormant" disease and prevent relapse are administered. The duration of scheduled postinduction therapy for girls is approximately 2 years and for boys, 3 years.

6. Prognosis

a. The 5-year survival rate for children younger than 20 years of age is 72%.

b. Prognostic factors

(1) Age and WBC count at diagnosis: Favorable for ages 1 to 9 years and WBC count less than 50,000/mm³

(2) Race: Survival rates for black children are lower than for white children.

(3) DNA index: Hyperdiploidy (>50 chromosomes) in blast cells favorable

(4) Cytogenetics
(a) t(9:22)—Philadelphia chromosome, poor outcome
(b) t(4:11)—MLL gene (11q23) rearrangement, poor outcome; high frequency in infants
(c) Immunophenotype (T-cell type ALL, high risk)
(d) CNS disease (adverse prognosis with ≥5 WBCs/mm³ CSF and blast cells)

ACUTE MYELOID LEUKEMIA

Acute myeloid leukemia (AML) represents 16% of the total cases of leukemia in children younger than 15 years of age and has an annual incidence of 6/1,000,000. Symptoms and signs of AML are similar to ALL, with some notable differences: gingival hyperplasia, leukemia cutis (yellow-brown to purple, nodular leukemic infiltrates of skin), chloroma (green leukemic masses associated with periosteum, usually seen in the scalp), and life-threatening hemorrhage and stroke or pulmonary infarcts due to leukostasis. AML is treated with induction chemotherapy (daunorubicin, cytarabine, etoposide, ± 6-thioguanine) and consolidation chemotherapy. CNS prophylaxis with intrathecal cytarabine is required. Overall survival rate is 42% for children younger than 20 years of age. Favorable prognostic factors include WBC count less than 100,000/mm³ at diagnosis, or AML-M3 type.

14.9 Neoplastic Tumors in Pediatrics

CENTRAL NERVOUS SYSTEM/BRAIN TUMOR

1. Epidemiology
   a. Astrocytic brain tumors (including pilocytic astrocytoma, all grades of astrocytoma, and glioblastoma multiforme) represent 52% of the total CNS tumors in patients younger than 20 years of age, followed in frequency by medulloblastomas/supratentorial primitive neuroectodermal tumors (includes intracranial neuroblastoma and pineoblastoma; 21%), other gliomas (includes oligodendrogliomas; 15%), ependymomas (9%), craniopharyngiomas, and choroid plexus tumors.
   b. CNS neoplasms are the most common solid tumors of childhood, accounting for approximately 17% of all malignancies in patients younger than 20 years of age, with an annual incidence of 30/1,000,000. Presenting signs usually secondary to increased intracranial pressure include cyclical vomiting, headache, ataxia, visual changes, and changes in personality/behavior. CNS tumors in children are treated with combined-modality therapy, including surgery, radiation therapy, and chemotherapy. The 5-year survival rate for all CNS tumors in children from 1985 to 1994 was 67%, with the best survival rates seen with astrocytomas in adolescents.

LYMPHOMA

1. Hodgkin's disease (HD)
   a. Pathology: The Reed-Sternberg (RS) cell, believed to arise from a germinal-center B cell, is the malignant cell in HD; the RS cells account for only a small percentage of the tumor mass.

    b. Epidemiology: HD represents 57% of the total cases of lymphoma in patients younger than 20 years of age and has an annual incidence of 12.1/1,000,000.

    c. Clinical features: Painless localized or regional lymph node enlargement with or without contiguous lymphatic spread. Constitutional symptoms (30% of patients) include unexplained fever, drenching night sweats, or weight loss of more than 10% body weight occurring in the previous 6 months.

    d. Staging (Ann Arbor Staging Classification)

       (1) Stage I: Involvement of a single lymph node region or of a single extralymphatic organ/site

       (2) Stage II: Involvement of two or more lymph node regions on the same side of the diaphragm or localized involvement of an extralymphatic organ or site and one or more lymph node regions on the same side to the diaphragm

       (3) Stage III: Involvement of lymph node regions on both sides of the diaphragm ± involvement of the spleen ± localized involvement of an extralymphatic organ or site, or both

       (4) Stage IV: Disseminated involvement of one or more extralymphatic organs or tissues with or without lymph node involvement

    e. Management: Combined-modality therapy is stratified for stage of disease and presence of constitutional symptoms and includes chemotherapy, radiation therapy, and surgery.

    f. Prognosis is good: The 5-year survival rate for patients younger than 20 years of age with HD is 91%. This is altered by the size of the mass, severity of constitutional symptoms, and lymphocyte predominance.

2. Non-Hodgkin's lymphoma (NHL): Malignant neoplasms arising from cellular components of the immune system include Burkitt's and Burkitt-like lymphoma and other T-cell lymphomas. NHL represents 41% of the total cases of lymphoma in patients younger than 20 years of age and has an annual incidence of 10.5/1,000,000. Symptoms and signs of NHL are similar to those in HD except noncontiguous spread and extranodal involvement is much more common, including jaw, maxillary, orbital tumors (endemic Burkitt's lymphoma), nasopharyngeal (Waldeyer's lymphoid tissue) or paranasal tumors (Burkitt-like lymphoma), intrathoracic (mediastinal) tumors (lymphoblastic lymphoma) causing dysphagia, dyspnea, and superior vena cava (SVC) syndrome, and GI tumors. Management includes multiagent chemotherapy and surgery. The overall 5-year survival rate for patients younger than 20 years of age with NHL is 72%, and for those with stage I or II NHL, greater than 90%

NEUROBLASTOMA

1. Etiology and pathophysiology: Neuroblastoma (NB) is a neoplasm arising from primitive adrenergic neuroblasts of neural crest tissue in the adrenal medulla, paravertebral sympathetic ganglia, or sympathetic paraganglia. It is one of the four "small, blue, round cell" tumors of childhood.

2. Epidemiology: NB represents approximately 8% of all cancer in children younger than 15 years of age and has an annual incidence

of 9.1/1,000,000. NB is the most common cancer of infancy; mean age of occurrence is in the second year of life, with more than 75% of cases diagnosed before 4 years of age.

3. Clinical features
   a. Symptoms and signs depend on the location of primary tumor and metastases and paraneoplastic effects:
      (1) Adrenal gland (35% of primary tumors): Large, firm abdominal mass
      (2) Retroperitoneal (paraspinal; 25%): Abdominal mass; radicular pain or paraplegia secondary to nerve root or spinal cord compression
      (3) Thorax (posterior mediastinum; 15%): Respiratory distress; spinal cord compression
      (4) Head and neck (cervical; 5%): May present with Horner's syndrome
      (5) Pelvis (5%): Pelvic mass; disturbance of bowel or bladder function
      (6) Metastatic disease: To bone, bone marrow, liver, lung, or skin is common at the time of diagnosis (in over 50% of cases). Proptosis and periorbital ecchymoses may be seen secondary to retrobulbar metastatic disease and bone pain with associated limping and irritability may be related to bone metastases. Occasionally, intractable secretory diarrhea is seen secondary to secretion of vasoactive intestinal peptide.
   b. Laboratory findings
      (1) Blood chemistries: LDH and serum ferritin levels elevated
      (2) Urinary catecholamine metabolites: Vanillylmandelic acid and homovanillic acid are elevated in 90% of cases.
      (3) CBC: Abnormal with bone marrow involvement
   c. Radiologic findings: Plain radiograph may show mass with calcifications.

4. Staging (International Neuroblastoma Staging System)
   a. Stage 1: Localized tumor with complete resection
   b. Stage 2: Localized tumor with incomplete resection
      (1) 2A: Lymph nodes negative
      (2) 2B: Regional lymph nodes positive
   c. Stage 3: Unresectable tumor infiltrating across midline
   d. Stage 4: Any tumor with metastatic disease (except as defined for stage 4S)
   e. Stage 4S: Localized primary tumor with metastasis to skin, liver, or bone marrow in infants (<12 months of age)

5. Management: Combined-modality therapy is stratified according to risk groups.
   a. Low-risk disease: Surgery alone
   b. Intermediate-risk disease
      (1) Multiagent chemotherapy (doxorubicin, cyclophosphamide)
      (2) Surgical excision of primary tumor
      (3) Radiation therapy to primary tumor bed controversial
   c. High-risk disease
      (1) Multiagent chemotherapy (doxorubicin, cyclophosphamide, cisplatin, etoposide)

(2) Surgical excision of primary tumor
(3) Double autologous bone marrow transplantation
(4) Radiation therapy to primary tumor bed and bulky metastatic sites

6. Prognosis: The 5-year relative survival rate for infants with NB is 83%, compared with 55% for children 1 to 4 years of age.

GERM CELL TUMOR/TERATOMA

Germ cell tumor (GCT) is a benign or malignant neoplasm arising from pluripotential primordial germ cells that undergo differentiation. GCT variants may arise as gonadal or extragonadal tumors. GCT represents approximately 7% of all cancer in patients younger than 20 years of age and has an annual incidence of 12.0/1,000,000. GCT usually presents as a mass in the gonads (61% of cases: abdominal mass in girls; scrotal mass in boys) or sacrococcygeal area: palpable presacral mass with or without extension to the buttock (external mass) or pelvis and abdomen (internal mass), with constipation and neurologic abnormalities of the bladder and lower extremities. The most common location of extragonadal tumor in infants is the mediastinum and intracranium. Laboratory findings include elevated α-fetoprotein or β-human chorionic gonadotropin. Management includes combined-modality therapy that is stratified for stage and location (testicular, ovarian, extragonadal), with chemotherapy, surgery, and radiation therapy. The 5-year survival rate for patients younger than 20 years of age with GCT is 87%; relative survival rates are better for gonadal tumors (94%) than for extragonadal tumors (71%).

WILMS' TUMOR (NEPHROBLASTOMA)

1. Pathology: Wilms' tumor (WT) is a neoplasm apparently arising from embryonic kidney cells or nephrogenic rests. Microscopic classification is based on the extent of anaplasia.
2. Epidemiology: WT represents approximately 6% of all cancer in children younger than 15 years of age. The mean age of occurrence is in the third year of life, with over 75% of cases diagnosed before the age of 5 years. WT is by far the most common form of renal cancer in children, representing approximately 95% of cases.
3. Clinical features
   a. Symptoms: Change in bowel habits, abdominal pain, vomiting, and constitutional symptoms of weight loss
   b. Signs: Palpable abdominal mass (often without associated pain), hypertension, and microscopic hematuria
      (1) Hereditary WT associated with congenital nonfamilial aniridia, genitourinary abnormalities, and mental retardation (WAGR syndrome); hemihypertrophy, Beckwith-Wiedemann syndrome, and Denys-Drash syndrome have been reported in approximately 20% of cases; bilateral WT (both kidneys involved) is reported in hereditary tumors (5% of WT cases).
      (2) Metastatic disease to the lung may be present at diagnosis.
      (3) Rare cases of extrarenal WT have been reported.
   c. Laboratory findings
      (1) CBC: Hemoglobin elevated secondary to increased erythropoietin production

(2) Blood chemistries: paraneoplastic calcemia

(3) Coagulation studies: acquired von Willebrand's disease

4. Management: Combined-modality therapy is stratified by stage and degree of anaplasia:

   a. Surgery: Radical nephrectomy is indicated for all cases of unilateral WT.

   b. Multiagent chemotherapy: Vincristine with actinomycin D or with doxorubicin and actinomycin D ± etoposide, cyclophosphamide

   c. Radiation therapy in the postoperative setting is given except for patients with stage 1 and stage 2 WT with favorable histology.

5. Prognosis: The 5-year survival rate for children younger than 15 years of age with WT is 92%.

14.10 Work-Up of the Child with a Suspected Malignancy

1. Presenting symptoms and signs in the child with cancer

   a. Table 14-6 lists signs and symptoms that warrant urgent evaluation and possible referral to a pediatric oncology center.

   b. Abnormal CBC: Only 20% of new cases of acute leukemia in children have a WBC count greater than 50,000/mm^3. Half of new cases present with a WBC count less than 10,000/mm^3. Remember to check the smear! Bone marrow examination is usually the most appropriate study for a child with an abnormal CBC. Bone marrow aspiration with or without trephine biopsy from the posterior iliac crest is a relatively benign and simple invasive procedure in children (Box 14-9).

   c. Differential diagnosis of abnormal CBC

      (1) Leukemoid or "leukemia form" reactions (WBC count in excess of 50,000/mm^3 with immature granulocytes or "left shift") may occur with infections due to *Streptococcus*, *Staphylococcus*, and *H. influenza*, and some viral, fungal, protozoa, and spirochete infections.

      (2) Atypical lymphocytosis may be seen with infectious mononucleosis–associated EBV and CMV infection and mumps, varicella, adenovirus, and pertussis infections.

      (3) Isolated thrombocytopenia (platelet count <50,000/mm^3) or severe anemia may be seen with ITP or TEC, respectively.

   d. Lymphadenopathy: Enlarged lymph nodes (>1 cm in diameter) in children are usually related to infections or granulomatous diseases. Supraclavicular and lower neck adenopathy is more suggestive of malignancy (HD). Note: Any enlarged lymph node that persists longer than 30 days should be sampled for biopsy unless a clear cause has been identified (e.g., TB, atypical TB, etc.).

2. Differential diagnosis of pediatric malignant tumors: Age and site are important factors when evaluating a child with a suspected malignant tumor (Table 14-7).

3. Approach to a child with a suspected malignancy: Proper treatment of a child with cancer requires accurate pathologic, and in some cases genetic and molecular diagnosis as well as assessment of extent of

Symptoms/Signs	Laboratory, Imaging Studies, and Consultations	Major Associated Tumors
Hypertension	Labs, CXR, abdominal sonogram	Renal or adrenal tumor, neuroblastoma
Weight loss, sudden onset	Labs, abdominal sonogram	Any malignancy
Petechiae/bruising and pallor	CBC, plt, diff	Leukemia, neuroblastoma
Adenopathy unresponsive to antibiotics	Surgical consultation, CXR, CBC, diff	Leukemia, lymphoma
Endocrine abnormalities		
Growth failure	Hormonal assays	Pituitary and hypothalamic tumors
Electrolyte disturbance	CT hypothalamic area	Hepatoblastoma
Sexual abnormalities	Abdominal CT	Gonadal tumors
Cushing's syndrome	Endocrine consult	Adrenal tumors
Brain	Neurology or neurosurgery consultation followed by imaging studies	Brain tumor
Headache, vomiting early AM		
Cranial nerve palsy, ataxia		
Dilated pupil, papilledema		
Afebrile seizures		
Hallucinations, aphasia		
Unilateral weakness, paralysis		
Eyes	Ophthalmologist consultation	Retinoblastoma, metastatic rhabdomyosarcoma, neuroblastoma
Leukocoria, proptosis, blindness		
Wandering eye		
Intraorbital hemorrhage		

Symptoms/Signs	Laboratory, Imaging Studies, and Consultations	Major Associated Tumors
Ears		
Bulging mass external canal	CBC, diff, imaging studies	LCH; rhabdomyosarcoma
Horner's syndrome	CBC, diff, imaging studies	Neuroblastoma
Puffy face and neck (superior vena cava syndrome)	CBC, diff, imaging studies	Mediastinal tumors
Pharyngeal mass	CBC, diff, imaging studies	Rhabdomyosarcoma, lymphoma, neuroblastoma, osteosarcoma
Periodontal mass, loose teeth	Dental consultation, imaging studies	LCH; Burkitt's lymphoma, neuroblastoma, osteosarcoma
Thorax		
Extrathoracic: mass	CBC, diff, imaging studies	Soft tissue sarcomas, mediastinal tumors, metastatic tumors
Intrathoracic: chronic cough, shortness of breath without fever or no history of asthma, allergies		
Abdomen/pelvis/intraabdominal mass	CBC, diff, lab, imaging studies	Wilms' tumor, soft tissue sarcoma, neuroblastoma, hepatoblastoma, hepatocarcinoma
Genitourinary: scrotal or vaginal mass/ swelling	Urinalysis, CBC, diff, sonogram of pelvis/abdomen	Germ cell tumor, rhabdomyosarcoma
Musculoskeletal: soft tissue/bone mass, or pain, limp	CBC, diff, imaging studies	Osteosarcoma, Ewing's sarcoma, leukemia, neuroblastoma, soft tissue sarcoma

CBC, complete blood cell count; CT, computed tomography; CXR, chest radiograph; diff, differential; labs, laboratory studies, usually hepatic and renal function and electrolytes; LCH, Langerhans cell histiocytosis.
Modified from Pizzo PA, Poplack DG: Principles and Practice of Pediatric Oncology, 4th ed. Philadelphia, Lippincott Williams & Wilkins, 2002.

Box 14-9   Indications for Bone Marrow Examination

Common Clinical Indications

Abnormal CBC with "blast forms"*
Abnormal CBC with unexplained adenopathy or hepatosplenomegaly
Cytopenia of more than one blood cell line (pancytopenia)
Leukoerythroblastosis (immature granulocytes and red blood cells on
   peripheral smear) without an identifiable cause (e.g., infection or
   acute blood loss).

Less Common Clinical Indications

Isolated cytopenia
Evaluation of mediastinal mass
Evaluation of solid tumor
Evaluation of fever of unknown origin
Megaloblastic anemia
Evaluation of suspected storage disease

---

*Leukemia may be diagnosed from peripheral blood samples if the white blood cell
count is greater than 30,000/mm^3 with greater than 75% leukemic blasts.
CBC, complete blood count.

disease (staging). Table 14-8 summarizes diagnostic action plans for a
child with a suspected malignancy.

14.11 Supportive Care In Pediatric Oncology: Oncologic Emergencies, Infections, and Treatment of Nausea

ONCOLOGIC EMERGENCIES

1. Respiratory distress and superior vena cava (SVC) syndrome
   a. Etiology: Obstruction of trachea or SVC from mediastinal tumors in
      lymphoma (HD and NHL), leukemia (T-ALL cases), germ cell
      tumors, and NB
   b. Management
      (1) Control airway
      (2) Emergent systemic chemotherapy (empirical): Corticosteroids,
          cyclophosphamide
      (3) Radiation therapy
2. Spinal cord compression
   a. Etiology: Epidural compression of spinal cord, conus medullaris, or
      cauda equina from extension of a paravertebral tumor through the
      intervertebral foramina or subarachnoid space metastases. Common
      tumors include sarcoma (Ewing's sarcoma, osteosarcoma, rhabdo-
      myosarcoma), neuroblastoma, lymphoma, CNS primary tumors with
      metastases.

Site	Under 1 Year	1 to 3 Years	3 to 11 Years	12-15 Years
Central nervous system	Astrocytoma Medulloblastoma Ependymoma Other gliomas* sPNET Choroid plexus tumor	Astrocytoma Medulloblastoma Ependymoma Other gliomas sPNET Choroid plexus tumor Glioblastoma multiforme Pineocytoma	Astrocytoma Other gliomas Glioblastoma multiforme Medulloblastoma Craniopharyngioma Ependymoma sPNET Pineocytoma	Astrocytoma Craniopharyngioma Other gliomas Glioblastoma multiforme Medulloblastoma Primary germ cell tumor
Head and neck	Neuroblastoma Retinoblastoma Rhabdomyosarcoma	Neuroblastoma Retinoblastoma Rhabdomyosarcoma Lymphoma (non-Hodgkin's)	Lymphoma (non-Hodgkin's, Hodgkin's) Rhabdomyosarcoma Neuroblastoma Osteosarcoma Ewing's sarcoma	Lymphoma (non-Hodgkin's, Hodgkin's) Osteosarcoma Rhabdomyosarcoma Ewing's sarcoma
Thorax	Neuroblastoma Germ cell tumor Rhabdomyosarcoma	Neuroblastoma Germ cell tumor Rhabdomyosarcoma Lymphoma (non-Hodgkin's)	Lymphoma (non-Hodgkin's, Hodgkin's) Neuroblastoma Rhabdomyosarcoma Osteosarcoma Ewing sarcoma	Lymphoma (non-Hodgkin's, Hodgkin's) Osteosarcoma Rhabdomyosarcoma Ewing's sarcoma

Abdomen/ retroperitoneal/ genitourinary	Neuroblastoma Germ cell tumor Wilms' tumor Rhabdomyosarcoma Hepatoblastoma	Neuroblastoma Wilms' tumor Rhabdomyosarcoma Germ cell tumor Lymphoma (non-Hodgkin's) Hepatoblastoma	Lymphoma (non-Hodgkin's, Hodgkin's) Neuroblastoma Wilms' tumor Rhabdomyosarcoma Germ cell tumor Ewing's sarcoma	Lymphoma (non-Hodgkin's, Hodgkin's) Germ cell tumor Rhabdomyosarcoma Ewing's sarcoma Hepatocellular carcinoma
Extremity	Rhabdomyosarcoma Fibrosarcoma	Rhabdomyosarcoma Fibrosarcoma	Rhabdomyosarcoma Osteosarcoma Ewing's sarcoma Fibrosarcoma	Osteosarcoma Rhabdomyosarcoma Fibrosarcoma Ewing sarcoma

*Other gliomas includes oligodendroglial tumors and mixed gliomas.
sPNET, supratentorial primitive neuroectodermal tumors (includes cerebral neuroblastoma, pineoblastoma).

Suspected Malignancy	Diagnostic, Laboratory, and Imaging	Tissue Diagnosis	Staging Studies
Leukemia	CBC with differential, uric acid, LDH, prothrombin time, partial thromboplastin time, fibrinogen, peripheral blood immunophenotyping	Bone marrow aspirational biopsy; tissue for immunophenotyping, cytogenetic studies, molecular studies (RT-PCR, FISH)	CXR, CSF cell count with differential
Brain/central nervous system tumors	MRI scan with contrast imaging	Surgical biopsy with excision if feasible	Spinal imaging, CSF cytology, audiogram, endocrine evaluation, neurologic examination
Lymphoma	CT/MRI scan of primary site/neck/chest/abdomen/pelvis, marrow aspiration/biopsy (should be done before tumor biopsy to rule out leukemia if NHL suspected), CBC, uric acid, LDH, erythrocyte sedimentation rate, serum copper (Hodgkin's disease)	Incisional nodal biopsy; tissue for immunophenotyping	Gallium PET scan, CXR, bone marrow aspiration/biopsy*; CSF cell count with differential and cytology (NHL); bone scan (optional)
Neuroblastoma	CT/MRI scan of primary tumor, urinalysis for vanillylmandelic acid/homovanillic acid (random urine specimen), CBC, uric acid, LDH, serum ferritin	Surgical biopsy with excision if feasible; tissue for biology studies (MYCN amplification)	Bone marrow biopsy/aspirate*, CT scan of liver*, CT scan of chest*, CXR, bone scan*, metaiodobenzylguanidine (MIBG) scan (if available)

Tumor	Imaging/Laboratory Studies	Surgery	Staging Evaluation
Rhabdomyosarcoma/other undifferentiated soft tissue sarcoma	CT/MRI scan of primary tumor	Surgical biopsy with excision if feasible	CT scan of chest and liver, CXR, CT scan/MRI of brain* and CSF cytology (for parameningeal tumors), bone scan, bone marrow aspiration/biopsy
Wilms'/renal tumor	CT scan/sonogram of abdomen with excretory urography, CBC, urinalysis, renal function tests, serum calcium	Surgical biopsy with excision and nephrectomy (except for bilateral Wilms' tumor)	CT scan of chest, CXR, bone scan (clear cell sarcoma), CT/MRI scan of brain (clear cell sarcoma and rhabdoid tumor of the kidney), bone marrow aspirate/biopsy (clear cell sarcoma)
Osteosarcoma	Plain radiograph of involved bone, CT/MRI scan of involved bone, bone scan, serum alkaline phosphatase, LDH	Surgical biopsy with excision (amputation) if feasible	CT scan of chest*, CXR
Ewing's sarcoma/primitive neuroectodermal tumor	MRI scan of primary site, plain radiograph of involved bone (if bone involved)	Surgical biopsy; tissue for molecular studies (RT-PCR, FISH)	CT scan of chest*, CXR, bone marrow aspiration/biopsy, bone scan
Germ cell tumor	CT/MRI of primary site, α-fetoprotein, β-human chorionic gonadotropin, LDH	Surgical biopsy and excision if feasible	CT scan of chest*, CXR, CT/MRI scan of brain (if clinically indicated), bone scan (if clinically indicated)

*May have been performed before tissue diagnosis.

CBC, complete blood count; CT, computed tomography; CSF, cerebrospinal fluid; CXR, chest radiograph; FISH, fluorescence in situ hybridization; LDH, lactate-dehydrogenase; MRI, magnetic resonance imaging; NHL, non-Hodgkin's lymphoma; PET, positron emission tomography; RT-PCR, reverse transcriptase polymerase chain reaction.

b. Presentation: Back pain (local or radicular), progressive weakness, sensory abnormalities, change in bowel/bladder function, paresis

c. Management
   (1) Emergent neurosurgical consultation
   (2) Dexamethasone 2 mg/kg/day divided every 6 hours (maximum 16 mg/day)
   (3) Radiation therapy

3. Increased intracranial pressure
   a. Etiology: Obstruction of cerebrospinal fluid flow by tumor causing hydrocephalus or mass effect and swelling caused by a CNS tumor or metastases
   b. Management
      (1) Emergent neurosurgical consultation
      (2) Dexamethasone 2 mg/kg first dose, then 0.5 mg/kg/dose every 6 hours (maximum 16 mg/day).

4. Tumor lysis syndrome
   a. Etiology: Tumor lysis syndrome from tumor cell catabolism and increased synthesis of uric acid is defined by the classic triad of hyperuricemia, hyperphosphatemia, and hyperkalemia; hypocalcemia can develop secondary to hyperphosphatemia. Risk factors:
      (1) ALL with leukocytosis (WBC >50,000/mm^3) and LDH greater than twice the upper limit of normal
      (2) NHL, high grade with significant tumor burden (LDH greater than twice the upper limit of normal)
      (3) Other pediatric malignant neoplasms with significant tumor burden
   b. Presentation
      (1) Elevated uric acid (>8 mg/dL), phosphorus, potassium
      (2) Symptomatic hypocalcemia (tetany, cramps)
      (3) Acute renal failure (oliguria, creatinine >1.5 mg/dL)
   c. Management
      (1) Hydration at 3000 mL/m^2/day (without potassium-containing solutions) ± alkalinization (20 to 40 mEq/L to maintain urine pH >6.5, but <8.0 to avoid calcium phosphate precipitation).
      (2) Uric acid reduction
         (a) Allopurinol 300 mg/m^2/day (oral or IV) divided every 8 hours
         (b) Urate oxidase 0.2 mg/kg/day (IV) once a day (*contraindicated in patients with G6PD deficiency*)
      (3) Hyperkalemia
         (a) Sodium polystyrene sulfonate (Kayexalate 1 g/kg/dose every 6 hours, maximum 60 g/day); administer as 25% sorbitol solution
         (b) Insulin 0.1 U/kg with glucose 25% solution 2 mL/kg
         (c) Dialysis
      (4) Hyperphosphatemia
         (a) Aluminum hydroxide 15 mL every 4 to 8 hours
         (b) Diuresis with furosemide 1 mg/kg (avoid with hypovolemia)
         (c) Dialysis

INFECTION

1. Fever and neutropenia (work-up and management)
   a. Definition: ANC 500/mm^3 or less, or less than 1000/mm^3 and falling after recent myelosuppressive chemotherapy, and fever greater than 38.5° C (orally) or three temperature elevations between 38° C and 38.5° C within a 24 hour period
   b. Diagnosis
      (1) Physical examination: Careful attention to oral cavity, perineum, central venous access site, and cutaneous wounds
      (2) Laboratory and radiologic evaluation
         (a) CBC with manual differential, basic metabolic profile, liver function panel
         (b) Blood culture(s) from all central venous catheter lumens/ports
         (c) Urinalysis/urine culture (do not catheterize)
         (d) Plain radiograph of chest if clinically indicated (dyspnea, tachypnea, rales, decreased breath sounds)
   c. Management: Empirical antimicrobial therapy (deliver first dose antibiotic within 30 to 60 minutes of arrival/registration in emergency department or clinic; consider local bacterial sensitivities and previous blood culture isolates)
      (1) Ceftazidime 50 mg/kg/dose (maximum dose is 2 g) IV every 8 hours
         (a) *For children with penicillin/beta-lactam allergy:* gentamicin 2 to 2.5 mg/kg/dose IV every 8 hours and clindamycin 10 mg/kg/dose (maximum dose 1.2 g) IV every 6 hours
      (2) Consider adding vancomycin if skin infection suspected, there are gram-positive bacteria isolates on blood culture, or the patient is seriously ill.
      (3) Consider adding gentamicin if there are gram-negative bacteria isolates on blood culture.
      (4) Consider IV amphotericin in children with persistent fever and neutropenia (4 to 7 days) for possible fungal infection.
2. Prevention of infection in patients with cancer
   a. Antimicrobial prophylaxis
      (1) *Pneumocystis carinii:* Indicated in children receiving immunosuppressive chemotherapy for hematologic malignancies, sarcomas, NB, WT, or CNS tumors
   b. Expectant therapy for prevention (options)
      (1) Co-trimoxazole (Bactrim, Septra) 150 mg/m^2 (maximum 160 mg) of the trimethoprim component orally two times a day, three sequential days per week
      (2) Dapsone 1 to 2 mg/kg/day (maximum 100 mg) orally once a day
      (3) Pentamidine aerosolized every 2 to 4 weeks
      (4) Atovaquone 30 mg/kg/day (maximum 1500 mg) for children older than 24 months of age and 45 mg/kg/day for children between 3 months and 24 months of age orally once a day
   c. Varicella
      (1) Indication: Children receiving immunosuppressive chemotherapy with exposure to chickenpox or zoster (susceptible patients or those with uncertain or unknown immunity)

(2) Management: Varicella-zoster immune globulin 125 U/10 kg (maximum 625 U) intramuscularly within 72 hours of exposure.

CHEMOTHERAPY-INDUCED NAUSEA AND VOMITING

1. Etiology: The emetic reflex has three key components: visceral afferents from the GI tract, emetic or vomiting center in the brain stem, and the area postrema or chemoreceptor trigger zone. Chemotherapy drugs used in children vary in their emetogenicity (Box 14-10). Emesis may be acute (within 24 hours after administration of chemotherapy) or delayed.
2. Management
   a. Medications: Serotonin (5-HT3) receptor antagonist (ondansetron, granisetron, dolasetron), dexamethasone (DXM), neurokinin-1 receptor antagonist (NK-1; aprepitant), metoclopramide (MCP)
   b. Pretreatment for acute nausea/vomiting (administered before each dose of chemotherapy)

Box 14-10   Emetogenicity of Selected Chemotherapeutic Agents

High

Cisplatin
Cyclophosphamide (>1000 mg/m²)
Cytarabine (>1000 mg/m²)
Moderate

Cyclophosphamide (<1000 mg/m²)
Ifosfamide
Doxorubicin
Etoposide
Cytarabine
Methotrexate (>1000 mg/m²)
Carboplatin
Low

Asparaginase
Methotrexate (<50 mg/m²)
Etoposide
Bleomycin
Vinblastine
Minimal

Corticosteroids
Vincristine
Mercaptopurine
Hydroxyurea

   (1) High emetogenicity: 5-HT3 + DXM ± NK-1 (in older children)
   (2) Moderate emetogenicity: 5-HT3 + DXM
   (3) Low emetogenicity: DXM or 5-HT3
   (4) Minimal emetogenicity: None
  c. Second-line therapy for acute nausea/vomiting: Phenothiazines (promethazine, chlorpromazine) or butyrophenones (droperidol, haloperidol)
  d. Management for delayed emesis
   (1) MCP 2 mg/kg/dose (maximum 30 mg) oral or IV every 6 hours as needed
    (a) Diphenhydramine 1 mg/kg/dose (maximum 25 mg) oral or IV given with MCP to prevent extrapyramidal reactions
   (2) DXM 1 mg/kg/dose (maximum 6 mg) oral or IV every 6 hours as needed
  e. Adjunctive therapy: Cannabinoids (dronabinol)

SUGGESTED READING

Aprikyan A, Dale DC: Mutations in the neutrophil elastase gene in cyclic and congenital neutropenia. Curr Opin Immunol 13:535-538, 2001.

Buchanan GR: ITP: How much treatment is enough? Contemp Pediatr 17:112-121, 2000.

Bussel JB: Immune thrombocytopenia purpura. In Michelson AD (ed): Platelets. San Diego, Elsevier Science, 2002.

Cohen ME, Duffner PK (eds): Brain Tumors in Children: Principles of Diagnosis and Treatment, 2nd ed. New York, Raven Press, 1994.

Constine LS, Paidas C, Schwartz CL, Korones DN: Pediatric solid tumors. In Rubin P (ed): Clinical Oncology: A Multidisciplinary Approach for Physicians and Students, 8th ed. Philadelphia, WB Saunders, 2001.

Cools J, DeAngelo DJ, Gotlib J, et al: A tyrosine kinase created by fusion of the PDGFRα and FIP1L1 genes as a therapeutic target of imatinib in idiopathic hypereosinophilic syndrome. N Engl J Med 248:1201-1214, 2003.

Elghetany MT, Davey FR: Erythrocytic disorders. In Henry JB (ed): Clinical Diagnosis and Management by Laboratory Methods, 19th ed. Philadelphia, WB Saunders, 1996.

George JN, Woolf SH, Raskob GE, et al: Idiopathic thrombocytopenia purpura: A practice guideline developed by explicit methods for the American Society of Hematology. Blood 88:3-40, 1996.

Heyworth PG, Cross AR, Curnutte JT: Chronic granulomatous disease. Curr Opin Immunol 15:578-584, 2003.

Huisman THJ, Carver MFH, Efremov GD: A syllabus of human hemoglobin variants (1996). Augusta, Ga, The Sickle Cell Anemia Foundation, 1996. Available at http://globin.cse.psu.edu/.

Knight PJ, Mulne AF, Vassy LE: When is lymph node biopsy indicated in children with enlarged peripheral nodes? Pediatrics 69:391-396, 1982.

Levy GG, Nichols WC, Lian EC, et al: Mutations in a member of the ADAMTS gene family cause thrombotic thrombocytopenic purpura. Nature 413:488-494, 2001.

Moake JL: Thrombotic microangiopathies. N Engl J Med 347:589-600, 2003.

National Heart, Lung and Blood Institute, Division of Blood Diseases and Resources: The Management of Sickle Cell Disease, 4th ed. NIH publication no. 02-2117. Bethesda, Md, National Institutes of Health, 2002. Available at www.nhlbi.nih.gov/health/prof/blood/sickle/index.htm.

Ries LAG, Smith MA; Gurney JG, et al (eds): Cancer Incidence and Survival among Children and Adolescents: United States SEER Program 1975-1995. National Cancer Institute, SEER Program. NIH publication no. 99-4649. Bethesda, Md, 1999. Available at http://seer.cancer.gov/publications/childhood/.

Vietti TJ, Steuber CP: Clinical assessment and differential diagnosis of the child with suspected cancer. In Pizzo, PA, Poplack DG (eds): Principles and Practice of Pediatric Oncology, 4th ed. Philadelphia, Lippincott Williams & Wilkins, 2002.

Vipul NM: Thalassemia syndromes. In Miller DR, Baehner RL (eds): Blood Diseases of Infancy and Childhood: In the Tradition of C. H. Smith, 7th ed. St. Louis, Mosby-Year Book, 1995.

WEBSITE

National Cancer Institute: www.cancer.gov

Cardiovascular Disorders

15

Shelley D. Miyamoto and Lloyd R. Felt

15.1 Approach to the Cardiovascular Evaluation: History and Physical Examination

1. Perinatal history
   a. In utero teratogenic exposure (e.g., phenytoin, rubella, alcohol)
   b. Gestational age, mode of delivery, transition to extrauterine life
   c. Complications (diabetes, pregnancy-induced hypertension)
   d. Associated congenital malformations or chromosomal abnormalities
2. Family history
   a. Family members with childhood cardiac illness (especially congenital heart disease [CHD] or cardiomyopathies)
   b. Genetic conditions or syndromes known to predispose to heart disease (e.g., Marfan's syndrome, Noonan's syndrome, Turner's syndrome, DiGeorge's syndrome, Down syndrome, Duchenne's muscular dystrophy, glycogen storage diseases)
   c. Sudden death (especially at an early age)
3. Present history
   a. Feeding pattern and feeding tolerance
   b. Growth and development
   c. Signs of heart failure: Tachycardia, tachypnea, diaphoresis, irritability, vomiting, peripheral edema, dyspnea on exertion
   d. Cyanosis or episodes of poor coloring
   e. Palpitations, chest pain (inciting and relieving factors)
   f. Syncope
   g. Exercise tolerance
4. Physical examination: See Chapter 1

15.2 Diagnostic Tests

ELECTROCARDIOGRAM

1. In the pediatric population, electrocardiogram (ECG) norms are age related (Fig. 15-1; see Appendix I-B). An important distinguishing characteristic is the gradual transition of right ventricular (RV) dominance of the fetus and newborn to the typical adult pattern of left

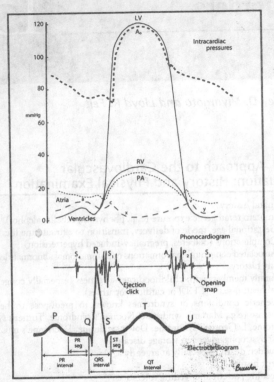

Figure 15-1 The cardiac cycle. A$_O$, aorta; LV, left ventricle; PA, pulmonary artery; RV, right ventricle. (From Robertson J, Shilkofski N: The Harriet Lane Handbook, 17th ed. Philadelphia, Elsevier Mosby, 2005.)

ventricular (LV) dominance. When interpreting an ECG, use a methodical, consistent approach to assure completeness:

   a. Rate

   b. Rhythm

   c. Axis (P wave, QRS, T wave)

   d. Conduction intervals (PR, QRS, QTc)

   e. Chamber enlargement

2. Rate: A rapid method for determining rate is achieved by measuring the R-R interval and using Figure 15-2, allowing that one "big box" corresponds to 0.20 second (at a paper speed of 25 mm/sec). Remember to measure *both* the atrial and ventricular rate, especially when atrioventricular (AV) block or dissociation is suspected. Normal age-specific heart rate (HR) ranges (beats per minute) and ECG parameters can be found in Appendix I-B.

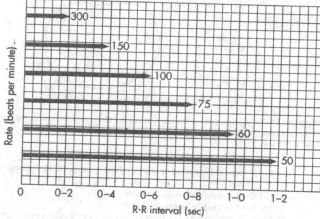

Figure 15-2 Estimation of the rate based on the R-R interval. (From Johnson KB: The Harriet Lane Handbook, 14th ed. St. Louis, Mosby, 1996.)

3. Rhythm: Normal sinus rhythm implies the presence of a normal sino-atrial (SA) node, which is located at the right atrium–superior vena cava (SVC) junction. Atrial depolarization results in a P-wave axis of 0 to 90 degrees. Therefore, sinus rhythm is defined by a P-wave axis of 0 to 90 degrees and a P wave preceding each QRS complex, and a QRS complex following each P wave.

4. Axis: The hexaxial reference is used to determine net depolarization/repolarization vectors of various chambers (atria or ventricles; Fig. 15-3). The simplest method is initially to determine the quadrant by evaluating the net QRS amplitude in leads I and aVF (Fig. 15-4). Next, identify the lead that is equiphasic (the R wave is roughly the same amplitude as the S wave). The net QRS vector or QRS axis will be perpendicular to this equiphasic lead and within the quadrant identified earlier. Normal values are age-related and listed in Appendix I-B.

   a. The relationship of the T-wave axis to the QRS axis (the QRS-T angle) should not deviate by more than 90 degrees. An abnormal QRS-T angle is associated with severe ventricular hypertrophy with strain, conduction system disease, or significant myocardial dysfunction.

5. Conduction intervals: Intervals are generally measured in lead II.

   a. The age-related range of PR intervals is shown in Appendix I-B.

   b. QRS intervals vary less with age and range from 0.05 second (50 msec) in the newborn to 0.10 second (100 msec) in the adolescent.

   c. QTc interval is calculated by measuring the QT interval directly, then correcting for HR using Bazett's formula: $QTc = QT \sqrt{R\text{-}R \text{ interval}}$. Use the R-R interval immediately preceding the measured QT interval.

      (1) Normal QTc intervals are

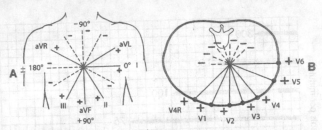

Figure 15-3 A, Hexaxial reference system. B, Horizontal reference system. (From Robertson J, Shilkofski N: The Harriet Lane Handbook, 17th ed. Philadelphia, Elsevier Mosby, 2005.)

        (a) 0.45 to 0.49 second or less in infants younger than 6 months of age

        (b) 0.44 second or less in children

        (c) 0.43 second or less in adolescents

    (2) Note: A prolonged QTc interval in isolation does not make the diagnosis of long QT syndrome. For information on the long QT syndrome, refer to the Suggested Reading list at the end of this chapter.

  d. Conduction disturbances

    (1) *Bundle branch block* implies slowed conduction in either of the two major branches of the infra-His conduction system. Right bundle branch block (RBBB) is most commonly associated with

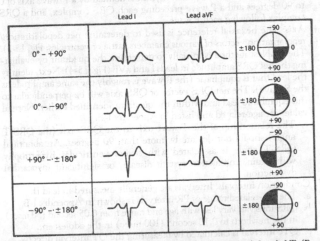

Figure 15-4 Locating quadrants of mean QRS axis from leads I and aVF. (From Park MK, Guntheroth WG: How to Read Pediatric ECGs, 3rd ed. Chicago, Year Book Medical Publishers, 1992.)

heart defects that cause a volume load of the right ventricle (such as an atrial septal defect [ASD]) or after cardiac surgery involving a right ventriculotomy in which the right bundle branch is physically disrupted. Left bundle branch block (LBBB) is rare in children, although it may be seen with metabolic disorders or dilated cardiomyopathy. Left anterior hemiblock (LAHB) is most commonly associated with AV canal defect or the postoperative setting.

- (a) RBBB criteria
    - (i) Right axis deviation (may be limited to terminal portion of QRS)
    - (ii) QRS duration greater than upper limit of normal for age
    - (iii) Slurring of the terminal portion of the QRS complex (i.e., wide, slurred S wave in leads I, V_5, V_6; wide, slurred R′ in leads aVR, V_4R, V_1, V_2).
- (b) LBBB criteria
    - (i) QRS duration greater than upper limit of normal for age
    - (ii) Absence of Q wave in V_6, monophasic R in V_1
- (c) LAHB criteria
    - (i) Normal QRS duration
    - (ii) Left axis deviation, qR pattern in lead I, aVL; rS in lead III
- (2) *Preexcitation* is the term used to describe the early ventricular depolarization seen in patients with Wolff-Parkinson-White (WPW) syndrome. An accessory pathway (bundle of Kent) allows conduction to bypass normal delay at the AV node, depolarizing the ventricular myocardium directly. This bypass tract acts as an important component of the A-V reentry circuit in some patients with supraventricular tachycardia. Criteria for the ECG diagnosis of WPW syndrome include
    - (a) Short PR interval (below the lower limit of normal for age).
    - (b) Delta wave: slurred upstroke of QRS that represents slower conduction velocity of ventricular myocardium.
    - (c) Note: In Lown-Ganong-Levine syndrome, patients have an accessory pathway that bypasses the AV node (short PR) but connects directly to the normal His-Purkinje system, allowing for normal ventricular depolarization (narrow QRS without a delta wave).
6. Chamber enlargement
    a. *Atrial enlargement* is diagnosed by evaluation of P-wave morphology, particularly in lead II.
        - (1) Right atrial enlargement (P-pulmonale): tall P waves (>2.5 to 3 mm)
        - (2) Left atrial enlargement (P-mitrale): Wide P waves with duration over 0.08 second; many are biphasic or bifid ("notched"), especially in leads V_3R and V_1, where the terminal negative P-wave deflection is prominent.
    b. *Ventricular hypertrophy* is diagnosed by the amplitude of R or S waves in the precordial leads. Age-related norms are listed in Appendix I-B. It is important to remember that ventricular hypertrophy is virtually impossible to diagnose in the presence of conduction abnormalities

such as bundle branch block. Cardiac malposition also precludes accurate estimation of chamber enlargement.

(1) Criteria for right ventricular hypertrophy (RVH)
   (a) R in V_1 greater than the 98th percentile for age
   (b) S in V_6 greater than the 98th percentile for age
   (c) Upright T wave in V_1 after 1 week of life
   (d) qR pattern in V_3R or V_1
   (e) Wide QRS-T angle, suggesting RVH with strain

(2) Criteria for left ventricular hypertrophy (LVH)
   (a) R in V_6 greater than the 98th percentile for age
   (b) S in V_1 greater than the 98th percentile for age
   (c) R leads in I, II, III, aVL, aVF greater than the 98th percentile for age
   (d) Deep Q waves (≥ 5 mm) in V_5, V_6
   (e) Wide QRS-T angle, suggesting LVH with strain

(3) Criteria for combined ventricular hypertrophy
   (a) Positive criteria (above) for both RVH and LVH in the absence of bundle branch block
   (b) Katz-Wachtel criteria: large amplitude (55 to 60 mm or more) equiphasic complexes in the mid-precordial leads (V_2 to V_5).

CHEST RADIOGRAPH

Information that can be gleaned from a good chest radiograph (CXR) includes heart size, specific chamber enlargement, pulmonary blood flow (as suggested by pulmonary vascular markings), situs determination, and other anomalies (Fig. 15-5).

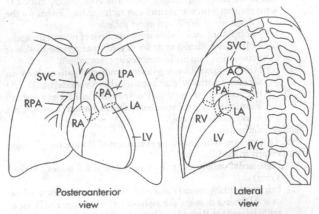

Posteroanterior view   Lateral view

Figure 15-5 Posteroanterior and lateral projections of normal cardiac silhouette. AO, aorta; IVC, inferior vena cava; LA, left atrium; LPA, left pulmonary artery; LV, left ventricle; PA, pulmonary artery; RA, right atrium; RPA, right pulmonary artery; RV, right ventricle; SVC, superior vena cava. (From Park MK: The Pediatric Cardiology Handbook, 3rd ed. Philadelphia, Mosby, 2003.)

1. Heart size: Evaluate the cardiothoracic (CT) ratio; a CT ratio of 0.55 or more suggests significant cardiomegaly. Pay attention to film quality and inspiratory effort (with poor inspiration, the CT ratio can be falsely elevated).

2. Specific chamber enlargement
   a. Right atrium (RA): Seen in the right lateral portion of the antero-posterior (AP) frontal radiograph
   b. Left atrium (LA): Best seen in the lateral film as a posterior displacement of the cardiac shadow, often displacing the air column of the left lower lobe bronchus. Bronchial compression may cause left lower lobe atelectasis in marked LA enlargement.
   c. RV: Best seen in the lateral projection as filling of the "retrosternal clear space." Sometimes, long-standing RVH may tip up the cardiac apex, contributing to the "boot-shaped heart" of tetralogy of Fallot (TOF).
   d. LV: Best seen in the frontal projection, where the cardiac apex is displaced downward and leftward

3. Great vessels
   a. Evaluate the laterality of the aortic arch by noting the indentation of the tracheal air column (right aortic arch is seen in 25% of patients with TOF).
   b. A narrow cardiac waist suggests transposition of the great arteries (TGA), either alone or in conjunction with other anomalies.
   c. Prominence of either great vessel suggests valvar stenosis with resultant poststenotic dilation.

4. Pulmonary blood flow
   a. Prominent pulmonary vascular markings may indicate increased pulmonary blood flow due to a L-R shunt (ventricular septal defect [VSD], ASD, patent ductus arteriosus [PDA]). They are present when vessels are seen well into the peripheral third of the lung fields or seen well in the lung apices.
   b. Diminished pulmonary markings demonstrated by thin spidery vessels in conjunction with black lung fields suggest decreased pulmonary blood flow, as can occur with various types of CHD (e.g., TOF, tricuspid atresia).
   c. Pulmonary venous congestion is seen as hazy, reticular vascular markings that are often horizontal and very indistinct. This should indicate abnormalities of LV inflow (heart failure with diastolic dysfunction, mitral stenosis, hypertrophic obstructive cardiomyopathy, total anomalous venous return with obstruction).

5. Situs abnormalities
   a. Location of the cardiac apex (levocardia, mesocardia, dextrocardia)
   b. Laterality and position of the abdominal organs (stomach bubble and liver)
   c. Branching pattern of the mainstem bronchi. The right bronchus takes a more vertical course than the left, with the right upper lobe bronchus superior to the right pulmonary artery (RPA).
   d. Note: Situs inversus totalis is not associated with an increased risk of CHD, but isolated segment situs abnormalities (inversus—stomach on the right, liver on the left or ambiguous—stomach on either side,

midline liver) are usually indicative of heterotaxy syndromes (polysplenia or asplenia) and have a high incidence of associated structural cardiac malformations.

6. Skeletal abnormalities
    a. Vertebral anomalies are seen in syndromes associated with CHD (vertebral, anal, tracheo-esophageal, and renal [VATER] complex).
    b. Rib notching is seen in chronic coarctation of the aorta secondary to dilation of intervertebral collateral vessels.
    c. Sternal anomalies (double manubrium in Down syndrome, pectus deformity)

ECHOCARDIOGRAM

An echocardiogram is an important noninvasive diagnostic modality that can provide valuable information regarding cardiac structure and function. The following is a brief description of the variable components of a typical "echo" (Fig. 15-6).

1. M-mode echocardiography: An "ice-pick" view of the motion of cardiac structures in real time. It is used primarily to
    a. Measure cardiac dimensions (chamber size, wall thickness)
    b. Determine ventricular function such as shortening fraction (normal is 28% to 44%) and ejection fraction (normal is 64% to 83%)

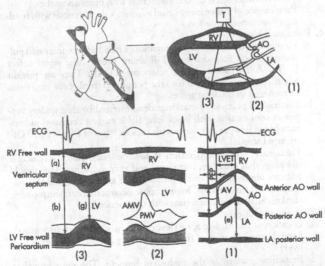

Figure 15-6 Cross-sectional view of the left side of the heart along the long axis (*top*) through which "ice pick" views of the M-mode echo recordings are made (*bottom*). AMV, anterior mitral valve; AV, aortic valve; ECG, electrocardiogram; LVET, left ventricular ejection time; PEP, pre-ejection period; PMV, posterior mitral valve; T, transducer; other abbreviations as in Figure 15-5. (From Park MK: Pediatric Cardiology for Practitioners, 3rd ed. Chicago, Year Book Medical Publishers, 1996.)

2. Two-dimensional echocardiography: A tomographic cross-sectional ultrasound beam. Obtained in a set of standard transthoracic views, it provides the greatest amount of information on cardiac structure (Figs. 15-7 through 15-10). Transesophageal echo has become an integral part of the evaluation and management of patients difficult to image via the thorax and during intraoperative repair of many heart defects.

3. Doppler echocardiography (pulsed, continuous, and color flow): Uses the Doppler shift in frequency of sound bounced off a moving object to calculate velocity and direction of blood flow within cardiac chambers, across valves, and through defects. It is used to predict hemodynamic effects of various lesions and is particularly useful in estimating transvalvular gradients and evaluating pulmonary hypertension.

CARDIAC MAGNETIC RESONANCE IMAGING

Cardiac magnetic resonance imaging (MRI) is particularly useful in the assessment of vascular structures within the chest cavity (e.g., coarctation of the aorta, aortic dilation in Marfan's syndrome or aortic stenosis). Quantification of regurgitant or shunt volume and assessment of ventricular function are other common indications for this important noninvasive tool.

CARDIOPULMONARY STRESS TESTING

Exercise testing by treadmill or bicycle protocol is an important aspect of the assessment of a child with known heart disease and in those with normal hearts undergoing evaluation for symptomatology that may be cardiac in origin (e.g., chest pain, syncope, palpitations, easy fatigue). Monitoring of HR and blood pressure (BP) response, ECG changes, maximum oxygen consumption, and ventilation properties can be helpful in assessing the cardiovascular health of a child and in monitoring the effectiveness of therapy.

CARDIAC CATHETERIZATION

Because of the evolution of more sophisticated noninvasive diagnostic tools such as echocardiography and MRI, cardiac catheterization is now less frequently used as a diagnostic tool and more often as a therapeutic option (i.e., angioplasty for coarctation, valvuloplasty for pulmonic stenosis, PDA coil closure, device occlusion of ASD). However, cardiac catheterization remains an invaluable tool for direct assessment of hemodynamics, cardiac output, and structural anatomy, as well as for obtaining biopsies of ventricular myocardium in the setting of myocarditis or cardiac transplantation.

15.3 Murmurs: Innocent or Pathologic

Heart murmurs are probably detected in 75% to 90% of all children at some point in their lifetime. The critical issue is to be able to identify the very few that are indicative of heart disease. When describing benign murmurs, one should use the term *innocent* versus *functional* because the former has an important calming effect on anxious parents, patients, and caretakers. It is important to remember that high-output states such as fever or anemia often intensify even the most benign murmur.

15—Cardiovascular Disorders

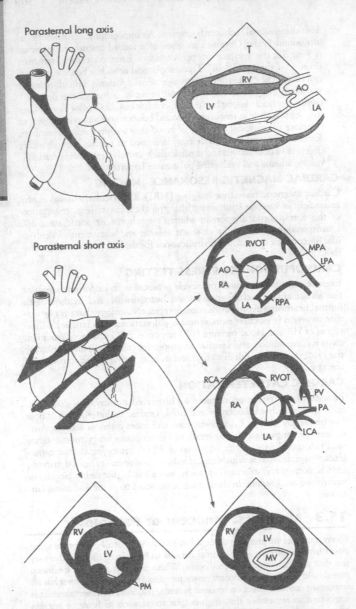

Parasternal long axis

T

RV

AO

LV

LA

Parasternal short axis

RVOT

MPA

AO

LPA

RA

LA

RPA

RCA

RVOT

RA

PV

PA

LA

LCA

RV

LV

PM

RV

LV

MV

Figure 15-7 Diagrammatic illustration of important two-dimensional echo views obtained from the parasternal transducer (T) position. LCA, left coronary artery; MPA, main pulmonary artery; MV, mitral valve; PM, papillary muscles; PV, pulmonary valve; RCA, right coronary artery; RVOT, right ventricular outflow tract; other abbreviations as in Figure 15-5. (From Park MK: Pediatric Cardiology for Practitioners, 3rd ed. Chicago, Year Book Medical Publishers, 1996.)

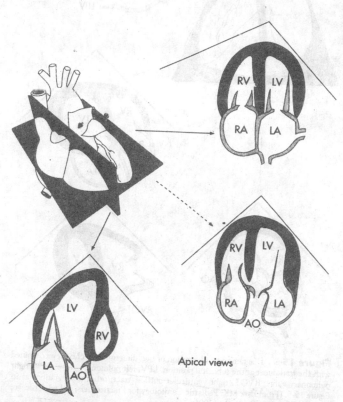

Apical views

Figure 15-8 Diagrammatic illustration of two-dimensional echo views obtained with the transducer at the apical position. Abbreviations as in Figure 15-5. (From Park MK: Pediatric Cardiology for Practitioners, 3rd ed. Chicago, Year Book Medical Publishers, 1996.)

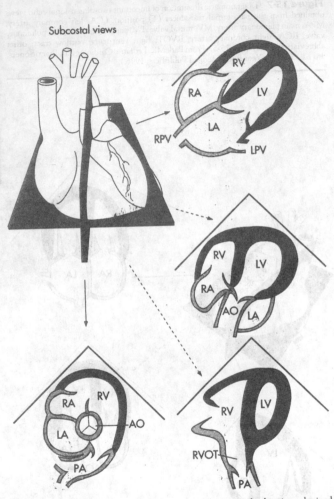

Figure 15-9 Diagrammatic illustration of two-dimensional echo views obtained with the transducer at the subcostal position. LPV, left pulmonary valve; RPV, right pulmonary valve; RVOT, right ventricular outflow tract; other abbreviations as in Figure 15-5. (From Park MK: Pediatric Cardiology for Practitioners, 3rd ed. Chicago, Year Book Medical Publishers, 1996.)

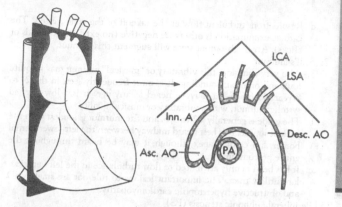

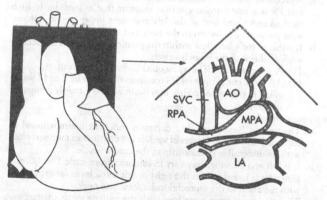

Suprasternal notch views

Figure 15-10 Diagrammatic illustration of two-dimensional echo views obtained with the transducer at the suprasternal notch. Asc. AO, ascending aorta; Desc. AO, descending aorta; Inn. A, innominate artery; LCA, left coronary artery; LSA, left subclavian artery; MPA, main pulmonary artery; other abbreviations as in Figure 15-5. (From Park MK: Pediatric Cardiology for Practitioners, 3rd ed. Chicago, Year Book Medical Publishers, 1996.)

TYPICAL INNOCENT MURMURS

1. Basal flow murmur (pulmonary and aortic flow murmur)
   a. Found in all age groups, it is probably the most common of all innocent murmurs.
   b. Usually it is a grade 2/6 systolic ejection murmur (SEM) heard best at either the left (pulmonic) or right (aortic) upper sternal border.

    c. Results from turbulent flow at the takeoff of the great vessels. The cardiac examination is otherwise negative (no extra heart sounds or clicks). Any high-output state will augment this murmur.

2. Still's murmur
    a. Also very common, this vibratory or "musical" murmur may be quite loud and ominous sounding. It is most frequently seen in the 2- to 8-year-old range but may be heard at any age. It is a low-pitched systolic murmur, with a vibratory or musical quality.
    b. The grade is generally a 2 to 3/6, and the murmur is loudest with the patient supine. It is best heard midway between the left lower sternal border and cardiac apex, though it may be heard throughout the entire precordium.
    c. It has been mainly attributed to flow turbulence in the left ventricular outflow tract. The important lesions to rule out are small VSD and obstructive hypertrophic cardiomyopathy.

3. Peripheral pulmonic stenosis (PS)
    a. A common innocent murmur of newborns and young infants, peripheral PS is a mid-systolic ejection murmur that is medium to high pitched and heard best at the left and right upper sternal borders, with prominent radiation to the back and both axillae.
    b. It is due to turbulent flow within the pulmonary artery at the acutely angled takeoff of the branch vessels.
        (1) An associated ASD may be quite difficult to rule out.
        (2) All innocent peripheral PS murmurs disappear by 8 to 12 weeks of life (a protracted course may occur among formerly premature infants).

4. Venous hum
    a. The venous hum is another common innocent murmur heard in early childhood (2 to 5 years of age). It is a continuous murmur, often with no discernible relationship to the cardiac cycle.
    b. It is soft and blowing, may vary in intensity from grade 1 to 3/6, and generally is heard best in the right or left infraclavicular area, often with radiation to the supraclavicular fossa and neck.
    c. This murmur is often quite loud with the patient in the sitting position, but it virtually disappears when the patient is supine with the neck rotated toward either shoulder. Similarly, it will disappear when the jugular veins are compressed by manual pressure.
    d. It is due to turbulent flow through the jugular and superficial veins as they traverse the clavicles.
    e. Important lesions in the differential are those that present with a continuous murmur, specifically PDA and arteriovenous malformations (AVMs).

5. Supraclavicular bruit
    a. Most prevalent in mid-childhood and adolescence, this murmur is heard best in the supraclavicular area and may radiate slightly to the lower neck.
    b. It is a high-pitched SEM that may be slightly harsh, usually grade 1 to 3/6. This murmur may be accentuated with light pressure on the subclavian artery. Typically it also is abolished when the patient raises the chin and throws back the shoulders.

   c. It is thought to be due to turbulence of flow at the takeoff of the brachiocephalic vessels from the aortic arch.
      (1) Pathologic lesions with similar-sounding murmurs that should be excluded include valvar aortic or pulmonic stenosis.
      (2) Abolition of the murmur with the previously discussed maneuvers, lack of an associated ejection click, and minimal radiation strongly suggest the diagnosis of an innocent supraclavicular bruit.
6. Mammary souffle
   a. This murmur is usually continuous but may occasionally be systolic ejection in nature. It is heard best in the second or third interspace in the mid-clavicular line on either the left or right hemithorax and is occasionally appreciated in pregnant/lactating young women.
   b. It may be accentuated with light pressure of the stethoscope, abolished with firm pressure (thought to be secondary to increased blood flow to developing or highly metabolic breast tissue).
   c. Because of the continuous nature of the murmur, it must be distinguished from a PDA or AVM.

CHARACTERISTICS OF PATHOLOGIC MURMURS

Listed here are some typical findings that help identify a murmur as "pathologic" (i.e., suggestive of cardiac disease) and one whose work-up should be pursued (see also Chapter 1 for location and type of murmurs).
1. Significant history of heart disease or congenital abnormality
2. Loud, harsh quality of murmur
3. Any diastolic murmur
4. Any holosystolic murmur
5. Any heart murmur appreciated in association with other abnormal cardiac findings (e.g., loud, single S2; diminished femoral pulses; ejection click; cyanosis)
6. Heart murmur in association with failure to thrive, congestive heart failure (CHF), or other significant systemic illness.

15.4 Heart Failure

DEFINITION AND PATHOPHYSIOLOGY

1. Heart failure occurs when cardiac output (systemic oxygen delivery) is insufficient for the metabolic requirements of the body. Children with heart failure may present with growth failure, irritability, diaphoresis with feeds, fatigue, or exercise intolerance.
2. The term congestive heart failure should be used carefully because many patients with significant cardiac dysfunction and limiting symptoms lack findings consistent with congestion.
3. The compensatory mechanisms invoked in the setting of heart failure and the physiologic consequences that can ensue are as follows:
   a. Decreased renal perfusion results in activation of the renin–angiotensin system, producing retention of sodium and water that will increase circulating preload and cardiac output. However, systemic and pulmonary edema can result.
   b. Decreased perfusion of the adrenal medulla causes release of catecholamines that improve cardiac contractility. However, catecholamine

release also results in an increase in HR and systemic vascular resistance (increased afterload), both of which are detrimental in that they result in an increase in myocardial oxygen demand.

c. Hypertrophy of cardiac muscle improves contractility but also increases myocardial oxygen consumption.

ETIOLOGY OF HEART FAILURE

1. *Systolic* pump failure (primary myocardial disease, myocarditis, idiopathic dilated cardiomyopathy, ischemic myocardium [coronary artery anomaly])
2. *Diastolic* pump failure (hypertrophic or restrictive cardiomyopathy)
3. Primary arrhythmia (supraventricular, junctional or ventricular tachycardia)
4. High-output states (anemia, thyrotoxicosis)
5. Volume overload lesions (L-R shunts—VSD, PDA)
6. Pressure overload lesions (critical aortic stenosis, coarctation of the aorta)

CLINICAL MANIFESTATIONS OF HEART FAILURE

1. The clinical picture of heart failure is variable and age dependent. As in adults, initial symptoms manifest as dyspnea on exertion. The history should therefore include questions to ascertain symptomatology during *age-appropriate* exertion:
   a. Physical activity at school for the older child and adolescent
   b. Normal play/keeping up with peers for toddlers
   c. Feeding for infants, for which a detailed history is crucial. Infants with heart failure manifest tachypnea or diaphoresis with feeds, diminished volume of each feeding, or a prolonged time needed to finish a normal volume. They exhibit poor weight gain because of decreased caloric intake and increased metabolic requirements.
2. Physical findings generally reflect the physiologic compensatory processes mentioned previously:
   a. Failure to thrive with low weight and preserved length
   b. Pulmonary venous congestion with pulmonary edema presenting as tachypnea, retractions, wheezing, rales (unusual in infants), and occasionally hypoxemia
   c. Systemic venous congestion, manifested primarily as an engorged and palpable liver, lower extremity edema, and jugular venous distention may be appreciated in older children.
   d. Tachycardia and hyperdynamic precordium (when cardiac contractility is intact) due to increased catecholamines
   e. Direct manifestations of diminished cardiac output such as cool extremities, poor distal perfusion, decreased urine output, or silent precordium (if due to primary pump failure) usually occur in decompensated heart failure.
   f. Specific cardiac findings such as a VSD murmur may help elucidate the *cause* of heart failure, but do not make the diagnosis of the clinical syndrome.
3. Laboratory findings in heart failure
   a. CXR: Cardiomegaly is invariably present (except in the rare case of restrictive cardiomyopathy or total anomalous venous return with

obstruction). Its absence should make the diagnosis of heart failure suspect.

b. ECG: As with the general cardiac examination, an ECG may give clues to the etiology (arrhythmia; low voltage in myocarditis; left atrial enlargement [LAE], biventricular hypertrophy [BVH] in VSD; Q waves and ST segment abnormalities in anomalies of the coronary artery), but there is no characteristic ECG diagnostic of heart failure.

MANAGEMENT

Goals of therapy are twofold: To treat the underlying causes of decreased cardiac output and to manage the symptoms produced by excessive compensatory mechanisms.

1. Diuretics to treat pulmonary and venous congestion
   a. Furosemide (0.5 to 2.0 mg/kg/dose orally or intravenously [IV] depending on severity of illness) repeated every 4 to 24 hours as needed is the drug of first choice and most commonly used for congestive signs and symptoms. *Care must be used at initiation of therapy if severe myocardial dysfunction is suspected.* Overaggressive diuresis may result in a sharp reduction in preload and cardiac output and should be undertaken with an IV line in place for prompt restoration of circulating volume if needed. Pay careful attention to urinary sodium and potassium losses, especially with concomitant use of digoxin.
   b. Spironolactone is often used in conjunction with higher doses of furosemide (more than 2 to 4 mg/kg/day) for its potassium-sparing and mild diuretic effects. The dosage range for spironolactone is 1 to 4 mg/kg/day divided two to four times a day (max 200 mg/day). Although there are no clinical studies in children, when added to the standard medical regimen for adults in severe heart failure spironolactone is associated with left ventricular remodeling and improved life expectancy.
2. Inotropic support is used to enhance cardiac contractility. The route of administration is again determined by severity of illness.
   a. Digoxin is a positive inotrope that can be used at a dose of 10 μg/kg/day in two divided doses. A stable level will be reached in about 2 to 3 days. There is no mortality benefit to digoxin in adult studies, but it may decrease rates of heart failure–related hospitalizations in that population.
   b. If the patient is sick enough to require prompt inotropic support, then IV therapy should be strongly considered because digitalization has fallen out of favor owing to risks of digoxin toxicity.
   c. For acute therapy, dopamine or dobutamine infusion at 5 to 10 μg/kg/min can be used.
3. Afterload reduction is of utmost importance in the management of heart failure.
   a. Milrinone is an IV phosphodiesterase inhibitor that improves cardiac contractility while also decreasing pulmonary and systemic vascular resistance.
   b. Angiotensin-converting enzyme (ACE) inhibitors such as captopril and enalapril are oral agents used in the outpatient setting.
4. Beta blockers have been well studied in adult patients with heart failure, but pediatric data are lacking.

  a. Excessive circulation catecholamines resulting from heart failure may lead to myocardial fibrosis, myocyte hypertrophy, and eventually apoptosis.
  b. Beta blockers (carvedilol, metoprolol) may antagonize this sympathetic nervous system activity and limit these deleterious effects.
5. Fluid and salt restriction is almost never used and, in fact, is often detrimental because it curtails appropriate caloric intake necessary for growth. It is reserved for the patient with severe heart failure in whom the underlying etiology is not treatable. Fluid overload is usually managed with diuretics.
6. Treatment of underlying cause (e.g., arrhythmia, anemia, surgical repair of CHD) may be necessary.
  a. Remember, the goal of therapy is the resumption of normal growth and development and preservation of quality of life with minimal risk and invasiveness.
  b. *Caution must be exercised when considering oxygen therapy for respiratory difficulty (even hypoxemia) in heart failure.* Oxygen is a strong pulmonary vasodilator. In those patients with heart failure due to L-R shunt lesions, it may precipitate a sudden increase in L-R flow, with acute aggravation of pulmonary edema, hypoxemia, and potential respiratory failure.
7. Mechanical circulatory support consisting of extracorporeal membrane oxygenation and ventricular assist devices can be used for severe, refractory cardiac failure secondary to cardiomyopathies or myocarditis, or after cardiac surgery. These mechanical devices can support the circulation pending myocardial recovery, or serve as a bridge to cardiac transplantation.

15.5 Arrhythmias

GENERAL APPROACH

1. Identifying the appropriate diagnosis before initiating therapy is critical in the management of arrhythmias.
  a. One must consider the setting of the suspected arrhythmia (mild intermittent palpitations versus aborted sudden death) and whether it is associated with potential hemodynamic compromise.
  b. The arbitrary range of 60 to 100 bpm for normal sinus rhythm is not always applicable to the pediatric patient, especially infants (see Appendix I-B).
2. Palpitations
  a. A common problem, especially among adolescents, nonspecific extrasystoles are benign, sometimes associated with stimulant use such as caffeine.
  b. Outpatient management is indicated if the episodes are brief and nonsustained and not associated with other symptomatology (pallor, diaphoresis, syncope).
  c. Use of a Holter monitor or transtelephonic event monitor, depending on the frequency of symptoms, may be necessary to arrive at an accurate diagnosis before the initiation of therapy.

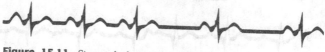

Figure 15-11 Sinus arrhythmia. (From Park MK: The Pediatric Cardiology Handbook. 3rd ed. Philadelphia, Mosby, 2003.)

CLASSIFICATION OF ARRHYTHMIAS

One approach in the classification of arrhythmias is to categorize based on rate.

Normal Rate (Including Extrasystoles)

1. Sinus arrhythmia
   a. Phasic variation in HR related to alteration in cardiac output during respiratory cycle. The HR increases slightly during inspiration, slows with expiration (Fig. 15-11).
   b. Clinical significance and management: This is a normal finding requiring no therapy.
2. Wandering atrial pacemaker
   a. Variation of P-wave morphology or axis without associated pauses or premature beats (Fig. 15-12).
   b. Clinical significance: This is usually a normal variant, although it may rarely be associated with structural abnormalities of the atria.
3. Premature atrial contraction (PAC)
   a. A premature beat caused by early depolarization of an ectopic focus in either atrium. The P-wave morphology is distinctly different from that of the sinus beat, but the QRS is *identical* to the normal sinus beat. A nonconducted PAC is seen when atrial depolarization occurs during the relative refractory period of the AV node and does not conduct through to the ventricle. *This may initially be thought to be a pause; look carefully for the abnormal P wave in the preceding T wave* (Fig. 15-13).
   b. Clinical significance: PACs are often seen in normal children (especially neonates), but may be associated with electrolyte abnormalities, digoxin toxicity, indwelling central catheters, or structural/surgical abnormalities of the atria.
   c. Management: Management is required only if an associated underlying abnormality is discovered.
4. Premature ventricular contraction (PVC)
   a. A premature beat caused by early depolarization of an ectopic focus within either of the ventricles. There may or may not be a visible P wave. The hallmark for recognition is the wide and bizarre configuration of the QRS complex representing slowed conduction of the

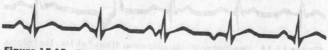

Figure 15-12 Wandering pacemaker. (From Park MK: The Pediatric Cardiology Handbook, 3rd ed. Philadelphia, Mosby, 2003.)

15—Cardiovascular Disorders

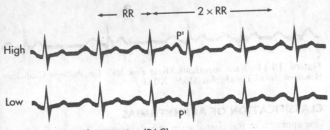

A Premature atrial contraction (PAC)

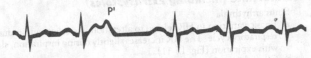

B Nonconducted PAC

Figure 15-13 A, Premature atrial contraction (PAC). B, Nonconducted PAC. (From Park MK: The Pediatric Cardiology Handbook, 3rd ed. Philadelphia, Mosby, 2003.)

impulse through the ventricular myocardium (Fig. 15-14). Note that there is a full compensatory pause. The length of the two cycles including the PVC is equal to the length of the preceding two normal cycles.

b. Clinical significance: PVCs are commonly seen in normal children, especially during sleep when the intrinsic sinus pacemaker slows. Occasionally, the adolescent patient may perceive single PVCs as a "skipped beat." Bigeminy (every other beat being a PVC) or trigeminy (every third) may also occur normally and requires no therapy. Important causes include hypoxemia, acidosis, electrolyte abnormalities, myocarditis, postoperative heart surgery, and secondary reactions to medications (catecholamines, anesthetic agents, theophylline).

c. Management: For simple infrequent and unifocal PVCs, especially those that decrease or disappear with faster HRs (e.g., resolve with exercise), reassurance is all that is needed. Those associated with symptoms of pallor or syncope or occurring during exercise ought to have a full cardiac evaluation.

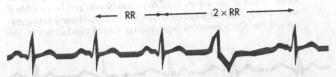

Figure 15-14 Premature ventricular contraction. (From Park MK: The Pediatric Cardiology Handbook, 3rd ed. Philadelphia, Mosby, 2003.)

Tachyarrhythmias

1. Supraventricular tachycardia (SVT)
   a. By strict definition, this refers to all tachyarrhythmias originating within the atria, although it is usually used in reference to reentrant tachycardia (WPW syndrome) or AV nodal reentrant tachycardia. This is the most common tachyarrhythmia seen in pediatric patients, especially infants. The HR is regular and fast (usually 230 bpm or more) with a normal (narrow) QRS complex. (Less than 5% may have rate-related bundle branch block with aberrant conduction, which can be confused for ventricular tachycardia.) Retrograde P waves may be visible (Fig. 15-15).
   b. The rate of SVT is usually slower in older children. This may make it more difficult to distinguish from sinus tachycardia or the more uncommon ectopic atrial tachycardia (typically 140 to 180 bpm) due to a rapidly depolarizing ectopic atrial focus.
   c. It is not associated with a significantly increased incidence of CHD. WPW-type AV reentrant tachycardia is associated with certain structural malformations (Ebstein's anomaly, L-TGA, some forms of hypertrophic cardiomyopathy).
   d. Clinical significance: Severity of symptoms is related to the rate and duration of tachycardia. Hemodynamic compromise in the older child is unusual because they will experience palpitations and seek treatment before the development of circulatory disturbance. Infants present with pallor, poor feeding, and vomiting that may progress to lethargy and shock if SVT persists unrecognized.
   e. Management: Hemodynamics and circulatory status *must* be assessed. If shock or hypotension is present, this is a medical emergency requiring *immediate* direct current (DC) synchronized cardioversion at 0.5 to 2 J/kg.
      (1) *Do not wait for IV access, sedation, or intubation for the infant in shock because it will dangerously delay potentially life-saving therapy.*
      (2) When cardioverting any patient already on digoxin, consider pretreatment with lidocaine to prevent ventricular fibrillation.
      (3) Always record the ECG during attempts at SVT termination.
      (4) For the patient with normal hemodynamics, there are a multitude of therapeutic options:
         (a) Vagal maneuvers: Carotid massage, gag reflex, rectal temperature, or Valsalva maneuvers (with the thumb in a closed mouth, have the older child "blow up" his or her hand); the diving reflex (a bag of ice placed across the nasal bridge)

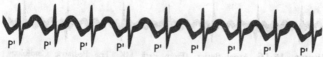

Figure 15-15 Atrial tachycardia. (From Park MK: The Pediatric Cardiology Handbook; 3rd ed. Philadelphia, Mosby, 2003.)

works well in infants, but be cautious of hypothermia if done repeatedly.

(b) Adenosine works extremely well to slow conduction at the AV node, breaking the reentry cycle. Although adenosine works immediately on infusion, it is very short acting (half-life of 9 seconds), which prevents its use as a preventive medication. Dose: 50 to 100 µg/kg rapid IV bolus, followed by normal saline flush. This dose can be doubled and repeated if the first dose does not work. The maximum adult dose is 6 mg. (See also the Appendix.)

(c) Medications that slow conduction at the AV node can be used for conversion in patients who are hemodynamically stable:

  (i) Digoxin: IV or oral digitalization (20 to 40 µg/kg, depending on age) usually results in conversion to sinus rhythm within 4 to 8 hours.

  (ii) Propranolol: Oral dosage of 1 to 4 mg/kg/day, with expected termination of SVT within 4 to 6 hours. IV administration must be carefully monitored for severe hypotension and bradycardia. As a negative inotrope, *it should be avoided if there is any suggestion of cardiovascular compromise.*

  (iii) Verapamil: Generally not used in infants younger than 1 year of age, and *contraindicated* at any age if heart failure or shock is present.

  (iv) The need for prophylaxis against recurrence depends on many factors, including patient age, symptomatology, and patient/parental anxiety.

(d) Maintenance therapy is generally indicated for the first 6 to 12 months of life in infants with maintenance digoxin or propranolol. In older verbal children, initiation of prophylactic medicine mainly depends on the frequency and severity of symptomatic episodes.

(e) If medical management fails, radiofrequency catheter ablation has been very successful at abolishing the reentrant circuit or ectopic focus.

2. Atrial flutter

  a. Rapid, regular atrial rate (250 to 500 bpm) with variable ventricular response. The rapid P waves have a typical "sawtooth" pattern; the QRS morphology is narrow and normal. The ventricular response (effective HR) determines cardiac output (Fig. 15-16).

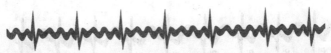

Figure 15-16 Atrial flutter. (From Park MK: The Pediatric Cardiology Handbook, 3rd ed. Philadelphia, Mosby, 2003.)

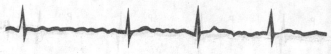

Figure 15-17 Atrial fibrillation with a slow ventricular response. (From Park MK: The Pediatric Cardiology Handbook, 3rd ed. Philadelphia, Mosby, 2003.)

    b. Clinical significance: Atrial flutter is often associated with structural abnormalities of the atria or prior atrial surgery. It may be idiopathic in the fetus and newborn.

    c. Management: If ventricular response is rapid, control may be obtained with digoxin. Alternatively, DC cardioversion is often required (especially in the newborn) to convert to normal sinus rhythm.

3. Atrial fibrillation

    a. Rapid, irregular, disorganized atrial depolarization with irregular ventricular response. The P waves are variable in morphology, if at all discernible. The QRS complex is narrow and normal (Fig. 15-17).

    b. Clinical significance: It is often associated with structural abnormalities of the atria or prior atrial surgery.

    c. Management: If ventricular response is rapid, control may be obtained with digoxin. Quinidine or amiodarone may be useful in preventing recurrence.

4. Ventricular tachycardia (VT)

    a. Wide, complex tachyarrhythmia with rapid and bizarre complexes, usually at rates of 130 to 200 bpm (Fig. 15-18).

    b. Clinical significance: Diminished cardiac output results from poor cardiac function or uncoordinated ventricular filling. Usually associated with structural cardiac disease, both preoperatively and postoperatively. Other etiologies include myocarditis, hypoxemia, acidosis, and electrolyte abnormalities. Long QT syndrome (congenital or acquired) must always be ruled out, especially in the setting of torsades de pointes (VT with shifting-axis QRS complexes).

    c. Management: DC synchronized cardioversion (1 to 2 J/kg) is immediately indicated if there is hemodynamic compromise. Otherwise, in hemodynamically stable patients, IV amiodarone (5 mg/kg) or lidocaine (1 mg/kg) followed by an infusion of lidocaine (20 to 50 μg/kg/min) should be administered.

Bradyarrhythmias

1. Sinus bradycardia

    a. Normal P wave and QRS morphology, occurring at an unusually slow rate

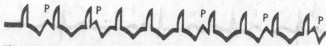

Figure 15-18 Ventricular tachycardia. (From Park MK: The Pediatric Cardiology Handbook, 3rd ed. Philadelphia, Mosby, 2003.)

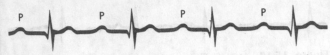

Figure 15-19 First-degree atrioventricular block. (From Park MK: The Pediatric Cardiology Handbook, 3rd ed. Philadelphia, Mosby, 2003.)

   b. Clinical significance: This condition is rarely myocardial in origin and more often reflects a high vagal tone, nutritional deficiency (anorexia nervosa), or central nervous system abnormality (especially increased intracranial pressure).
   c. Management: Treat underlying causes. If hemodynamic compromise is present, attempt increasing HR with atropine, transcutaneous pacing, or isoproterenol infusion.
2. First-degree AV block
   a. Not actually a slow rhythm but characterized by prolongation of the PR interval due to abnormal conduction at the AV node (Fig. 15-19)
   b. Clinical significance: Can be seen with digoxin toxicity, present in some forms of TGA, ASD, or other CHD in which atrial dilation is present; it also may be a manifestation of carditis in acute rheumatic fever or Lyme disease. It is occasionally seen in normal children.
   c. Management: Address underlying cause if evident; otherwise, no specific therapy is required.
3. Second-degree AV block
   a. Mobitz type I with progressive AV nodal dysfunction that manifests as gradual prolongation of the PR interval until a QRS is dropped (Wenckebach phenomenon; Fig. 15-20)
   b. Mobitz type II in which sudden loss of conduction through the AV node results in a P wave without a following QRS (Fig. 15-21)
   c. Clinical significance: This block may be a normal finding (especially Mobitz type I) in adolescents during sleep or in other states with high resting vagal tone. Mobitz type II is associated with a high incidence of CHD, including TGA, left atrial isomerism, and neonatal lupus syndrome.
   d. Management: Usually no therapy is needed unless bradycardia results in symptoms from decreased cardiac output. A pacemaker may eventually be necessary to modulate the ventricular rate.
4. Third-degree (complete) heart block
   a. No atrial impulses are conducted through to the ventricles. The ventricular rate (QRS) is completely independent of and slower than the atrial rate (Fig. 15-22).

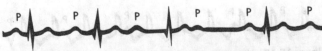

Figure 15-20 Second-degree atrioventricular block (Mobitz type I). (From Park MK: The Pediatric Cardiology Handbook, 3rd ed. Philadelphia, Mosby, 2003.)

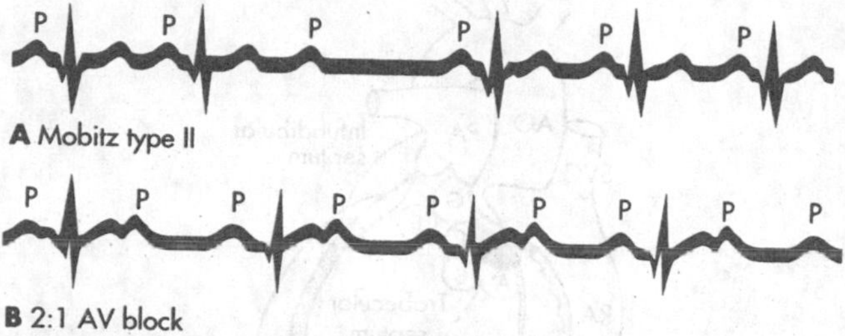

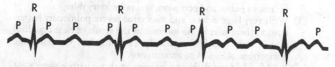

A Mobitz type II

B 2:1 AV block

Figure 15-21 A, Second-degree atrioventricular (AV) block (Mobitz type II). B, 2:1 AV block. (From Park MK: The Pediatric Cardiology Handbook, 3rd ed. Philadelphia, Mosby, 2003.)

  b. Clinical significance: High incidence of CHD, including TGA, left atrial isomerism, or in structurally normal hearts as part of the neonatal lupus syndrome or due to Lyme carditis.
  c. Management: Pacemakers are indicated for hemodynamic compromise, associated heart failure, and in the postoperative setting. Congenital complete heart block does not automatically require pacing if the ventricular escape rate is adequate to allow for hemodynamic stability and normal growth and development.

15.6 Congenital Malformations/Congenital Heart Disease

Congenital heart disease (CHD) may be broadly categorized into four distinct groups based on the clinical physiology:
1. Left-to-right (L-R) shunts (VSD, ASD, PDA)
2. Right-to-left (R-L) shunts (TOF)
3. Obstructive lesions (aortic or pulmonic stenosis/atresia, coarctation of the aorta)
4. Transposition physiology (TGA)

LEFT-TO-RIGHT SHUNTS

These are characterized by pulmonary overcirculation and the potential for development of Congestive Heart Failure (CHF). The onset of congestive symptoms is variably dependent on the specific lesion and is related to the normal postnatal fall in pulmonary vascular resistance. The magnitude

Figure 15-22 Complete (third-degree) atrioventricular block. (From Park MK: The Pediatric Cardiology Handbook, 3rd ed. Philadelphia, Mosby, 2003.)

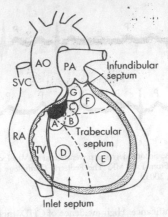

Figure 15-23 Classification of ventricular septal defect (VSD) location. A, B, C, Perimembranous VSD; D, inlet muscular VSD; E, trabecular muscular VSD; F, G, outlet muscular, subarterial, or supracristal VSD. TV, tricuspid valve; other abbreviations as in Figure 15-5. (From Park MK: The Pediatric Cardiology Handbook, 3rd ed. Philadelphia, Mosby, 2003.)

of the shunt is determined by two critical factors: the size of the defect, and the balance of pulmonary and systemic vascular resistance.

1. Ventricular Septal Defect (VSD): The most common heart malformation, it accounts for about 25% of all CHD. A VSD is classified depending on the location within the septum (Fig. 15-23).
   a. History: Small defects are detected only by the murmur, with no other abnormalities on physical examination. If defects are large enough, gradual development of CHF (tachypnea and poor feeding) may occur over the first 2 to 6 weeks of life. Very large defects may present with pulmonary hypertension if the diagnosis is delayed.
   b. Physical examination findings
      (1) Small to moderate defects cause a coarse, 2 to 4/6 holosystolic murmur heard best at the left lower sternal border. The systolic murmur represents the pressure differential across the defect from LV to RV.
      (2) If the shunt is large, there will also be an apical diastolic rumble (a low-pitched filling sound representing increased flow across the mitral valve) and signs of CHF such as hepatomegaly, decreased pulses and perfusion, and pulmonary rales.
      (3) With very large defects and associated severe pulmonary hypertension there may be no murmur as the result of near equalization of right and left ventricular pressures, but the pulmonic component of S_2 will be accentuated.
   c. ECG: LAE, LVH, or BVH can be seen in those with a significant shunt.

d. CXR: Cardiomegaly (LA, LV) and engorged pulmonary vessels, sometimes with overt pulmonary edema, can be visualized.

e. Management: The goal of therapy is to ensure normal growth and development.

   (1) Enhanced caloric intake, with either nasogastric supplementation or high-caloric density formula (24 to 30 calories/oz), is often necessary because of increased metabolic demands.

   (2) Anticongestive therapy with furosemide (usually 1 mg/kg/dose two to three times a day), and ACE inhibitors have been used. However, improvement in surgical technique and morbidity has resulted in earlier surgical repair in the place of medical management in those with large shunts.

   (3) If normal growth cannot be readily achieved or if the defect is large and unlikely to spontaneously close over time, surgical repair is indicated.

2. Atrial Septal Defect (ASD): This defect accounts for 5% to 10% of all CHD. ASD classification is based on the location of the defect within the atrial septum: Secundum (most common), primum, sinus venosus, and coronary sinus defects.

   a. History: Usually asymptomatic until the third or fourth decade of life (pulmonary hypertension, atrial arrhythmia). There may be increased frequency of lower respiratory infections owing to chronically increased pulmonary blood flow.

   b. Physical examination findings: Mildly active parasternal tap/heave (RV dilation). Grade 2/6 SEM heard best at the left upper sternal border (LUSB), which represents increased flow through a normal pulmonic valve ("relative" pulmonic stenosis). *There is a fixed and widely split second heart sound.*

   c. ECG: Most commonly shows RV conduction delay early (notched QRS or rsR′ in the right precordial leads), but occasionally shows first-degree AV block, right axis deviation, and RVH

   d. CXR: May show mild cardiomegaly (especially RA, RV) and prominent main pulmonary artery (MPA) segment

   e. Management: If spontaneous closure does not occur, elective closure is indicated to prevent long-term complications. Device closure in the catheterization laboratory can be performed for most secundum-type defects, even in some symptomatic infants. If the child is doing well, closure can ideally be electively performed around the age of 2 years. Surgical repair is now reserved mostly for those with extremely large defects, for types other than secundum ASDs, or in those requiring surgery for associated defects.

3. Persistent or Patent Ductus Arteriosis (PDA)

   a. History: Noted most commonly in premature infants and occasional term newborns, may cause CHF if large; usually asymptomatic in the older child

   b. Physical examination findings: Typically described as a 2 to 4/6 continuous murmur with systolic accentuation ("machinery murmur"), best heard in the left infraclavicular area or LUSB, radiates to the back

   c. ECG: May show LAE, LVH, if shunt is large

    d. CXR: Cardiomegaly (especially LA, LV), increased pulmonary blood flow
    e. Management: In a premature infant, closure is recommended for the symptomatic PDA causing CHF, either pharmacologically (indomethacin) or with surgical ligation. In the older infant or child, transcatheter coil occlusion is recommended for the prevention of subacute bacterial endocarditis (SBE). Surgery is rarely necessary in the older child.

RIGHT-TO-LEFT SHUNTS

These are characterized by the presence of desaturated blood in the systemic circulation because of obligate intracardiac R-L shunting. These lesions are often associated with variable obstruction to pulmonary blood flow. Visible cyanosis occurs when there is 5 g/dL desaturated hemoglobin in the systemic circulation. The degree of cyanosis depends on the severity of obstruction to pulmonary blood flow and intracardiac mixing. The prototype lesion to describe R-L shunting is Tetralogy of Fallot (TOF).

1. The most common of all cyanotic lesions, TOF represents about 10% of all CHD.
    a. Four basic anatomic defects are associated with TOF:
       (1) Malalignment VSD (large)
       (2) Overriding aorta (the aorta receives flow from both ventricles)
       (3) Pulmonic stenosis (valvar or infundibular)
       (4) RVH
    b. History: Variable depending on the degree of RV outflow tract (RVOT) obstruction—if this is minimal or absent, the patient may not be cyanotic, with flow at the VSD occurring L-R (so-called "pink tet," physiology is similar to that of a large VSD). Obstruction to pulmonary blood flow causes R-L intracardiac shunting from RV to the aorta through the malalignment VSD. As the RVOT obstruction worsens, cyanosis becomes more pronounced.
    c. Physical examination findings: Usually cyanotic, with peripheral oxygen saturations of 75% to 85%; loud 2 to 3/6 SEM due to RVOT obstruction that radiates to the back and axillae; prominent RV tap, there may be clubbing if cyanosis is long-standing
    d. ECG: Right-axis deviation (RAD) and RVH
    e. CXR: RVH with small or absent MPA segment; variable pulmonary oligemia is reflective of degree of cyanosis.
    f. Management: Significant cyanosis in neonates with TOF is treated with prostaglandin E_1 (PGE1) infusion to maintain patency of the ductus arteriosus for pulmonary blood flow. Improvements and advancements in neonatal cardiovascular surgical techniques have made primary repair of TOF in the neonatal period possible for some patients. Alternative options include surgical palliation with a modified right Blalock-Taussig shunt (see Glossary of Surgical Procedures section, later, and Fig. 15-24) or balloon dilation of the pulmonary valve, followed by complete repair (VSD closure and RVOT reconstruction) at about 4 to 6 months of age or sooner.
2. Hypercyanotic or "tet spell": The pathophysiology of these "spells" is incompletely understood, but may be related to spasm of the RVOT

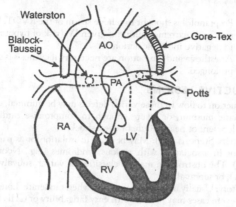

Figure 15-24 Palliative surgical procedures for patients with cyanotic congenital heart defects resulting in decreased pulmonary blood flow. Abbreviations as in Figure 15-5. (From Park MK. The Pediatric Cardiology Handbook, 3rd ed. Philadelphia, Mosby, 2003.)

(infundibulum) or an acute change in the balance of pulmonary vascular resistance (PVR) and systemic vascular resistance (SVR), favoring increased R-L shunt. Increasing cyanosis leads to progressive hypoxemia and metabolic acidosis, and it may progress to hemodynamic collapse, seizures, and possibly death. Spells typically occur at 2 to 4 months of age.

a. Physical examination findings: Deep cyanosis, hyperpnea, limpness, decreased murmur (due to diminution of flow across the narrowed RVOT)

b. Management: Intervention needs to be urgent because a vicious cycle can easily ensue as hypoxemia further promotes increased PVR and decreased SVR. The following steps should be undertaken in order of ease and related to the severity of the spell, with the primary goal of increasing pulmonary blood flow:

   (1) Supplemental oxygen may decrease PVR (may be of limited value because of baseline anatomic RVOT obstruction).

   (2) Knee-chest position results in decreased venous return (preload) and increases SVR with the goal of decreasing the R-L shunt and improving pulmonary blood flow.

   (3) Sedation with morphine (0.1 to 0.2 mg/kg subcutaneously or intramuscularly) is probably the most effective therapy in most cases. It decreases venous return, depresses respiratory center, and relaxes infundibulum.

   (4) IV fluid infusion may augment flow through the constricted RVOT.

   (5) Peripheral arterial constriction with phenylephrine may favor the balance of flow from left to right.

(6) Propranolol is thought to relieve spasm of the RVOT. It must be used with extreme caution if given IV (risk of hypotension due to negative inotropic actions).

(7) Anesthesia and intubation are necessary if cyanosis is severe and prolonged.

OBSTRUCTIVE LESIONS

The obstruction to flow in these varied defects may be minimal, causing an asymptomatic murmur, or severe enough to compromise cardiac output with development of heart failure or even shock.

1. Pulmonary Stenosis (PS): May be seen in isolation or as part of other CHD or in association with various syndromes (e.g., Noonan's syndrome). The obstruction may be classified as valvar, subvalvar (infundibular), or supravalvar.
   a. History: Usually asymptomatic, even when moderate. Long-standing or severe cases may present with easy fatigability or CHF. Newborns with critical PS may be quite cyanotic.
   b. Physical examination findings: Variable 2 to 5/6 SEM is heard best at LUSB and radiating to the back. There may be an ejection click or muffled pulmonic second sound (P_2). A variable systolic thrill is felt.
   c. ECG: Moderate to severe cases will show RAD and RVH.
   d. CXR: May demonstrate RVH (though rarely cardiomegaly) or poststenotic dilation of the MPA
   e. Management: Mild PS requires no therapy other than SBE prophylaxis and longitudinal follow-up. Moderate PS (transvalvular gradient 30 to 50 mm Hg) is usually well tolerated and requires intervention only if associated with symptoms. Severe PS (transvalvular gradient of ≥60 mm Hg) requires therapy with pulmonary balloon valvuloplasty or surgical valvotomy.

2. Aortic stenosis: May be classified as valvar (usually due to a congenitally bicuspid or dysplastic valve), supravalvar (e.g., Williams' syndrome), or subvalvar (e.g., subaortic membrane or hypertrophic cardiomyopathy). Valvar aortic stenosis is often seen in combination with other left-sided obstructive lesions (e.g., coarctation of the aorta, mitral stenosis).
   a. History: Usually asymptomatic, even when moderate. Long-standing or severe cases may present with easy fatigability, dizziness, or syncope. Newborns with critical aortic stenosis will present with severe LV dysfunction and shock.
   b. Physical examination findings: An ejection click is usually audible, sometimes heard best in the suprasternal notch or at the apex. There is a variable 2 to 5/6 harsh SEM best heard at the right upper sternal border, radiating to the suprasternal notch and neck. *This pattern of radiation is very helpful in distinguishing aortic stenosis from PS in the smaller child.* There may be a systolic thrill, displaced point of maximal impulse, or hemihypertrophy of the left chest if LVH is severe.
   c. ECG: May demonstrate LVH (with strain if severe)
   d. CXR: May show a prominent LV shadow or poststenotic dilation of the ascending aorta
   e. Management: Mild cases require only subacute bacterial endocarditis (SBE) prophylaxis. Balloon valvuloplasty is indicated in moderate

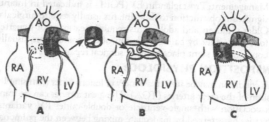

Figure 15-25 The Ross procedure (pulmonary root autograft). A, B, The aortic valve is excised and replaced by the native pulmonary valve with coronary reimplantation. C, A conduit or homograft is then placed in the right ventricle to pulmonary artery position. Abbreviations as in Figure 15-5. (From Park MK: The Pediatric Cardiology Handbook, 3rd ed. Philadelphia, Mosby, 2003.)

cases (mean transvalvular gradient of <40 mm Hg) without significant aortic insufficiency (which may worsen during the procedure). Surgical valvotomy is indicated for those unresponsive to balloon dilation. Because of size limitations, valve replacement is delayed as long as possible to allow the largest prosthesis to be used. In addition, because anticoagulation is not benign in young patients, some infants and young children with severe stenosis may undergo the Ross procedure (Fig. 15-25) instead of prosthetic valve replacement. Isometric exercise such as weight training is contraindicated in the setting of aortic stenosis because it increases the transvalvular gradient and puts the hypertrophied myocardium at risk.

3. Coarctation of the aorta: Usually a discrete narrowing of the juxtaductal aorta, it is commonly seen in conjunction with other left-sided obstructive lesions (especially bicuspid aortic valve).

a. History: The presentation is extremely age dependent. The infant presents with increased work of breathing and signs of poor cardiac output, such as feeding intolerance, renal failure due to poor renal perfusion, or necrotizing enterocolitis. If coarctation is not recognized, the infant will progress to shock and hemodynamic collapse within the first 2 to 8 weeks of life. Older children and adolescents are usually asymptomatic and are noted to have hypertension on routine BP screening (>20 mm Hg systolic BP in arms vs. legs). They may occasionally have abdominal pain or leg pain because of transient lower body ischemia.

b. Physical examination findings: The hallmark of this diagnosis is diminished, delayed, or absent femoral pulses. In addition, there is a continuous murmur in the left axilla, and prominent brachial pulses. These findings may not be reliably present in the newborn with a PDA supplying descending aortic blood flow.

c. ECG: Infant—RAD, RVH; older child—normal or LVH

d. CXR: Infant—cardiomegaly, pulmonary edema; older child—LV enlargement, rib notching (secondary to dilated intercostal arteries)

e. Management: Prostaglandin E1 (PGE1) is indicated in infants with significant obstruction to flow. Infants usually require surgical repair. Older children and adolescents require treatment of hypertension, followed either by balloon dilation of the coarctation, usually with concomitant stent placement, or surgical repair.

TRANSPOSITION PHYSIOLOGY

1. This condition may be seen in a variety of lesions other than simple transpositon of the great arteries (TGA). The great arteries can be transposed in association with single-ventricle or double-outlet RV variants. This defect is characterized by inadequate mixing between the pulmonary and systemic circulations, preventing desaturated blood from reaching the lungs and oxygenated blood from reaching the peripheral organs. The circulations are said to be in *parallel* rather than the usual *series* (Fig. 15-26).

2. TGA: The aorta arises anteriorly from the RV, the pulmonary artery posteriorly from the LV. Survival depends on the degree of mixing, which may occur at various levels (ASD, VSD, PDA). Definitive management varies depending on the presence of associated lesions (VSD or PS). We will discuss TGA without other associated defects.

   a. History: Infants (more commonly boys) are often quite blue, with Po_2 levels in the 20 to 30 mm Hg range. There may be hypoxemia-induced hyperpnea and acidosis.

   b. Physical examination findings: Profound cyanosis without respiratory distress and unresponsive to supplemental oxygen. There is no murmur, and a loud, single S_2 is present.

   c. ECG: Often normal; may show RAD, RVH.

   d. CXR: Narrow cardiac "waist" reflecting anterior-posterior relationship of the great arteries; this may produce the characteristic "egg on a string" appearance.

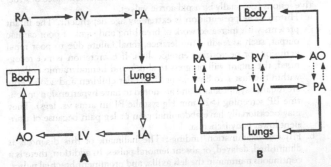

Figure 15-26 Circulation pathways of normal "in series" (A) circulation and "in parallel" (B) circulation seen in transposition of the great arteries. *Open arrows* indicate oxygenated blood and *closed arrows* desaturated blood. Abbreviations as in Figure 15-5. (From Park MK: The Pediatric Cardiology Handbook, 3rd ed. Philadelphia, Mosby, 2003.)

e. Management: If the level of arterial oxygen saturation is sufficient to maintain a normal serum pH (usually 70% or higher), then no urgent therapy is needed. If hypoxemia is severe and metabolic acidosis becomes manifest, then attempts to improve mixing must be initiated immediately. The procedure of choice is balloon atrial septostomy (Rashkind procedure). This bedside procedure is designed to improve atrial level mixing of oxygenated and deoxygenated blood. Alternative therapies that may be useful include PGE1 infusion, sedation, intubation, or transfusion to augment mixing. This is usually followed by arterial switch operation (see Glossary of Surgical Procedures section, following) as soon as possible.

15.7 Glossary of Surgical Procedures

SHUNTS

1. Blalock-Taussig (BT) shunt (see Fig. 15-24): Classically, this consisted of a turndown* of the subclavian artery to the ipsilateral branch pulmonary artery for augmentation of pulmonary blood flow in cyanotic defects. The *modified* BT shunt is more routinely used today and consists of a synthetic (Gore-Tex) interposition graft between the right innominate or subclavian artery and ipsilateral branch pulmonary artery.

2. Glenn shunt: The classic Glenn is an end-to-end anastomosis of the SVC to the RPA, which has been transected from the MPA. This has been replaced more commonly with a "bidirectional" Glenn (Fig. 15-27A), with the SVC anastomosed end-to-side to the RPA, which retains continuity with the MPA/left pulmonary artery.

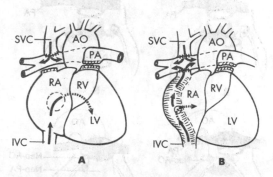

Figure 15-27 A, Bidirectional Glenn procedure with anastomosis of the superior vena cava to the right pulmonary artery. B, Fontan procedure with baffling of the superior and inferior vena cava flow into the right pulmonary artery, done with or without a fenestration into the right atrial cavity. Abbreviations as in Figure 15-5. (From Park MK: The Pediatric Cardiology Handbook, 3rd ed. Philadelphia, Mosby, 2003.)

OPEN HEART PROCEDURES

1. Modified Fontan (Fig. 15-27B): Used for single-ventricle variants to systematically separate the systemic and pulmonary circulations. There are generally three stages to completing the Fontan operation:
   a. Modified BT shunt in the neonatal period
   b. Bidirectional Glenn with takedown of the BT shunt at 4 to 6 months of age
   c. Intra-atrial baffling of the inferior vena cava return to the RPA (2 to 3 years of age). This is usually fenestrated to allow a "pop-off" in the case of postoperative elevated PVR.
2. Norwood procedure: Staged surgical palliation for hypoplastic left-heart syndrome. The approach is similar to the modified Fontan, except that the first stage includes reconstruction and augmentation of the hypoplastic ascending aorta and aortic arch with the root of the MPA and pericardium. It includes an atrial septectomy.
3. Arterial switch operation (Fig. 15-28): This procedure is performed in the setting of TGA. Both great vessels are transected above the valves and reanastomosed to the physiologically correct ventricle. This is accompanied by individual transplantation of the coronary arteries to the neoaorta.

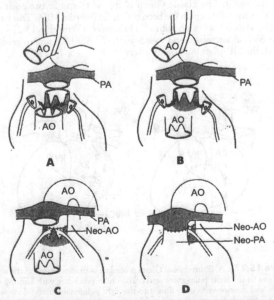

Figure 15-28 Arterial switch operation for transposition of the great arteries. AO, aorta; PA, pulmonary artery. (From Park MK: The Pediatric Cardiology Handbook, 3rd ed. Philadelphia, Mosby, 2003.)

15.8 Common Problems of Concern

CHEST PAIN

This is a frequently encountered symptom that generates concern regarding a possible cardiac pathologic process. A complete history and physical examination are essential for an accurate diagnosis.

1. Etiology (Box 15-1)
   a. The majority of chest pain in pediatrics is musculoskeletal in origin, primarily costochondritis (about 50%). Reproducibility with palpation of the costochondral junction is diagnostic.
   b. Symptoms that may indicate a cardiac etiology include exertional angina (crushing substernal pain as opposed to the more typical stabbing, sharp pain usually reported) and positional pain (worse when supine), which suggests pericarditis. Younger children may perceive palpitations as chest pain.
2. Diagnosis and management
   a. Work-up may include an ECG and CXR; however, care should be used because these may feed into the patient's and family's anxiety

---

Box 15-1 Etiologies of Pediatric Chest Pain

Musculoskeletal

Costochondritis (Tietze's syndrome)
Precordial catch (Texidor's twinge)
Chest wall trauma
Slipping rib syndrome

Pulmonary

Spontaneous pneumothorax
Pleuritis, pleural effusion, pleurodynia
Lobar pneumonia (especially with sympathetic effusion)
Severe cough, bronchitis (may be musculoskeletal)
Pulmonary hypertension
Acute pulmonary infarction (sickle cell disease)

Cardiac

Pericarditis, myocarditis
Coronary insufficiency (especially due to anomalous origin of the left
   coronary artery; also in cocaine abuse)
Arrhythmia
Pulmonary vascular obstructive disease (pulmonary hypertension)
Mitral valve prolapse

Psychological

Conversion disorder
Hyperventilation, panic attack
Depression

regarding the possibility of a cardiac origin of the chest pain. Firm reassurance and a trial of nonsteroidal anti-inflammatory agents are effective for most cases of musculoskeletal chest pain.

b. Patients with hyperventilation/panic syndromes in addition to rapid, shallow breathing may display muscular rigidity/spasm equivalent to "hypocalcemic" tetany as a rapid fall in carbon dioxide tension (and subsequent alkalosis) enhances binding of free calcium to bone, rendering it unavailable for muscle contraction. Breathing into a paper bag or a rebreathing mask will correct the problem. Sometimes anti-anxiety agents may be needed. For all patients, concerns of the patient and family regarding etiology and risk of sudden death must be addressed directly.

SYNCOPE

This condition is defined as a transient loss of consciousness, usually due to diminution in delivery of a vital substrate (usually oxygen) to the brain (Box 15-2). It is common in pediatrics, especially in the adolescent. Syncope often engenders tremendous anxiety in patients, parents, and caretakers owing to a fear of sudden death.

Box 15-2   Etiology of Syncope

Autonomic
Vasovagal (most common cause of syncope in children)
Excessive vagal tone (athletes, adolescents)
Reflex
Situational (e.g., cough, micturition, hair grooming)
Pallid breath holding
Orthostatic (dehydration, blood loss)

Cardiac
Obstructive lesions (aortic stenosis, hypertrophic obstructive cardiomyopathy, primary pulmonary hypertension)
Arrhythmia (supraventricular tachycardia, ventricular tachycardia, heart block)
Hypercyanosis ("tet spells")
Miscellaneous (pump dysfunction, myocardial infarction, anomalous coronary anatomy)

Noncardiac
Neurologic (seizures, migraine)
Metabolic (hypoglycemia)
Hyperventilation
Hysterical (audience, complete absence of trauma)
Vascular (cervical anomalies, vertebrobasilar insufficiency)

1. Etiology
   a. The most common etiology for syncope in children and adolescents is innocent vasovagal (vasodepressor, neurocardiogenic) syncope, along with other autonomic causes.
   b. Important cardiac etiologies in which a loss of consciousness may identify otherwise healthy patients at risk of sudden death include hypertrophic (obstructive) cardiomyopathy, congenital long QT syndrome, and occult arrhythmias.
2. Diagnosis and management
   a. A careful neurologic and cardiac examination, as well as a screening ECG, should identify the majority of patients with possible life-threatening illness. A family history of premature sudden death and syncope occurring during exercise are important red flags. Referral to a cardiologist or other specialist should be made for the following:
      (1) Exertional syncope
      (2) Syncope associated with chest pain or palpitations
      (3) Any cardiac abnormality on physical examination or ECG
      (4) Family history of sudden death
      (5) Family history of seizures
      (6) Any neurologic abnormality or residua
      (7) Unexplainable or atypical episodes
      (8) Recurrent episodes
   b. Firm but simple reassurance, along with avoidance of known triggers (e.g., prolonged standing, blood drawing) and recognition of presyncopal symptoms with appropriate intervention (sitting or lying down), are sufficient in most cases. Both conscious increased fluid and solute (salt) intake and treatment with mineralocorticoids (fludrocortisone) are effective in those prone to orthostasis.

SUGGESTED READING

Garson A, Bricker JT, Fisher DJ, Neish SR (eds): The Science and Practice of Pediatric Cardiology, 3rd ed. Philadelphia, Lippincott Williams & Wilkins, 2005.

Park MK: The Pediatric Cardiology Handbook, 3rd ed. Philadelphia, Mosby, 2003.

Robinson B, Anisman P, Eshaghpour E: A primer on pediatric ECGs. Contemp Pediatr 11:69-96, 1994.

Schwartz PJ, Moss AJ, Vincent GM, Crampton RS: Diagnostic criteria for the long QT syndrome: An update. Circulation 88:782-784, 1993.

WEBSITE

PediHeart: www.pediheart.org (provides information specific to pediatric cardiology, including diagrams of congenital heart defects)

Pulmonary and Allergic Diseases

16

Robert B. Klein, Anthony J. Alario,
and Michael S. Schechter

16.1 Anaphylaxis

1. Pathophysiology: Anaphylaxis is a potentially fatal medical emergency related to an acute, usually unexpected, generalized reaction caused by the release of potent biochemical mediators (e.g., histamine, platelet-activating factor, eosinophil chemotactic factors). This reaction may be mediated by immunoglobulin E (IgE) and induced by a specific allergic interaction with previously sensitized cells, or it may be non-IgE mediated. The target organs of the chemical mediators are primarily the blood vessels (increased permeability) and smooth muscle (contraction). Atopic individuals do not seem to experience anaphylaxis more frequently, although in such patients reactions may be more severe and asthma is a specific risk factor. Fatal reactions in children are uncommon.

2. Etiology: Foods (e.g., peanuts, tree nuts, seeds, egg, shellfish, milk, fish, fruits) are the most common cause. Other major causes include penicillin and all other antibiotics, insulin, gamma globulin, foreign serums, enzymes, biologics, and nonsteroidal anti-inflammatory drugs (aspirin and others). Hymenoptera venom (yellow jacket, wasp, hornet, honeybee, fire ant), local anesthetics, radiographic contrast materials, sulfites (preservatives), semen, and latex also can be associated with anaphylaxis.

3. Clinical features
   a. Onset: Symptoms have an explosive onset within seconds/minutes of exposure of the triggering agent, or they can be delayed for several hours. Late-phase or biphasic reactions occur 4 to 8 hours after the initial exposure and comprise 5% to 20% of reactions. Over 50% of fatal reactions happen within the first hour.
   b. Severity: Mild cutaneous allergic symptoms to severe and life-threatening
      (1) Mild to moderate allergic reactions: Generally local reactions limited to specific target organs
         (a) Skin (majority of reactions): Local redness, edema, hives, angioedema, urticaria (e.g., after a mild insect bite)
         (b) Gastrointestinal (GI) tract: Nausea, vomiting, cramping abdominal pain
         (c) Upper airway: Sneezing, cough, intense rhinorrhea

(2) Severe allergic reaction: Characterized by the following sequence of signs and symptoms
    (a) Generalized flush
    (b) Urticaria
    (c) Paroxysmal coughing
    (d) Scratchy sensation in the back of the throat
    (e) Tongue swelling
    (f) Severe anxiety
    (g) Dyspnea, stridor
    (h) Wheezing
    (i) Orthopnea
    (j) Vomiting
    (k) Cyanosis
    (l) Shock
4. Diagnosis: Based on a history of exposure to a precipitating agent and characteristic clinical features. Laboratory studies generally are not necessary.
5. Management
    a. Severe reaction: In severe, life-threatening reactions, the prompt institution of therapy is imperative. Rapid assessment of airway, breathing, circulation, and mental status is essential.
        (1) Epinephrine: 0.01 mL/kg of 1:1000 solution, subcutaneously; and repeat every 20 minutes if needed. If there is a site of entry on an extremity (insect sting, allergy injection) a tourniquet can be used and epinephrine can be injected directly into the area on the extremity (with this method, an additional dose of epinephrine should also be given for systemic therapy, above the tourniquet—for example, on the other arm).
        (2) Oxygen: Administer by mask and, if wheezing, coadminister a beta agonist.
        (3) Medications
            (a) Diphenhydramine 1 to 2 mg/kg intravenously (IV), intramuscularly (IM), or orally (PO) every 4 to 6 hours for 24 to 48 hours
            (b) Corticosteroids (to help prevent late symptoms)
        (4) Secondary treatments
            (a) Histamine antagonist: Ranitidine 1.5 mg/kg can be administered PO or IV.
            (b) Glucagon 0.1 mg/kg IV can be administered if the patient is refractory to initial treatment or is receiving beta-blocking agents.
    b. Mild to moderate local reaction (swelling, hives, pruritus)
        (1) Apply tourniquet (as previously) if entry of causative agent is on an extremity.
        (2) Medicate: Administer an oral antihistamine (e.g., diphenhydramine 1 to 2 mg/kg IV/IM with additional doses orally every 6 hours for 24 to 48 hours).
        (3) Applying ice to the site may help temporarily.
    c. Prophylaxis: To prevent recurrences of severe reactions, prophylactic measures should be instituted.

(1) Avoidance of the precipitating agent and use of a Medic-Alert bracelet
(2) An epinephrine autoinjector device (e.g., Epi-Pen) should be provided to patients (families) and schools for children with severe insect or food reactions.
(3) Immunotherapy is beneficial for severe insect venom anaphylaxis. It is *not* needed for mild cutaneous reactions.

6. Pretreatment prophylaxis: Giving corticosteroids or diphenhydramine *before* exposure may prevent a severe reaction if there is unavoidable exposure to offending agent (e.g., radiocontrast material).

16.2 Allergic Rhinitis

1. Etiology and pathophysiology
   a. A chronic inflammatory response is produced based on an excessive T-cell release of interleukin-4 (and other mediators), stimulating B-cell production of IgE.
      (1) Allergens react with antigen-specific IgE on the patient's nasal mast cells.
      (2) Mast cells are activated to release histamine, leukotrienes, and prostaglandins, which promote vasodilation and edema and trigger neural reflexes, including hypersecretion and sneezing.
   b. In young children (<4 years), the condition is often perennial. Causes include house dust mites, animal dander, and molds.
   c. In older children (>4 years), seasonal symptoms occur from tree and grass pollens in the spring and ragweed pollen in the fall.
   d. Aggravating factors include cigarette smoke, pollutants, and changes in humidity.
   e. A family history of atopy is often found.

2. Epidemiology: Allergic rhinitis is the most common cause of *chronic* rhinitis, affecting 8% to 10% of U.S. children. Allergic rhinitis has a major impact on quality of life for children (e.g., school problems, sleep disturbances).

3. Clinical features
   a. Chronic symptoms include sneezing accompanied by nasal and conjunctival congestion with watery discharge; conjunctival injection and pruritus are seen. A history of mouth breathing, snoring, and upward rubbing of the nose ("allergic salute") is often identified.
   b. An examination reveals the presence of "allergic shiners" (edema and stasis leads to gray-bluish discoloration and puffiness under lower eyelids); fine creases under lower lids (Dennie's lines); horizontal creases (allergic creases) across bridge of nose; pale, boggy nasal mucosa; and pharyngeal follicular hypertrophy.
   c. Other signs or symptoms include eczema, hypernasal speech, malocclusion, and recurrent otitis media, sinusitis, and epistaxis.

4. Diagnosis and laboratory findings
   a. Diagnosis depends on historical and examination findings already noted.
   b. Nasal cytology (Hansel staining secretions for eosinophils) can be helpful. Greater than 10% eosinophils suggests allergy.

c. Computed tomography scans can help to rule out sinusitis, or radiographs can be obtained to evaluate for foreign body, if clinically indicated.

d. Skin tests or radioallergosorbent test (RAST) can help identify the offending antigen, which must be correlated clinically.

5. Differential diagnosis: Many of these conditions may coexist in a child with allergic rhinitis:

a. Recurrent, low-grade viral upper respiratory tract infection (usually not associated with nasal eosinophilia, or history or signs of atopy)

b. Foreign body (unilateral, purulent, foul-smelling discharge)

c. Chronic sinusitis

d. Adenoidal hypertrophy

6. Management

a. Avoid precipitating allergens and eliminate allergens from the environment:

(1) Encase the mattress and box spring in airtight plastic (to avoid mites).

(2) Remove "dust collectors" (including carpets) from the bedroom

(3) Exclude pets from bedrooms.

(4) High-efficiency particulate air (HEPA) filters for environmental causes and air conditioners for pollen-induced allergies can be helpful.

b. Pharmacotherapy

(1) Antihistamines: Use nonsedating agents such as fexofenadine, loratadine, desloratadine, or cetirizine, when age-appropriate. Begin in lower doses and increase until desired effects occur. (Side effects are infrequent and include sedation, restlessness, dry mouth, constipation, and urinary retention.)

(2) Decongestants: Pseudoephedrine is most commonly used and can be used orally along with antihistamines to reduce the swelling; try to avoid excessive topical (nasal) use because of "rebound" effects resulting in rhinitis medicamentosa, which can itself be very difficult to treat.

(3) Cromolyn sodium: Administer every 4 to 6 hours by nasal route. It has few side effects and is best for prophylaxis and as adjunct therapy to antihistamines, or alone for very confined cases of seasonal pollenosis.

(4) Ipratropium bromide: 0.03% or 0.06% can reduce the volume of watery secretions, but has little effect on other symptoms.

(5) Corticosteroids: Effective short-term anti-inflammatory therapy for exacerbations, with few side effects (local irritation, epistaxis). Beclomethasone, flunisolide, fluticasone, mometasone, or budesonide may be used topically daily or twice a day by nasal route.

c. Immunotherapy: Consider if the previous treatments become ineffective. Immunotherapy is most effective for a skin test– or RAST-identified, seasonal, pollen-related allergy. It is also effective for allergies to dust mites, animal (especially cat) dander, pollens, and molds. Therapy may continue for 3 years or longer.

d. Follow-up: Visit should be scheduled within 2 to 4 weeks to review environmental control, the efficacy of drug therapy, and the resolution of comorbid disorders (e.g., otitis media with effusion).

16.3 Asthma

1. Definition: Reversible airways obstruction due to airway inflammation and increased airway hyperresponsiveness. Clinically, these characteristics translate into recurrent episodes of wheezing, dyspnea, and cough that have both acute and chronic manifestations in most patients.

2. Pathophysiology

   a. Airway obstruction: Figure 16-1 outlines the pathogenesis of bronchial inflammation and airway hyperresponsiveness that, in turn, leads to airway obstruction, the final common pathway for the symptoms and signs of asthma.

   b. Air trapping and hyperinflation: Small airways obstruction (secondary to bronchospasm, secretions, and mucus plugging) produces air trapping. As air is trapped, the functional residual capacity rises, and the patient is breathing at or near total lung capacity—the result is hyperinflation.

   c. Accessory muscles: To maintain oxygenation in the face of hyperinflation, accessory muscles of respiration are used. It is the extent of accessory muscle use rather than the degree of wheezing that predicts the severity of impairment in pulmonary function during an acute exacerbation.

   d. Hypoxia and ventilation/perfusion ($\dot{V}/\dot{Q}$) mismatch: Hypoxemia in a severe exacerbation occurs mostly from a mismatch of ventilation (due to obstruction) and perfusion (i.e., $\dot{V}/\dot{Q}$ mismatch). As airflow obstruction progresses, oxygen saturation (SaO_2) falls, PcO_2 rises, and the peak expiratory flow rate (PEFR) falls to below 25% of that predicted. As hypoxemia and hyperinflation increase, pulmonary vascular resistance rises, thus creating a vicious cycle that perpetuates hypoxia.

   e. Cardiovascular: Negative pleural pressures become more negative. Progressive hyperinflation leads to increased left ventricular afterload, which clinically produces a pulsus paradoxus (a fall in systolic blood pressure during each inspiration, normally 10 to 15 mm Hg or less). The presence of a pulsus paradoxus indicates the attack is severe and that the PEFR will be 50% or less of predicted.

   f. An asthma exacerbation may occur in two phases.

      (1) Acute: Immediate phase (within 4 to 8 hours) is triggered by an allergen or antigen and biochemical mediators that result in immediate bronchoconstriction.

      (2) Delayed: A later response (8 hours or more) is characterized by progressive airways inflammation and hyperresponsiveness. During the later phase, obstruction to airflow may be mechanical (i.e., mucus plugging) and consequently more difficult to treat.

3. Epidemiology: Asthma is one of the most prevalent and clinically significant childhood conditions. It is estimated that between 5% and

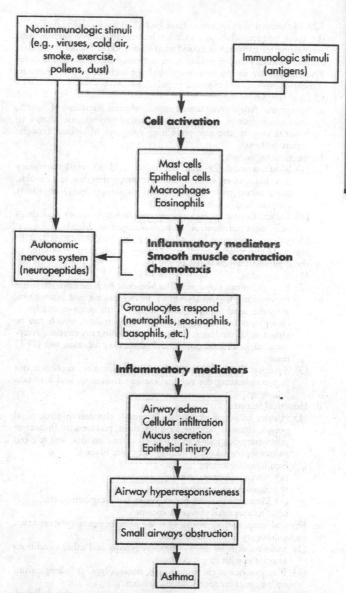

Figure 16-1 Pathophysiology of asthma.

10% of children have asthma or have had wheezing episodes. Asthma is the most frequent chronic condition leading to school absenteeism, accounting for 23% of days missed from school. Over the last 3 decades, asthma morbidity and mortality have increased by 40% each decade. The changes are driven by a relatively large increase in prevalence in African-American and Hispanic populations.

4. Clinical features
   a. Symptoms: Acute or recurrent cough, wheeze, shortness of breath, and chest tightness. A nocturnal cough that persists more than 2 to 3 weeks may be the sole presenting symptom of asthma (cough-variant asthma).
   b. Aggravating factors
      (1) Most common: Exercise (see later), cold air, viral respiratory infections, or exposure to environmental allergens (e.g., molds, dust, mites, cockroaches, animal dander, pollens) or airway irritants (e.g., smoke, pollutants)
      (2) Other: Emotional factors: personal/family stressors and drugs (e.g., aspirin, nonsteroidal anti-inflammatory drugs)
   c. Patterns of symptoms: It is clinically helpful to determine certain aspects of symptom occurrences. Treatment can then be tailored to those patterns, which include
      (1) Seasonality
      (2) Episodic versus persistent: The National Asthma Education and Prevention Program (NAEPP) divides asthma into *intermittent*, with the need for episodic treatments with quick-acting bronchodilators (rescue medications), and *persistent*, which can be either mild, moderate, or severe, depending on daytime symptoms, nighttime symptoms, and pulmonary function test (PFT) results.
      (3) Severity: The severity of previous episodes is an important risk factor indicating the need to escalate treatment and maintain follow-up.
   d. Historical features
      (1) History of atopic dermatitis (eczema), chronic rhinitis, nasal polyps, sinusitis, adverse food reactions, prematurity (bronchopulmonary dysplasia), recurrent croup/pneumonia, and rule out gastroesophageal reflux disease and cystic fibrosis
      (2) Family/social history
         (a) Atopy, allergies, asthma
         (b) Smokers in household
         (c) Living conditions, pet exposure, mold exposures, etc.
         (d) Occupational allergen exposure
   e. Physical examination: Focuses on the skin, upper respiratory tract, and pulmonary examination (Box 16-1)
      (1) Examine skin for signs of flexural eczema and other conditions associated with atopic dermatitis.
      (2) The presence of chronic rhinitis, nasal polyps, or "allergic shiners" suggests an allergic/atopic tendency.
      (3) Pulmonary examination: Bilateral wheezing is the hallmark of asthma but may not be a reliable marker of disease severity

Box 16-1   Important Pulmonary Features on Physical Examination

1. The rate, depth, and rhythm of respirations (including retractions, accessory muscle use) are important indicators of asthma.
2. The degree of breathlessness and inability to speak in sentences suggest hypoxemia from a severe exacerbation.
3. In an infant, paradoxical abdominal wall motion (i.e., with the abdomen rising on inspiration) suggests significant distress.
4. A prolonged expiratory phase on forced exhalation is characteristic of airflow obstruction.
5. Grunting (the body's way of producing physiologic positive end-expiratory pressure to keep small airways open) and flaring of the alae nasi are signs of air hunger. These are *not* commonly seen in most asthma exacerbations, so their presence suggests severe impairment or another diagnosis (e.g., grunting is sometimes seen in acidotic infants).
6. A pulsus paradoxus above 15 mm Hg suggests significant pulmonary (and possible cardiovascular) compromise.

    (i.e., an extremely "tight" asthmatic patient may not move enough air to wheeze). Predominantly small airways disease may result in more cough and dyspnea rather than wheeze.

f. Laboratory findings
   (1) PEFR: A useful measure to assess severity and follow the course of asthma on a regular basis, the PEFR is the maximum flow rate generated during a forced expiratory maneuver, measured in liters/minute.
     (a) Its primary limitation is that a reliable measurement is effort dependent. Therefore it is usually recommended for use in children 5 years of age or older. Proper instruction is essential.
     (b) A baseline personal best needs to be established for every patient. Home measurements should be made at least twice daily (ideally, early morning and evening). The PEFR can also be measured before and after bronchodilator therapy as a guide to assess severity as well as the response to treatment. Figure 16-2 provides a nomogram for calculating PEFRs (values determined by patient's height).
     (c) Interpretation: The emphasis is not on an isolated reading but on trends from a predetermined baseline, the so-called personal best.
       (i) A drop of 20% from personal best may predict an exacerbation within 12 to 24 hours. The institution or change of medication may thwart an attack.
      (ii) A measurement of 50% to 80% of personal best suggests an acute exacerbation may be present, and an increase or addition of medication (e.g., prednisone) may be needed.

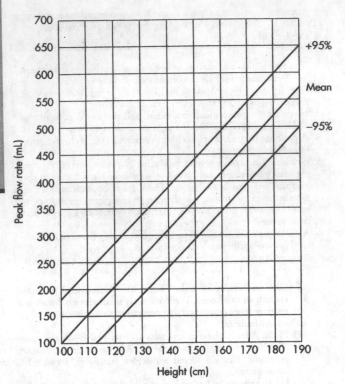

Figure 16-2 Nomogram for calculating peak expiratory flow rate based on height (mean ± 95th percentile). (Data from Godfrey S, Kamburoff PL, Nairn JR: Spirometry, lung volumes and airway resistance in normal children aged 5 to 18 years. Br J Dis Chest 34:15-24, 1970.)

        (iii) A measurement below 50% indicates a medical alert: Immediate bronchodilators and anti-inflammatory therapy are needed, and the physician should be notified.

    (2) Chest radiograph (CXR): The CXR is not a generally useful or indicated study in most patients with asthma. Consideration for obtaining a CXR in an acute exacerbation should be given to patients who

        (a) Have clinical findings suggestive of another diagnosis (e.g., foreign body, pneumonia)

        (b) Do not respond as expected to aggressive asthma therapy

        (c) Have *focal* findings: Wheezing, fine crackles, or localized decreased breath sounds (i.e., pneumonia, pneumothorax)

(d) Have a temperature 39° C or higher (to rule out pneumonia); or
(e) Have had prior history of pneumothorax.

(3) Complete PFTs: PFTs should ideally be obtained in all asthmatic patients at some point in their disease course or whenever other conditions are entertained, because they may reveal the presence of upper or lower airway problems. Improvement of 12% in the peak flow or forced expiratory flow in 1 second (FEV_1) after bronchodilators in a large airway is helpful in establishing the diagnosis of asthma. Inability to improve airway measures can have important prognostic implications and be a sign of persistent airway "remodeling" (basement membrane fibrosis).

(4) Other laboratory studies occasionally obtained to confirm the diagnosis or to rule out other diagnoses include
(a) Complete blood count (for eosinophilia)
(b) Nasal or sputum for eosinophils
(c) Sinus radiographs or computed tomography scan (for sinusitis)
(d) Allergy testing, bronchoprovocation, and exhaled nitrous oxide measures

5. Diagnosis
   a. Diagnosis is based on clinical features and PFT results. Underdiagnosis of asthma is a concern; children with recurrent wheezing episodes are much more likely to have asthma than pneumonia, bronchitis, or some other condition.
   b. *Exercise-induced asthma*: Can occur in almost all patients with chronic asthma but also may be the only presentation for a smaller subset of patients. Diagnosis suggested by the clinical features of wheezing, cough, shortness of breath, chest tightness, and problems with endurance during exercise. Confirmation of the diagnosis can be made by finding a decrease in PEFR (or FEV_1) by 15% or more within 10 minutes after exercising during an exercise challenge test. Baseline spirometry should be normal when not exercising, or the child has underlying chronic asthma.

6. Differential diagnosis: "All that wheezes may not be asthma." Many other conditions may produce focal or generalized wheezing (sometimes accompanied by stridor) in infants and children, including the following:
   a. Obstruction involving major airways
      (1) Foreign body in trachea, bronchus, or esophagus
      (2) Vascular rings
      (3) Laryngotracheomalacia
      (4) Enlarged lymph nodes or tumor
      (5) Laryngeal webs
      (6) Tracheostenosis or bronchostenosis
   b. Obstructions involving both large and small airways
      (1) Viral bronchiolitis
      (2) Cystic fibrosis
      (3) *Chlamydia trachomatis* infection
      (4) Bronchopulmonary dysplasia
      (5) Aspiration (from dysfunction in swallowing or gastroesophageal reflux)

(6) Vascular engorgement

(7) Pulmonary edema

7. Management

a. Introduction

(1) The *basic goal of asthma therapy* is to maintain control as close to normal baseline functioning as possible and to avoid the peaks and valleys in symptoms associated with suboptimal asthma care. Evidence suggests that a lack of control may result in more permanent "airway remodeling."

(2) It is imperative that the asthma patient and family be attuned to

(a) the triggers that produce acute or worsening symptoms;

(b) the remedies, medical as well as psychobehavioral (e.g., stress reduction, relaxation) that ameliorate or control symptoms; and

(c) the use and abuse of medications and therapies.

(3) Much of medically centered asthma care is guided by clinical response to interventions, with the use of a graduated or "step-up" and "step-down" approach, adding medications or changing doses or frequency contingent on patient symptoms or PEFR measurements.

(4) Algorithms for asthma management formulated by the National Heart, Lung, and Blood Institute (NHLBI) and the NAEPP are presented in the following sections.

b. Acute exacerbation management

(1) Estimation of severity: As a guide to management, an *estimation of the severity* of the exacerbation is critical. Table 16-1 provides criteria to determine the severity of an acute exacerbation. These criteria can be applied in virtually any setting.

(2) Home management: The key to successful home management of an acute exacerbation begins with prior education of the patient and family as well as provider availability. The algorithm in Figure 16-3 adapted from the 1997 NHLBI guidelines outlines a strategy for home management.

(3) Office or emergency department management: In an acute exacerbation, knowledge of the patient's past and current asthma history is crucial: Is this a "brittle" asthmatic with frequent, severe exacerbations? Is the patient currently on prednisone or maximal home management? How close is this patient to impending respiratory failure? *Immediate* assessment of vital signs and key clinical asthma parameters to determine severity is warranted for all patients ill enough to seek acute care. Figure 16-4 (adapted from the 1997 NHLBI guidelines) outlines office or emergency department management.

(4) Patients discharged to home after acute exacerbation: The treating physician should provide:

(a) A detailed treatment plan for the next 3 to 5 days. This may or may not include a 7-day (or longer) course of prednisone (1 to 2 mg/kg/day every morning).

(b) Contingency plans for what to do should symptoms recur (e.g., escalating the frequency of treatments or the institution of prednisone). Notify the primary care physician.

	Mild	Moderate	Severe	Respiratory Arrest Imminent
Symptoms				
Breathlessness	While walking Can lie down	While talking (infant—softer, shorter cry; difficulty feeding) Prefers sitting	While at rest (infant—stops feeding) Sits upright	
Talks in	Sentences	Phrases	Words	
Alertness	May be agitated	Usually agitated	Usually agitated	Drowsy or confused
Signs				
Respiratory rate†	Increased	Increased	Often >30/min	
Use of accessory muscles; suprasternal retractions	Usually not	Commonly	Usually	Paradoxical thoracoabdominal movement
Wheeze	Moderate, often only end expiratory	Loud; throughout exhalation	Usually loud; throughout inhalation and exhalation	Absence of wheeze
Pulse/minute‡	<100	100-120	>120	Bradycardia
Pulsus paradoxus	Absent; <10 mm Hg	May be present: 10-25 mm Hg	Often present: >25 mm Hg (adult); 20-40 mm Hg (child)	Absence suggests respiratory muscle fatigue
Functional Assessment				
Peak expiratory flow (% predicted or % personal best)	>80%	Approximately 50%-80% or response lasts <2 hr	<50%	

	Mild	Moderate	Severe	Respiratory Arrest Imminent
Functional Assessment				
Pa_{O_2} (on air)	Normal (test not usually necessary)	>60 mm Hg (test not usually necessary)	<60 mm Hg; possible cyanosis	
Pc_{O_2} (on air)	<42 mm Hg (test not usually necessary)	<42 mm Hg (test not usually necessary)	>42 mm Hg; possible respiratory failure	
Sa_{O_2}% (on air) at sea level§	>95%	91-95%	<91%	

*The presence of several parameters, but not necessarily all, indicates the general classification of the exacerbation. Many of these parameters have not been systematically studied, so they serve only as general guides.

†Guide to rates of breathing in awake children:

Age	Normal Rate
<2 mo	<60/min
2-12 mo	<50/min
1-5 yr	<40/min
6-8 yr	<30/min

‡Guide to normal pulse rates in children:

Age	Normal Rate
2-12 mo	<160/min
1-2 yr	<120/min
2-8 yr	<110/min

§Hypercapnia (hypoventilation) develops more readily in young children than in adults and adolescents.

Adapted from National Heart, Lung, and Blood Institute: Guidelines for the Diagnosis and Management of Asthma. NIH publication no. 97-4051. Bethesda, Md, National Institutes of Health, 1997.

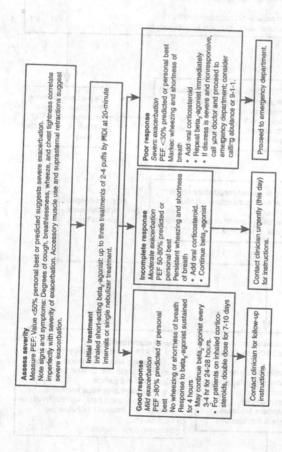

Assess severity
Measure PEF: Value <50% personal best or predicted suggests severe exacerbation.
Note signs and symptoms: Degrees of cough, breathlessness, wheeze, and chest tightness correlate imperfectly with severity of exacerbation. Accessory muscle use and suprasternal retractions suggest severe exacerbation.

Initial treatment
Inhaled short-acting beta₂-agonist: up to three treatments of 2-4 puffs by MDI at 20-minute intervals or single nebulizer treatment.

Good response
Mild exacerbation
PEF >80% predicted or personal best
No wheezing or shortness of breath
Response to beta₂-agonist sustained for 4 hours
• May continue beta₂-agonist every 3-4 hr for 24-28 hours.
• For patients on inhaled corticosteroids, double dose for 7-10 days.

Contact clinician for follow-up instructions.

Incomplete response
Moderate exacerbation
PEF 50-80% predicted or personal best
Persistent wheezing and shortness of breath
• Add oral corticosteroid.
• Continue beta₂-agonist

Contact clinician urgently (this day) for instructions.

Poor response
Severe exacerbation
PEF <50% predicted or personal best
Marked wheezing and shortness of breath
• Add oral corticosteroid
• Repeat beta₂-agonist immediately
• If distress is severe and nonresponsive, call your doctor and proceed to emergency department; consider calling ambulance or 9-1-1.

Proceed to emergency department.

Note:
Patients at high risk of asthma-related death should receive immediate clinical attention after initial treatment.
Additional therapy may be required.

Figure 16-3 Algorithm for home management of an acute asthma exacerbation. MDI, metered-dose inhaler; PEF, peak expiratory flow. (From National Heart, Lung, and Blood Institute: Guidelines for the Diagnosis and Management of Asthma. NIH publication no. 97-4051. Bethesda, Md, National Institutes of Health, 1997.)

Initial assessment
History, physical examination (ausculation, use of accessory muscles, heart rate, repiratory rate), PEF or FEV_1, oxygen saturation, and other tests as indicated

FEV_1 or PEF >50%
• Inhaled beta$_2$-agonist by metered-dose inhaler or nebulizer, up to three doses in first hour
• Oxygen to achieve O_2 saturation ≥90%
• Oral corticosteroids if no immediate response

FEV_1 or PEF <50% (severe exacerbation)
• Inhaled high-dose beta$_2$-agonist and anticholinergic by nebulization every 20 minutes or continuously for 1 hour
• Oxygen to achieve O_2 saturation ≥90%
• Oral systemic corticosteroid

Repeat assessment
Symptoms, physical examination, PEF, O_2 saturation, other tests as needed

Impending or actual respiratory arrest
• Intubation and mechanical ventilation with 100% O_2
• Nebulized beta$_2$-agonist and anticholinergic
• Intravenous corticosteroid

Admit to hospital intensive care
(see box below)

Moderate exacerbation
FEV_1 or PEF 50-80% predicted/personal best
Physical exam: moderate symptoms
• Inhaled short-acting beta$_2$-agonist every 60 minutes
• Systemic corticosteroid
• Continue treatment 1-3 hours, provided there is improvement

Severe exacerbation
FEV_1 or PEF <50% predicted/personal best
Physical exam: severe symptoms at rest, accessory muscle use, chest retraction
History: high-risk patient
No improvement after initial treatment
• Inhaled short-acting beta$_2$-agonist, hourly or continuous + inhaled anticholinergic
• Oxygen
• Systemic corticosteroid

Continued

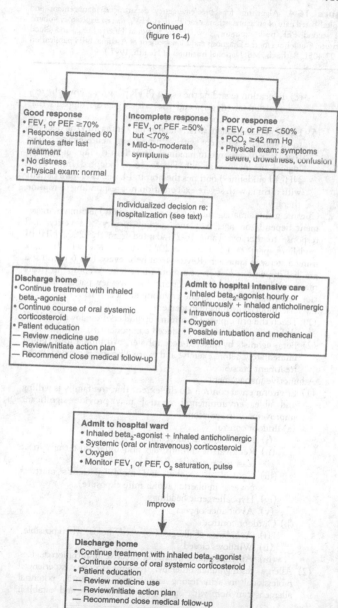

Continued
(figure 16-4)

Good response
- FEV$_1$ or PEF ≥70%
- Response sustained 60 minutes after last treatment
- No distress
- Physical exam: normal

Incomplete response
- FEV$_1$ or PEF ≥50% but <70%
- Mild-to-moderate symptoms

Poor response
- FEV$_1$ or PEF <50%
- PCO$_2$ ≥42 mm Hg
- Physical exam: symptoms severe, drowsiness, confusion

Individualized decision re: hospitalization (see text)

Discharge home
- Continue treatment with inhaled beta$_2$-agonist
- Continue course of oral systemic corticosteroid
- Patient education
  — Review medicine use
  — Review/initiate action plan
  — Recommend close medical follow-up

Admit to hospital intensive care
- Inhaled beta$_2$-agonist hourly or continuously + inhaled anticholinergic
- Intravenous corticosteroid
- Oxygen
- Possible intubation and mechanical ventilation

Admit to hospital ward
- Inhaled beta$_2$-agonist + inhaled anticholinergic
- Systemic (oral or intravenous) corticosteroid
- Oxygen
- Monitor FEV$_1$ or PEF, O$_2$ saturation, pulse

Improve

Discharge home
- Continue treatment with inhaled beta$_2$-agonist
- Continue course of oral systemic corticosteroid
- Patient education
  — Review medicine use
  — Review/initiate action plan
  — Recommend close medical follow-up

Figure 16-4 Algorithm for office/emergency department management and hospital-based care of an acute asthma exacerbation. FEV_1, forced expiratory volume in 1 second; PEF, peak expiratory flow. (From National Heart, Lung, and Blood Institute: Guidelines for the Diagnosis and Management of Asthma. NIH publication no. 97-4051. Bethesda, Md, National Institutes of Health, 1997.)

      (c) Education regarding the use of PEFR measurements, the recognition of triggers, and the critical signs/symptoms that would require contacting a physician.

    (5) Hospital management: Many factors may enter into the decision to hospitalize a patient with asthma in an acute exacerbation (e.g., lack of response to maximal outpatient therapy or psychological or social reasons). Figure 16-4 (adapted from 1997 NHLBI guidelines) outlines the hospital-based care for a patient with asthma with severe exacerbation not responding to routine therapy.

  c. Chronic asthma management: Chronic (i.e., daily) asthma management depends on age, past and current history of severity, and response to therapy. Table 16-2 (adapted from the 2002 NHLBI guidelines update on selected topics 2002) outlines treatment strategies using a stepwise approach. Review treatment every 1 to 6 months; a gradual stepwise reduction or a more immediate "step-up" in treatment may be necessary. It is important first to review patient medication technique, adherence, and environmental control.

  d. Exercise-induced asthma management

    (1) Teach the principles of "warming up and cooling down" with all children with an exercise-induced component.

    (2) Beta$_2$ agonists by metered-dose inhaler, two inhalations (puffs) immediately before exercise and every 4 hours, as needed, is the treatment of choice.

  e. Adjunctive management

    (1) Environmental control: To the extent that the family is willing and able, environmental control may provide significant improvement in symptoms.

      (a) Indoor control

        (i) No smoking in household

        (ii) Removal of curtains/rugs and other dust traps in at least the patient's room

        (iii) Control of roaches and molds; patient's mattress covered in plastic (avoids mite exposure)

        (iv) Hypoallergenic bedding

        (v) Avoidance of pets

      (b) Outdoor control

        (i) Avoidance of allergies (ragweed, molds) when possible

        (ii) Windows closed

        (iii) Air-conditioned interior or effective air filtration devices

    (2) Allergy testing/immunotherapy: Referral to an experienced professional in skin testing and RAST to identify potential allergens can help with environmental controls and establish

| Severity | Clinical Features before Treatment or Adequate Control | | Daily Medications Required to Maintain Long-Term Control |
	Symptoms/Day (PEF or FEV₁)	Symptoms/Night (PEF Variability)	
Step 4: severe persistent	Continual (≤60%)	Frequent (>30%)	*Preferred treatment:* High-dose inhaled corticosteroids *and* Long-acting beta₂ agonists *and* (if needed) Corticosteroid tablets or syrup long term (2 mg/kg/day, generally do not exceed 60 mg/day) (Make repeat attempts to reduce systemic corticosteroids and maintain control with high-dose inhaled corticosteroids)
Step 3: moderate persistent	Daily (>60%<<80%)	>1 night/wk (>30%)	*Preferred treatment:* low- to medium-dose inhaled corticosteroids and long-acting beta₂ agonists *Alternative treatment:* increase inhaled corticosteroids within medium-dose range *or* Low- to medium-dose inhaled corticosteroids and either leukotriene modifier or theophylline *If needed (particularly in patients with recurring severe exacerbations):* Preferred treatment: increase inhaled corticosteroids within medium-dose range and add long-acting beta₂ agonists Alternative treatment: increase inhaled corticosteroids within medium-dose range and add either leukotriene modifier or theophylline

Continued

Severity	Clinical Features before Treatment or Adequate Control		Daily Medications Required to Maintain Long-Term Control
	Symptoms/Day (PEF or FEV₁)	Symptoms/Night (PEF Variability)	
Step 2: mild persistent	>2/wk but <1/day (≥80%)	>2 nights/mo (20%-30%)	*Preferred treatment:* low-dose inhaled corticosteroids *Alternative treatment (listed alphabetically):* cromolyn, leukotriene modifier, nedocromil, *or* sustained-release theophylline to serum concentration of 5-15 μg/mL
Step 1: mild intermittent	≤2 days/wk (≥80%)	≤2 nights/mo (<20%)	*No daily medication needed:* Severe exacerbations may occur, separated by long periods of normal lung function and no symptoms. A course of systemic corticosteroids is recommended.

Quick Relief: All Patients

Short-acting bronchodilator: Two to four puffs short-acting beta₂ agonists as needed for symptoms.
Intensity of treatment will depend on severity of exacerbation; up to three treatments at 20-minute intervals or a single nebulizer treatment as needed. Course of systemic corticosteroids may be needed.
Use of short-acting beta₂ agonists more than twice a week in intermittent asthma (daily, or increasing use in persistent asthma) may indicate the need to initiate (increase) long-term control therapy.

*Small children may require some variation/changes to management.
Adapted from National Heart, Lung, and Blood Institute: Guidelines for the Diagnosis and Management of Asthma—Update on Selected Topics 2002. NAEPP Expert Panel Report. NIH publication no. 02-5075; Bethesda, Md, National Institutes of Health, 2003.

prognosis (worse with higher specific allergy level and total IgE level). Allergen immunotherapy may be helpful in refractory cases. An allergist or pulmonologist may also be helpful for patients with severe exacerbations or those refractory to standard therapies.

(3) Medication dosages: Tables 16-3 to 16-5 outline the medication dosages for current acute and maintenance therapy. New medications for asthma include a combination of a long acting beta-agonist, formoterol fumarate with a corticosteroid, budesonide (Symbicort) and omalizumab (Xolair), an IgE blocking immunoglobulin.

16.4 Cystic Fibrosis

1. Epidemiology: Cystic fibrosis (CF) is the most common life-shortening genetic disease in whites, affecting 30,000 Americans, with an incidence of 1/3200 among whites (who make up 96% of the U.S. CF population), 1/17,000 among African Americans, and 1/90,000 among Asians and Native Americans.

2. Etiology/genetics
   a. CF is an autosomal recessive disease caused by an abnormal gene on the long arm of chromosome 7. The gene product, called *cystic fibrosis transmembrane conductance regulator* (CFTR), locates to the apical cell membrane and regulates ion transport by a blend of Na^+ absorption and Cl^- secretion.
   b. There are more than 1000 known CFTR mutations, but 50% of patients with CF are homozygous for the ΔF508 mutation, and 35% are compound heterozygotes with one ΔF508 mutation.
   c. There are several different classes of gene mutation leading to different types of abnormality in the CFTR protein (defective protein production; defective protein processing within the cytoplasm; defective regulation; and defective ion conduction). These, in turn, are associated with different degrees of functional compromise in CFTR and corresponding differences in disease severity.

3. Pathophysiology
   a. Abnormalities in ion transport lead to excessive salt content in the sweat, and decreased water in pancreatic and male reproductive tract secretions, leading in turn to ductal obstruction (pancreatic insufficiency and congenital bilateral absence of the vas deferens).
   b. In the airways, the decreased water–mucin ratio of the airway surface liquid compromises ciliary clearance of mucus, leading to bronchial infections.
   c. The ensuing inflammatory response is associated with release of toxic mediators (e.g., cytokines, elastase) and a vicious cycle of cellular events leading to obstruction and bronchiectasis, persistence of infection and inflammation, and eventual respiratory failure (Fig. 16-5).

4. Clinical features: CF is a multisystem disorder that primarily affects the reproductive tract, sweat glands, gastrointestinal tract, and respiratory tract (see Fig. 16-5).
   a. Meconium ileus at birth with or without an associated ileal atresia: All infants with documented meconium ileus should be evaluated for CF.

Medication	Dosage Form	Adults	Children	Duration	Comments
Short-Acting Beta₂ Agonists					
MDI					
Albuterol (e.g., Proventil, Ventolin)	0.09 mg	2 puffs 5 min before exercise	1-2 puffs 5 min before exercise	4-6 hr	May double dose for mild exacerbations
		1-2 puffs every 4-6 hr	1-2 puffs every 4-6 hr		
Terbutaline (e.g., Brethine)	0.20 mg	1-2 puffs every 4-6 hr		4-6 hr	
Dry Particle Inhalers (CFC Free)					
Albuterol (Rotacaps)	0.20 mg/capsule	1-2 capsules every 4-6 hr and before exercise		4-6 hr	
Nebulizer Solutions					
Albuterol	5 mg/mL	1.25-5 mg every 4-8 hr	0.05 mg/kg (1.25-2.5 mg) every 4-6 hr	4-6 hr	Mix with 2-3 mL normal saline; may be premixed May mix with cromolyn or ipratropium Continuous nebulization (10-15 mg/hr)

Anticholinergics (MDI)

Ipratropium (Atrovent)	0.018 mg	2-4 puffs every 6 hr	1-2 puffs every 6 hr	4-6 hr	Additional benefit if used with beta$_2$ agonist therapy *not* established. Slower acting than beta$_2$ agonists

Combination Agents (MDI)

Albuterol/ipratropium (Combivent)	Same formulation as individual drug	1-4 puffs every 6 hr	1-2 puffs every 6 hr	4-6 hr	

Class effects, beta$_2$ agonists: Rapid (5-15 min) onset of action except bitolterol (30-120 min).
Class adverse effects, beta$_2$ agonists: Tremor, tachycardia, tachyarrhythmias, palpitations, hypokalemia, insomnia. Tachyphylaxis with prolonged use. Nonselective agents (e.g., epinephrine, isoproterenol, metaproterenol, isoetharine) not recommended because of potential for excess cardiac stimulation. Paradoxical bronchospasm rare, but reported with all inhaled medications; (?) related to medication preservatives (benzalkonium chloride) or other medication components.

MDI, metered-dose inhaler.

Medication	Dosage Form	Adults/Teens	Children	Comments
Systemic Corticosteroids				
Prednisone (Deltasone, Liquid Pred)	Tablets: 1, 2.5, 10, 20, 25, 50 mg Solution, syrup, concentrate solution: all 5 mg/1 mL	7.5-60 mg/day "Burst": 40-60 mg once or twice daily for 3-10 days	0.25-2 mg/kg/day one to four times per day "Burst": 1-2 mg/kg/day; max. 60 mg/day for 3-10 days	1. Long-term control; daily dose in morning or alternate day 2. Burst for establishing control or during deterioration, continue until 80% peak expiratory flow or symptoms resolve 3. No evidence that tapering steroids prevents relapse
Prednisolone (e.g., Pediapred, Prelone, Ovapred)	Tablets: 5 mg Solutions: 5 mg/mL (240, 480 mL) Solutions: 15 mg/5 mL	Same as prednisone	Same as prednisone	Same as prednisone
Inhaled Corticosteroids See Table 16-5				
Anti-inflammatory Drugs				
Cromolyn (Intal)	MDI: 0.8 mg/puff Nebulizer solution: 20 mg/2 mL ampule (60, 120 mL)	2-4 puffs every 6-8 hr 1 ampule every 6-8 hr	1-2 puffs every 6-8 hr 1 ampule every 6-8 hr	1. Not recommended for patients <2 yr of age 2. Not for acute exacerbations 3. 10-60 min before exercise or allergen exposure; protective for 1-2 hr 4. May require 6-wk trial to assess effectiveness
Nedocromil (Tilade)	MDI: 1.75 mg/puff	2-4 puffs every 6-12 hr	1-2 puffs every 6-12 hr	Same as cromolyn

Medication	Formulation	Dose	Dose	Comments
Montelukast (Singulair)	Tablets: 4 or 5 mg chewable; 10 mg film-coated	10 mg every evening (adults and children ≥15 yr)	6-14 yr: 5 mg every evening; 2-5 yr: 4 mg every evening	1. Leukotriene receptor antagonist 2. Not affected by food 3. No clinically important drug interactions reported to date
Combined Medications: Long-Term Beta$_2$ Agonists and Corticosteroids				
Fluticasone/salmeterol (Advair)	DPI 100, 250, or 500 μg/50 μg per inhalation	1 inhalation twice daily; dose depends on severity of asthma	1 inhalation twice daily; dose depends on severity of asthma	
Methylxanthines†				
Theophylline (Slo-Phyllin, Slo-bid, Theo-Dur)	Liquids, sustained-release tablets, and capsules	Starting dose 10 mg/kg/day up to 300 mg max.; usual max. 800 mg/day	Starting dose 10 mg/kg/day Usual max.: <1 yr of age: 0.2 × age (in weeks) + 5 = mg/kg/day ≥1 yr of age: 16 mg/kg/day	
Long-Acting Beta$_2$ Agonists				
Salmeterol (Serevent)	MDI: 0.21 mg/puff DPI: 0.05 mg/blister	2 puffs every 12 hr 1 blister every 12 hr	1-2 puffs every 12 hr 1 blister every 12 hr	1. Not for acute exacerbations 2. One or two puffs nightly for nocturnal symptoms 3. Must have concurrent quick-relief medication
Albuterol (Proventil, Repetabs, Volmax)	Sustained-release tablet 4, 8 mg	4-8 mg every 12 hr Max. dose 32 mg	Not recommended	1. More systemic adverse effects 2. Shorter-acting oral formulations available (tablets, syrup), but not recommended

*Not intended as "quick-relief" medication.
†Serum monitoring is important (serum concentration of 5-15 μg/mL at steady state).
DPI, dry powder inhaler; MDI, metered-dose inhaler.

Inhaled Corticosteroid	Dosage Form	Low Dose	Medium Dose	High Dose	Comments
MDI (Dose/Puff)					
Beclomethasone dipropionate (Vanceril, Beclovent, Vanceril DS)	42 µg 84 µg	84-336 µg 42 µg (2-8 puffs) 84 µg (1-4 puffs)	336-672 µg 42 µg (8-16 puffs) 84 µg (4-8 puffs)	>672 µg 42 µg (>16 puffs) 84 µg (>8 puffs)	Possible association with posterior subcapsular cataracts
Triamcinolone acetonide (Azmacort)	100 µg	400-800 µg (4-8 puffs)	800-1200 µg (8-12 puffs)	>1200 µg (>12 puffs)	Spacer included with MDI
Flunisolide (AeroBid, AeroBid-M)	250 µg	500-700 µg (2-3 puffs)	1000-1250 µg (4-5 puffs)	>1250 µg (>5 puffs)	Regular and mint flavor (contains menthol)
Fluticasone (Flovent)	44 µg 110 µg 220 µg	88-176 µg 44 µg (2-4 puffs)	176-440 µg 44 µg (4-10 puffs) or 110 µg (2-4 puffs)	>440 µg 110 µg (>4 puffs) or 220 µg (>2 puffs)	Most potent topical corticosteroid

Nebulizer Suspension					
Budesonide (Pulmicort Respules)	0.25 mg/2 mL 0.5 mg/2 mL	0.25 mg total daily dose	0.5 mg total daily dose	1 mg total daily dose	Recommended for use with jet nebulizer
DPI (Dose/Spray)					
Fluticasone (Flovent)	50 µg 100 µg 250 µg	50 µg (2-4 inhalations)	100 µg (2-4 inhalations)	100 µg (>4 inhalations) or 250 µg (>2 inhalations)	Distributed in blister packs: 4 blisters/disk; 60 blisters/box
Budesonide (Pulmicort Turbuhaler)	200 µg	100-200 µg (1 inhalation)	520-400 µg (1-2 inhalations)	>400 µg (>2 inhalations)	1. Dose indicator 2. Possible association with posterior subcapsular cataracts

Class effects, inhaled steroids: Anti-inflammatory benefit not evident for 2-4 wk; potential for hypothalamic-pituitary axis suppression.
Class adverse effects, inhaled steroids: Dysphonia, nasal congestion, oral candidiasis, caution if underlying adrenal insufficiency or immunocompromise, exposure to varicella. (?) Delayed growth, otherwise no growth effect. Adverse effects minimized by use of spacer, rinsing of mouth after inhaler use. Paradoxical bronchospasm rare, but reported with all inhaled medications; (?) related to medication preservatives or other medication components.
*Some doses may be outside package labeling.

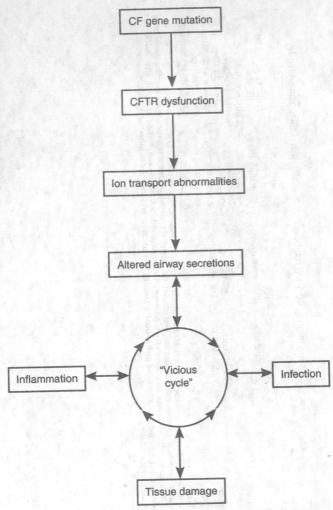

Figure 16-5 Pathogenesis of cystic fibrosis (CF). CFTR, cystic fibrosis transmembrane conductance regulator.

b. Failure to thrive secondary to pancreatic insufficiency.
c. Hypoelectrolytemia and heat prostration secondary to sweat electrolyte losses (especially common in young infants during hot summer months): Any young child with hypochloremic metabolic alkalosis and hyponatremia should be evaluated for CF.

d. "Pulmonary exacerbations" are common and characterized by
  (1) Increased symptoms: Cough, dyspnea, chest tightness, hemoptysis, or anorexia
  (2) Signs: New wheezes or crackles, or weight loss
  (3) Laboratory: Decreased FEV_1, or new CXR changes
e. Chronic wheezing and airway obstruction evidenced by PFT results with or without a reversible component. Any "asthmatic" patient not responding to usual therapy should be evaluated for CF.
f. Chronic cough secondary to recurrent bacterial sinusitis or lower respiratory tract infection
g. CXR with hyperinflation or characteristic increased bronchial markings; "train tracks" from thickened, fibrosed airways
h. Nasal polyps
i. Chronic pansinusitis
j. Clubbing of digits (late finding)
k. Recurrent abdominal pain secondary to pancreatitis, recurrent intestinal obstruction due to inspissated stool in the ileocecal region (meconium ileus equivalent), cramping from malabsorption, or recurrent intussusception
l. Hepatosplenomegaly with serum evidence of biliary obstruction
m. Fat-soluble vitamin deficiency

5. Diagnosis and laboratory findings
  a. The median age at diagnosis is 6 months, but the mean age at diagnosis is 3 years because many patients are diagnosed later in childhood or even in adulthood.
  b. The most common symptoms suggesting the diagnosis are
    (1) Respiratory symptoms: 50%
    (2) Failure to thrive/malnutrition: 34%
    (3) Steatorrhea/abnormal stools: 26%
    (4) Meconium ileus: 21%
  c. Family history leads to the diagnosis in 16% of patients. Less than 5% of new cases are currently diagnosed by newborn screening, a number that will increase in the future as newborn screening becomes more widespread. Newborn screening is accomplished by measuring immunoreactive trypsin (IRT) in the blood; high IRTs are followed up by genotyping, and the diagnosis is confirmed by sweat test.
  d. Laboratory diagnosis
    (1) Measurement of chloride concentration in sweat obtained by pilocarpine iontophoresis is the definitive diagnostic test.
    (2) Sweat testing can be reliably performed after 72 hours of age.
    (3) Sweat chloride of less than 40 mEq/L is normal, and more than 60 mEq/L is abnormal.
    (4) Sweat chlorides in the 40- to 60-mEq/L range are considered indeterminate, but are often due to the presence of mild CF mutations.
    (5) CF genotyping is a specific, but not a sensitive test (approximately 7% of CF mutations are unidentified).

6. Management
  a. *Nutrition*: Patients with CF are at risk for malnutrition because of the combination of protein-fat malabsorption (in the 93% of patients

with pancreatic insufficiency) and increased metabolic requirements consequent to chronic airway inflammation and increased work of breathing. A clear relationship between nutritional adequacy and maintenance of lung function has been documented. Treatment regimen includes

(1) Pancreatic enzyme supplementation with all food intake. Dosing is standardized according to the lipase activity of the enzyme preparation. The typical dose is between 2000 and 3000 units of lipase per kilogram at each meal and snack. Very high doses (>6000 U/kg) have been associated with a rare complication, *fibrosing colonopathy*. Pancreatic enzyme preparations are not completely acid stable, and patients who appear to need relatively high doses will also commonly use a proton pump inhibitor or histamine type 2 antagonist to suppress gastric acidity.

(2) Fat-soluble vitamin supplements

(3) High-calorie nutritional supplements

b. *Lung disease management:* Airway infection and inflammation generally begin in the first year of life, often in the absence of any signs or symptoms. PFT is not sensitive to these early changes, and the average FEV_1 at 5 years of age is 100% predicted. It drops, on average, by about 2% to 2.5% per year throughout childhood. The early institution of preventative and aggressive therapeutic strategies slows the progression of symptomatic lung disease (see Fig. 16-5).

(1) *Bronchial obstruction*

(a) Airway clearance augmentation techniques: These are typically used twice daily for 20 minutes when patients are well, and more often during pulmonary exacerbations (see later). The most commonly used approaches are chest percussion, high-frequency chest wall oscillation (the Vest), and devices such as the Flutter or Acapella valves.

(b) Bronchodilators: About 25% of CF patients have consistent bronchodilator responsiveness, and most have it intermittently. The use of bronchodilators (e.g., albuterol and salmeterol) is common but of unproven efficacy.

(c) Dornase alfa (recombinant human DNase [Pulmozyme]): When neutrophils participating in the inflammatory response undergo necrosis, they release DNA that increases viscoelasticity and adhesiveness of CF sputum. Dornase alfa breaks down extracellular DNA, improving mucus clearance. The dose is 2.5 mg once daily, by inhalation.

(2) *Infection:* Airway infection can be controlled but not eradicated.

(a) Potential organisms to target with antimicrobial treatment include

(i) *Pseudomonas aeruginosa* (PA) and other species: PA may be present in the first year of life, and becomes increasingly prevalent with age. As the organism persists in the airway, it develops the ability to produce alginate, which gives it a "mucoid" phenotype, making it ineradicable and leading to accelerated progression of lung disease.

(ii) *Staphylococcus aureus*

(iii) *Haemophilus influenzae*

(iv) *Burkholderia cepacia*: *B. cepacia* is an uncommon organism that uniquely infects patients with CF and has worrisome implications because it is multiresistant, can cause fulminant disease, and is transmissible.

(b) Intermittent flare-ups of infection occur, and are treated with discrete courses of systemic antibiotic therapy. Antibiotics are chosen based on cultures of airway secretions. Table 16-6 lists antibiotic choices.

(c) Specific anti-PA therapy is used as indicated.

   (i) Patients with chronic PA airway infection are treated with chronic inhaled antibiotics (most typically, tobramycin [TOBI] 300 mg twice daily on alternating months). Aerosolized antibiotics achieve high concentration in the airway, have minimal systemic effects/toxicity, and are convenient (compared with IV); however, penetration into obstructed airways is less, causing decreased effectiveness during exacerbations.

   (ii) When initially acquired, PA can often be eliminated. Thus, frequent surveillance airway cultures are performed, and at initial detection, inhaled ± systemic antibiotics are prescribed to eradicate PA (even in asymptomatic individuals).

(3) *Inflammation*: a number of anti-inflammatory agents have been shown to be beneficial in CF, but there is some controversy regarding their use.

Table 16-6 **Intravenous Antibiotic Choices for Treating Patients with Cystic Fibrosis**		
Antibiotic	**Child Dose**	**Adolescent Dose**
Vancomycin	15 mg/kg every 6 hr	500 mg every 6 hr or 1 g every 12 hr
Linezolid	10 mg/kg every 8 hr	600 mg every 12 hr
Rifampin	10 mg/kg every 12 hr	600 mg every 12 hr
Amikacin	7.5 mg/kg every 8 hr	7.5 mg/kg every 12 hr
Tobramycin	10 mg/kg every day	10 mg/kg every day
Aztreonam	50 mg/kg every 8 hr	2 g every 8 hr
Ceftazidime	50 mg/kg every 8 hr	2 g every 8 hr
Meropenem	40 mg/kg every 8 hr	2 g every 8 hr
Piperacillin, piperacillin/ tazobactam	100 mg/kg every 6 hr	3 g every 6 hr
Ticarcillin, ticarcillin/ clavulanate	100 mg/kg every 6 hr	3 g every 6 hr
Ciprofloxacin	15 mg/kg every 12 hr	400 mg every 12 hr

(a) Systemic steroids are used in selected patients to improve airway function.

(b) Inhaled corticosteroids are used commonly, particularly in patients with apparent airway reactivity, but their benefit has not been clearly demonstrated.

(c) Ibuprofen, when given in high doses (20 to 30 mg/kg twice daily to a maximum 1600 mg/dose), leads to long-term benefits in lung function, particularly in children between 6 and 12 years of age.

(d) Macrolide antibiotics (especially alternate-day azithromycin 250 mg if weight <40 kg or 500 mg if weight ≥40 kg) have been shown to lead to improved lung function possibly through secondary anti-inflammatory effects.

c. *Admission orders:* Box 16-2 lists typical orders for inpatient admission and treatment of a pulmonary exacerbation of CF.

Box 16-2   Routine Orders for Patients with Cystic Fibrosis Admitted with Pulmonary Exacerbation

*Diet: high-calorie diet with snacks, supplements as per nutritionist
*Consults
  *Nutrition
  *Respiratory therapy (airway clearance assistance four times daily—chest physiotherapy, Flutter valve, positive expiratory pressure valve, vest, etc.)
  *Physical therapy (to facilitate activity and exercise)
  *Teachers, child life specialist (for prolonged stays)
  †Endocrinology (for patients with CF-related diabetes)
  †Gastroenterology (for patients with gastrointestinal issues)
*IV to heparin or saline lock in between antibiotic administrations (to facilitate activity)
*Laboratory testing: Initial blood work may be done with first aminoglycoside level
  *Complete blood count, electrolytes, glucose, creatinine, U/A, liver enzymes, albumin, PT, PTT
  †Total IgE (a screen for allergic bronchopulmonary aspergillosis)
  †Prealbumin (a screen for nutritional status)
  †Vitamin A and E levels
  †HbA$_{1C}$ (if >10 years of age)
  †Sputum culture (CF protocol)
    †Bacterial culture
    †Fungal culture
    †Acid-fast bacilli smear and culture
  †Aminoglycoside levels (peak and trough) around third or fourth dose and with every dosage change

---

Box 16-2   Routine Orders for Patients with Cystic Fibrosis Admitted with Pulmonary Exacerbation—cont'd

†Oral glucose tolerance test—fasting and 2 hours after 1.75 g/kg of glucose solution

†72-hour stool fat collection

†Chest radiograph (if not done just before admission)

†Spirometry (simple) in pulmonary function testing laboratory (if not done just before admission)

†Audiometry on admission (if >6 years of age and receiving aminoglycosides)

*Medications

  *ADEK vitamins (tablets or drops)

  *Vitamin K 5 mg orally

  *Pancreatic enzymes (as per home routine)

  †Actigall (ursodeoxycholic acid)

  †Insulin for pancreatic insuffciency

  †Dornase alfa (recombinant human DNase [Pulmozyme]) 2.5 mg by aerosol once daily

  †Albuterol

  †Hypertonic saline (7%) 4 mL by aerosol twice daily

  †Tobramycin 300 mg by aerosol twice daily

  †Antibiotics (usually a combination of aminoglycoside and beta-lactam) based on sensitivities of most recent sputum culture (see text for choices and doses)

*Applies to all patients.
†Applies to some patients.
CF, cystic fibrosis.

---

   d. *Immunizations:* Patients with CF should receive all the age-appropriate immunizations recommended for normal children. Annual influenza vaccine is given each fall.

7. Genetic counseling and prognosis
   a. For parents who have a child with CF, each pregnancy has a 1 in 4 chance that the fetus will have CF and a 1 in 2 chance that it will be a carrier.
   b. The life expectancy and quality of life for patients with CF have improved steadily over the last 5 decades. Unfortunately, the end result of infection and inflammation is irreversible bronchiectasis and eventual respiratory failure. At this point, the only remaining option is bilateral lung transplantation. The 5-year survival after lung transplantation is approximately 50%, with bronchiolitis obliterans due to chronic rejection an ongoing problem. The current expected median age at death is 33.5 years.

16.5 Noisy Breathing in Infants and Children

DEFINITIONS OF NOISES

Noises are those that are generally heard without a stethoscope. The most important distinguishing characteristic of these noises is the phase of respiration in which they occur. Continuous sounds that are heard best on inspiration locate the point of air turbulence to the extrathoracic airway; those that are heard best on expiration suggest intrathoracic obstruction and turbulence.

STRIDOR

Acute Stridor

If not related to foreign body aspiration, most causes of acute stridor are infectious and discussed in Chapter 19 (e.g., croup).

Chronic Stridor

Chronic stridor usually presents in the first few months of life, sometimes later depending on the causes (Table 16-7).

Table 16-7 Definitions and Associations of Chronic Airway Noises

Noise	Implication	Clinical Association
Stridor: continuous loud, harsh sound heard predominantly on inspiration	Implies *extrathoracic* obstruction	Laryngomalacia Gastroesophageal reflux disease Subglottic stenosis (congenital) Tracheomalacia (congenital or vascular sling/ring) Other: webs, cysts, papilloma, foreign body
Wheezing: musical, continuous (>250 msec) sound heard predominantly on expiration	Implies *intrathoracic* obstruction	Asthma Cystic fibrosis Foreign body
Stertor: snoring; inspiratory noise of irregular quality	Implies *nasopharyngeal* obstruction	Craniofacial anomalies (e.g., Pierre Robin, Down syndromes) Primary obstructive sleep apnea (obesity) Neuromuscular disorders (spinal muscular atrophy)

CHRONIC STERTOR (SNORING) AND OBSTRUCTIVE SLEEP APNEA SYNDROME

1. *Infant* obstructive sleep apnea syndrome (OSAS) may be associated with:
   a. Craniofacial abnormalities
      (1) Example: Pierre Robin syndrome
      (2) Congenital nasal obstruction
         (a) Choanal stenosis and atresia
         (b) Nasal stenosis syndromes
   b. Chromosomal abnormalities (e.g., Down syndrome)
   c. Neuromuscular disease (e.g., spinal muscular atrophy)
2. *Childhood* OSAS: Although children with the aforementioned syndromes may present later in life with obstructed breathing, the primary cause of OSAS and nighttime snoring in childhood is adenotonsillar hypertrophy and obesity.
   a. About 6% to 10% of children regularly snore at night, and about 2% have OSAS.
   b. Complications of OSAS
      (1) Excessive daytime sleepiness in less than 50%
      (2) Neurobehavioral abnormalities (including attention deficit hyperactivity disorder)
      (3) Systemic hypertension
      (4) Growth failure
      (5) Nocturnal enuresis (especially secondary)
      (6) Pulmonary hypertension and cor pulmonale—late
   c. Diagnosis of OSAS is based on overnight polysomnography.
   d. Treatment of OSAS
      (1) Tonsillectomy and adenoidectomy (T&A) is first-line treatment, even in the presence of "normal-sized" tonsils or obesity.
      (2) When obesity is present, weight loss is essential but difficult to obtain.
      (3) When T&A fails, continuous positive airway pressure or bilevel positive airway pressure may be used.

SUGGESTED READING

American Academy of Pediatrics: Clinical practice guideline: Diagnosis and management of childhood obstructive sleep apnea syndrome. Pediatrics 109:704-712, 2002.

Gibson RL, Burns JL, Ramsey BW: Pathophysiology and management of pulmonary infections in cystic fibrosis. Am J Respir Crit Care Med 168:918-951, 2003. Available at http://ajrccm.atsjournals.org/cgi/content/full/168/8/918.

National Heart, Lung, and Blood Institute: Guidelines for the Diagnosis and Management of Asthma. NIH publication no. 97-4051. Bethesda, Md, National Institutes of Health, 1997.

National Heart, Lung, and Blood Institute: Guidelines for the Diagnosis and Management of Asthma—Update on Selected Topics 2002. NAEPP Expert Panel Report. NIH publication no. 02-5075, Bethesda, Md, National Institutes of Health, 2003. Available at www.nhlbi.nih.gov/guidelines/asthma/execsumm.pdf.

Leung KC, Chung H: Diagnosis of stridor in children. Am Fam Physician 60:40-48, 1999. Available at www.aafp.org/afp/991115ap/2289.html.

Schechter MS, Barker PM: GER and respiratory disease associated with reflux in childhood. Clin Pulm Med 6:178-186, 1999.

WEBSITES

Cystic Fibrosis Medicine: www.cysticfibrosismedicine.com

eMedicine, articles on pediatric pulmonology: www.emedicine.com/ped/PULMONOLOGY.htm

Gastrointestinal Disorders

17

Albert M. Ross IV, Sulaiman Bharwani,
Chandan N. Lakhiani, and Idris Dahod

17.1 Gastroesophageal Reflux

1. Definition: Gastroesophageal reflux (GER) is the retrograde passage of gastric or duodenal contents into the esophagus. It occurs normally but becomes pathologic when acidified gastric contents damage the esophageal mucosa or the lower esophageal sphincter (LES), or if it leads to pain, malnutrition through caloric loss, aspiration, or asthma.
2. Etiology and pathophysiology: Unknown, may be an exaggeration of a physiologic condition. Contributing factors include delayed emptying, increased abdominal pressure, and decreased LES tone (medications, etc.)
3. Clinical manifestations
   a. The generalized manifestations of GER are shown in the following. Note that symptoms of GER are nonspecific and mimic many other conditions.
   b. Age-related manifestations
      (1) Infants
         (a) Irritability
         (b) Interrupted feeding
         (c) Failure to thrive (emesis with malnutrition)
         (d) Apnea of infancy: Sudden infant death syndrome or acute life-threatening events
         (e) Recurrent pneumonia (i.e., aspiration)
         (f) Rumination
         (g) Infant "spells"; seizure-like events
      (2) Older children
         (a) Anorexia
         (b) Chronic cough/reactive airway disease/nocturnal cough
         (c) Dysphagia
         (d) Hematemesis
         (e) Iron-deficiency anemia
         (f) Esophageal strictures
         (g) Barrett's esophagus
4. Diagnosis
   a. The diagnosis can often be made by careful history taking, despite the variability and nonspecificity of symptoms (as noted previously).

b. Barium swallow (barium esophagram) helps rule out structural anomalies that may cause GER. The diagnosis of reflux itself should be made with caution with this method because of a high rate of false-positive results. Barium swallow does not quantify reflux but may locate obstructions, webs, or intestinal malrotation.

c. Esophageal pH probe and six-channel pneumogram entails continuous monitoring of distal esophageal pH for 18 to 24 hours. This test has now become the standard to evaluate reflux and acid clearance. It gives a graphic printout of esophageal pH versus time and provides the percentage of elapsed time where the pH is under 4.0, the total number of reflux events, the number of episodes lasting more than 5 minutes, and the duration of the long reflux episodes.

d. Esophageal scintiscan (milk scan; Tc-99m) measures the gastric emptying time and may allow detection of aspiration of gastric contents.

e. Esophageal manometry may be a useful adjunct to the evaluation of GER. Reduced LES pressure and abnormal peristaltic activity characteristic of specific diseases may be detected.

f. Endoscopy and biopsy are direct tests used to diagnose esophagitis secondary to reflux and structural/mucosal abnormalities, including hiatal hernia, webs, and other infectious causes of esophagitis.

5. Management

a. Conservative therapy includes dietary modifications and positioning, but it is usually of modest effectiveness at best. Small, frequent feedings, thickened feedings with cereals (generally 15 mL of cereal in 30-mL formula), and prone positioning at 30 degrees or more during sleep and after feedings are among the maneuvers that may be used.

b. Medical therapy

(1) A combination of a histamine type 2 (H_2) receptor antagonist (acid secretion blocker) such as ranitidine (2 to 4 mg/kg/dose twice daily) or a proton pump inhibitor such as omeprazole (20 mg once a day) or lansoprazole (15 mg once a day) with an agent that enhances gastric emptying or lowers sphincter pressure (e.g., cisapride, starting dose 0.1 mg/kg/dose every 6 hours; or metoclopramide [Reglan], starting dose 0.1 mg/kg/dose every 6 hours) is usually instituted for moderate to severe symptomatic reflux. Central nervous system side effects of metoclopramide such as tardive dyskinesia and dystonic symptoms mandate judicious use.

(2) Agents to increase sphincter pressure, such as bethanechol chloride (Urecholine; 0.4 mg/kg/24 hours, every day, before meals and at bedtime), may be used when the reflux is associated with severe LES hypotonia or hiatal hernia. Respiratory side effects limit its use.

(3) Antacids are used occasionally as an adjunct to other treatment for acute dyspeptic symptoms.

c. Surgical therapy—specifically, fundoplication—is recommended for the following cases:

(1) Infants with severe intractable apnea or neurologically based feeding problems with dangerous reflux

(2) Certain children requiring gastrostomies for feeding who have severe reflux

(3) Children with intractable asthma associated with GER who do not respond to medical management

(4) Chronic intractable discomfort, although this is unlikely now with proton pump inhibitors

17.2 Acid Peptic Disorders

1. Definitions

   a. *Reflex esophagitis* generally occurs in the lower part of the esophagus and may extend proximally. The endoscopic appearance is either normal or the esophagus may appear reddened or "heaped up," or have nonconfluent erosions appearing as red patches or striae above the Z line. In severe cases, longitudinal erosions may occur with mucosal friability and hemorrhage. Frank ulceration and well-formed strictures are unusual in children. Biopsies are necessary for diagnosis and may show hyperplasia of the basal cell zone of the esophageal squamous epithelium and increased stromal papillary length as well as an eosinophilic infiltrate. The clinical features, diagnosis, and therapy of GER-associated esophagitis are discussed in the previous section. Long-term sequelae include strictures and Barrett's esophagus, with a greatly increased cancer risk.

   b. *Helicobacter pylori* infection may be found colonizing the fundic and body gastric mucosa; it usually causes inflammation in the gastric antrum, which provides an optimum pH for its activity. The antral gastritis caused by *H. pylori* in children has a characteristic nodular appearance on endoscopy. It may be the precursor to the ulcer disease commonly seen in adulthood.

   c. *Peptic ulcer* is a well-defined, circumscribed loss of tissue occurring in those parts of gastrointestinal (GI) tract that are exposed to pepsin and acid, primarily the stomach and duodenum. It is caused by the loss of equilibrium between the destructive forces of luminal acid and pepsin and protective forces of gastric and duodenal mucosal defense (Box 17-1). There is strong evidence suggesting an association between *H. pylori* infection and duodenal ulcer. These ulcers tend to be chronic and have been found to be associated with *H. pylori* infection in over 90% of cases in adults. There is weaker evidence for an association of *H. pylori* with gastric ulcer. Both duodenal and gastric ulcers are far less common in children compared with adults. Gastric ulcers tend to be transient and may resolve spontaneously; they are mostly seen in infants and very young children.

   d. Active *duodenitis* is found in a majority of patients with duodenal ulcers and as an isolated finding in occasional children. However, the relationship of *H. pylori* to duodenitis is not very clear. It has been suggested that luminal acid may induce gastric metaplasia in the duodenum, allowing *H. pylori* colonization and producing an acute inflammatory reaction.

   e. *Stress ulcers* and *stress-related ulcers* are often referred to as *secondary peptic ulcers* and may have a variety of associated causes.

> ## Box 17-1   Factors Involved in Ulcerogenesis
>
> *Aggressive Factors*
>
> *Helicobacter pylori* infection
> Peptic activity
> Bile acids
> Medications (e.g., nonsteroidal anti-inflammatory drugs)
> Alcohol, coffee
> Smoking
> Stress
> Acid
>
> *Protective Factors*
>
> Extraepithelial: mucus, bicarbonate, hydrophobic layer
> Epithelial: cell turnover, protein synthesis, prostaglandins
> Subepithelial: blood flow, bicarbonate

From George DE, Glassman M: Peptic ulcer disease in children. Gastrointest Endosc
Clin North Am 4:23-37,1994.

      (1) Shock, respiratory failure, sepsis, hypoglycemia, severe burns
         (Curling's ulcer), and intracranial lesions (Cushing's ulcer) may
         cause stress ulcers. Chronic systemic diseases may also be causes.
      (2) Use of aspirin, nonsteroidal anti-inflammatory drugs (NSAIDs),
         and steroids have been associated with gastritis and gastric
         ulcers.

2. Clinical manifestations: Age-specific symptoms
  a. Newborns: Abrupt hemorrhage or perforation—"stress ulcer" of the
     newborn—may occur.
  b. Older infants: Vomiting, poor feeding, and irritability may occur.
  c. Toddlers and preschool-age children: Poorly localized abdominal
     pain, vomiting, and bleeding may be present.
  d. Older children and adolescents: Signs and symptoms are similar to
     those for adults, including hematemesis, melena, recurrent abdomi-
     nal pain, loss of appetite, postprandial pain, nocturnal pain, epigas-
     tric pain, and recurrent vomiting. There may be a positive family
     history or a history of use of ulcerogenic medications.

3. Diagnosis
  a. Physical examination may show signs of blood loss (tachycardia,
     pallor, hypotension, or underlying systemic disease). Examination
     may also reveal epigastric tenderness or localized periumbilical ten-
     derness and guarding. A rectal examination should be performed on
     all patients to look for occult blood.
  b. Diagnostic modalities for acid-peptic disorders
    (1) If *H. pylori* infection is suspected, "indirect" tests include
       (a) Serologic testing for anti-*H. pylori* antibody immunoglobu-
          lin G (IgG; 95% sensitive)
       (b) ^{13}C urea breath testing (95% sensitive)

(2) Endoscopy with biopsy of suspicious-appearing mucosal areas is the investigation of choice, with 90% to 95% accuracy for diagnosing ulcers, esophagitis, gastritis, and duodenitis, but this test often is overused for functional abdominal pain.

    (a) Endoscopy is often used to detect *H. pylori*-associated inflammation (antral gastritis, duodenal ulcers, and duodenitis). Histologic diagnosis can be confirmed by Warthin-Starry silver stain and Giemsa stain. The urease activity of *H. pylori* can be detected in the CLO-test, a commercially available test with a sensitivity of 80% to 90% that gives the results within 2 to 3 hours.

    (b) Endoscopy is also helpful for therapeutic purposes (e.g., for electrocautery of bleeding ulcers).

(3) If Zollinger-Ellison syndrome is being considered, fasting and 60-minute postprandial serum gastrin levels should be sent.

(4) An upper GI series is a barium study that identifies 70% to 80% of peptic ulcer disease but has now been largely replaced by endoscopy because it is relatively insensitive in childhood and will often miss gastritis.

  c. Differential diagnosis is shown in Box 17-2.

4. Complications of acid-peptic disease

  a. GI bleeding is a relatively common complication.

  b. Perforation

    (1) Severe abdominal pain, epigastric pain with radiation to back or right upper quadrant (if penetrating ulcer)

    (2) Physical examination: Boardlike abdomen, rebound tenderness, severe epigastric tenderness, absent bowel sounds

    (3) Diagnosis: Free air in the peritoneal cavity or biliary tree evident from radiographic studies of abdomen

    (4) Therapy: Surgery

Box 17-2 Differential Diagnosis of Ulcer Disease

Gastrointestinal Tract

Recurrent abdominal pain (functional pain)
Crohn's disease
Parasites (*Giardia*)
Eosinophilic gastroenteritis
Spinal cord lesions

Non–Gastrointestinal Tract/Others

Gallbladder/biliary tract
Pancreatitis
Urinary tract infection
Henoch-Schönlein purpura

From George DE, Glassman M: Peptic ulcer in children. Gastrointest Endosc Clin North Am 4:23-37, 1994.

  c. Gastric outlet obstruction
    (1) Nausea, vomiting of undigested or partially digested food, epigastric pain unrelieved by food or antacids
    (2) Physical examination: Large amount of air and fluid in the stomach
  d. Posterior penetration or perforation: Manifested by severe back pain and pancreatitis
5. Management
  a. Medical therapy should be aimed at eradicating H. pylori infection, if present, by a combination of antibiotics (e.g., metronidazole, clarithromycin) and omeprazole (to neutralize gastric acidity). If H. pylori is absent, general strategies to reduce acid production (H_2 blocker, proton pump inhibitors, or misoprostol), increase mucosal protection (sucralfate, misoprostol), and decrease certain risk factors (e.g., cigarette smoking) should be considered.
    (1) H_2 receptor antagonists: Ranitidine is given in a dosage of 2 mg/kg/dose twice a day or cimetidine in a dosage of 20 to 40 mg/kg over 24 hours—four divided doses with meals and at bedtime for 8 weeks—or famotidine in a dosage of 1 to 1.2 mg/kg/24 hours divided every 8 to 12 hours.
    (2) Proton pump inhibitors (e.g., omeprazole [Prilosec], lansoprazole [Prevacid]): These suppress gastric acid secretion by specific inhibition of the hydrogen/potassium-ATPase at the secretory surface of the gastric parietal cell. They are indicated for the treatment of severe reflux-associated esophagitis with erosions. The dose is 20 mg orally every day for omeprazole and 15 mg orally every day for lansoprazole.
    (3) Proton pump inhibitors like omeprazole or lansoprazole in combination with antibiotics like amoxicillin and metronidazole have been shown to eradicate H. pylori infection.
    (4) Antacids: These reduce the hydrogen ion concentration. The recommended dose is 0.5 to 1.5 mg/kg 1 and 3 hours after each meal and at bedtime. Alternating aluminum- and magnesium-containing antacids has been shown to decrease the incidence of diarrhea and constipation in some patients.
    (5) Sucralfate is a nonabsorbed sulfated disaccharide that acts locally to form a barrier for irritated mucosa in the esophagus, stomach, or duodenum. The recommended dose is 1 g/1.73 m^2, given a half hour before meals and at bedtime for 4 to 6 weeks.
    (6) Misoprostol is a synthetic prostaglandin E_1 analog; it decreases gastric acid production and increases mucus and bicarbonate secretion. It is indicated for the prevention of NSAID-induced gastric ulcers. Therapy with misoprostol should be continued for the duration of NSAID therapy.
    (7) Special diets have not been associated with ulcer development or healing; however, foods that directly cause symptoms of pain and discomfort should be avoided.
  b. Surgical therapy is very rarely indicated in children but is used under the following circumstances:
    (1) As an alternative for children with chronic ulcers, refractory to medical therapy
    (2) Children with pyloric obstruction

(3) Unremitting or recurrent hemorrhage, unresponsive to therapeutic endoscopy
(4) Perforation

17.3 Inflammatory Bowel Disease

EPIDEMIOLOGY, ETIOLOGY, AND PATHOGENESIS

1. Epidemiology: Ulcerative colitis and Crohn's disease, often grouped under inflammatory bowel disease (IBD), are chronic, spontaneously relapsing disorders of the GI tract. They are characterized by a set of clinical, endoscopic, and histologic characteristics. IBD is frequently diagnosed in children; 24% to 30% of all patients with Crohn's disease and about 20% with ulcerative colitis present before they are 20 years of age.

2. Etiology and pathogenesis: The initial causes and the precise immunomodulatory defects of IBD are not known. General opinion is that an initial inciting cause, possibly infectious, sets up a permanent, deranged immunologic response in persons who have a genetic susceptibility to responding in this fashion. The GI mucosal immune system seems to be central in this complex interplay of genetic susceptibility, environmental influences, diet, enteric flora, and specific infectious agents (e.g., virus, bacteria, toxin). This interplay promotes the chronic pathologic participation of plasma cells (via antibodies), T cells, macrophages (via cytokines and monokines), and polymorphonuclear leukocytes (production of reactive oxygen metabolites). The resultant immunoregulatory abnormalities lead to tissue destruction, chronic inflammation, and fibrosis of the area involved.

3. Differential diagnosis is given in Box 17-3.

CROHN'S DISEASE (REGIONAL ENTERITIS)

1. Definition: Crohn's disease is a chronic *transmural* and frequently *submucosal* inflammatory disease that can affect any part of the GI tract from mouth to anus; it most commonly involves the terminal ileum and colon.

2. Clinical manifestations depend on the areas of intestinal involvement and the severity of the disease process at the time of presentation.
   a. Weight loss and growth failure (insidious onset), due to either inadequate nutrient intake or chronic nutrient malabsorption
   b. Fever, usually low grade
   c. Abdominal discomfort, periumbilical or right lower quadrant abdominal pain
   d. Diarrhea: Frequently postprandial (small bowel and colonic Crohn's)
   e. Vomiting, anorexia, nausea, and epigastric distress (stomach and esophagus involvement)

3. Extraintestinal manifestations
   a. Arthritis, erythema nodosum, uveitis, aphthous ulcers
   b. When presenting with growth failure, rule out
      (1) Endocrine causes, growth hormone deficiency, pituitary dysfunction, and thyroid dysfunction
      (2) Malignancies: Intestinal lymphoma presents with weight loss, fever, or increased erythrocyte sedimentation rate.

Box 17-3   A General Differential Diagnosis of Inflammatory Bowel Disease

Abdominal Pain May Be Caused By

Lactose intolerance with cramps
Constipation
Acid-peptic disease
Psychosocial stress
Irritable bowel syndrome
Appendicitis
Biliary tract disease
Pancreatitis
Hepatitis
Peritonitis
Tumor
Urinary tract problems
Renal stones/renal disease
Henoch-Schönlein purpura
Pneumonia
Gastroenteritis
Intussusception
Volvulus
Sickling syndromes
Incarcerated hernia
Pelvic inflammatory disease

Diarrhea May Be Due To

Infectious etiology (bacterial, viral, parasitic)
Toddler's diarrhea
Lactose intolerance
Sucrase-isomaltase deficiency
VIPoma (vasoactive intestinal peptide–producing tumor)
Malabsorptive states
Ileal resection
Cystic fibrosis

Rectal Bleeding May Signify

Polyps
Meckel's diverticulum
Rectal fissure
Hemorrhoids
Hemolytic-uremic syndrome (increased levels of blood urea nitrogen and creatinine, evidence of hemolysis)
Arteriovenous malformation
Tumor
Brisk upper gastrointestinal bleed
Henoch-Schönlein purpura

(3) Perianal disease, renal calculi, and gallstones. Complications include adhesions, strictures, or intramural abscesses; free perforation, abscesses; fistulae from one organ to another, bowel to bowel, bowel to skin, or bowel to vagina/bladder; and perianal disease.

4. Diagnosis
   a. Complete history should include family history, growth pattern, appetite, and bowel habit.
   b. Physical findings may help establish the correct diagnosis (e.g., aphthous stomatitis, digital clubbing, abdominal mass, perianal skin tags, abscesses, fissures). Height and weight measurements, long-term growth curves, and anthropometrics should never be omitted.
   c. Laboratory evaluation is outlined in Box 17-4.
   d. Stool may be positive for leukocytes and show occult blood. Stool cultures should be consistently and repeatedly negative for bacteria and negative for ova and parasites. If positive, the infectious agent should be treated first.
   e. Plain abdominal radiographs may show colitis with or without evidence of intestinal obstruction or inflamed bowel.
   f. An upper GI series and small bowel follow-through may show fixed deformities, mucosal irregularity, nodularity, or thickened, separated loops of bowel.
   g. Colonoscopy with biopsy may show rectal sparing or terminal ileum/cecum involvement with evidence of crypt abscess formation and granulomata.
   h. A computed tomography (CT) scan should be done if abdominal abscess is suspected. Ultrasonography may also identify abscesses.

Box 17-4   Laboratory Evaluation of the Child with Inflammatory Bowel Disease

Laboratory Tests

Complete blood count and differential (anemia, leukocytosis, thrombocytosis), prothrombin time, sedimentation rate (elevated)
Urinalysis
Stool guaiac, cultures for bacteria; smears for ova, parasites and fat; assay for *Clostridium difficile* toxin
Serum total proteins, albumin (low), transferrin, immunoglobulins
Serum electrolytes, calcium, magnesium, phosphate, iron, zinc
Serum folate, vitamins A, E, D, B_{12}
Serum aspartate aminotransferase (AST) and alanine aminotransferase (ALT), alkaline phosphatase, bilirubin

Special Tests

Fecal α_1-antitrypsin
Lactose breath test
Colonoscopy with biopsies

5. Management
   a. Pharmacologic therapy (Table 17-1): Steroids are the mainstay for inducing remission, salicylate compounds for maintaining remission, and 6-mercaptopurine or azathioprine for maintaining remission in steroid-dependent patients.
   b. Correction of nutritional deficiencies
      (1) Correct existing electrolyte disorders, anemia, and vitamin deficiencies.
      (2) Total parenteral nutrition (TPN) with bowel rest may be necessary in severe cases. TPN also promotes growth.
      (3) The long-term use of elemental formula supplementation may be helpful in growth failure.
   c. Psychiatric or social work consultation may be helpful with assisting the patient and family in coping with this chronic disease. Teenagers may have compliance problems because of weight gain and other steroid side effects. Psychosocial assessment has a crucial role in children with IBD.
   d. Surgical therapy when needed is guided by the goal of saving as much bowel as possible; 70% of patients with Crohn's disease require surgery at some point during their life. Indications include the following:
      (1) Perforation
      (2) Obstruction
      (3) Extensive perianal or rectal disease unresponsive to other therapeutic modalities
      (4) Severe growth failure in which a localized segment may be removed and growth restored

ULCERATIVE COLITIS

1. Definition: Ulcerative colitis is confined to the colonic mucosa. The process involves the rectum, with proximal extension. Pancolitis is the most common form (62%), whereas less extensive disease localized to the left colon (22%) and rectum (15%) occurs less frequently.
2. Clinical manifestations may present as early as infancy, but prevalence increases around puberty, with a peak onset at 16 to 20 years of age.
   a. Diarrhea and lower abdominal cramping, which is intensified before and during defecation and relieved by the passage of stool and flatus
   b. Presence of bright red blood and mucus mixed with feces
   c. Increased urgency, frequency of stools
   d. Low-grade fevers
   e. Iron-deficiency anemia
   f. Tenesmus
   g. Note: Extraintestinal manifestations are found somewhat less frequently than in Crohn's disease, but overlap greatly with those seen in Crohn's disease.
3. Complications
   a. Toxic megacolon: This occurs in a small percentage of children with pancolitis and is usually precipitated by colonic distention (barium enema or extensive endoscopy), anticholinergic medication, or hypokalemia. The colonic diameter exceeds 6 cm. There is a greatly increased risk of sepsis, shock, and perforation.

Crohn's Disease

Acute Exacerbation

Methylprednisolone 1-2 mg/kg/day of prednisone-equivalent dose intravenously (IV) divided two to four times a day over 7-10 days. Once clinical improvement is achieved, therapy may be changed to oral prednisone at the same dose divided twice a day. Taper to 1 mg/kg/day, daily, and then to every other day over 4-6 wk depending on clinical response. When remission is achieved, taper and discontinue.

Remission

Olsalazine 30-40 mg/kg/day orally divided twice a day (250-mg tablets)

Folate supplement 1 mg every day

Mesalamine 250- or 400-mg tablets; approximately 50 mg/kg divided two or three times a day

Perianal Disease or Fistula

Metronidazole 15 mg/kg/day divided every 8 hours (1 g maximum)

Refractory Disease

Azathioprine 1-2 mg/kg/day divided twice a day

or

6-Mercaptopurine 1.5 mg/kg/day divided twice a day

or

Methotrexate 10 mg/m², weekly, PO, SC

or

Infliximab 5-10 mg/kg week 0, 2, 6 and as needed

Ulcerative Colitis

Severe to Moderate Colitis

Methylprednisolone 1-2 mg/kg/day of prednisone-equivalent dose IV divided two to four times a day over 7-10 days. Once clinical improvement is achieved, therapy may be changed to oral prednisone at the same dose divided twice a day. Taper to 1-2 mg/kg/day, daily, and then to every other day over ≤6 wk depending on clinical response. When remission is achieved, taper and discontinue.

Mild or Localized Distal Colitis

Olsalazine 30-40 mg/kg/day divided twice a day

Folate 1 mg every day

Hydrocortisone enemas

Mesalamine 250- or 400-mg tablets; approximately 50 mg/kg/day divided two or three times a day

Mesalamine enemas or rectal suppositories

Refractory Disease

Azathioprine 2 mg/kg/day

6-Mercaptopurine 1.5 mg/kg/day divided twice a day

Cyclosporine continuous IV infusion started as a dose of 1-2 mg/kg/day and then switched to the oral form at 4-8 mg/kg/day

or

FK506 (tacrolimus)—clinical trials have proved beneficial

Folate 1 mg daily if on sulfasalazine

Note: Fulminant colitis may require up to 3 mg/kg/day of methylprednisolone or prednisone or Methotrexate or Infliximab

   b. Colonic carcinoma: The cumulative risk has been shown to be as high as 20% per decade after 10 years of disease process in children diagnosed with pancolitis before the age of 10 years and a cumulative risk of about 0.5% to 1% per year with later onset disease, mandating constant, lifelong awareness and surveillance.
   c. Sclerosing cholangitis involving the biliary tree
4. Laboratory findings
   a. Laboratory evaluation is described in Box 17-3.
   b. Fecal blood and leukocytes
   c. Stool cultures (including *Salmonella, Shigella, Campylobacter, Yersinia, Aeromonas hydrophilia, Clostridium difficile, Entameba histolytica,* and *Escherichia coli* 0157-H7) should be negative.
   d. Plain abdominal/pelvic radiograph may indicate perforation or toxic megacolon.
   e. Sigmoidoscopy/colonoscopy reveals uniform confluent colitis, confirmed by biopsies that may show goblet cell depletion, cryptitis, crypt abscesses, and derangements of mucosal architecture, without submucosal involvement or granulomata.
   f. A barium enema, preferably double contrast, may show a pattern of spiculation, mucosal irregularities, ulceration, pseudopolyp, and loss of haustrations.
   g. An upper GI series and small bowel follow-through are conducted to exclude any evidence of small-bowel disease.
   h. The key radiographic and endoscopic differences between Crohn's disease and ulcerative colitis are shown in Boxes 17-5 and 17-6, respectively.
5. Management

Box 17-5   Radiographic Differences between Crohn's Disease and Ulcerative Colitis

Crohn's Disease

Deep ulcerations (often longitudinal and transverse)
Segmental lesions (skip lesions)
Strictures
Fistulae
Cobblestone appearance of mucosa (caused by submucosal inflammation)
"Thumbprinting" common

Ulcerative Colitis

Fine, superficial ulceration
Continuous involvement (including rectum)
Shortening of the bowel
Symmetric bowel contour
Decreased mucosal pattern
Pseudopolyp

Modified from Feldman S: Gastroenterology. In Ferri F (ed): Practical Guide to the Care of the Medical Patient, 3rd ed. St. Louis, Mosby, 1955.

> ### Box 17-6 Endoscopic Features of Crohn's Disease and Ulcerative Colitis
>
> #### Crohn's Disease
>
> Asymmetric and discontinuous process
> Deep, longitudinal fissures
> Cobblestone appearance
> Mucosal edema
> Mucosal friability not usually present
> Strictures
>
> #### Ulcerative Colitis
>
> Uniform involvement beginning at anorectal junction; very friable mucosa
> Diffuse, uniform erythema replacing the usual mucosal vascular pattern
> Rectal involvement invariably present if disease is active
> Pseudopolyps in advanced active disease

Modified from Feldman S: Gastroenterology. In Ferri F (ed): Practical Guide to the Care of the Medical Patient, 3rd ed. St. Louis, Mosby, 1955.

a. Pharmacologic therapy: See Table 17-1.
b. Nutritional support: Parenteral nutrition does not seem to be effective in inducing disease remission in ulcerative colitis (40%) compared with Crohn's disease (70%).
c. Counseling for the patient and family helps with adjustment to the disease and medications.
d. Surgical therapy: Proctocolectomy is curative in ulcerative colitis. Pull-through surgical procedures can restore "normal" anatomy, without necessitating a permanent ileostomy. If surgery is avoided, long-term monitoring of ulcerative colitis is essential to prevent adenocarcinoma of the colon. Usual indications for surgery are as follows:
   (1) Toxic megacolon and systemic toxicity
   (2) Perforation
   (3) Uncontrollable bleeding
   (4) Growth failure
   (5) Steroid dependency
   (6) Medical intractability

17.4 Diarrhea

The chief complaint of diarrhea can mean either loose stools or increased frequency of bowel movements. Diarrhea can be divided into acute or chronic symptoms. Acute diarrhea is of 2 weeks' duration or less.

ACUTE DIARRHEA

See Chapter 19 (Infectious Diseases), Section 19.10.

CHRONIC DIARRHEA

1. Definition: Diarrhea lasting over 4 weeks is chronic. It can harm through malnutrition or blood loss, but often is due to functional or annoying causes that, although a problem, are not a danger to the patient.
2. Etiology
   a. Major causes of chronic diarrhea are listed in Box 17-7.
   b. Many causes overlap; for example, although Crohn's disease is an inflammatory disease, it can cause malabsorption, and celiac sprue results from inflammation of the mucosa, but is typically thought of as a malabsorptive illness.

Box 17-7   Major Causes of Chronic Diarrhea

In Infants

Intractable diarrhea of infancy/postinfectious diarrhea
Cow's milk and soy protein intolerance
Protracted infectious enteritis
Microvillus inclusion disease
Immune enteropathy–celiac disease
Hirschsprung's disease
Congenital transport defects
Short bowel syndrome
Nutrient malabsorption
Munchausen's syndrome by proxy

In Toddlers

Toddler's diarrhea
Congenital sucrose sucrose-isomaltase deficiency
Pancreatic insufficiency (cystic fibrosis, Shwachman-Diamond syndrome)
Chronic nonspecific diarrhea (excessive simple sugar intake)
Protracted viral enteritis
Giardiasis
Tumors (secretory diarrhea; e.g., neuroblastoma, VIPoma)
Celiac disease
Ulcerative colitis and Crohn's disease
Eosinophilic gastroenteritis
Immunodeficiency

In School-Aged Children

Inflammatory bowel disease
Appendiceal abscess
Primary lactase deficiency
Constipation with encopresis
Irritable bowel syndrome
Laxative abuse
Giardiasis

---

    c. The more common causes are annoying but not life-threatening, such as toddler's diarrhea, irritable bowel syndrome, excess fruit juice intake, or lactose intolerance.

    d. Different causes are more common in different age groups.

       (1) IBD is more common in the preteen or teen.

       (2) Celiac sprue more often presents in toddlers, but can arise at any age after wheat gluten has been introduced into the diet.

       (3) Congenital sucrase-isomaltase deficiency will not be demonstrated until sucrose is introduced into the diet.

3. Evaluation and management (Fig. 17-1)

    a. Laboratory evaluation is outlined in Box 17-8.

    b. If a child has profuse, watery diarrhea, especially if the child is experiencing electrolyte problems or dehydration, a trial of bowel rest with no food or drink while intravenous (IV) fluid is supporting the patient may be helpful in determining the cause of the diarrhea. If the diarrhea stops when the child is NPO, it is an osmotic diarrhea, and once this is determined, you can evaluate the diet for the source of the osmotic substance.

    c. If bowel rest does not stop the diarrhea, you have to look for causes of secretory diarrhea or inflammatory diarrhea, or for Munchausen's syndrome by proxy.

    d. An easy way to think of therapy for chronic diarrhea is to treat inflammation and correct malabsorption. Chronic diarrhea puts the child at risk for malnutrition either through nutrient and blood loss secondary to inflammation or through poor absorption of needed calories, fats, protein, and minerals. Monitoring growth provides an important measurement of therapeutic success. In addition, depending on the cause, one needs to follow hemoglobin, iron, fat-soluble vitamins, essential fatty acids, and serum albumin.

    e. Cow-soy protein allergy

       (1) Discontinue cow's milk protein formula or, if breast-feeding, remove milk products from the mother's diet. The mother should receive nutritional counseling to ensure she receives adequate calcium and protein without cow's milk.

       (2) Because there is a good chance that a child allergic to cow's milk will also be allergic to soy protein, use a protein hydrolysate formula such as Alimentum or Nutramigen.

       (3) If no improvement with a protein hydrolysate formula, try a single–amino acid protein source formula such as Neocate or Elecare.

       (4) Reintroduce cow's milk protein between 1 and 2 years of age. This should usually be done in the clinic (or if the reaction was anaphylaxis rather than diarrhea, then in the hospital with an IV line in place). Often, some well-meaning relative will have challenged the child in an uncontrolled manner with ice cream, yogurt, or other milk products, and this will give you a good idea of the likelihood of a nonreactive challenge.

    f. IBD: See Section 17.3.

    g. Pancreatic insufficiency

       (1) Pancreatic enzyme replacement

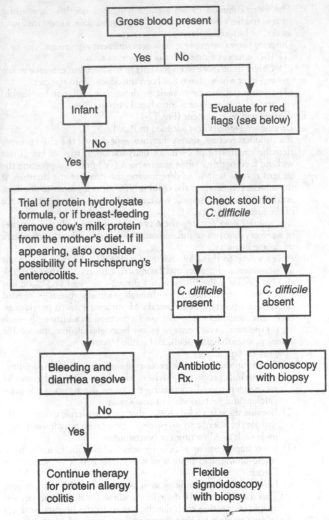

Figure 17-1 Evaluation of chronic diarrhea.

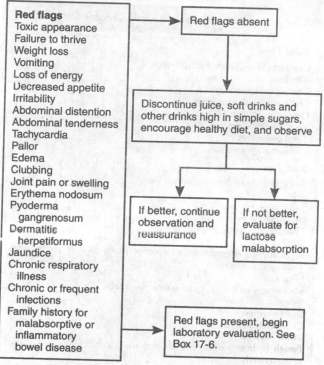

Red flags
Toxic appearance
Failure to thrive
Weight loss
Vomiting
Loss of energy
Decreased appetite
Irritability
Abdominal distention
Abdominal tenderness
Tachycardia
Pallor
Edema
Clubbing
Joint pain or swelling
Erythema nodosum
Pyoderma
  gangrenosum
Dermatitis
  herpetiformis
Jaundice
Chronic respiratory
  illness
Chronic or frequent
  infections
Family history for
  malabsorptive or
  inflammatory
  bowel disease

Red flags absent

Discontinue juice, soft drinks and other drinks high in simple sugars, encourage healthy diet, and observe

If better, continue observation and reassurance

If not better, evaluate for lactose malabsorption

Red flags present, begin laboratory evaluation. See Box 17-6.

Figure 17-1, cont'd

    (2) Fat-soluble vitamin supplementation: A, D, E, K
    (3) Trial of predigested formula, or formula with a high percentage of fat as medium-chain triglycerides
    (4) Tube feedings, especially nighttime supplementation
    (5) Involvement of a center for cystic fibrosis
  h. Lactase deficiency
    (1) Lactase enzyme supplements (LactAid)
    (2) Lactose-free milk
    (3) Lactose-free diet. Calcium supplements may be needed.
  i. Sucrase-isomaltase deficiency: Sucraid (sacrosidase), and avoid sucrose
  j. Celiac sprue
    (1) Gluten-free diet (lifelong)
    (2) Avoid products containing gluten that at first glance might seem harmless. Examples include vinegar, hydrogenated vegetable protein, malt, and caramel coloring.

Box 17-8   Laboratory Evaluation of Chronic Diarrhea

Blood Tests

Complete blood count with differential
Albumen
Test for inflammation
Erythrocyte sedimentation rate
C-reactive protein
Tests for celiac sprue
Total serum IgA
Tissue transglutaminase

Stool Tests

Tests for carbohydrate malabsorption
pH
Reducing substances
Nonreducing substances
Tests for pancreatic insufficiency
Fecal elastase
Fecal fat 72-hour quantitative collection preferred over spot fecal fat
Tests for inflammation
Hemoccult
Microscopic examination for white blood cells
Tests for infection
Giardia antigen
Clostridium difficile toxin
Sweat chloride
Breath hydrogen tests for carbohydrate malabsorption or bacterial overgrowth

---

  k. Short bowel syndrome: Therapy depends on both the measured length and the functional length remaining, and includes TPN, continuous drip feedings, and vitamin B_{12} injections.
  l. Toddler's diarrhea: Remove simple sugars from the diet, encourage a normal diet, and monitor growth and weight gain.

17.5 Celiac Disease

1. Etiology/epidemiology: Celiac disease (CD) is a permanent (lifelong) sensitivity to gluten in wheat and related proteins found in barley and rye and is an immune-mediated enteropathy. CD occurs in about 1 in 100 to 1 in 200 of the general population.
2. Clinical manifestations
   a. GI symptoms predominate, typically beginning between 6 months and 2 years of age, after the introduction of gluten into the diet. Onset is usually insidious and characterized by diarrhea or even frank

steatorrhea accompanied by poor weight gain or weight loss, progressive abdominal distention, and muscle wasting, typically involving the buttocks and proximal limb muscles. The child becomes anorexic, fussy, and listless.

   b. Non-GI symptoms (50%) may include short stature, delayed puberty, megaloblastic anemia due to malabsorption of vitamin B, and folate, osteopenia (calcium and vitamin D deficiency), and stomatitis/glossitis (vitamin A deficiency).

   c. A number of autoimmune and nonautoimmune conditions are strongly associated with CD. These include type 1 diabetes (4% to 8% of patients with insulin-dependent diabetes also have CD), Down syndrome (12% of patients also have CD), Turner's syndrome, and Williams' syndrome. Selective IgA deficiency is strongly associated with CD (1:50).

3. Diagnosis: Early diagnosis and treatment of CD is important because untreated CD is associated with a greater risk of malignancy—in particular, small intestine lymphoma in adults.

   a. Pretreatment: Biopsy of the small intestine for histologic examination remains the best way to make a definitive diagnosis.

   b. The endomysial antibody (EMA) and tissue transglutaminase (TTG) tests are two serologic test choices, each with a sensitivity and a specificity that generally exceed 95%. Note that an EMA or TTG test result in the IgA-deficient patient may be falsely negative, so obtain IgA levels at the same time as testing for CD.

4. Management

   a. The only treatment for CD is a strict gluten-free diet for life (i.e., a diet that excludes all products that contain proteins derived from wheat, rye, and barley).

   b. Safe alternative sources of starch includes rice, corn, potato, amaranth, legumes, quinoa, and soy.

   c. If the serologic test was positive before diagnosis, repeat the test after 6 months for monitoring purposes. If the child has remained strictly gluten free, the test result is usually negative by 6 months after the start of treatment.

17.6 Acute Pancreatitis

1. Definition: *Acute pancreatitis* is defined as a single attack or discrete but recurrent attacks of abdominal pain, usually severe, often with vomiting, associated with elevated pancreatic enzyme levels in the blood. There is acute focal or diffuse swelling of the pancreas. Resolution of all aspects follows the acute attack. Recurrent attacks of acute pancreatitis may ultimately give rise to chronic pancreatitis.

2. Etiology: The causes of acute pancreatitis are listed in Box 17-9. Most cases of acute pancreatitis in childhood result from viral infection or are idiopathic.

3. Pathogenesis: The pathogenesis of acute pancreatitis is unknown. One view is that an unchecked activation of enzymes in the pancreas leads to local parenchymal destruction, inflammation, and extrapancreatic tissue injury. The extent of destruction is limited by the body's own

Box 17-9   Causes of Acute Pancreatitis

Obstruction/Anatomic

Choledocholithiasis
Tumor
Worms or foreign bodies
Pancreas divisum with accessory duct obstruction
Anomalous union of the pancreaticobiliary ducts
Choledochal cyst
Periampullary duodenal diverticula
Hypertensive sphincter of Oddi

Toxins

Ethyl alcohol
Methyl alcohol
Scorpion venom
Organophosphate insecticides

Metabolic Abnormalities

Hypertriglyceridemia
Hypercalcemia
Organic acidemia
Refeeding syndrome
Malnutrition: juvenile tropical pancreatitis

Infection

Parasitic: ascariasis, clonorchiasis, malaria
Viral: mumps; rubella; hepatitis A, B, C; coxsackievirus B; echovirus;
    adenovirus; cytomegalovirus; varicella; Epstein-Barr virus; human
    immunodeficiency virus
Bacterial: mycoplasmas, *Campylobacter jejuni, Mycobacterium tuber-
    culosis, Mycobacterium avium-intracellulare* complex, legionella,
    leptospirosis

Vascular Abnormalities

Vasculitis: hemolytic-uremic syndrome, Henoch-Schönlein purpura,
    Kawasaki's disease, systemic lupus erythematosus, polyarteritis
    nodosa, malignant hypertension

Miscellaneous Abnormalities

Penetrating peptic ulcer
Crohn's disease
Reye's syndrome
Familial pancreatitis

Idiopathic

Adapted from Steinberg W, Tenner S: Acute pancreatitis. N Engl J Med 330:
1198-1210, 1994.

protective mechanisms to counteract the activation of various enzymes.

4. Clinical manifestations
   a. Abdominal pain is the clinical hallmark of acute pancreatitis. The pain is often epigastric or diffuse and not relieved by a change in body position. It may radiate to the back.
   b. Nausea and vomiting are commonly present and may be associated with intestinal ileus.
   c. Physical findings include a distressed patient with a tender and often distended abdomen (due to pancreatic swelling, ascites, or dilated bowel with ileus).
   d. Signs of peritoneal irritation may be evident.
   e. Signs of hemorrhagic necrosis
      (1) A bluish discoloration of the flanks (Grey Turner's sign)
      (2) A bluish discoloration of the umbilicus (Cullen's sign)
   f. Fever, tachycardia, dyspnea, and hypotension due to hypovolemia, infection, pleural effusion, and acute respiratory distress syndrome are possible.
   g. Confusion and mental status changes with multisystem involvement may occur. An acute attack of pancreatitis without complications and without multisystem disease usually resolves within a week, and mortality is rare in children with this disease.

5. Complications
   a. Shock
   b. Coagulopathy
   c. Renal and respiratory insufficiency
   d. Encephalopathy
   e. Pancreatic necrosis and pseudocyst formation
   f. Abscess

6. Diagnosis
   a. Serum pancreatic amylase and lipase: These are specific pancreatic enzymes—the turnover of amylase may be more rapid and may normalize before lipase.
   b. Complete blood count (CBC) may show leukocytosis and anemia.
   c. Glucose and electrolytes may be abnormal; acidosis may be present.
   d. Serum calcium and albumin must be checked.
   e. Liver aminotransferases and bilirubin may be elevated, with hepatic and biliary system involvement.
   f. Serum triglyceride level should be checked to rule out triglyceridemia.
   g. A sweat chloride test may be done to rule out cystic fibrosis.
   h. Blood and urine screens for possible drug/toxin ingestion may be performed when suspected.
   i. Abdominal ultrasonography is the most useful noninvasive imaging modality. It is useful to:
      (1) Examine the parenchyma and duct of pancreas
      (2) Look at other organs for cause (e.g., cholelithiasis)
      (3) Look for complications (e.g., ascites, pseudocyst)
   j. A CT scan can provide greater cross-sectional anatomic detail, and, unlike ultrasonography, it is not limited by interference of bowel gas.

k. Endoscopic retrograde cholangiopancreatography offers the best anatomic detail of the pancreatic and biliary ducts. It has both diagnostic and therapeutic benefits, especially in stone removal.

7. Management
   a. The treatment of acute pancreatitis is guided by two principles:
      (1) Reduce or eliminate factors contributing to the disease.
      (2) Provide good supportive care to the patient.
   b. Discontinue all unnecessary drugs.
   c. Perform early endoscopic therapy in selected cases for obstructing lesions like common bile duct stone or ascariasis.
   d. Correct electrolyte abnormalities, hypoalbuminemia, and hypovolemia.
   e. Use transfusion for severe anemia.
   f. Stop enteral feeding to reduce stimulation of the pancreas.
   g. Initiate TPN early on during the illness to avoid superimposed nutritional deficiencies.
   h. Nasogastric suction may be necessary for frequent incessant vomiting.
   i. Analgesics or narcotics may be required.
   j. Somatostatin/octreotide has been used in trials. It reduces pancreatic activity.
   k. Consider peritoneal lavage in severe pancreatitis.
   l. Surgical debridement may be required in some cases.

17.7 Acute Viral Hepatitis

BACKGROUND

1. Primary acute viral infection of the liver is most commonly caused by five distinct viruses: Hepatitis A, B, C, D, and E. The five viruses cause similar acute clinical illnesses:
   a. Hepatitis A virus (HAV), an RNA enterovirus, causes 30% of hepatitis in the United States.
   b. Hepatitis B virus (HBV), a DNA virus, causes 50% of hepatitis in the United States.
   c. Hepatitis C virus (HCV), an RNA virus, causes 20% of hepatitis in the United States.
   d. Hepatitis D virus (HDV, type D, delta), a defective virus consisting of RNA nucleoprotein, is found only in association with HBV infection.
   e. Hepatitis E virus (HEV, type E) is a picornavirus similar to HAV, an RNA virus.
2. Other viruses reported in association with hepatitis (as part of a generalized illness) in children include cytomegalovirus, herpes virus, varicella-zoster virus, Epstein-Barr virus, rubella, coxsackievirus, and adenovirus.

HEPATITIS A VIRUS

1. Epidemiology: HAV infection has worldwide distribution. Its seroprevalence is close to 100% in underdeveloped countries; somewhat lower frequencies are found in developed countries.
   a. Transmission
      (1) Fecal-oral (household, intimate contacts, institutional contacts)
      (2) Common source of transmission by contaminated food, water, shellfish

    (3) Nosocomial transmission

    (4) Parenteral transmission—uncommon

  b. Source

    (1) No known carrier state

    (2) Maintenance through person-to-person spread

  c. High-risk exposure

    (1) Low socioeconomic status

    (2) Endemic areas throughout the world

    (3) Attack rates are known to be highest among children of primary and nursery school age (day care centers, institutionalized children).

  d. Incubation period of 2 to 6 weeks

2. Clinical manifestations

  a. The typical course of HAV infection is shown in Figure 17-2.

  b. Symptoms

    (1) In 90% to 95% of children younger than 5 years of age, cases are asymptomatic.

    (2) An abrupt onset of nonspecific features occurs, such as fever, headache, anorexia, nausea, right upper quadrant abdominal pain, and jaundice; leukopenia, hepatomegaly, and splenomegaly are common.

    (3) Illness is usually self-limited.

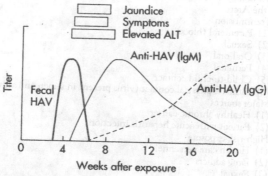

Figure 17-2 Hepatitis A sequence of events. After exposure there is a brief period of viremia, which occurs during the incubation phase (2 to 6 weeks). The period of fecal hepatitis A virus (HAV) excretion overlaps this prodromal phase and continues into the early part of the symptomatic phase. Frank jaundice may occur up to 6 weeks after exposure but is not present in all cases, especially young children. The alanine aminotransferase (ALT) elevation also precedes the development of clinical symptoms; ALT usually remains abnormal even after serum bilirubin returns to normal. Anti-HAV becomes detectable early in the acute symptomatic phase of the illness; the initial response is anti-HAV (immunoglobulin M [IgM]), which peaks shortly after the onset of symptoms and progressively declines. This is succeeded by a gradual rise in anti-HAV (IgG), which peaks after the symptomatic phase and remains detectable indefinitely. (Modified from Balistreri WF: Viral hepatitis. Emerg Med Clin North Am 9:365-399, 1991.)

3. Diagnosis: Clinical suspicion plus serologic markers form the diagnosis. Also, IgM antibody to HAV begins to rise at the time symptoms appear and continues to persist for about 4 months, and then IgG antibody develops, which tends to persist for many years.
4. Complications: Rare cases of fulminant hepatitis have been reported. There is no known chronic form of the disease, but it may take a prolonged, relapsing course.
5. Management
   a. Acute illness
      (1) Bed rest as needed for early symptomatic stage, then as tolerated; general symptomatic treatment with hydration
      (2) Intensive supportive care may be required for rare cases of fulminant hepatitis; consider liver transplantation.
   b. Prevention
      (1) Measures for proper hygiene and isolation procedures
      (2) Passive immunization with immunoglobulin should be given before exposure or during the incubation period of hepatitis A.
      (3) Active immunization: Vaccine against HAV is currently available. Indications include high-risk groups, such as day care center clientele, military personnel, travelers, and institutionalized children.

HEPATITIS B VIRUS

1. Epidemiology: It is highly endemic in Africa, Asia, the Pacific Islands, and the Arctic.
   a. Transmission
      (1) Parenteral (blood)
      (2) Sexual
      (3) Oral-oral
      (4) Perinatal
      (5) Child-to-child contact
      (6) Intimate physical contact (virus present in semen and saliva)
   b. Major sources
      (1) Healthy chronic carrier
      (2) Patient with acute hepatitis infection
   c. High-risk exposure
      (1) Health care personnel
      (2) Drug addicts
      (3) Sexual
      (4) Perinatal
      (5) Renal hemodialysis
      (6) Clinical laboratory personnel
      (7) Institutionalized persons
   d. Incubation period of 2 to 6 months
2. Clinical features
   a. The typical course of HBV infection is shown in Figure 17-3.
   b. Symptoms
      (1) Symptoms range from clinically asymptomatic to fulminant hepatitis.
      (2) With icteric HBV, the onset is more insidious and the course more prolonged than with HAV infection.

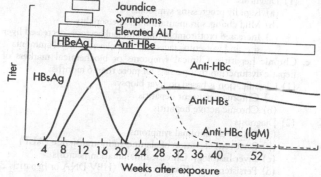

Figure 17-3 Typical course of acute hepatitis B virus (HBV) infection. The earliest detectable serum maker of HBV infection after exposure is a rise in HBsAg (hepatitis B surface antigen), which may appear from 1 to 10 weeks after exposure; HBeAg (hepatitis B e antigen) and HBV-DNA follow closely. HBsAg is detectable 2 to 8 weeks before the symptomatic phase, during which alanine aminotransferase (ALT) levels and serum bilirubin concentration rise, and constitutional signs appear. Clearance of HBsAg, which is neutralized by anti-HBs (antisurface antibody), occurs by 6 to 8 months; those who fail to clear are termed *HBsAg carriers*. Anti-HBc (anticore antibody), which appears just before the symptomatic phase, is the first host-induced immunologic response to hepatitis B infection. Anti-HBc may be the only marker of HBV after clearance of HBsAg but before the rise in anti-HBs. (Modified from Balistreri WF: Viral hepatitis. Emerg Med Clin North Am 9:365-399, 1991.)

    (3) Atypical features include a serum-sickness–like illness, membranous nephropathy, and Gianotti-Crosti syndrome, a papular rash associated with nonicteric hepatitis.

3. Diagnosis is based on suggestive clinical features plus either or both of these serologic markers:
    a. HBsAg (hepatitis B surface antigen)
    b. IgM antibody to core antigen
    c. Like other acute hepatitides, the clinical picture alone is not sufficient for diagnosis.

4. Clinical sequelae/complications
    a. Hepatitis B carrier state: A persistent infection without clinical evidence of disease. The risk of carrier state is highest in neonates. There is an inverse relationship between the age at which HBV infection is acquired and the chances of becoming a chronic carrier. Only 3% of patients with a prior history of hepatitis B infection go on to develop chronic carrier state.
    b. Fulminant hepatitis (1% to 5%): Rapid progression to coma occurs after the onset of hepatitis in some patients; in others, it is insidious over a week to 10 days. Fulminant hepatitis has a 60% to 90% mortality rate.

(1) Diagnosis
  (a) Rapidly progressing symptoms
  (b) Mild changes in mentation and personality
  (c) Increased prothrombin time and leukocytosis, decreased liver size, and worsening jaundice, with elevated blood ammonia
c. Chronic hepatitis: Clinical symptoms or biochemical markers of hepatic dysfunction that persists for more than 6 months
  (1) Classification is based on liver biopsy.
    (a) Chronic persistent hepatitis
    (b) Chronic active hepatitis
  (2) Diagnosis
    (a) Relatively minimal symptoms
    (b) Persistent elevation of alanine aminotransferase (ALT)
    (c) Liver histology: Chronic inflammation/necrosis
    (d) Persistence of HBsAg and HBV (HBV DNA or hepatitis B e antigen [HBeAg]) in serum
d. Cirrhosis of the liver
e. Hepatocellular carcinoma: More than 80% of cases of hepatocellular carcinoma can be associated with HBV infection. It occurs several years after the acquisition of HBV infection.

5. Management
  a. Acute illness
    (1) Symptomatic therapy for hydration, fever, vomiting, weakness, and nutrition
    (2) Hospitalization with intensive supportive care for fulminant hepatitis or if the patient has coagulopathy and protracted vomiting. Treatment modalities include low-protein diet, TPN, lactulose, management of electrolyte imbalance, and coma. Plasmapheresis has been attempted on occasion, as well as liver transplantation (see later).
  b. Prevention
    (1) Passive immunization: Hepatitis B immune globulin (HBIG) and HBV vaccine should be administered as soon as possible after exposure (Table 17-2).
    (2) Universal administration of hepatitis B vaccine to infants at 0 to 2 days, 1 to 2 months, and 6 to 8 months of age and to selected high-risk groups (Table 17-3).
    (3) Universal screening of pregnant women should be undertaken.
  c. Treatment of chronic hepatitis
    (1) Interferon alpha has been shown to have limited efficacy in resolving the chronic infection, but it has been less effective for chronic infections acquired during infancy and early childhood. There are no definitive recommendations because of a lack of proven long-term effects and the high cost of the treatment. Negative prognostic parameters for success with interferon include high HBV DNA level, serum aminotransferase levels less than 2.5 times normal, and infection acquired at an early age.
    (2) Lamivudine may be of benefit to patients with interferon resistance and chronic hepatitis.

Table 17-2 Hepatitis B Postexposure Prophylaxis

Groups at Risk	Treatment
Neonate of HBsAg-positive mother	HBIG + HBV vaccine*
Contact with acute hepatitis B	
Intimate	HBIG + HBV vaccine
Household (no blood exposure)	None
Casual	None
Infants (<12 mo with acute case in primary care)	HBIG + HBV vaccine
Household with identifiable blood exposure	HBIG + HBV vaccine
Contact with chronic hepatitis B	
Intimate	HBV vaccine
Household	HBV vaccine
Casual	None
HBsAg-positive needle-stick to Q HBsAg-negative person	HBIG + HBV vaccine

*Dose is 0.5 mL HBIG within 12 hr of birth; 0.5 mL HBV vaccine within first week of birth and at 1 and 6 mo.
HBIG, hepatitis B immune globulin; HBsAg, hepatitis B surface antigen; HBV, hepatitis B virus.
Modified from Snyder J: Expanding alphabet of viral hepatitis. Semin Pediatr Gastroenterol Nutr 2(2):4-8, 1991.

(3) Liver transplantation: HBsAg persists after solid organ transplantation in almost all patients who are infected with HBV. In the post-transplantation liver, hepatitis and graft failure are caused in most cases by recurrent HBV infection. Treatment with interferon before liver transplantation has been shown to

Table 17-3 Recommendation for the Administration of Hepatitis B Virus Vaccines

Population	Recombivax HB (mL)	Energix-B (mL)
Infants of HBsAg-negative mothers and children <11 yr	0.25	0.50
Infants of HBsAg-positive mothers (should receive HBIG 0.5 mL within 12 hr of birth)	0.5	0.5
Children 11–19 yr	0.5	1
Adults	1	1
Patients on dialysis or immunosuppression	1	2

From Romero R, Lavine JE: Viral hepatitis in children. Semin Liver Dis 14:289-302, 1994.

improve the outcome by delaying the recurrence of infection in the graft.
(4) Clinical sequelae of hepatitis B infection are similar to those of delta hepatitis (Fig. 17-4).

HEPATITIS C VIRUS

1. Epidemiology: HCV is responsible for causing up to 90% of the non-A, non-B hepatitis in the United States. Three important risk factors for non-A, non-B hepatitis in the United States are use of IV drugs (40%), transfusions (10%), and occupational and sexual exposures (10%). Approximately 40% of cases of non-A, non-B hepatitis have not been associated with any risk factor. The pediatric HCV population includes the following:
   a. Patients with hemophilia or thalassemia, other post-transfusion patients
   b. Childhood cancer survivors
   c. Patients with a liver transplant
   d. Patients on dialysis
   e. IV drug exposures
   f. Sexual exposures
   g. Perinatal exposure (less common than earlier thought, but possible)

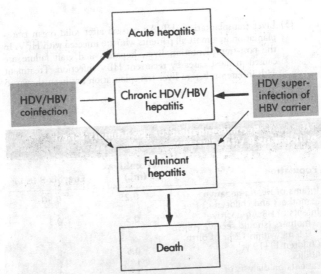

Figure 17-4 The clinical sequelae of hepatitis D virus (HDV) and hepatitis B virus (HBV) infection. (From Balistreri WF: Viral hepatitis. Emerg Med Clin North Am 9:365-399, 1991.)

2. Clinical manifestations and course
   a. The typical sequence of events in acute post-transfusion HCV infection is shown in Figure 17-5.
   b. Symptoms
      (1) Mostly asymptomatic; presents with abnormal aminotransferases on routine blood screening; may present as a typical viral hepatitis
      (2) May present as hepatic failure and cirrhosis
      (3) May present with hepatocellular carcinoma
      (4) May present as fulminant hepatitis
3. Diagnosis is based on clinical suspicion plus serologic markers.
   a. Anti-HCV (IgG): There is a delay of 1 to 6 months between the onset of acute infection and the appearance of the antibody; therefore, anti-HCV is not useful for early diagnosis.
   b. "Second-generation" assays for hepatitis C:
      (1) Enzyme-linked immunosorbent assay
      (2) Radioimmunoblot assay
      (3) Direct detection of HCV RNA by polymerase chain reaction
   c. Fluctuating pattern of serum aminotransferase levels
4. Clinical sequelae/complications
   a. Half of infected patients go on to develop chronic hepatitis (compared with about 10% of patients with HBV infection); 10% go on to develop cirrhosis of the liver.
   b. A small portion of patients with HBsAg-negative hepatocellular carcinoma are anti-HCV–positive.
5. Management: Currently there are no effective preventive measures for HCV infection. Immunoglobulin has no proven benefit, and there is no vaccine. Interferon alpha may be of some benefit in children, but relapse is very frequent. Approximately 15% of patients develop HCV infection after orthotopic liver transplantation, and a significant number of those previously infected with HCV will reinfect the graft. Ribavirin also can be used, especially in cases without spontaneous resolution of hepatitis within 2 and 4 months of onset.

DELTA HEPATITIS

1. Epidemiology: HDV is an infectious particle that can cause infection only in the presence of active HBV infection (coinfection with acute HBV, or superinfection in HBsAg carrier).
2. Clinical manifestations
   a. HBV/HDV coinfection, which would be serologically identical to HBV acute infection (antigens and antibodies in hepatitis B) with presence of HDV Ag and anti-HDV (IgM; see Fig. 17-4)
3. Management is identical to that of HBV infection.
4. Clinical sequelae of delta hepatitis and hepatitis B are similar.

HEPATITIS E VIRUS

1. One percent of non-A, non-B hepatitis in the United States is caused by HEV.
2. Epidemiology: Predominantly a fecal or water-borne infection present in developing countries, especially in areas with inadequate public sanitation, malnutrition, and extensive flooding. Hepatitis E is endemic to Southeast Asia and the Indian subcontinent.

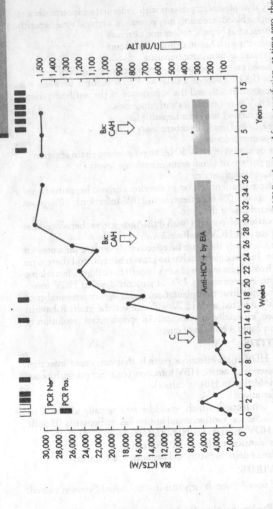

Figure 17-5 Typical sequence of events in acute post-transfusion hepatitis C virus (HCV) infection. After a transfusion, at time zero, there is a slow, progressive rise in the alanine aminotransferase (ALT) level (gray area; upper limit of normal, 44 IU/L), indicating the onset of hepatitis at week 9. The solid circles indicate the appearance and duration of antibody to HCV (anti-HCV) as measured by radioimmunoassay (RIA; in counts per minute). The bar indicates the appearance and duration of anti-HCV as measured by enzyme immunoassay (EIA). Polymerase chain reactivity (PCR) was noted 2 weeks after exposure and 9 weeks before the first appearance of anti-HCV. C, infectivity established by chimp inoculation; Bx, liver biopsy; CAH, chronic active hepatitis. (Data from Alter JH, Purcell RK‡, Shih JW, et al: Detection of antibody to hepatitis C virus in prospectively followed transfusion recipients with acute and chronic non-A, non-B hepatitis. N Engl J Med 321:1494-1500, 1989.)

3. Clinical manifestations and pathologic features of hepatitis E are remarkably similar to those of hepatitis A; however, the incubation period is longer (6 weeks). The attack rates for HEV infections are highest in adolescents and young adults. The mortality rate is higher than in HAV and much higher in pregnant women with fulminant hepatitis. There does not appear to be a chronic form of hepatitis E.
4. Diagnosis is based on the detection of anti-HEV antibody in serum by enzyme-linked immunoassays.
5. Management and prevention
   a. Hygiene: Avoid potentially contaminated food and water.
   b. Pooled immunoglobulins from endemic areas may be effective in controlling this infection.

17.8 Gastrointestinal Hemorrhage

Gastrointestinal bleeding in children can present in several distinct ways. The clinical presentation ranges from occult blood in stools to acute, life-threatening hemorrhage and shock.
1. Definitions
   a. Hematemesis: Vomiting of blood, either "coffee-ground" color and texture or bright red, usually indicates bleeding is proximal to the ligament of Treitz.
   b. Melena: Dark, tarry stool; may have foul or sickeningly sweet odor; usually indicates bleeding from the upper GI tract
   c. Hematochezia: Bright red blood per rectum; usually indicates bleeding from the left colon or anorectal region. However, major upper GI hemorrhage may also present as hematochezia.
2. Reaction to hemorrhage
   a. Ten to 15% loss of blood volume
      (1) Contraction of the venous system
      (2) Movement of the extravascular fluid into the intravascular space
      (3) Blood flow shunted to the heart and brain
   b. Fifteen percent loss of blood volume
      (1) Increased inotropy and increased chronotropy seen secondary to sympathetic stimulation
      (2) Increased peripheral vasoconstriction
      (3) Increased secretion of antidiuretic hormone and aldosterone
      (4) Secondary effects: elevated glucose and fatty acid levels, elevated lactate levels secondary to tissue hypoxia
   c. Thirty percent loss of blood volume
      (1) Hypotension
      (2) Metabolic acidosis
      (3) Shock (Box 17-10)
3. Diagnosis
   a. General questions
      (1) Is it really blood? (rule out bright red foods, drinks)
      (2) Is it from the GI tract? (rule out nosebleed, menstruation)
      (3) How significant is the bleed?
   b. History
      (1) Past bleeding

> **Box 17-10   Treatment of Patients with Hypovolemic Shock Secondary to Gastrointestinal Hemorrhage**
>
> Establish adequate intravenous (IV) access by placing IV catheters: for mild shock, one IV catheter; for moderate or severe shock, two IV catheters.
> Rapidly infuse saline, lactated Ringer's or Plasmanate (10 mL/kg/ 10 min until vital signs normalize).
> Carefully monitor pulse, blood pressure, and, if needed, central venous pressure to avoid fluid overload.
> Monitor urine output, skin perfusion, and orthostatic changes in pulse and blood pressure for early recognition of shock.
> Transfuse with packed red blood cells to return oxygen-carrying capacity to normal.
> Carefully record all fluids transfused, and estimate and record all recognized fluid losses.

Modified from Olson AD, Hillemeier AC: Gastrointestinal hemorrhage. In Wyllie R, Hyams JS (eds): Pediatric Gastrointestinal Disease: Pathophysiology, Diagnosis, and Management. Philadelphia, WB Saunders, 1993.

(2) Quality and quantity of blood loss
(3) Drug history (aspirin, steroids, NSAIDs)
(4) Prior GI surgery
(5) Ongoing symptoms of peptic disease
(6) Protracted retching and vomiting (consider gastroesophageal tear—Mallory-Weiss)
(7) Associated diseases (diabetes, hematologic disorders, renal failure)
(8) Color and character of stool—presence or absence of hematemesis
c. Physical examination
(1) Pulse, blood pressure (lying and sitting). A pulse increase of more than 20 bpm or a postural fall in systolic blood pressure greater than 10 to 15 mm Hg indicates significant blood loss with orthostatic changes.
(2) Oropharynx and nasal examination for evidence of bleed
(3) Abdominal examination
(a) Masses, tenderness, distention
(b) Bowel sounds, abdominal bruits
(c) Evidence of liver disease (hepatomegaly, splenomegaly, ascites, caput medusa)
(4) Digital rectal examination: Hemorrhoids, polyps, fissures, color of stool, and occult blood testing
(5) Skin: Jaundice (liver disease), ecchymoses (coagulation abnormality), cutaneous telangiectasia (Rendu-Osler-Weber disease), labial and buccal pigmentation (Peutz-Jeghers syndrome), and other mucocutaneous changes (Ehlers-Danlos syndrome)

(6) Insert nasogastric (NG) tube to determine whether bleeding is from the upper GI tract (absence of bright red blood, clots, or coffee-ground–like guaiac-positive material does not necessarily rule out upper GI bleeding because it could have subsided or the patient could be bleeding from the duodenal bulb without reflux into the stomach); make note of the presence of bile in the aspirate. An indwelling NG tube placement with periodic lavage and aspiration may help estimate the rate of bleeding

d. Initial laboratory work-up: After stabilizing the patient with fluid resuscitation and necessary volume replacement (see Box 17-10), the following laboratory work should be sent:

(1) Type and cross-match for several units of packed red blood cells (PRBC; depending on the estimated blood loss) and transfuse as needed. A rough guideline used in most infants and children is that administration of 5 mL of PRBC/kg will raise the hematocrit three points and the hemoglobin 1 g/dL.

(2) CBC (with differential and platelet count) and reticulocyte count should be done. The initial value of hemoglobin and hematocrit should be considered to be falsely high until blood volume is replaced. After bleeding ceases, the hemogram may continue to fall for up to 6 hours, and full equilibration may require 24 hours.

(3) Prothrombin time, partial thromboplastin time, and bleeding time (if there is a high degree of suspicion) should be done to exclude bleeding disorders.

(4) Liver enzymes (ALT, aspartate aminotransferase, gamma-glutamyltranspeptidase), glucose, and electrolytes should be checked to exclude liver disease and electrolyte abnormalities.

(5) Elevation of blood urea nitrogen out of proportion to creatinine suggests that the bleeding site is in the upper GI tract.

e. Diagnostic maneuvers

(1) Esophagogastroduodenoscopy may be used for numerous purposes. With upper GI endoscopy, the cause and location of bleeding can be identified in well over 80% of cases.

(a) Active bleeding documented by NG lavage for diagnosis and treatment

(b) History of prior upper GI bleed or varices

(c) History of chronic GI complaints (vomiting, GER, heartburn, ulcer disease, H. pylori infections)

(d) Therapy: in situ coagulation, sclerotherapy, variceal ligation, and so forth

(2) Colonoscopy: More specific and accurate than a barium enema. In chronic colonic bleeding, the cause of the bleeding can be identified in most patients. It allows access for procedures such as polypectomy, electrocoagulation, laser therapy, and biopsies to confirm colitis. Polyethylene glycol by NG tube is usually used to empty the colon of blood before the colonoscopy if the procedure is done during active bleeding.

(3) Meckel's scan should be considered whenever significant lower GI bleeding has occurred. Technetium pertechnetate is used,

often after gastrin administration, to localize ectopic gastric mucosa in a Meckel's diverticulum or other intestinal duplication. Bleeding from a Meckel's diverticulum is usually painless.

(4) Bleeding scans: The Tc-99m pertechnetate–labeled red blood cell scan may be considered when a small intestinal source of bleeding is suspected or when no source can be found by endoscopy. It is sensitive and accurate in localizing the site of active GI bleeding provided it is at a rate of 0.5 mL/min or higher. The half-life of the isotope enables imaging to continue for up to 24 hours.

(5) Selective angiography is effective in localizing the source of bleeding in 40% to 85% of patients with lower GI bleeding. An advantage is that the catheter can be left in position for therapeutic reasons, including infusion of vasopressin or direct embolization of vascular malformations.

(6) Upper GI radiography has a secondary role in GI bleeding. The upper GI series is particularly helpful in defining anatomic defects such as esophageal strictures, malrotation of the bowel, and deep ulcerations.

(7) Barium enema is often needed in neonates and infants presenting with signs of obstruction along with GI bleeding:

(a) Volvulus (diagnostic only)

(b) Intussusception (diagnostic and therapeutic)

(c) It is also effective in defining the location of polyps.

4. The common and uncommon causes of upper and lower GI bleeding as a function of age are listed in Tables 17-4 and 17-5, respectively.

5. Management

a. Stabilize cardiovascular status; correct shock.

b. For upper GI bleeds, use normal saline lavages (not ice water) with reasonable volume to provide adequate stomach lavage; continue lavage until fluid is clear. Avoid using excessive lavage volumes so that vomiting will not result. Leaving the NG tube in place can be helpful in monitoring for resumption of bleeding.

c. Correct bleeding abnormalities by administering fresh frozen plasma (10 mg/kg) or vitamin K (5 to 10 mg, intramuscular or IV) if the patient has coagulopathy, and platelets if the patient is severely thrombocytopenic.

d. Decrease gastric acidity with H_2 receptor antagonist (ranitidine 0.5 mg/kg/dose intravenously every 6 hours) or proton pump inhibitors (omeprazole or lansoprazole) in cases of probable peptic ulcer or gastritis. The gastric pH may be monitored to keep it above 4 with the use of antacids.

e. Vasoactive agents may be used in consultation with a gastroenterologist. Vasopressin in the form of a continuous IV drip of 0.2 to 0.4 U/min has been used to decrease blood flow through the celiac and mesenteric vessels to decrease variceal bleeding. It has also been used in stress ulcers, focal or diffuse gastritis, and Mallory-Weiss tears. Reported complications include abdominal pain, diarrhea, decreased urine output, and hyponatremia.

f. More recently, somatostatin or its synthetic analog (octreotide) has been used effectively to decrease variceal hemorrhage. It has the dual

Table 17-4 **Causes of Upper Gastrointestinal Bleeding, by Age**

Age Group	Common	Less Common
Neonates (0-30 days)	Swallowed maternal blood Gastritis Duodenitis	Coagulopathy Vascular malformations Gastric/esophageal duplication Leiomyoma
Infants (30 days-1 yr)	Gastritis and gastric ulcer Esophagitis Duodenitis	Esophageal varices Foreign body Aortoesophageal fistula
Children (1-12 yr)	Esophagitis Esophageal varices Gastritis and gastric ulcer Duodenal ulcer Mallory-Weiss tear Nasopharyngeal bleeding	Leiomyoma Salicylates Vascular malformation Hematobilia Nonsteroidal anti-inflammatory drugs
Adolescents (12 yr-adult)	Duodenal ulcer Esophagitis Esophageal varices Gastritis Mallory-Weiss tear	Thrombocytopenia Dieulafoy's ulcer Hematobilia

Modified from Olson AD, Hillemeier AC: Gastrointestinal hemorrhage. In Wyllie R, Hyams JS (eds): Pediatric Gastrointestinal Disease: Pathophysiology, Diagnosis, and Management. Philadelphia, WB Saunders, 1993.

effect of reducing GI blood flow and inhibiting gastric acid secretion. The dose of octreotide acetate (Sandostatin) is as follows:

(1) Loading: 1 to 2 µg/kg IV over 2 to 5 minutes
(2) Maintenance: 1 to 2 µg/kg/hr continuous IV infusion

g. Beta blocker: Propranolol is used chronically to prevent rebleeding of varices once the acute bleeding is under control. The dose is adjusted to reduce the heart rate by 20% to get optimum results. It should be used with caution because of respiratory and cardiac side effects.

h. Sclerotherapy involves injecting a sclerosing agent directly into the varix or alongside it. Repeated injections may be needed to obliterate the varices; complications include esophageal ulceration, stricture, and perforation.

i. Ligation of esophageal varices is possible; endoscopically placed elastic bands are used for this purpose. The success rate has been reported to be higher than with sclerotherapy, with fewer complications.

j. Balloon tamponade of varices is also possible.

k. Laser photocoagulation and thermal coagulation are used endoscopically to treat localized bleeding lesions, including "visible vessels" in peptic ulcers, esophageal tears, and arteriovenous malformations.

Table 17-5 **Causes of Lower Gastrointestinal Bleeding, by Age**

Age Group	Common	Less Common
Neonates (0-30 days)	Anorectal lesions Swallowed maternal blood Milk allergy Necrotizing enterocolitis Midgut volvulus	Vascular malformations Hirschsprung's enterocolitis Intestinal duplication Coagulopathy
Infants (30 days-1 yr)	Anorectal lesions Midgut volvulus Intussusception Meckel's diverticulum Infectious diarrhea Milk protein allergy	Vascular malformations Intestinal duplication Acquired thrombocytopenia
Children (1-12 yr)	Juvenile polyps Meckel's diverticulum Intussusception (<3 yr) Infectious diarrhea Anal fissure Nodular lymphoid hyperplasia	Henoch-Schönlein purpura Hemolytic-uremic syndrome Vasculitis (systemic lupus erythematosus) Inflammatory bowel disease
Adolescents (12 yr-adult)	Inflammatory bowel disease (any age) Polyps Hemorrhoids Anal fissure Infectious diarrhea	Arteriovascular malformation Adenocarcinomas Henoch-Schönlein purpura Pseudomembranous colitis

Modified from Olson AD, Hillemeier AC: Gastrointestinal hemorrhage. In Wyllie R, Hyams JS (eds): Pediatric Gastrointestinal Disease: Pathophysiology, Diagnosis, and Management. Philadelphia, WB Saunders, 1993.

l. Reserve surgery for specific conditions:
  (1) Meckel's diverticulum
  (2) Duplication of small bowel
  (3) Hirschsprung's disease
  (4) Exploration in a patient requiring multiple transfusions (e.g., more than 1.5 times their blood volume), but usually with poor results

SUGGESTED READING

Balistreri WF: Viral hepatitis. Pediatr Clin North Am 35:637-669, 1988.

Bingley PJ, Williams AJ, Norcross AJ, et al: Undiagnosed coeliac disease at age seven: Population-based birth cohort study. BMJ 328:322-323, 2004.

Case S: The gluten-free diet: How to provide effective education and resources. Gastroenterology 128(4 Suppl 1):S128-S134, 2005.

Fasano A, Catassi C: Current approaches to the diagnosis and treatment of celiac disease: An evolving spectrum. Gastroenterology 120:636-651, 2001.

Fox V: Acute pancreatitis. Semin Pediatr Gastroenterol Nutr 4(2), 1995.

Freeman KB, Adelson JW: Chronic pancreatitis. Semin Pediatr Gastroenterol Nutr 4(2), 1995.

George DE, Glassman M: Peptic ulcer disease in children. Gastrointest Endosc Clin North Am 4:23-37, 1994.

Grand RJ, Ramakrishna J, Calenda KA: Inflammatory bowel disease in the pediatric patient. Gastroenterol Clin North Am 24:613-632, 1995.

Hatch TF: Encopresis and constipation in children. Pediatr Clin North Am 35: 257-280, 1988.

Hill ID, Dirks MH, Liptak GS, et al: Guideline for the evaluation and treatment of celiac disease in children. J Pediatr Gastroenterol Nutr 40:1-19, 2005

Kupper C: Dietary guidelines and implementation for celiac disease. Gastroenterology 128(4 Suppl 1):S121-S127, 2005.

Nowicki MJ, Balistreri WF: The hepatitis C virus: Identification, epidemiology, and clinical controversies. J Pediatr Gastroenterol Nutr 20:248-274, 1995.

Orenstein SR: Controversies in pediatric gastroesophageal reflux. J Pediatr Gastroenterol Nutr 14:338-348, 1992.

Rewers M: Epidemiology of celiac disease: What are the prevalence, incidence and progression of celiac disease? Gastroenterology 128(4 Suppl 1):S47-S51, 2005.

Romero R, Lavine JE: Viral hepatitis in children. Semin Liver Dis 14:289-302, 1994.

Silverman A, Roy CC (eds): Pediatric Clinical Gastroenterology. St. Louis, Mosby, 1995.

Snyder JD: Expanding alphabet of viral hepatitis. Semin Pediatr Gastroenterol Nutr 2(2):4-7, 1991.

Steinberg W, Tenner S: Acute pancreatitis. N Engl J Med 330:1198-1210, 1994.

Suchy FJ: Chronic viral hepatitis in children. Semin Pediatr Gastroenterol Nutr 2(2), 1991.

Wyllie R, Hyams JS (eds): Pediatric Gastrointestinal and Liver Disease: Pathophysiology, Diagnosis, and Management, 3rd ed. Philadelphia, Saunders, 2006.

Walker WA, Durie PR, Hamilton JR (eds): Pediatric Gastrointestinal Disease: Pathophysiology, Diagnosis, Management, 2nd ed. Hamilton, Ontario, BC Decker, 1995.

Urologic Conditions

18

Jeffrey M. Becker and Anthony A. Caldamone

18.1 Hernias and Hydroceles

1. Etiology and pathophysiology: Pediatric hernias and communicating hydroceles share a common etiology: incomplete obliteration of the processus vaginalis. They differ only in the contents of the processus vaginalis and the extent of the patency:
   a. Hernias contain solid tissue (e.g., bowel, omentum, ovary).
   b. Hydroceles contain peritoneal fluid.
2. Anatomy/embryology
   a. Five to 6 weeks' gestation: Gonads appear on genital ridge in upper abdomen.
   b. Ten to 12 weeks: The trunk of the embryo elongates, causing an apparent descent of gonads to the internal inguinal ring.
   c. Twelve weeks: Processus vaginalis appears as a sac protruding from the peritoneal cavity into the internal ring.
   d. Twenty-seven to 28 weeks: The testis along with intraperitoneal pressure pushes the processus vaginalis down through the inguinal canal into the scrotum, creating an open channel between the scrotum and abdomen.
   e. Forty weeks: Shortly before birth and after testicular descent, the processus vaginalis fuses to itself, becoming a fibrous cord, thereby cutting off communication between the scrotum and peritoneal cavity.
3. Classification
   a. Hernias
      (1) Reducible: Hernia contents can be pushed back into abdomen.
      (2) Incarcerated: Hernia contents cannot be pushed back into abdomen.
      (3) Strangulated: The blood supply of hernia contents is compromised, usually resulting in bowel ischemia or infarction.
   b. Hydroceles
      (1) Communicating: Free communication of fluid between scrotum and abdomen due to patent processus vaginalis
      (2) Noncommunicating
         (a) Fluid present in scrotum (usually from fetal period)

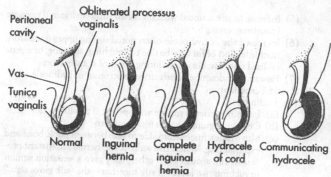

Figure 18-1 Different forms of inguinal hernia and hydrocele arising from failure of the processus vaginalis to obliterate completely. (From Rowe MI, Lloyd DA: Inguinal hernia. In Welch KJ, Randolph JG, Ravitch MM, et al. [eds]: Pediatric Surgery, 4th ed. Chicago, Year Book Medical Publishers, 1986, pp 779-791.)

      (b) Does not reduce into abdomen because processus vaginalis has already closed

      (c) Common in newborns (Fig. 18-1)

   (3) Hydrocele of cord: Fluid trapped in a segmental patency of the processus vaginalis

4. Epidemiology

  a. In the general pediatric population, there is a 1% to 2% incidence of inguinal hernia.

  b. In premature infants with birth weight less than 1000 g, there is a 30% incidence.

  c. Incidence is increased if family member affected.

  d. Hernias: Right sided in 60%, left sided in 30%, bilateral in 10%

  e. Male-to-female prevalence of 4:1

  f. Associated genitourinary (GU) conditions

   (1) Ambiguous genitalia

   (2) Hypospadias

   (3) Cryptorchidism

   (4) Epispadias-exstrophy

  g. Fluid in peritoneal cavity from ventriculoperitoneal shunt, peritoneal dialysis, or ascites predisposes to inguinal hernia by causing increased intra-abdominal pressure.

5. Clinical features

  a. History

   (1) This condition usually appears as an intermittent bulge in groin or scrotum.

   (2) Fluctuation in the size of the scrotum indicates communicating hydrocele or hernia.

   (3) Most often it is detected by parents or during well-baby check.

   (4) If the hernia is large, it may be painful.

      (5) Increase in size is noted with increased intra-abdominal pressure (coughing, crying).

      (6) Increased size of hydrocele often noted during upper respiratory tract infection or flu may be due to coughing, sneezing, or a generalized serositis; also seen during bouts of constipation.

      (7) Parents may describe bluish tinge to scrotum in hydrocele.

  b. Physical examination

    (1) Technique

      (a) Examine patients supine and upright if possible.

      (b) Observe inguinal region for asymmetry.

      (c) Move index finger from side to side between pubic bone and external ring. When the walls of the hernia sac (patent processus) rub against each other, they give a sensation similar to rubbing two layers of silk together—the "silk glove sign."

    (2) Specific findings

      (a) Hernia: Often can feel continuity between mass and inguinal canal

      (b) Hydrocele

        (i) Able to palpate above the mass

        (ii) No continuity felt between mass and inguinal canal

      (c) Attempt to reduce mass into the abdomen if patient appears nontoxic.

6. Laboratory findings: None required

7. Management and prognosis

  a. Hernia

    (1) Reducible hernias should be electively repaired regardless of age.

    (2) Incarcerated hernias require more urgent surgery.

    (3) Strangulated hernias require an emergency operation.

  b. Hydrocele

    (1) Most infants will spontaneously close their patent processus vaginalis within the first year.

    (2) Repair is usually reserved for hydroceles persisting beyond the first year of life.

  c. Because of the risk of a subsequent hernia in opposite groin, contralateral exploration and repair may be performed under the following circumstances:

    (1) Boys younger than 1 year of age (assuming the first side was repaired without difficulty)

    (2) Girls of all ages (low risk of injury to gonads)

    (3) Patients with ventriculoperitoneal shunts, continuous ambulatory peritoneal dialysis catheters, and ascites

18.2 Acute Scrotal Swelling

1. Acute scrotal swelling is a potential urologic emergency. There is a wide differential diagnosis, ranging from the rare idiopathic scrotal wall edema, which resolves spontaneously, to testicular torsion that requires urgent surgical correction and can have catastrophic sequelae if not detected and treated early in its course.

2. Differential diagnosis (Box 18-1)

Box 18-1   Differential Diagnosis of the Acutely
Swollen Scrotum

Common

Hernia
Hydrocele
Testicular torsion
Torsion of testis/appendix epididymis
Epididymitis
Orchitis
Varicocele
Trauma

Rare

Acute idiopathic scrotal wall edema
Henoch-Schönlein purpura of scrotal wall
Idiopathic fat necrosis of scrotum
Spontaneous gangrene of scrotal wall
Peritonitis
Tumor

3. Clinical features
   a. Symptoms
      (1) Testicular torsion
         (a) Acute onset, severe testicular pain
         (b) Often with associated nausea and vomiting
         (c) Pain may radiate to abdomen
      (2) Epididymitis
         (a) More gradual onset of pain
         (b) Often associated urinary tract symptoms (dysuria, urethral discharge)
         (c) Pain may radiate to inguinal region
   b. Age
      (1) Newborn and adolescent: Higher incidence of testicular torsion
      (2) Mid-childhood: Higher incidence of appendiceal torsion
      (3) Postpubertal: Higher incidence of epididymitis
4. Physical examination
   a. Examine uninvolved testis to establish normal baseline.
   b. Cremasteric reflex: Gentle stroking of inner thigh skin causes contraction of the cremaster muscle and causes ipsilateral testicle to retract toward the inguinal canal. The presence of a cremasteric reflex on the affected side strongly suggests the diagnosis is *not* testicular torsion.
   c. Involved testis
      (1) High riding suggests testicular torsion.
      (2) Isolated upper pole tenderness suggests torsed appendix testis or epididymitis.

d. Blue dot sign: Small, discrete blue discoloration of scrotum represents torsed appendix testis or epididymis.
5. Diagnostic studies
   a. Urinalysis: Pyuria (white blood cell [WBC] count) or bacteriuria more likely in infectious etiology (epididymitis or orchitis; see Chapter 19 for urinary tract infection [UTI])
   b. Scrotal ultrasonography (US) with color Doppler
      (1) Diagnostic test of choice
      (2) Accurately detects presence or absence of blood flow to testis
      (3) Reliability depends on sonographer
6. Specific causes of acute scrotal swelling.
   a. Testicular torsion (torsion of the spermatic cord)
      (1) Etiology and pathophysiology
         (a) Vessels of the spermatic cord twist, compromising blood supply to the testis.
         (b) Testicular torsion occurs in 1 in 4000 men or boys younger than 25 years of age
         (c) Two thirds of cases occur in boys aged 12 to 18 years.
      (2) Embryology/etiology (Fig. 18-2)
         (a) Intravaginal torsion
            (i) Most common *after* neonatal period
            (ii) Twist takes place within tunica vaginalis and results from an abnormally high insertion of the tunica on the spermatic cord (bell-clapper deformity), allowing excessive testicular mobility within the scrotum.
         (b) Extravaginal torsion
            (i) Most common in neonates
            (ii) Testis and cord twist because of nonfixation of tunica vaginalis within scrotum.

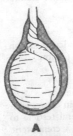
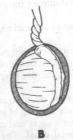
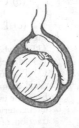

Figure 18-2 Types of torsion of the testis. A, Intravaginal torsion (torsion within the attachment of the tunica vaginalis). B, Extravaginal torsion (torsion of the cord). C, Torsion between the epididymis and testis. (From Leape L: Torsion of the testis. In Welch KJ, Randolph JG, Ravitch MM, et al. [eds]: Pediatric Surgery, 4th ed. Chicago, Year Book Medical Publishers, 1986.)

(3) Clinical features
  (a) Pain
    (i) Usually it is of sudden onset and increasing severity.
    (ii) It may radiate to the abdomen.
    (iii) One third have had similar episodes that resolved (suggests intermittent torsion).
  (b) Associated symptoms may include nausea and vomiting.
  (c) Twenty percent have incidental history of testicular trauma.
(4) Physical examination
  (a) Pain at rest (without palpation) occurs.
  (b) Affected scrotum is erythematous, edematous.
  (c) Testis may have transverse lie (instead of normal vertical lie).
  (d) Testis itself is exquisitely tender.
  (e) Cremasteric reflex is usually absent.
(5) Diagnostic studies
  (a) Scrotal US with color Doppler
  (b) Testicular scan (if US not available)
  (c) Scrotal exploration: If the diagnosis is fairly certain from history and physical examination, immediate surgical exploration, detorsion, and testicular fixation should be performed without diagnostic tests.
(6) Management and prognosis: The goal of treatment is testicular salvage, which depends on the duration and degree of torsion.
  (a) Duration of torsion
    (i) Salvage likely if less than 4 to 6 hours
    (ii) Increased incidence of atrophy at more than 8 hours
    (iii) Essentially no salvage after 24 hours
  (b) Degree of torsion
    (i) One twist (360 degrees) or less of cord may not result in complete ischemia.
    (ii) Two twists (720 degrees) usually result in complete ischemia.
  (c) Manual detorsion: In experienced hands, manually untwisting the torsion in the emergency department can buy some time before surgery, as in the situation where a child has recently eaten. Affected testis is detorsed by external rotation of one or two full turns of the testis (left clockwise, right counterclockwise). If successful, the patient experiences relief of pain but needs surgery within 24 hours to prevent retorsion. This is done under sedation.
  (d) Surgery
    (i) Parents must know that the testis may need to be removed.
    (ii) After torsed cord/testis is untwisted, if viable, testis is fixed to its tunica vaginalis to prevent recurrence (scrotal orchidopexy).
    (iii) If nonviable, an orchiectomy is performed.
    (iv) A contralateral scrotal orchidopexy is performed as a preventive measure.
b. Epididymitis: Acute or chronic inflammation of the epididymis

(1) Etiology and pathophysiology
  (a) May result from UTI with retrograde spread along vas deferens
  (b) *Escherichia coli, Chlamydia, Neisseria gonorrhoeae* common (see Chapter 19)
(2) Epidemiology
  (a) Peak incidence in adolescence
  (b) More common in boys with
    (i) UTIs
    (ii) Structural lesions of GU tract (urethral strictures, posterior urethral valves)
    (iii) Previous GU tract reconstruction
    (iv) Indwelling urethral catheters
(3) History
  (a) Onset of pain is usually more gradual than in testis torsion.
  (b) Pain may radiate to ipsilateral groin.
  (c) The patient may have symptoms of UTI (dysuria, frequency, urethral discharge).
(4) Clinical features
  (a) May have fever
  (b) Enlarged, tender epididymis (located posterior, superior, and inferior to testis)
  (c) Adjacent ipsilateral testis normal, nontender
  (d) Prehn's sign: Relief of pain with elevation of involved hemiscrotum more consistent with epididymitis than torsion; unreliable in children
(5) Diagnostic studies
  (a) Complete blood count: Leukocytosis or normal
  (b) Urinalysis, culture and sensitivity: Pyuria (present in 46% boys with epididymitis), bacteriuria occasionally present if associated with UTI
  (c) Scrotal US or nuclear scan if torsion cannot be excluded; often see *increased* flow to affected epididymis/testis
  (d) Boys with associated UTI: US and voiding cystourethrogram (VCUG)
(6) Management
  (a) Antibiotics (treat as if treating UTI)
  (b) If sexually active, need to treat as if a sexually transmitted disease
  (c) Scrotal elevation and bed rest
  (d) Analgesics/nonsteroid anti-inflammatory drugs
c. Torsion of testicular and epididymal appendages
  (1) Etiology, pathophysiology, and embryology
    (a) Small vestigial appendages, most commonly attached to upper pole of testis (appendix testis) and epididymis (appendix epididymis)
    (b) If on a small stalk, can twist and infarct, causing acute scrotal pain and swelling (Fig. 18-3)
    (c) Occurs most commonly between 7 and 12 years of age
  (2) Clinical features
    (a) Acute onset of scrotal pain

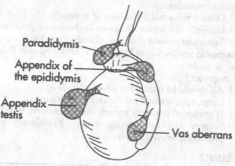

Figure 18-3 Torsion of the appendix testis. In addition to the appendix testis (hydatid of Morgagni), torsion may involve the paradidymis, the appendix epididymis, and the vas aberrans. (From Leape L: Torsion of the testis. In Welch KJ, Randolph JG, Ravitch MM, et al. [eds]: Pediatric Surgery, 4th ed. Chicago, Year Book Medical Publishers, 1986, pp 1396-1398.)

(b) Usually not as painful as testicular torsion

(c) Nausea/vomiting usually absent

(3) Physical examination

(a) If examined early, there may be localized tenderness over twisted appendix with nodule.

(b) If examined late, the degree of swelling may preclude accurate diagnosis.

(c) Torsed appendix may be visible as "blue dot sign" through scrotal skin.

(d) Remainder of testis is nontender.

(4) Diagnostic studies: Color Doppler US if unable to distinguish from testicular torsion

(5) Management and prognosis

(a) Supportive measures (analgesics, elevation)

(b) Resolves spontaneously (rarely requires surgical excision)

(c) If unable to exclude epididymitis, give empiric oral antibiotics.

d. Varicocele: Dilated veins in the spermatic cord

(1) Etiology, pathophysiology, and embryology

(a) Results from incompetent valves of spermatic vein

(b) Ninety percent are left sided, presumably because spermatic vein enters left renal vein at right angle compared with the oblique junction of the right spermatic vein with the inferior vena cava.

(c) Compromise of sperm production by testis may result from hyperthermia/hypoxia.

(2) Epidemiology: Rare before puberty, it can be present in up to 10% to 20% of postpubertal boys.

(3) Clinical features: Often asymptomatic, with a dull ache in affected scrotum

    (4) Physical examination
      (a) Dilated veins feel like a "bag of worms."
      (b) It usually resolves or decreases in the supine position.
      (c) Testicular volume is measured with an orchidometer.
    (5) Diagnostic studies: Color Doppler US obtained only if diagnosis still in doubt.
    (6) Management
      (a) All should be referred to a urologist.
      (b) Large, symptomatic varicoceles require surgery.
      (c) If ipsilateral testicular growth stunted, surgery is indicated.
      (d) Surgery involves ligating (tying off) dilated veins but preserving arterial supply.

18.3 Trauma

Genitourinary trauma (occurring in 5% to 10% of injured children) may range from a self-limited process to a potentially life-threatening or disfiguring injury requiring emergency intervention.

OVERVIEW

1. Clinical features
  a. Previous GU history (i.e., anatomic anomalies, solitary kidney). Twenty to 25% of renal injuries may be associated with preexisting anomalies.
  b. Mechanism of injury
    (1) Blunt or penetrating
    (2) Details (e.g., speed of car, type of weapon)
  c. Gross hematuria: Voiding discomfort may signify urethral injury.
2. Physical examination
  a. Vital signs: Severe tachycardia and hypotension may signify life-threatening bleeding from renovascular trauma or bleeding from pelvic veins secondary to pelvic fracture.
  b. Chest
    (1) Rib fracture may cause renal injury.
    (2) Rib fracture is suspected if pneumothorax or subcutaneous air is present.
  c. Abdomen
    (1) Suprapubic distention with an inability to void may signify urethral injury.
    (2) Suprapubic tenderness can be associated with bladder contusion/ rupture.
    (3) Diffuse tenderness may be seen with an intraperitoneal bladder rupture.
  d. Flank: Ecchymosis or tenderness may reflect renal/ureteral injury.
  e. Rectal examination: Elevated (high-riding) or tender prostate—suspect urethral injury.
  f. External genitalia
    (1) Blood at meatus indicates a possible urethral injury (*do not attempt catheterization*).
    (2) Perineal hematoma: Suspect urethral injury.
    (3) Determine whether scrotal/penile skin is intact.

g. Vagina
   (1) Examine for laceration into urethra, bladder, rectum, or peritoneal cavity.
   (2) This can be a life-threatening injury if missed.
3. Diagnostic studies: Specific studies should be tailored to suspected injury (see later).
   a. Blood work: Complete blood count, electrolytes, blood urea nitrogen, creatinine
   b. Urinalysis
   c. Imaging: Intravenous pyelography (IVP), computed tomography (CT; abdomen/pelvis), cystogram, retrograde urethrogram. CT is the study of choice.

KIDNEY TRAUMA

1. Pathophysiology and epidemiology
   a. Most common GU organ injured
   b. Usually result of blunt trauma (motor vehicle accident, falls, sports injuries)
   c. More common in boys than girls
   d. May be associated with previously undetected anatomic anomaly (especially ureteropelvic junction [UPJ] obstruction)
   e. Kidney is more commonly injured in pediatric age group (compared with adults) because in children the kidney is larger in proportion to abdominal size, with less protective fat and lower ribs that are not completely ossified.
2. Diagnosis (staging)
   a. All children with trauma and hematuria (gross or microscopic) need a work-up.
   b. The degree of hematuria does not necessarily correlate with the degree of injury.
   c. The extent of the work-up depends on the stability of the patient.
      (1) Unstable patient (shock) or patient already in operating room: "One-shot IVP" may help make diagnosis of GU trauma and confirms presence of normally functioning contralateral kidney in case nephrectomy is necessary on injured side.
      (2) Stable patient
         (a) CT abdomen/pelvis
         (b) CT cystogram with postdrainage plain film (kidney, ureter, and bladder) if bladder injury suspected
3. Classification of renal injuries
   a. Minor (85%)
      (1) Renal contusion: No break in renal capsule
      (2) Minor laceration: Extends into the superficial cortex but not the collecting system
   b. Major (15%)
      (1) Major laceration: Extends deep into parenchyma and/or collecting system
      (2) Complete UPJ disruption
      (3) Vascular injuries: Tears or occlusions of renal artery, vein, or major branches

4. Management of blunt renal trauma
   a. Minor injuries (contusions, minor lacerations)
      (1) Observation and bed rest in hospital until gross hematuria resolves
      (2) No heavy activity for 2 to 4 weeks
      (3) Follow-up study (IVP, CT, or US) in 6 to 8 weeks
      (4) Repeat urinalysis in 6 to 8 weeks
      (5) Blood pressure check, urinalysis 1 year after injury
   b. Major injuries (major lacerations/vascular injuries)
      (1) Observation may be adequate for injuries associated with only
         (a) Small amount of urinary extravasation
         (b) Minor perirenal hematoma
      (2) Surgical correction or exploration required in the following situations:
         (a) Expanding or uncontrolled hematoma
         (b) Pulsatile hematoma
         (c) Extensive urinary extravasation
         (d) UPJ disruption
         (e) Nonviable renal parenchyma (>30%)
         (f) Falling hematocrit during observation
         (g) Vascular injury (usually requires nephrectomy)

URETERAL TRAUMA

1. Pathophysiology and epidemiology
   a. Injuries to ureter are uncommon in children, usually secondary to blunt ureteral trauma (avulsion of ureter, laceration from bony fracture, crush injury).
   b. Diagnosis often delayed: May present with urinary extravasation (urinoma). Observe for butterfly "hematuria" in groin or ureteral obstruction. Hematuria not always present.
   c. Operative repair usually is needed.

BLADDER TRAUMA

1. Pathophysiology and epidemiology
   a. The pediatric bladder is intra-abdominal and thus more susceptible to blunt injury.
   b. Suspect injury in any blunt or penetrating trauma to lower abdomen, pelvis, or perineum.
   c. Ninety percent of bladder ruptures are associated with pelvic fracture.
   d. Ten to 15% of pelvic fractures have associated bladder rupture.
2. Diagnosis: Cystogram or CT cystogram (always obtain postvoid plain film)
   a. Requires complete filling of bladder to capacity: bladder capacity estimate = (age in years + 2) × 30 mL
   b. Contrast should be instilled under gravity; it should *not* be forcefully injected.
3. Classification and management of bladder rupture
   a. Extraperitoneal (most common)
      (1) Management: Catheter drainage (urethral or suprapubic) with a follow-up cystogram 1 to 2 weeks to see if healed
   b. Intraperitoneal: Often results from blunt trauma to a full bladder
      (1) Management involves operative repair with primary closure and suprapubic catheter drainage.

SCROTAL TRAUMA

1. Testicle
   a. It is infrequently injured secondary to its mobility.
   b. Direct blunt trauma may cause testicular rupture; US is useful in diagnosis. Testicular rupture/fracture implies a break in the tunica albuginea and requires surgical repair.
   c. Consider testicular torsion as etiology of pain even with history of trauma.
2. Scrotal skin: If repair is needed, the redundancy of scrotal skin avoids requiring grafting.

PENILE TRAUMA

1. Toilet seat injury occurs when a boy is voiding and hurries to finish, slamming down the seat and resulting in a contusion or laceration. Management is conservative.
2. Zipper injury (also known as the "Something About Mary" injury)
   a. Penile skin (usually foreskin) gets caught in zipper, more common in uncircumcised boys.
   b. The zipper is released by cutting the median bar of zipper mechanism with bone cutters.

18.4 Hypospadias

1. Definition: Hypospadias is an abnormal opening of the urethra on the ventral side of the penis, scrotum, or perineum proximal to its normal location on the tip of the glans penis.
2. Embryology: The urethra forms on the ventral aspect of the penis as two tubes growing toward each other, meeting at the corona. Urethral folds fuse in the midline, creating a tunnel that becomes the urethra. Hypospadias results when the edges of the urethral folds fail to unite (Fig. 18-4).

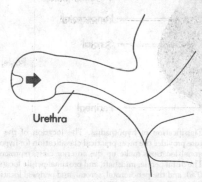

Urethra

Figure 18-4 Formation of the glanular urethra. (From Bellinger MF: Embryology of the male genitalia. Urol Clin North Am 8:375-382, 1981.)

3. Etiology: Multifactorial mode of inheritance and defect in androgen action locally at genital tissue level implicated
4. Epidemiology
   a. Incidence is between 1:125 and 1:300 for boys.
   b. Incidence increases if the father or a sibling is affected (14% of siblings will be affected).
5. Associated anomalies
   a. Undescended testis (9%)
   b. Hydrocele/hernia (9%)
   c. No significant increase in other urinary tract abnormalities. Upper tract (i.e., kidney) screening is *not* necessary, unless there is a scrotal meatus or associated undescended testis.
6. Classification (Fig. 18-5)
7. Physical examination
   a. Position/size of meatus
   b. Formation of foreskin
   c. Amount of ventral skin
   d. Presence or absence of chordee (penile curvature)
   e. Examine for hernia/hydrocele/cryptorchidism

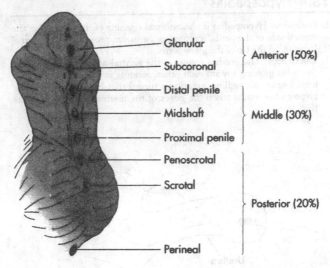

Figure 18-5 Classification of hypospadias. The location of the meatus *after* correction of curvature provides the most practical classification for hypospadias. The glanular and subcoronal locations make up the anterior class, representing 50% of hypospadias cases. The distal penile, midshaft, and proximal penile locations make up the middle class (30%), and the penoscrotal, scrotal, and perineal locations make up the posterior class (20%). (From Duckett JW Jr: Modern hypospadias. In Seidmon EJ, Hanno PM [eds]: Current Urologic Therapy, 3rd ed. Philadelphia, WB Saunders, 1994.)

8. Diagnostic studies: None are necessary, unless hypospadias is present with one or both testes nonpalpable, in which case an intersex condition must be excluded. For several degrees of hypospadias (i.e., penoscrotal), US of the urinary tract should be obtained.
9. Management
    a. A plethora of hypospadias repairs have been described. They vary depending on the preference of the urologist, position and size of the meatus, presence or absence of chordee, and amount of available foreskin.
    b. Hypospadiac boys should not be circumcised at birth.
        (1) The foreskin may be required for the repair.
        (2) If a circumcision is started and abnormal position of the meatus is suspected, the procedure should be abandoned and urologic consultation sought.
    c. Boys with chordee *should not be circumcised at birth.* The foreskin may be necessary for the repair.
    d. Repair is usually done at 6 to 18 months of age.
    e. All repairs have the following in common:
        (1) Straighten penile bend if present.
        (2) Create urethra that will allow normal voiding (standing instead of sitting).
        (3) Usually performed on an outpatient basis
10. Complications of hypospadias repair
    a. Urethrocutaneous fistula (most common reason for second operation)
    b. Urethral stricture
    c. Residual chordee
    d. Meatal stenosis
    e. Urethral diverticula

18.5 Epispadias

1. Definition
    a. In epispadias, the urethra and meatus are on the dorsal aspect (top side) of the penis.
    b. The spectrum of the disease ranges from glanular epispadias, in which the urethra opens on the dorsal aspect of the glans, to the exstrophy-epispadias complex, in which the urethral anomaly is associated with a ventral defect of the midline abdominal wall through which an open, exposed bladder protrudes.
2. Incidence
    a. Complete epispadias: 1 in 120,000 boys; 1 in 450,000 girls
    b. Exstrophy-epispadias complex: 1 in 40,000 live births (male-to-female ratio is 2:1)
3. Management: Surgical repair, which may require multistage repair, especially if associated with bladder exstrophy

18.6 Cryptorchidism

1. Definition and significance: Literally translated as "hidden testicle," cryptorchidism is a common pediatric urologic problem that requires

careful management. Potential ramifications of an undescended testicle are as follows:

- a. Infertility
- b. Testicular malignancy
- c. Psychological stress

2. Embryology
   a. Two phases of normal testicular descent
      (1) Intra-abdominal descent at 5 to 27 weeks: From upper abdomen to internal inguinal ring
      (2) Intracanalicular descent at 27 to 30 weeks: From internal inguinal ring to scrotum
   b. Many theories exist to explain testicular descent, although none has definitively been proved.

3. Epidemiology
   a. Incidence
      (1) Full-term newborns: 3%
      (2) Premature infants: 33% (varies depending on degree of prematurity)
   b. Other factors that increase incidence of cryptorchidism
      (1) Low birth weight
      (2) First-born boy
      (3) Maternal estrogen exposure
   c. At 1 year of age, the incidence of cryptorchidism is only 0.8%. Many cryptorchid testes undergo spontaneous descent during the first year of life (usually during the first 3 months).

4. Classification
   a. Retractile testis
      (1) Not truly undescended
      (2) Retract vigorously due to active cremasteric reflex
      (3) Can be manipulated into the scrotum and stay there when released
      (4) No increased risk for infertility or malignancy
   b. Absent testis
      (1) The testis is absent on physical examination and after diagnostic work-up.
      (2) Twenty to 40% of impalpable testes are absent.
      (3) It likely results from intrauterine testicular torsion.
   c. Ectopic testis
      (1) The testis is present but followed an abnormal path of descent during intrascrotal descent.
      (2) The most common location is superficial inguinal pouch.
   d. Truly undescended testis
      (1) The testis is present along the normal line of descent but has not reached scrotum.
      (2) It may be inguinal, abdominal, or suprascrotal.
   e. Latent or acquired undescended testis
      (1) Testis once descended (probably retractile), now "stuck" in an undescended position
      (2) Usually located in upper scrotum or lower inguinal canal

Laparoscopic Findings	Significance	Incidence
Blind-ending cord structures at internal inguinal ring	Absent testis (likely intrauterine torsion)	59%
Testicular vessels enter internal inguinal ring	Inguinal or prescrotal testis	19%
Testis seen in abdomen	Intra-abdominal testis	22%

5. History: If the testis was ever documented to be in the scrotum, retractile testis is more likely. If there is a history of inguinal bulging, undescended testis is most likely.
6. Clinical features
   a. Is testis palpable or impalpable?
   b. Technique: Block the internal ring with one hand. With the other, beginning at internal ring, walk fingers down along spermatic cord and attempt to palpate testis and milk it into the scrotum.
7. Diagnosis
   a. Laboratory studies are not necessary unless bilateral anorchia is suspected.
   b. US and CT are unreliable in the localization of a cryptorchid testis because of a high false-negative rate.
   c. Laparoscopy is the gold standard. One of the three situations described in Table 18-1 will be seen.
8. Management (Table 18-2)
   a. Orchidopexy
      (1) Brings testis down into scrotum and fixes it in place
      (2) May be done laparoscopically or open, depending on location of testis
      (3) One- or two-stage operation
          (a) Identify testis; separate processus vaginalis from spermatic cord.

Testis Location	Treatment
Absent testis	Contralateral scrotal orchidopexy Hormonal replacement if bilateral (rare)
Retractile testis	Hormonal (hCG/GnRH) popular in Europe Follow-up examination to make sure not undescended
Undescended testis	Orchidopexy if persists past 6 mo of age Usually performed at 1 yr of age

GnRH, gonadotropin-releasing hormone; hCG, human chorionic gonadotropin.

      (b) Mobilize testis and spermatic cord to achieve enough length to bring testis into scrotum.

      (c) Fix (suture) testis into scrotum or place in a pouch between dartos and scrotal skin.

9. Prognosis
   a. Fertility
      (1) Cryptorchid testes histologically abnormal as early as 1 year of age
      (2) Paternity rates after orchidopexy for
          (a) Unilateral cryptorchidism: 71% to 92%
          (b) Bilateral cryptorchidism: 43% to 62%
      (3) Only one study demonstrates progressive decline in fertility with increasing age of orchidopexy; however, most advocate performing the operation before 1 year of age.
   b. Malignancy
      (1) Twenty to 40 times increased risk of cancer developing in an undescended testis (even after orchidopexy).
      (2) A contralateral testis is also at an increased risk (one fourth of all tumors develop in the contralateral testis).
      (3) Orchidopexy allows easier testicular examination, but *does not lower risk for cancer*.

18.7 Urinary Tract Infections

A UTI in a child may be an isolated, nonrecurrent illness of childhood, or it may be the first clue to an anatomic or functional disturbance of the GU system.

1. Definitions
   a. *Pyuria* (i.e., WBCs in urine specimen): 10 WBCs/mm³ or more of urine in an *uncentrifuged* specimen is defined as pyuria. Pyuria alone is poorly correlated with UTI. The following are associated with pyuria *without* bacteriuria:
      (1) Concentrated urine (dehydration)
      (2) Irritation from topical agents
      (3) Inflammation of neighboring structures, (e.g., acute appendicitis)
      (4) Trauma
      (5) Instrumentation
      (6) Calculi (may also have bacteriuria)
      (7) Acute glomerulonephritis
      (8) Interstitial nephritis
      (9) Oral polio vaccine
      (10) Renal tubular acidosis
      (11) *Note*: If WBC count is 10/mm³ or more *and* Gram stain is positive, then 90% of patients will have a positive urine culture (i.e., UTI).
   b. Bacteriuria (i.e., bacteria in urine specimen)
      (1) The condition of bacteriuria depends on the method of collection (Table 18-3).
      (2) Bacteriuria *without* pyuria may be an asymptomatic condition *or* secondary to contamination.

Method	Colony Count
Suprapubic aspiration	Any bacteria
Urethral catheter	>10,000 CFU/mL
"Clean catch"	≥50,000 CFU/mL

CFU, colony-forming units.

   c. UTI: Most often symptomatic infection in association with positive urine culture of *appropriately* obtained specimen (i.e., by suprapubic aspiration or urethral catheterization)

2. Epidemiology
   a. Incidence
     (1) During the first year of life, 0.3% to 1.2% of infants have symptomatic UTI.
     (2) Boys are affected more commonly than girls during first 3 months.
     (3) Girls are affected more commonly than boys after 1 year of age.
     (4) Cumulative incidence for UTI by 10 years of age: boys, 1%; girls, 5% (*E. coli* is by far the most common organism, especially in first infections)
     (5) Circumcision decreases the incidence of UTI among male infants.
     (6) Thirty to 40% of patients with UTI demonstrate some GU anomaly (on imaging studies) that has contributed to the UTI.
   b. Recurrence
     (1) Thirty to 40% of children have a recurrence after first UTI.
     (2) Seventy-five percent recur after the third UTI.

3. Etiology and pathophysiology
   a. Most UTIs are considered to be ascending in origin, often related to predisposing factors. Other processes associated with UTI include hematogenous spread (especially in young infants), lymphogenous spread (e.g., from constipation), or extension from another organ (e.g., from abdominal infection such as appendicitis).
   b. Age
     (1) Neonates: Often the result of bacteremia
     (2) Non-neonates: Ascending infection from GI tract into urethra
   c. Bacteria
     (1) *E. coli*: 80% of UTIs; *Klebsiella* and *Enterobacter* are also common.
     (2) Non–*E. coli* infections are more common in patients with anatomic or functional abnormalities.
   d. Anatomic anomalies and variations .
     (1) Shorter urethral length and its proximity to anus explains the higher incidence of UTIs among girls.
     (2) Vesicoureteral reflux is the most common finding in association with UTI.

       (3) Functional (e.g., neurogenic bladder) or anatomic anomaly (e.g., vesicoureteral reflux, UPJ obstruction) predisposes to UTI because of urinary stasis.

   e. Constipation and soiling increase the incidence of lower-tract UTIs secondary to
     (1) Direct mechanical compression of the bladder
     (2) Increased bacterial contamination of the perineum
     (3) Decreased voiding frequency

4. Clinical features
   a. Clinical features vary according to the child's age (Table 18-4).
   b. "Clinical syndromes" associated with UTI
     (1) Bacteriuria (see earlier)
     (2) Cystitis: Suprapubic pain, frequency, urgency, no fever or low-grade fever (*Note:* Pinworm infection may ascend into the bladder and present in an asymptomatic manner [i.e., identified on routine urinalysis] *or* as symptoms of cystitis with pruritus vagina.)
     (3) Pyelonephritis: High fever (≥38° C), toxicity, flank or abdominal pain, costovertebral angle tenderness, vomiting
     (4) Urosepsis: Seen in newborn/young infants often with congenital anomalies, urosepsis is associated with bacteremia, fever, toxicity, electrolyte disturbances, and shock.
   c. Many patients have symptoms of a UTI (i.e., frequency, dysuria) *without* significant bacteriuria (Box 18-2).
   d. Evaluate history and predisposing factors (as noted earlier):
     (1) Frequency/urgency
     (2) Fever is common with upper-tract infections (pyelonephritis).
     (3) Flank tenderness usually indicates pyelonephritis.
     (4) Abdomen: Lower abdominal mass may indicate full bladder or colon "full of stool" seen in some patients who "hold it in."

Age	Signs/Symptoms
Neonate/infant	Hypothermia, hyperthermia, failure to thrive, vomiting, diarrhea, sepsis, irritability, lethargy, jaundice, malodorous urine
Toddler	Abdominal pain, vomiting, diarrhea, constipation, abnormal voiding pattern, malodorous urine, fever, poor growth
School age	Dysuria, frequency, urgency, abdominal pain, abnormal voiding pattern (including incontinence or secondary enuresis), constipation, malodorous urine, fever
Adolescent	Dysuria, frequency, urgency, abdominal pain, malodorous urine, fever

From Sherbotie JR, Cornfeld D: Management of urinary tract infections in children. Med Clin North Am 75:327-328, 1991.

Box 18-2   Causes of Urinary Tract Symptoms without Bacteriuria

Urethritis, nonspecific
Soaps, detergents, bubble bath
Medications, lotions
Vaginal foreign bodies
Candida
Emotional disturbances
Vulvovaginitis
Fabrics, laundry soaps, clothing dyes
Trauma (sexual abuse)
Pinworms
Trichomonas

---

   (5) Incontinence
   (6) Constipation
5. Physical examination
   a. Not useful to detect UTI in young infants
   b. Include the following:
      (1) Blood pressure measurement
      (2) Search for congenital malformations
      (3) Careful examination of abdomen, perineum, and genitalia
6. Localization of infection
   a. Upper tract (acute pyelonephritis)
      (1) Fever, abdominal or flank pain
      (2) Responsible for renal scarring (especially after recurrent episodes)
      (3) More likely to be associated with structural abnormality
   b. Lower tract (cystitis): Dysuria, incontinence, urgency, frequency, suprapubic or low back pain
7. Laboratory studies
   a. Rapid diagnostic assays performed by dipstick urinalysis on fresh specimens can suggest UTI.
      (1) Leukocyte esterase (an enzyme derived from neutrophils) is 74% to 76% sensitive and 71% to 98% specific for UTI.
      (2) Nitrites (reduction of dietary nitrates, nitrites by bacteria) assay is 70% to 90% sensitive, 90% to 100% specific.
   b. Urine microscopy (use appropriately obtained specimen)
      (1) One or more bacteria/oil field in Gram-stained specimen or 10 or more WBC/mm^3 correlates with a positive urine culture (i.e., 10^5 colony-forming units [CFU]/mL).
      (2) Note: Gross hematuria and proteinuria are uncommon in UTI.
   c. Urine culture
      (1) Unless contaminated, a catheterized urine specimen with greater than 10^5 CFU/mL defines a UTI in all children.

(2) Over 10^4 CFU/mL in neonates may indicate UTI.

(3) Serially obtained specimens will improve diagnostic precision.

(a) Single positive specimen is 80% accurate for UTI.

(b) Two consecutive positive specimens are 95% accurate.

(4) Most cultures that are positive for several species (usually <10^5 CFU/mL) are considered contaminated. To avoid contamination, refrigerate specimen at 4° C or culture promptly within 6 to 12 hours. Correlation with pyuria on urinalysis is helpful.

d. Blood cultures should be obtained in patients with suspected urosepsis or pyelonephritis and in very young neonates (<28 days of age) with UTI.

e. Blood urea nitrogen and creatinine should be obtained in select cases with complicated or chronic infection.

f. Radiographic evaluation

(1) All children with a febrile UTI require at least these:

(a) Upper-tract study (US)

(b) Lower-tract study (VCUG)

(2) Useful diagnostic imaging procedures in UTIs are given in Table 18-5.

8. Management

a. Uncomplicated UTI

(1) Initial antimicrobial therapy may include

(a) Oral antimicrobials (empiric to cover most common organisms)

(i) Trimethoprim/sulfamethoxazole (TMP/SMX; 8 to 10 mg/ kg/day TMP), orally every 12 hours for 7 to 10 days *or*

(ii) Amoxicillin-clavulanate (30 to 50 mg/kg/day) orally every day for 7 to 10 days *or*

(iii) Nitrofurantoin (5 to 7 mg/kg/day) orally every day for 7 to 10 days *or*

(iv) Newer-generation cephalosporin (e.g., loracarbef, cefprozil, cefixime)

(v) *Note:* Because of resistance, oral amoxicillin and first-generation cephalosporins are not recommended.

(b) Symptomatic medication (for pain and bladder spasms) in patients 6 to 12 years of age: Phenazopyridine (Pyridium) 12 mg/kg/day orally three times a day (maximum 200-mg dose for 2 days)

(2) Ongoing therapy is directed by clinical response, result of urine culture, and sensitivity of offending organisms. The optimal duration of antimicrobial therapy for uncomplicated UTI is unclear. Short courses of therapy (1 to 4 days) are not currently recommended because of insufficient evidence to demonstrate superiority over conventional therapy (7 to 10 days in children).

(3) The expectation is that clinical improvement (a decrease in fever, pain, and dysuria) will occur within 24 to 48 hours.

b. Pyelonephritis and complicated UTI

(1) These often require parenteral antibiotics, hydration, and hospitalization.

Table 18-5 **Diagnostic Imaging in Pediatric Urinary Tract Infections**

Examination	Evaluates	Comments
Ultrasonography	*Kidney:* hydronephrosis, scarring, interval growth, duplication *Ureter:* dilation *Bladder:* ureterocele, wall thickening	Be sure to order as "renal/bladder ultrasound" because many centers scan only the kidneys unless otherwise specified; does *not* demonstrate renal *function*
Voiding cystourethrogram	Vesicoureteral reflux; posterior urethral valves	Should not be performed during *acute* infection—only after negative culture documented (usually 2-4 wk post-urinary tract infection)
Technetium-DMSA scan or technetium-GH scan	Renal function; renal scarring	Often obtained after pyelonephritis to monitor for renal scarring
Furosemide (Lasix) technetium-DTPA scan	Renal excretion	Obtained when uretero-pelvic junction obstruction or obstructive megaureter are considered
Intravenous pyelography	Renal function; anatomic detail of urinary tract	Becoming an outmoded test

DMSA, dimercaptosuccinic acid; DTPA, diethylene triamine pentaacetic acid; GH, glucoheptonate.

    (2) Ampicillin (100 to 200 mg/kg/day every 4 hours IV) can be used as initial therapy. A previous history of pyelonephritis or infection with a resistant organism indicates the need for broad-spectrum coverage by adding gentamicin (3 to 7.5 mg/kg/day) or by using a cephalosporin alone.

    (3) Response to therapy (reduction in fever, toxicity, pain) should occur in 48 to 72 hours.

  c. Requirements for neonates with UTI

    (1) Hospitalization

    (2) Parenteral antimicrobials: ampicillin/gentamicin

    (3) Urologic evaluation (see later)

  d. Monitoring initial therapy (24 to 48 hours after antimicrobials initiated) is based on clinical response. In uncomplicated UTI, a urine culture obtained 24 to 48 hours after institution of therapy should be sterile ($<10^4$ CFU/mL). In addition, a Gram stain of an unspun specimen should show no organisms or be below 5 WBC/mm^3.

  e. *Note:* Failure of clinical response should suggest a lack of compliance, an underdiagnosed underlying medical condition, or an anatomic abnormality.

9. Follow-up and monitoring: Because infection tends to recur, often in asymptomatic form, the follow-up of a UTI should be carefully organized. Recurrence is most likely during the first 6 to 12 months after an infection.

  a. In a complicated infection, after a course of antimicrobial therapy is completed, a urine culture can be obtained in 1 week to ensure proof of care.

  b. Postinfection imaging studies (Fig. 18-6)

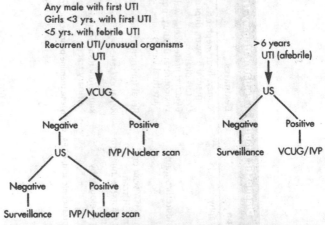

Figure 18-6 Algorithms for urinary tract infection (UTI) evaluation. IVP, intravenous pyelography; US, ultrasonography; VCUG, voiding cystourethrography. (Modified from Caldamone AA: Urinary tract infections in children. In Caldamone AA, Stein BS, Smith JA [eds]: Clinical Urologic Practice. New York, WW Norton, 1995.)

Table 18-6	Grades of Urinary Reflux
Grade	**Description**
I	Proximal ureter
II	Distal ureter
III	Mild dilatation
IV	Moderate dilatation, reflux to pelvis
V	Severe dilatation, reflux to pelvis

c. Among patients with significant reflux, recurrent infection is prevented by prophylactic antibiotic therapy, which is continued until the reflux resolves or is repaired.

d. Multiple recurrences of UTI can occur even with normal GU function. Patients should be carefully assessed for correctable contributing factors (see later). Prophylactic antibiotic therapy is often prescribed when infections are frequent, socially distressing, or associated with renal scarring. TMP/SMX (2 mg/kg/day TMP orally in 1 dose) or nitrofurantoin (2 mg/kg/day in 1 dose) may be used and continued for 6 to 12 months with serial monitoring of urine.

e. Home screening can assist in the follow-up of a UTI by using simple, inexpensive tests such as the nitrate chemical test for bacteria and agar-coated dip slides.

10. Complications of UTI
  a. Reflux
    (1) Grades of urinary reflux are classified in Table 18-6.
    (2) Reassess with radionuclide VCUG (less exposure to radiation) every 12 to 18 months.
    (3) Grade II or higher requires antibiotic prophylaxis (see later).
  b. Renal (within capsule) and perinephric (exterior to capsule) abscesses
    (1) Persistent fever, chills, toxicity, flank pain, despite appropriate therapy
    (2) May present with abdominal mass, extreme leukocytosis, high erythrocyte sedimentation rate, persistent pyuria/bacteriuria
    (3) US or abdominal CT for evaluation
    (4) Urologic consultation for percutaneous drainage (perinephric abscess)
    (5) Multiple antimicrobials as treatment
  c. Renal scarring: Scarring of the renal parenchyma from UTI/pyelonephritis or reflux is the most significant long-term sequela of UTIs because this can lead to a permanent loss of renal function.

11. Prevention/prophylaxis
  a. The goal is to prevent reflux-associated pyelonephritis.
  b. Use antibiotic prophylaxis for all grades of reflux.
  c. Antimicrobials (Table 18-7): TMP/SMX (2 mg/kg TMP) as a single bedtime dose or nitrofurantoin (1 to 2 mg/kg at bedtime), or sulfisoxazole (50 mg/kg at bedtime)
  d. Discontinue when reflux resolves.

18—Urologic Conditions

Table 18-7 Common Oral Antibiotics for Childhood Urinary Tract Infections

Antibiotic	How Supplied	Treatment	Prophylaxis
Amoxicillin	Suspension: 125 mg/5 mL, 250 mg/5 mL Chew tablets: 125 mg, 250 mg Capsules: 250 mg, 500 mg Infant (<8 kg) drops: 50 mg/mL	20-40 mg/kg/24 hr divided every 8 hr	5-10 mg/kg at bedtime if used
Sulfisoxazole*	Suspension: 500 mg/5 mL Syrup: 500 mg/5 mL Tablets: 500 mg	150 mg/kg/24 hr divided every 6 hr	40-50 mg/kg at bedtime
Nitrofurantoin†	Suspension (Furadantin): 25 mg/5 mL Capsule: 25 mg, 50 mg, 100 mg	5-7 mg/kg/24 hr divided every 6 hr	1-2 mg/kg at bedtime
TMP/SMX*	Suspension: 40 mg TMP/5 mL Single-strength tablets: 80 mg TMP Double-strength tablets: 160 mg TMP	8-10 mg TMP/kg/24 hr divided every 12 hr	2 mg TMP/kg at bedtime

*Contraindicated in infants younger than 2 months of age.
†Contraindicated in infants younger than 1 month of age.
TMP/SMX, trimethoprim/sulfamethoxazole.

e. Other preventive measures
  (1) Avoiding irritants
  (2) Wiping perineum area front to back
  (3) Increasing water intake
  (4) Emptying bladder every 3 to 4 hours
  (5) Wearing pure cotton underpants

SUGGESTED READING

Baker LA, Silver RI, Docimo DG: Cryptorchidism. In Gearhart JP, Rink RC, Mouriquand PDE (eds): Pediatric Urology. Philadelphia, WB Saunders, 2001.

Caldamone AA: Urinary tract infections in children. In Caldamone AA, Stein BS, Smith JA (eds): Clinical Urologic Practice. New York, WW Norton, 1995.

Canning DA, Pavlock C: Hernia and hydrocele in boys. In Resnick, Caldamone AA (eds): Atlas of the Urologic Clinics of North America. Philadelphia, Saunders-Elsevier, 2004, pp 1-13.

Keating MA, Rich MA: Hypospadiology. In Resnick, Caldamone AA (eds): Atlas of the Urologic Clinics of North America. Philadelphia, Saunders-Elsevier, 2004.

Kogan SJ, Hadziselimovic F, Howards SS, Huff D, Snyder HM III: The embryology and endocrinology of epididymal-testicular development and descent in humans. In Gillenwater JY, Grayhack JT, Howards SS, Mitchell ME (eds): Adult and Pediatric Urology, 4th ed. Philadelphia, Lippincott Williams & Wilkins, 2002.

Rabinowitz R, Hulbert WC Jr: Acute scrotal swelling. Urol Clin North Am 22: 101-105, 1995.

Shortliffe L: The management of urinary tract infection in children without urinary tract abnormalities. Urol Clin North Am 22:67-73, 1995.

Snyder HM, Caldamone AA: Genitourinary injuries. In Welch KJ, Randolph JG, Ravitch MM, et al. (eds): Pediatric Surgery, 4th ed. Chicago, Year Book Medical Publishers, 1986.

WEBSITES

American Academy of Family Physicians: Urinary Tract Infections in Children: www.aafp.org/afp/980515ap/heller.html

Children's Memorial Hospital: Hernia and Hydrocele: www.childrensmemorial.org/depts/urology/hernias.asp

Digital Urology Journal: Hypospadias: www.duj.com/hypospadias.html

Cryptorchidism: www.nlm.nih.gov/medlineplus/ency/article/000973.htm

Infectious Diseases 19

Anthony J. Alario, David Pugatch,
Emily C. Lutterloh, Stephen K. Obaro,
and Kelly L. Matson

19.1 Bacteremia and Sepsis

1. Definitions
   a. Bacteremia: Viable bacteria in the blood, documented by a positive blood culture. Bacteremia can be occult (described later), transient (e.g., dental procedures), or sustained (e.g., endocarditis, abscess).
   b. Sepsis: Suspicion of severe infection and systemic inflammatory response (ill or toxic appearance, hyperthermia or hypothermia, chills)
   c. Septic shock: Life-threatening, severe sepsis with hypotension that fails to respond promptly to routine fluid resuscitation. Etiology of sepsis/septic shock can be bacterial (discussed later) or viral.
   d. Multiple organ system dysfunction: Evidence of altered organ function (central nervous system [CNS], respiratory, cardiac) in a patient with septic shock
2. Pathophysiology: The pathophysiologic progression from bacteremia to multiple organ system failure is manifest through an interaction with the infecting organism, the body's defenses, and physiologic responses (Fig. 19-1).
3. Etiology
   a. Common bacterial causes of septic shock in children
      (1) *Streptococcus pneumoniae* (becoming less frequent with immunization)
      (2) *Neisseria meningitidis*
      (3) Group B streptococci
      (4) *Haemophilus influenzae* (becoming less frequent with immunization)
      (5) *Staphylococcus aureus*
      (6) *Escherichia coli*
      (7) *Listeria*
      (8) *Staphylococcus epidermidis*
      (9) *Streptococcus viridans*
   b. Factors predisposing children to bacteremia/sepsis (although on many occasions no underlying cause is identified)

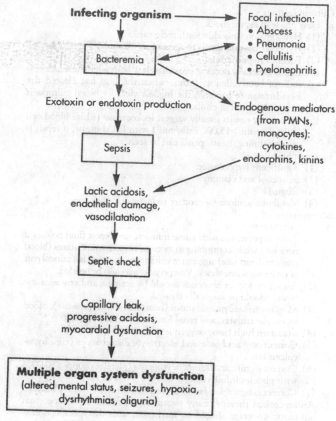

Pathophysiologic progression of bacterial infection. PMN, polymorphonuclear leukocyte.

(1) Trauma (including minor trauma)
(2) Burns
(3) Chronic illness (even without obvious immunocompromise)
(4) Complicated surgery
(5) Complicated urinary tract infection (UTI)
(6) Immunocompromise (human immunodeficiency virus [HIV], medications)
(7) Indwelling catheters
(8) Intra-abdominal conditions (obstruction, perforation)
(9) Malnutrition

4. Clinical features
   a. Early phase of septic shock
      (1) Hypotension (vasodilation), tachycardia
      (2) Hyperventilation (leads to respiratory alkalosis)
      (3) Fever or hypothermia
      (4) Chills generally occur approximately 1 hour after the acute episode of bacteremia at a time when the host has cleared the bloodstream of bacteria; the highest yield for blood cultures is before the onset of chills.
      (5) Laboratory results usually suggest leukocytosis (white blood cell [WBC] count >15,000 cells/mm^3) with left shift, or, if sepsis is overwhelming, neutropenia can be seen.
   b. Late phase
      (1) Significant hypotension
      (2) Skin cool and clammy
      (3) Oliguria
      (4) Metabolic acidosis (secondary to lactic acidosis)
5. Management
   a. Supportive care
      (1) Treat hypotension with saline infusion, and repeat fluid boluses if necessary while continuing to monitor hemodynamic status (blood pressure, heart rate); aggressive volume resuscitation is a critical part of reversing septic shock. Vasopressors may also be needed.
      (2) All septic foci or abscesses should be drained, and any necrotic bowel should be surgically treated.
      (3) Monitor hemodynamic status (heart rate, blood pressure), blood gases, electrolytes, and renal function (urinary output).
      (4) Maintain high tissue oxygen levels; avoid hypoxemia.
      (5) Correct any acid-base and electrolyte disturbances (e.g., hypocalcemia).
      (6) Correct significant thrombocytopenia (platelet counts ≤50,000) with platelet infusions.
      (7) Correct coagulation factor depletion with fresh frozen plasma.
   b. Antimicrobial therapy: Early treatment is crucial. Broad-spectrum antibiotic coverage should be instituted, with the specific agents depending on the suspected source of infection and underlying factors. Antibiotic coverage should be narrowed when the etiologic agent and its antibiotic sensitivities are determined.
      (1) Neutropenic patient: A beta-lactam (ceftazidime, cefepime) to cover *Pseudomonas* and other gram-negative organisms, and consider vancomycin for gram-positive coverage.
      (2) Suspected skin source: Vancomycin to cover methicillin-resistant *S. aureus* (MRSA), and clindamycin if a toxin-producing *Streptococcus* or *Staphylococcus* is suspected.
      (3) Suspected intra-abdominal process: Ampicillin (to cover enterococci), an aminoglycoside (gram-negative coverage), and clindamycin or metronidazole (anaerobic coverage).
      (4) Suspected pulmonary infection: A cephalosporin (cefuroxime, ceftriaxone), and consider vancomycin if staphylococcal pneumonia is suspected

(5) Suspected UTI (e.g., urosepsis, pyelonephritis, abscess): Ampicillin (to cover enterococci) and an aminoglycoside for additional gram-negative coverage.

19.2 Occult Bacteremia and Management of the Febrile Infant

1. Definition and etiology
   a. Occult bacteremia is unsuspected blood-borne bacterial infection; that is, the patient is sent home without the knowledge of the etiology of the infection and is later identified to have bacteremia.
   b. The most common organism has been S. pneumoniae. However, the number of invasive S. pneumoniae infections is decreasing with increasing use of pneumococcal conjugate vaccine.[2]
   c. Risk of meningitis is a major concern and is related to the causative organism. Risk is highest with meningococcal, intermediate with H. influenzae, and lower with pneumococcal bacteremia.
2. Clinical features and epidemiology
   a. It is most common in children 3 to 24 months of age, with a higher prevalence in urban poor; it is much less likely in suburban and rural populations unless predisposing factors are present.
   b. Overall, approximately 3% to 5% of febrile 3- to 24-month-olds have bacteremia (3% to 5% of those may develop meningitis).
   c. Poor appearance is often associated with serious bacterial illness, whereas well appearance does not exclude it.
   d. A temperature above 39.5° C, age under 18 months, and WBC count above 15,000 cells/mm³ are predictive of those children most likely to be bacteremic.
3. Identification and management of the infant with a temperature above 38.0° C but without a focus for infection: The vast majority of these infants will have viral infections as a source of their fever. The following are often termed the Rochester criteria and apply primarily to previously well infants. A chronically ill infant may merit a complete evaluation for sepsis if highly febrile or ill appearing.
   a. Neonates 0 to 28 days of age
      (1) It is often difficult to identify an infant this young who may be bacteremic. Observation, clinical assessment, or laboratory evaluations may not be reliable or helpful.
      (2) Work-up should be similar to that for infants 29 to 90 days of age (see later and Fig. 19-2) with the caveat that after a complete clinical and laboratory evaluation, hospital admission for observation should be considered, and presumptive antimicrobial treatment should be given for infants 0 to 28 days of age with fever.
   b. Infants 29 to 90 days of age
      (1) Identification of infants at low risk for bacteremia is a potentially helpful strategy in this age group.
         (a) Criteria to define low-risk infants between 29 days and 3 months of age
            (i) Good appearance (i.e., not toxic or septic appearing)

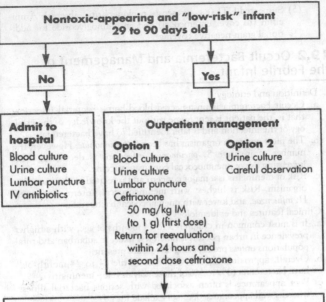

Figure 19-2 Management of febrile infant 29–90 days old. (Adapted from Baraff LJ: Practice guideline for the management of infants and children 0 to 36 months of age with fever without source. Ann Emerg Med 36:602–614, 2000.)

(ii) No past history of perinatal/neonatal complications/ illness
(iii) No focal signs of infection (except otitis media)
(iv) WBC count between 5000 and 15,000/mm^3
(v) Total band count under 1500/mm^3
(vi) Normal urinalysis (5 WBCs/high-power field [hpf]) or a negative Gram stain smear for bacteremia
(vii) If diarrhea is present, less than 5 WBCs/hpf in stool

(b) Note that this strategy will not exclude all infants with serious infection (i.e., even if all criteria are fulfilled, bacteremia, especially in early stages, can still be present).

(2) Management: Figure 19-2 illustrates strategies for the management of a previously healthy infant 29 to 90 days of age with fever (≥38.0° C) and no source.

c. Infants 91 days to 36 months of age
(1) General assessment: For older infants, illness severity (i.e., "toxicity") can be best assessed by observation of key clinical items.[1]
(a) Quality of cry (i.e., is cry strong or weak, moaning or high pitched?)
(b) Reaction to parent stimulation (i.e., is the child content/consolable or hardly responsive or irritable?)
(c) State variation (i.e., is the child awake/alert or awake only with prolonged stimulation?)
(d) Response to social overtures (i.e., does the child interact with observer and smile, or is the child dull, expressionless?).
(2) Management (Fig. 19-3)
(3) Antibiotic selection (Table 19-1)

19.3 Infections of the Central Nervous System

BACTERIAL MENINGITIS

1. Etiology of bacterial meningitis differs depending on age.
   a. Neonate to 28 days: Gram-negatives, group B streptococci, Listeria, S. pneumoniae, others
   b. 29 days to 24 months: S. pneumoniae, N. meningitidis, type b H. influenzae, S. aureus, gram-negatives, others
   c. Over 24 months: S. pneumoniae, N. meningitidis, other streptococci, type b H. influenzae, tuberculosis (TB), others
2. Clinical features
   a. Infants: In this age group the presenting symptoms and signs may be nonspecific.
   (1) High-pitched cry
   (2) Irritability
   (3) Anorexia
   (4) Vomiting
   (5) Lethargy
   (6) Full fontanelle
   (7) Meningeal signs are uncommon, and fever may not invariably be present.
   (8) Seizures may be an early manifestation of meningitis.

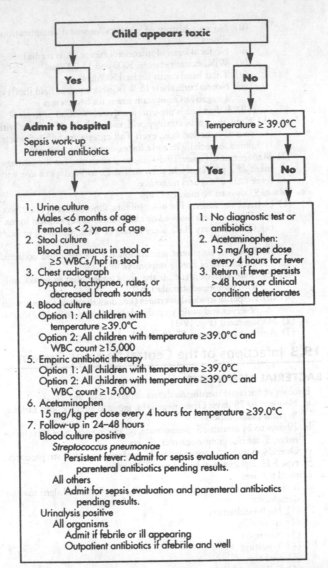

Figure 19-3 Management of febrile infant 92 days to 36 months of age. WBC, white blood cell count. (Adapted from Baraff LJ, Brass JW, Fleisher GR, et al: Practice guideline for the management of infants and children 0 to 36 months of age with fever without source. Ann Emerg Med 36:602–614, 2000.)

Table 19-1 **Antibiotics for Bacteremia**	
Situation	**Suggested Regimen**
Neonate (age ≤4 days) or community acquired	AMP + AG or CTX
Neonate (age >4 days)	Antistaph* + AG or CAZ
Infant (age 1-3 mo)	AMP + CTX or CRO
Older infants and children	CFX, CRO, or CTX
Immunocompromised or nosocomial	Vancomycin + AG or CAZ

*Antistaphylococcal agent based on expected susceptibility.
Many other regimens are possible depending on history, expected susceptibility, and condition. Amphotericin is added in 4 to 7 days if no response occurs in an immunocompromised patient.
AG, aminoglycoside; AMP, ampicillin; CAZ, ceftazidime; CFX, cefuroxime; CRO, ceftriaxone; CTX, cefotaxime.

b. Older children (≥12 months)
(1) Meningeal signs (stiff neck, nuchal rigidity) are more reliable in older children.
(2) Brudzinski's sign (passive flexion of the head on the chest with the patient supine causes involuntary flexion of the hips) may be present.
c. A lumbar puncture (LP) must be performed as soon as the diagnosis is suspected.
d. Papilledema, suggesting increased intracranial pressure (ICP), is a relative contraindication to LP. However, a patient may be pretreated with mannitol (0.25 to 1.0 g/kg intravenously [IV]) 15 to 30 minutes before performing an LP. If necessary, treat with antibiotics first, and then obtain an LP once the patient is stable.
(1) Papilledema is rare in acute bacterial meningitis, and its presence may suggest other diagnostic possibilities (e.g., brain abscess).
(2) Neurologic consultation should be considered.
3. Diagnosis
a. An LP must be performed as soon as the diagnosis is suspected if there are no obvious contraindications, such as papilledema.
b. Interpretation of the cerebrospinal fluid (CSF) in bacterial meningitis
(1) The CSF can be cloudy, under increased pressure, with more than 100 WBCs/mm³ (predominantly neutrophils). Elevated total protein, low glucose (less than one half blood glucose), and organisms on a Gram stain smear are also done.
(2) Classic features may be absent, and if meningitis is clinically suspected, treatment should not be delayed. A CSF culture will confirm the diagnosis.
c. Other diagnostic procedures include a complete blood count (CBC) with differential, blood culture, blood smear, and cultures from any purpuric lesions; cultures of other body fluids (e.g., stool, urine, joint fluid, abscess, middle ear); blood urea nitrogen (BUN); serum and urine electrolytes and osmolarity; and placing a tuberculin skin test (purified protein derivative [PPD]).

4. Management: Antimicrobial therapy must be initiated as soon as possible—immediately after bacteriologic specimens have been obtained (Table 19-2).
   a. Antimicrobials
      (1) The initial choice of antibiotics usually is based on the patient's age, the results of the CSF Gram stain smear, and other underlying conditions.
      (2) For patients who respond rapidly with appropriate antimicrobial agent, 7 to 10 days of therapy is sufficient. Longer duration of treatment is usually required for gram-negative bacteria (Table 19-3).
   b. Dexamethasone
      (1) The goal of steroid therapy is to reduce the incidence of short (elevated ICP) and long-term (hearing impairment) sequelae from meningitis.
      (2) Dexamethasone therapy has been shown to be most efficacious for H. influenzae meningitis; its efficacy in other forms of meningitis is unclear.
      (3) Consider its use in infants and children 6 weeks of age and older with suspected bacterial meningitis. Begin treatment as early as possible (i.e., 10 to 20 minutes before, or at least concomitant with, the first dose of antimicrobials; after 12 hours of antimicrobial therapy, it is unlikely to be effective).
      (4) Recommended dosing
          (a) 0.15 mg/kg/dose, given every 6 hours IV for 4 days
          (b) As above, but for 2 days is an alternative regimen
      (5) Not useful for "partially treated" or aseptic meningitis
      (6) Major adverse effect is gastrointestinal (GI) bleeding; monitor for bleeding with hemoglobin and stools for blood.
   c. Other aspects of management
      (1) In addition, attention must be paid to ensuring adequate peripheral perfusion and correcting fluid, electrolyte imbalance, and coagulopathies.
      (2) Frequent recording of vital signs and daily neurologic examinations, with measurement of head circumference in children with open fontanelles
      (3) Fluid status should be closely monitored. The Syndrome of Inappropriate Anti-Diuretic Hormone (SIADH) can occur secondary to cerebral edema injury within the first 72 hours.
      (4) A repeat LP should be obtained after 24 to 48 hours of therapy in patients who respond poorly to treatment. If treatment is effective, cultures and stains are usually negative after 48 hours.
      (5) Fever during the first 48 to 72 hours of therapy can occur and should not be surprising.
          (a) Once adequate therapy begins, the duration of fever typically varies between 4 to 6 days. H. influenzae meningitis is associated with relatively longer duration of fever.
          (b) Prolonged or secondary fever should prompt evaluation for inadequate treatment, nosocomial infection, phlebitis, immune-mediated arthritis, or suppurative complications

Predisposing Factor	Common Bacterial Pathogen	Antimicrobial Therapy
Age		
<1 mo	Group B streptococci, E. coli, L. monocytogenes, Klebsiella species	Ampicillin plus cefotaxime or ampicillin plus an aminoglycoside
1-23 mo	S. pneumoniae, N. meningitidis, Group B streptococci, E. coli, H. influenzae type b	Vancomycin plus a third-generation cephalosporin Vancomycin plus ampicillin plus a third-generation cephalosporin
>23 mo	N. meningitidis, S. pneumoniae	Vancomycin alone or vancomycin plus ceftazidime or vancomycin plus meropenem (if gram-negative agent suspected)
Cerebrospinal fluid shunt	Coagulase-negative staphylococci, S. aureus, Propionibacterium acnes, aerobic gram-negative bacilli (including P. aeruginosa)	
Post neurosurgery	S. aureus, coagulase-negative staphylococci, aerobic gram-negative bacilli (including P. aeruginosa)	Same as for cerebrospinal fluid shunt
Head trauma		
Basilar skull fracture	S. pneumoniae, H. influenzae, group A β-hemolytic streptococci	Vancomycin plus a third-generation cephalosporin
Penetrating trauma	S. aureus, coagulase-negative staphylococci, aerobic gram-negative bacilli (including P. aeruginosa)	Vancomycin plus cefepime, vancomycin plus ceftazidime, or vancomycin plus meropenem

Microorganism	Duration of Therapy (Days)
Group A streptococci	14-21
S. pneumoniae	10-14
N. meningitidis	7
H. influenzae	7
Aerobic gram-negative bacilli	21*
L. monocytogenes	≥21

*Neonates should be treated for 2 weeks beyond the first sterile cerebrospinal fluid culture, or more than 3 weeks, whichever is longer.

(e.g., abscess in the subdural space, bones, joints, pericardium, or pleural spaces). It may also be due to drug fever, but sometimes the cause is unknown.

(6) At the completion of antimicrobial therapy, children should be observed for 24 to 48 hours or longer before discharge from the hospital. (Relapse of bacterial meningitis generally occurs on the third day after completion of antimicrobial therapy). A routine LP at the end of adequate therapy is usually not necessary if the patient has had a satisfactory clinical course.

(7) Close household and day care center contacts of children with meningitis are at increased risk, especially from type b H. influenzae (the risk is about 0.5% for household contacts younger than 6 years of age) and N. meningitidis (the risk is about 0.5% for all persons). Observation for fever/illness is important, and prophylaxis should be considered for persons at risk (consult the Red Book, 27th edition [American Academy of Pediatrics, 2006]).

(8) All children with invasive disease due to N. meningitidis should receive rifampin therapy (10 mg/kg dose once daily for 2 days; maximum 600 mg/day) before discharge to eradicate carriage from the nasopharynx.

(9) Acute complications possibly affecting management include
  (a) Seizures, shock, disseminated intravascular coagulation
  (b) Subdural effusions (e.g., empyema)
  (c) Shift of brain contents due to increased ICP and cerebral edema with herniation or compression of brain tissue

5. Outcome
  a. Mortality: If detected and treated early and there are no secondary complications, the mortality rate is between 3% and 10% (higher in newborns and the elderly).
  b. Sequelae
    (1) Focal neurologic deficits: Vasculitis secondary to meningitis can lead to possible deficits, such as cortical vein thrombosis, cerebral infarction, cortical necrosis, hemiparesis, quadriparesis, spinal cord infarction, epilepsy, diabetes insipidus.

(2) Hydrocephalus: Secondary to obstruction of CSF flow
(3) Of children who survive, 20% to 30% or more may have long-term sequelae (e.g., loss of cognitive skills, deafness, perceptual handicaps).

ASEPTIC (BACTERIAL CULTURE–NEGATIVE) MENINGITIS

1. Etiology: Caused by enteroviruses, herpes simplex virus type 2 (HSV-2), *Borrelia burgdorferi* (Lyme disease; Table 19-4).
2. Clinical features
   a. Cases of viral meningitis outnumber bacterial 30 to 1.
   b. Viral meningitis is most prevalent from May to September.
   c. Photophobia, headaches, rash, and constitutional symptoms are presenting complaints.
   d. CSF evaluation
      (1) Cell count is usually below 500 total WBCs (although counts can be in the thousands).
      (2) Early in viral meningitis, polymorphonuclear leukocytes (PMNs) may predominate; later the majority of cells are lymphocytes, although conversion to lymphocytosis may not occur.
      (3) Glucose is over 50 mg/dL, and protein is under 100 mg/dL (with TB, an elevated protein may be seen).
3. Management
   a. Supportive measures include early restriction of fluids, fever control, analgesia, and bed rest.
   b. Antivirals are used depending on identified etiology (e.g., acyclovir for HSV meningoencephalitis, which has been associated with significant CNS sequelae such as seizures and visual and intellectual impairments).
   c. Sequelae from viral meningitis are unlikely, but seizures may occur early; some degree of hearing loss has been reported.

	Frequent Causes	**Infrequent Causes**
Viruses	Enteroviruses	Mumps
	Arboviruses	Lymphocytic choriomeningitis virus
	Herpes simplex virus type 2	Human immunodeficiency virus
Bacteria	*Borrelia burgdorferi* Partially treated bacterial meningitis	*Mycobacterium tuberculosis*
	Parameningeal focus	*Leptospira* species
Other		Fungi
		Mycoplasma pneumoniae

BRAIN ABSCESS

1. Pathophysiology and etiology: Brain abscess can develop through hematogenous or contiguous spread. Organisms are from upper airway or mouth flora and include aerobes (α-hemolytic streptococci, S. aureus), anaerobes (Peptococcus, Bacteroides), or some combination.
2. Clinical features
   a. History: Should uncover possible predisposing causes (Box 19-1)
      (1) Headache, seizures, confusion, disorientation, behavioral changes, and speech disturbances are common.
      (2) Fever is not often prominent.
   b. Physical examination: Identify extracranial foci of infection and neurologic impairment, which may be reflective of the anatomic site of the abscess (e.g., aphasia with temporal lobe lesion, or dizziness and ataxia with cerebellar lesions). The examination may also be entirely nonfocal. An LP should be done unless contraindicated (e.g., increased ICP).
   c. Laboratory: Blood cultures and neuroimaging studies (computed tomography [CT] or magnetic resonance imaging [MRI]), as well as examination of CSF if LP done
   d. Diagnosis: Neuroimaging is used to confirm an intracranial mass or small abscess.
3. Management
   a. Initial empirical antibiotic therapy usually includes ceftriaxone (100 mg/kg/day) and metronidazole (30 mg/kg/day IV) or sulbactam-ampicillin at least 200 mg/kg/day alone. This can be modified once a bacteriologic etiology is identified. In patients who have an underlying condition (e.g., a shunt) that predisposes to the development of brain abscesses, selection of antibiotic is based on most likely causative agent (see earlier).
   b. Aspiration and surgical drainage is helpful to identify a bacterial etiology and provide a cure.
   c. To control brain swelling, fluids should be restricted; mannitol and dexamethasone can be given in the presence of cerebral edema.
   d. Radionuclide or CT scans are helpful to monitor resolution of the abscess as well as to determine the duration of antibiotic therapy follow-up.

Box 19-1   Predisposing Conditions for Development of Brain Abscess

Cyanotic congenital heart disease
Chronic otitis media
Bacterial meningitis
Penetrating head injury
Sinusitis
Cystic fibrosis

19.4 Skin and Soft Tissue Infections

CELLULITIS OF THE HEAD AND NECK

1. Buccal cellulitis
   a. Pathophysiology and etiology
      (1) Buccal cellulitis is the result of inflammation of the soft tissues above the buccinator muscle of either cheek caused by bacteremic spread of either *S. pneumoniae* or *H. influenzae* type B.
      (2) Buccal cellulitis is most common in the child between 6 and 24 months of age.
   b. Clinical features: A bacteremic disease, it is associated with fever and an acutely tender, erythematous, indurated cheek with unilateral swelling. A break in the skin is usually not seen.
   c. Management
      (1) Blood cultures should always be obtained.
      (2) Empirical treatment for buccal cellulitis requires antibiotics active in tissues, blood, and CSF against *H. influenzae* and *S. pneumoniae*. Ceftriaxone (75 to 100 mg/kg/day IV every 8 hours [maximum 9 g/day]) or cefotaxime (100 to 150 mg/kg/day [maximum 2 g/day]) is appropriate. When meningitis is suspected, vancomycin should be added.
2. Facial cellulitis (not limited to preseptal or buccal areas)
   a. Etiology
      (1) Secondary to trauma that disrupts the integrity of the skin (e.g., foreign objects, insect bites, human bites). Causative organisms are *S. aureus* or group A β-hemolytic streptococci (GABHS).
      (2) Intraoral trauma or dental abscess: Causative organisms are anaerobic and *Streptococcus* species of the mouth.
      (3) Secondary to cervical lymphadenitis (look for history of lymph node swelling and tenderness on same side): Causative organisms are *S. aureus* or GABHS.
   b. Clinical features
      (1) The clinical presentation of facial cellulitis with an identified portal of skin entry (which may include the periorbital or buccal areas) is a gradual increase of swelling, erythema, and tenderness.
      (2) Facial cellulitis due to intraoral trauma or dental abscess may be slowly or rapidly progressive, depending on location and types of bacteria involved. Children frequently have difficulty swallowing or speaking.
   c. Management
      (1) Treatment of facial cellulitis for which a portal of skin entry is identified requires antibiotic treatment with activity against *S. aureus* and GABHS. A first-generation cephalosporin (e.g., cefazolin) or beta-lactam–stable penicillin (e.g., nafcillin) is usually sufficient. However, because of the increasing prevalence of community-associated MRSA, vancomycin should be considered in a child who presents with symptoms of toxicity.
      (2) Dental evaluation should be obtained for a child with an intraoral infection. Dental extraction is usually required for children

with dental abscesses associated with facial swelling. Antibiotic treatment with penicillin or clindamycin treats the usual offending organisms.

CELLULITIS OF THE EXTREMITIES AND TRUNK

1. Etiology: *S. aureus* and GABHS (erysipelas).
2. Clinical features
   a. Characteristically, the involved superficial skin is warm, erythematous, tender, and sometimes indurated. Noninfectious causes of localized skin erythema and swelling (i.e., urticaria, bug bites), may become secondarily infected and become sources for cellulitis.
   b. Streptococcal cellulitis (erysipelas) is suggested by an advancing, well-demarcated erythema with heaped-up borders; facial involvement may assume a "butterfly" distribution.
3. Diagnosis
   a. A CBC and erythrocyte sedimentation rate (ESR) should be obtained to assess the degree of systemic response.
   b. A blood culture should be performed on patients with cellulitis and systemic symptoms (fever, generalized toxicity) or in immunocompromised patients.
   c. *Warning*: The child with apparent cellulitis who has fever, toxic clinical appearance, and severe pain may have a deep soft tissue infection such as necrotizing fasciitis, which is a medical/surgical emergency.
4. Management
   a. Immobilization and elevation of the affected extremity and application of warm compresses, 10 to 20 minutes, four times or more a day, can be helpful.
   b. Incision and drainage of any primary suppurative focus may be necessary for refractory cases.
   c. Antimicrobials
      (1) Localized cellulitis of the extremity or trunk without fever usually responds well to oral antimicrobials such as first-generation cephalosporins (e.g., cephalexin).
      (2) Cellulitis with systemic toxicity (high fever, elevated WBC count and ESR)
         (a) Nafcillin or oxacillin, 100 to 200 mg/kg/day IV every 4 to 6 hours, maximum 12 g/day, *or*
         (b) Cefazolin (Ancef), 75 to 100 mg/kg/day, maximum 6 g/day
         (c) For communities where rates of community-associated MRSA are more than 10% to 15%, start empirical therapy with clindamycin or TMP/SMX; use vancomycin for seriously ill patients (i.e., toxic-appearing, immunocompromised, or patients with a limb-threatening infection).
      (3) Immunocompromised patients: Use an antibiotic effective against gram-negative enteric organisms and *Pseudomonas* (e.g., ceftazidime).
      (4) Streptococcal disease or erysipelas: Benzathine penicillin G (Bicillin) 0.6 to 1.2 MU intramuscularly (IM) 1 dose, or oral penicillin V 25 to 50 mg/kg/day orally every 6 hours for 10 days (tablets 125, 250, 500 mg; elixir, 125, 250 mg/5 mL), *or*

procaine penicillin G 600,000 to 900,000 U IM every 12 hours, or penicillin 100,000 U/kg/day IV every 4 hours. Treatment should be continued for 7 to 10 days.

NECROTIZING FASCIITIS

1. Pathophysiology and etiology
   a. Necrotizing fasciitis is a severe soft tissue infection involving the fascia and surrounding tissues. When muscle is involved, the terms *necrotizing bacterial myositis* or *myonecrosis* may be used.
   b. Necrotizing fasciitis may follow a wound or traumatic soft tissue injury, or may arise spontaneously.
   c. The causative organisms may be GABHS or *S. aureus* alone, or may involve a mixture of aerobic and anaerobic organisms.
   d. In neonates, omphalitis (infection around the umbilical stump) may present as a necrotizing fasciitis, and is usually due to a mixture of gram-positive, gram-negative, and anaerobic organisms.
2. Clinical features
   a. Erythema, tenderness, and edema may develop as early as 2 to 3 days and as late as 2 weeks after an initial traumatic injury.
   b. As the infection progresses, the overlying skin may develop discoloration, vesicles, blisters, or bullae.
   c. There may be crepitance on examination, and the skin may become gangrenous and slough.
   d. The child usually appears clinically "septic," especially as the disease progresses, although blood cultures are usually negative.
3. Diagnosis: An MRI scan of the involved tissues can help to confirm the diagnosis.
4. Management
   a. Necrotizing fasciitis require aggressive surgical and medical management. An emergent surgical consult should be obtained and immediate extensive surgical debridement is necessary, ensuring all devitalized tissue is removed. Gram stain and cultures of the wound tissues should be sent.
   b. Empirical antimicrobial treatment initially should be very broad in spectrum and include coverage for *S. aureus*, GABHS, clostridial species, and gram-negative organisms (e.g., a regimen of vancomycin plus ceftriaxone plus an aminoglycoside). Consider adding clindamycin if patient has associated toxic shock syndrome in addition to necrotizing fasciitis (decreases toxin production).

IMPETIGO

1. Pathophysiology and etiology: Staphylococci (*S. aureus*), streptococci
2. Clinical features
   a. Staphylococci (*S. aureus*) generally cause a *bullous* type of lesion that may denude, leaving a clean, eroded base of erythema.
   b. Streptococci are usually associated with *crusted*, "honey-colored," non-bullous lesions; they may be secondarily infected with staphylococci.
3. Diagnosis
   a. Usually made by clinical appearance: Multiple, usually circular lesions, sometimes coalesced, with or without regional lymphadenopathy

b. Gram stain and culture of fluid-filled bullae usually are not necessary.
4. Management: Depends on extent of cutaneous involvement
   a. Localized (i.e., minimal cutaneous involvement with few lesions)
      (1) Cleanse with 3% hexachlorophene soap.
      (2) Topical antibiotic ointment (e.g., mupirocin) can be applied to the lesions two to three times daily for 7 to 10 days.
      (3) If no prompt resolution, consider an alternative diagnosis or treat with systemic antimicrobials.
   b. Disseminated involvement: For multiple lesions (e.g., more than 8 to 10), systemic therapy with an antistaphylococcal agent (e.g., first-generation cephalosporin or beta-lactamase–resistant antibiotic) is indicated for 7 to 10 days.
      (1) Cephalexin (Keflex) 20 to 50 mg/kg/day orally every 6 hours or
      (2) Cefadroxil (Duricef) 30 mg/kg/day orally every 12 to 24 hours or
      (3) Amoxicillin/clavulanic acid (Augmentin) 20 to 40 mg/kg/day orally every 8 hours or 25 to 45 mg/kg/day orally every 12 hours
   c. In addition to systemic antimicrobial treatment, recurrences may be prevented by "decontamination" of colonized skin by having the child scrub in shower or bath with an antibacterial soap (neck to toes), twice a day for 3 straight days. Application of mupirocin 2% ointment twice a day to the nares for 5 days may help to decrease staphylococcal carriage in patients with recurrent infections.
   d. Persistent infections may be due to resistance (i.e., community-associated MRSA) and may warrant changing antimicrobial coverage to oral TMP/SMX or clindamycin.
   e. Pyogenic infections involving the hair follicle (e.g., folliculitis, furuncles, carbuncles)
      (1) Usual cause of furuncles and carbuncles is *S. aureus*. Infrequently, gram-negative organisms, including *Pseudomonas aeruginosa*, are isolated.
      (2) Because furuncles and carbuncles (a coalescence of several furuncles) are abscesses, incision and drainage is indicated for fluctuant lesions, in addition to antibiotics, as previously.
5. Complications: Impetigo caused by streptococci M-types 49 or 55 can result in poststreptococcal glomerulonephritis, but rheumatic fever is not a common sequela of skin infection.

STAPHYLOCOCCAL SCALDED SKIN SYNDROME AND STAPHYLOCOCCAL SCARLET FEVER

1. Pathophysiology and etiology: These represent a spectrum of dermatologic manifestations of staphylococcal infection related to the release of soluble toxins by *S. aureus*.
2. Clinical features
   a. Staphylococcal scalded skin syndrome (SSS) begins as a prodrome of abrupt onset of fever, irritability, and skin tenderness, followed by intense erythema beginning at the head and neck, and rapidly spreading distally.
   b. Large, flaccid bullae may appear.
   c. Exfoliation can occur in large sheets beginning in the flexure surfaces.

d. Nikolsky's sign (gentle rubbing of noninvolved skin results in slough-ing of the epidermis) is suggestive of SSS; its absence, however, does not exclude the diagnosis.

3. Diagnosis
   a. Cultures of the skin, nose, throat, and blood should be obtained.
   b. Differentiate direct staphylococcal skin invasion (i.e., impetigo) from toxin-mediated skin changes: aspirated fluid from intact bullae in bullous impetigo may contain organisms on culture and Gram stain, but will be sterile in SSS. However, in SSS, cultures of the nares, pharynx, or other source of infection may be positive.

4. Management
   a. A 7- to 10-day parenteral course of a penicillinase-resistant antimi-crobial: oxacillin or nafcillin 100 to 200 mg/kg/day IV every 4 hours, maximum 12 g/day. Because of the increasing problem of community-associated MRSA, vancomycin should be used for severe or life-threatening disease.
   b. After a good clinical response has been achieved, therapy may usu-ally be completed with an oral penicillinase-resistant agent.
   c. Apply saline compresses to denuded areas to decrease fluid loss.
   d. Hydration and maintenance of normal body temperature are impor-tant in patients with extensive skin losses. Unnecessary skin trauma (e.g., adhesive from tape) should be avoided.
   e. Topical antibiotics are not necessary.

BITES

1. Animal bites
   a. Epidemiology and etiology
      (1) Approximately 1 to 2 million Americans are bitten each year by animals.
      (2) The common pathogens causing bite-wound infections are S. *aureus*, anaerobic and microaerophilic streptococci, other anaerobic cocci, *Clostridium* species (including *Clostridium tetani*), *Pasteurella multocida*, *Corynebacterium* species, aerobic enteric gram-negative bacilli, *Bacteroides* species, *Streptobacillus moniliformis*, and *Spirillum minus* (the latter two are associated with rat bite fever).
   b. Management
      (1) Assess the extent of the wound (depth, amount of tissue destruc-tion) and the patient's immunity to tetanus.
      (2) Cleansing and local antisepsis help prevent bacterial complica-tions.
      (3) Surgical care of a deep, extensive bite includes irrigation, debridement, and in some cases antimicrobial therapy (Table 19-5).
      (4) Prophylactic measures for rabies or tetanus should be considered (Table 19-6 and section on tetanus prophylaxis).
      (5) Antimicrobial prophylaxis with oral amoxicillin-clavulanate (40 mg/kg/24 hours amoxicillin) or IV ampicillin/sulbactam (100 to 200 mg/kg/24 hours) should be considered, especially for bites on the face, hands, feet, or genitals.

| | Time from Injury | |
Category of Management	<8 Hours	≥8 Hours
Method of cleaning	Sponge away visible dirt. Irrigate with a copious volume of sterile saline solution by high-pressure syringe irrigation.* Do not irrigate puncture wounds.	Sponge away visible dirt. Irrigate with a copious volume of sterile saline solution by high-pressure syringe irrigation.* Do not irrigate puncture wounds.
Wound culture	No—unless signs of infection exist	Yes—except in wounds of >24 hr duration without signs of infection
Debridement	Remove devitalized tissue	Same as for wounds of <8 hr duration Remove devitalized tissue
Operative debridement and exploration	Yes, if one of the following: Extensive wounds (devitalized tissue) Involvement of the metacarpophalangeal joint (closed fist injury) Cranial bites by large animal†	Yes, if one of the following: Extensive wounds (devitalized tissue) Involvement of the metacarpophalangeal joint (closed fist injury) Cranial bites by large animal†
Wound closure	Yes, for nonpuncture bite wounds	No
Assess tetanus immunization status	Yes	Yes
Assess risk of rabies from animal bites	Yes	Yes
Assess risk of hepatitis B from human bites	Yes	Yes
Assess risk of HIV infection from human bites	Yes	Yes

Initiate antimicrobial therapy	Yes, for: Moderate or severe bite wounds, especially if edema or crush injury is present Puncture wounds, especially if penetration of bone, tendon sheath, or joint has occurred Facial bites Hand or foot bites Genital area bites Wounds in immunocompromised and asplenic people	Yes, for: Moderate or severe bite wounds, especially if edema or crush injury is present Puncture wounds, especially if penetration of bone, tendon sheath or joint has occurred Facial bites Hand or foot bites Genital area bites Wounds in immunocompromised and asplenic people
Follow-up	Inspect wound for signs of infection within 48 h	Same as that for wounds of <8 hr duration

*Use of an 18-gauge needle with a large-volume syringe is effective. Antimicrobial or anti-infective solutions offer no advantage and may increase tissue irritation.

†Radiographic studies in facial and head injuries are indicated if penetrating central nervous system injury is suspected.

HIV, human immunodeficiency virus.

Adapted from American Academy of Pediatrics; Pickering LK, Baker CJ, Long SS, McMillan JA (eds): Red Book: 2006 Report of the Committee on Infectious Diseases, 27th ed. Elk Grove, III, American Academy of Pediatrics, 2006.

Animal Type	Evaluation and Disposition of Animal	Postexposure Prophylaxis Recommendations
Dogs, cats, and ferrets	Healthy and available for 10 days of observation Rabid or suspected rabid Unknown (escaped)	Do not begin prophylaxis unless animal develops symptoms of rabies.* Immediate vaccination and RIG. Consult public health officials for advice.
Skunks, raccoons, bats, foxes, and most other carnivores; woodchucks	Regarded as rabid unless geographic area is known to be free of rabies or until animal is proven negative by laboratory tests	Immediate vaccination and RIG
Livestock, ferrets, rodents, and lagomorphs (rabbits and hares)	Consider individually	Consult public health officials. Bites of squirrels, hamsters, guinea pigs, gerbils, chipmunks, rats, mice, other rodents, rabbits, and hares almost never require anti-rabies treatment.

*During the 10-day holding period, treatment with RIG and vaccine should be initiated at the first sign of rabies in the biting dog or cat. The symptomatic animal should be killed immediately.

RIG, rabies immune globulin (human).

Adapted from American Academy of Pediatrics; Pickering LK, Baker CJ, Long SS, McMillan JA (eds): Red Book: 2006 Report of the Committee on Infectious Diseases, 27th ed. Elk Grove, Ill, American Academy of Pediatrics, 2006.

2. Rabies prophylaxis
   a. Diagnosis: The following should be considered before administering antirabies treatment.
      (1) Species of biting animal (see Table 19-6)
      (2) Vaccination status of the biting animal: A properly immunized adult animal (i.e., with one or more doses of rabies vaccine) has only a minimal chance of acquiring or transmitting the rabies virus.
      (3) Circumstances of the biting incident: An unprovoked attack is more suggestive of behavior of a rabid animal than is a provoked attack.

    (4) Type of exposure: Casual contact usually is not an indication for prophylaxis.

  b. Management: Postexposure prophylaxis

    (1) Immediately cleanse the wound with soap and water. Prophylactic antibiotics and tetanus toxoid are provided as indicated (see Table 19-6).

    (2) If prophylaxis is indicated, *both* rabies immune globulin (RIG), 1 dose of 20 IU/kg (as much of the dose as possible is used to infiltrate the wound[s], if present, and the rest given IM), *and* rabies vaccine (human diploid cell vaccine, rabies virus antigen, or purified chick embryo cell vaccine) should be given as soon as possible after exposure. Five doses of any of the three vaccines are given on days 0, 3, 7, 14, and 28. Ideally, immunization series should be initiated and completed with the same product vaccine.

3. Human bites

  a. Etiology: Usually mixed infections: staphylococci, gram-negative anaerobes and anaerobes from the mouth, aerobic streptococci, *Eikenella corrodens*, *Corynebacterium* species, *Haemophilus* species, and *Bacteroides* species

  b. Management

    (1) Evaluation is similar to that for animal bites, but human bites have a greater propensity to develop into a destructive deep tissue infection (especially those on the hand or involving joints).

    (2) Surgical management, including irrigation, debridement, and provision for drainage, plays a key role. These wounds are usually not sutured because of the potential for anaerobic infection.

    (3) Antimicrobial therapy should be provided prophylactically at the time of the bite with recommendations similar to those for animal bites (see Table 19-6).

4. Tetanus immunoprophylaxis

  a. Tetanus toxoid: 0.5 mL IM (diphtheria and tetanus [DT] in children <7 years of age; tetanus and diphtheria [Td] in those >7 years of age) is indicated in the following:

    (1) Clean, minor wounds: If the previously fully immunized child (three or more doses) has *not* received a booster dose in the last 10 years, *or* if the child is incompletely immunized (under three previous doses of toxoid)

    (2) Contaminated wounds (tetanus-prone wounds): If the previously immunized child has not received a booster dose in the last 5 years, or if the child is incompletely immunized

    (3) All wounds neglected for more than 24 hours

  b. Tetanus immune globulin human: 3000 to 6000 U IM should be given in the following situations:

    (1) Contaminated wounds or puncture wounds in the incompletely immunized child

    (2) Wounds resulting from missiles, crushing, avulsions, burns, and frostbite in the incompletely immunized child

9.5 Infections of the Eye and Surrounding Tissues

INFECTIONS OF EYELIDS AND LACRIMAL SYSTEM

Hordeolum (stye)

a. Etiology and clinical features: S. *aureus* infection of the sebaceous glands of eyelids with a painful swelling along lid margins

b. Management

   (1) Warm compresses three to four times a day

   (2) Rarely, antibiotic ointment and incision and drainage

c. Differential diagnosis

   (1) Chalazion: Retained meibomian gland secretions forming a granulomatous mass anywhere along the tarsus of the eyelid. Management is similar to that for a hordeolum.

Blepharitis

a. Etiology and clinical features

   (1) Usually secondary to seborrhea, sometimes superinfected with S. *aureus*

   (2) A buildup of yellow crusty scales on the eyelashes accompanied by erythema and edema of the lid margins

b. Management

   (1) Warm compresses should loosen scales that can then be removed with a soft cotton swab, moistened in sodium sulfacetamide eye solution, three times a day.

   (2) Seborrhea may be found elsewhere and should be treated.

Dacryocystitis

a. Etiology and clinical features

   (1) Seen most often in young infants with *dacryostenosis* (congenital stenosis of the lacrimal duct), which results in stasis of tears and mucus in the lacrimal sac. Secondary infection with pneumococci or staphylococci can occur.

   (2) Presents as purulent (green-yellow) discharge and swelling from the inferomedial canthus of the eye

b. Management

   (1) The sac may be "milked" by applying gentle pressure over the inflamed skin surface below the medial canthus, relieving swelling and discomfort.

   (2) Warm compresses and topical antibiotics help. Surgical probing and drainage may be necessary in difficult cases.

CONJUNCTIVITIS

The etiology, clinical manifestations, and management of childhood conjunctivitis (based on the age of child) are shown in Table 19-7.

PERIORBITAL CELLULITIS (PRESEPTAL CELLULITIS)

Pathophysiology and etiology

a. Infection can occur from contiguous spread after minor trauma (even without a break in the skin), an insect bite, hordeolum, or impetigo

Age	Possible Etiology	Clinical Manifestations	Management
<3 days	Silver nitrate/chemical conjunctivitis	Mild, rarely purulent	Self-limited
1 day–3 wk	N. gonorrhoeae (staphylococci, streptococci, fecal organisms)	Intense inflammation, copious, purulent yellow discharge, lid edema	Culture discharge Give systemic penicillin Screen for syphilis Topical sulfacetamide drops Goal is to prevent corneal ulceration, scarring
3–16 wk	C. trachomatis (may not be prevented by standard neonatal topical prophylaxis)	Inclusion conjunctivitis Mucopurulent discharge common Can be associated with pneumonitis (i.e., afebrile pneumonia with staccato cough, tachypnea, and wet crackles)	Obtain rapid detection antigen test (direct or indirect fluorescent antibody) Erythromycin (50 mg/kg/day orally, divided four times/day for 14 days) Topical antibiotics are not needed Evaluate and treat mother and partners for chlamydial infection
>16 wk–adult	S. pneumoniae Haemophilus aegyptius S. aureus H. influenzae (nontypeable) Moraxella lacunata	Conjunctival injection, mild mucopurulent discharge Begins unilaterally; may spread bilaterally	Cultures not usually needed or helpful Topical sulfacetamide drops (both eyes, two to three times/day for 10 days) Rule out foreign body, uveitis, corneal abrasion H. influenzae infection can be associated with ipsilateral otitis (conjunctivitis-otitis syndrome)

Continued

Age	Possible Etiology	Clinical Manifestations	Management
	Adenovirus Enteroviruses	Can be severe, with hemorrhagic discharge and pain May last weeks	Cool compresses Topical antibiotics if secondarily infected or course prolonged Examine for pharyngitis (i.e., pharyngoconjunctival fever = adenovirus)
	Herpes simplex virus	Variable in severity from superficial conjunctivitis to deep corneal involvement with dendritic keratitis ("branching coral", photophobia, foreign body sensation	Fluorescein dye will stain dendrites Consult ophthalmologist Topical vidarabine ointment (3%) or trifluridine drops (2%) four times/day for 14 days Possibly also oral acyclovir Avoid steroids
	Allergic reaction	Usually presents bilaterally mild conjunctival injection, pruritic, watery discharge, chemosis (corneal edema) History of atopy or contact with allergen	Topical anti-inflammatories (e.g., ketorolac) Topical steroids

(in these cases, *S. aureus* is the usual organism). Other etiologies include type b *H. influenzae* (now much less frequent), *S. pneumoniae*, *Streptococcus pyogenes*, or anaerobes.

   b. The preseptal space (between the skin of the eyelid and the orbital septum) rapidly accumulates inflammatory cells and edema.

   c. Usually this is a condition of young children (6 months to 5 years of age).

2. Clinical features
   a. Relatively acute onset of unilateral edema of the lids with erythematous or violaceous discoloration and tenderness
   b. Early in the infection there may be few systemic signs such as fever, and the eye itself usually is normal (i.e., little conjunctival injection, vision is normal, and eye movement is not painful).
   c. Later symptoms include fever, irritability, and marked upper and lower lid edema; conjunctival injection and discharge may occur.

3. Diagnosis and laboratory findings
   a. Diagnosis usually can be made from history and clinical findings.
   b. Leukocytosis may be present.
   c. ESR may be normal or very elevated.
   d. A blood culture should be obtained.
   e. An LP to rule out meningitis is necessary in infants (<6 months), especially if bacteremia is suspected.
   f. In toxic-appearing children without an obvious reason for periorbital infection, other sources of infection should be considered.

4. Differential diagnosis (Tables 19-8 and 19-9)

5. Management
   a. Mild cases: No fever, toxicity, or leukocytosis and low or normal ESR
      (1) High-dose oral amoxicillin-clavulanate or other antistaphylococcal agent for 10 days may be used if a careful follow-up at 12 to 24 hours can be assured.
      (2) Alternatively useful are ceftriaxone or cefotaxime, a single IM dose with careful follow-up, and either a repeat IM dose or completion of 7- to 10-day course with an oral agent.
   b. Moderate to severe infection
      (1) A patient with fever, leukocytosis (WBC count >15,000/mm^3), elevated ESR, and young age (<12 months) should be admitted for IV or IM antistaphylococcal therapy (e.g., nafcillin, clindamycin) for at least 24 to 48 hours pending resolution. Oral antimicrobials can then be given for 7 to 10 days.
      (2) Obtain orbital imaging studies if no improvement in 24 hours.

ORBITAL CELLULITIS

1. Pathophysiology and etiology
   a. Orbital cellulitis is an acute infection of the orbital space. The orbit is a pyramid-shaped bony cavity bounded anteriorly by the orbital septum and separated from the sinuses by three walls, one being the paper-thin medial wall, the lamina papyracea, separating the orbit from the ethmoid sinuses.
   b. The organisms responsible for orbital infection are similar to those related to skin, oral cavity (dental), and sinus infection.
   c. Rarely, fungal organisms can be involved.

Table 19-8 Features Distinguishing Preseptal (Periorbital) from Septal (Orbital) Cellulitis

	Preseptal (Periorbital) Cellulitis	Septal (Orbital) Cellulitis
Epidemiology/ risk factors	Trauma, skin infection, upper respiratory tract infection	Chronic sinusitis, trauma
Etiologic agents	S. aureus, S. pneumoniae (see Table 19-9)	S. aureus, S. pneumoniae, anaerobes
Clinical features		
Differential diagnosis	Allergic reaction, trauma, angioneurotic edema, sinusitis, child abuse, severe conjunctivitis	Orbital trauma, ruptured dermoid cyst, rhabdomyosarcoma, thyroid eye disease
Management	Hospitalize if age <2 yr for IV antibiotics (ampicillin-sulbactam or cefotaxime) Obtain orbital imaging studies if no improvement in 24 hr	An ophthalmic emergency Hospitalize in all cases IV—cefotaxime, cefuroxime, ceftriaxone, clindamycin, or ticarcillin-clavulanate Obtain orbital imaging studies Drain and culture abscess if present Indications for surgery Ophthalmoplegia with impaired visual acuity Globe displacement Progression of symptoms after 24 hr of antibiotics
Prognosis	Usually excellent if treated promptly	May be complicated by: Blindness from optic nerve or retinal vascular damage Spread to central nervous system (brain abscess) Cavernous sinus thrombosis Secondary glaucoma

Table 19-9 **Clinical and Laboratory Differences between Preseptal and Orbital Cellulitis**

Finding	Preseptal Cellulitis	Orbital Cellulitis
Fever	Present	Present
Lid edema	Moderate to severe	Severe
Chemosis	Absent or mild	Moderate or marked
Proptosis	Unusual	Present
Pain on eye movement	Absent	Present
Ocular mobility	Normal	Decreased
Vision	Normal	Diplopia on lateral gaze; diminished vision
Leukocytosis	Minimal or moderate	Marked
Erythrocyte sedimentation rate	Normal or elevated	Very elevated
Additional findings	Skin infection	Sinusitis; dental abscess

2. Clinical features
   a. Initial presentation is similar to that for preseptal cellulitis; often the signs and symptoms of sinusitis may also be present.
   b. Table 19-8 illustrates the clinical differences distinguishing preseptal from orbital cellulitis as the condition progresses.
3. Diagnosis and management
   a. The diagnosis is usually made on clinical manifestations.
   b. This infection is an otolaryngologic/ophthalmologic emergency. Subspecialist consultation is needed for timely management.
   c. CT or MRI scan of the orbit and sinuses can confirm the extent of the infection, evaluate the globe, and localize any foreign body.
   d. Surgical drainage of any abscesses or complicated sinusitis is usually undertaken.
   e. Initial antimicrobial therapy should include penicillinase-resistant penicillin (nafcillin) or ceftriaxone (50 mg/kg IM or IV once daily). Alternative antibiotics include cefuroxime, clindamycin, or ticarcillin-clavulanate. Antimicrobials are usually continued after drainage of any abscesses or until complete resolution.
   f. Ophthalmoplegia with impaired vision and globe displacement are indications for surgery.
4. Prognosis
   a. Prognosis in uncomplicated, promptly treated cases is excellent.
   b. Sequelae that can complicate course and outcome include
      (1) Spread to CNS (meningitis, brain abscess)
      (2) Septic thrombosis of the cavernous sinus
      (3) Blindness from optic nerve or retinal vascular involvement

19.6 Otolaryngologic Infections

ACUTE OTITIS MEDIA

1. Pathophysiology: Eustachian tube dysfunction occurs as a result of mucosal edema from an upper respiratory infection. Inadequate ventilation (drainage) of the middle ear then occurs, leading to negative middle ear pressure. A sterile transudate within the middle ear develops from persistent negative pressure. This middle ear transudate is then seeded by colonized organisms or infected nasopharyngeal contents during aspiration and insufflation from crying and nose blowing. This results in inflammation of mucosa lining the middle ear.

2. Epidemiology: One of the most common infections in pediatric practice, acute otitis media (AOM) occurs in 10% to 20% of children for each year of life up to 6 years of age, then decreases to below 1% by 12 years of age. As many as 10% will have AOM before 3 months of age.

3. Etiology: S. pneumoniae (40%), H. influenzae nontypeable (25% to 30%), GABHS (15%), and Moraxella catarrhalis (20%) are the major organisms associated with AOM. S. aureus and enteric gram-negative bacilli (in neonates) are less frequent causes. Viruses cause 10% to 40% of middle ear effusions.

4. Clinical features
   a. Fever, crying, sleep disturbance, ear pain, and pulling at ear are common.
   b. AOM is classically defined as a bulging, opacified, discolored tympanic membrane (TM) through which the landmarks are poorly visualized; mobility of the TM is decreased or absent.
   c. Early in AOM, changes may be seen first in the pars flaccida (anterior superior portion of the TM) with intense hyperemia and retraction or bulging. There is inability to visualize the short process of the malleus.
   d. Eventually the light reflex is lost and the TM becomes opaque.

5. Diagnosis
   a. Pneumatic otoscopy: The clinical standard for bedside diagnosis, in which the TM shows decreased mobility. With a bulb insufflator, a small amount of air is injected and withdrawn into a well-sealed external auditory canal. Normally the TM will "flick"; nonmovement signifies fluid, infection, or a poor seal.
   b. Tympanometry (see section on Auditory Screening, Chapter 2) can be helpful in confirming clinically suspect cases.
   c. Tympanocentesis: Aspiration of fluid from the middle ear is indicated for relief of severe pain, for etiologic diagnosis in neonates or immunocompromised children, for failed antibiotic treatment, and for treatment of mastoiditis.

6. Management (based on American Academy of Pediatrics [AAP] recommendations)
   a. Control pain with acetaminophen or ibuprofen. Consider topical benzocaine in children older than 5 years without perforation.
   b. In children younger than 6 months, treat with antibiotics.
   c. In children 6 months to 2 years of age and those with severe otalgia or temperature greater than 39° C, treat with antibiotics (Box 19-2).

Box 19-2   Recommended Treatment for Acute Otitis Media in Children

First-line drug: high-dose amoxicillin (80-90 mg/kg/day)
Duration of treatment: 5 days, treat for 10 days if younger than 2 years or with underlying medical condition, recurrent acute otitis media, or chronic suppurative otitis media
Alternative for treatment failure, amoxicillin allergy, or recurrent acute otitis media: amoxicillin-clavulanate (high dose), cefuroxime, cefdinir, ceftriaxone, clindamycin, or azithromycin

d. For children 2 years of age and older, consider initial observation without antibiotics if illness is not severe and offer antibiotics if there is no improvement within 48 to 72 hours. Up to 40% of bacterially associated cases of AOM may resolve spontaneously without antibiotics.

e. The patient should symptomatically improve (e.g., fever, otalgia, appetite) within 24 to 48 hours. A persistently symptomatic child requires reexamination or change to another antimicrobial.

f. A clinical reevaluation should occur in 15 to 30 days after starting therapy to determine whether a middle ear effusion persists (see the next section). If complete resolution has occurred, the patient is considered cured.

g. After AOM, asymptomatic fluid within the middle ear may normally be present for up to 30 days in 40% of children. Effusion that persists past 4 weeks is usually managed in the same manner as that for otitis media with effusion (see the next section).

h. Recurrent AOM: Repeated episodes of AOM may be prevented using the guidelines in Box 19-3. Periodic monitoring is necessary for patients with repeated episodes of otitis media.

OTITIS MEDIA WITH EFFUSION

1. Clinical features
   a. Persistence of fluid in the middle ear space for 4 to 8 weeks after an episode of AOM with sensation of fullness in head or ears or diminished hearing is indicative of otitis media with effusion (OME). Asymptomatic middle ear effusion of less than 4 weeks' duration can routinely follow AOM, usually is sterile, and resolves without specific treatment.
   b. The problem is compounded if the OME is bilateral because this may be associated with hearing loss.
2. Diagnosis: Persistence of middle ear effusion beyond 4 weeks after episode of AOM with the following characteristics:
   a. The TM is thickened with a gray or amber fluid–filled middle ear. Sometimes an air–fluid level, bubbles, or bluish fluid may be present.

Box 19-3   Prophylaxis to Prevent Recurrent Otitis Media

Candidates for Therapy
- Two episodes of otitis media in the first year of life
- Three episodes within 6 months (at any age)

Duration of Prophylactic Treatment (Any of the Following)
- Three months after an acute episode (if no breakthrough infection)
- The winter months (usually November to April)

Antimicrobial Regimen (Any of the Following)
- Sulfisoxazole 7 mg/kg divided twice a day
- TMP/SMX (4 mg TMP/20 mg SMX/kg) single daily dose
- Amoxicillin 125 mg (<2 years of age) or 250 mg (>2 years of age) single daily dose

---

   b. Decreased mobility of the TM is demonstrated by pneumatic otoscopy. Sometimes a cholesteatoma from long-standing eustachian tube dysfunction appears as a cream-colored mass behind the TM, in the area of the pars flaccida. A CT scan can help characterize this lesion.

   c. Tympanometry performed to corroborate otoscopy and provide baseline to follow the resolution of the OME. Tympanograms (see section on Auditory Screening, Chapter 2) show flattened (type C) or displaced (type B) curves, indicative of reduced TM compliance.

   d. Audiometry may be performed on children older than 3 years of age to assess for hearing deficits.

3. Management

   a. A child with OME and no difficulty hearing or developmental delay should be managed by watchful waiting for 3 months from the date of effusion onset (if known) or diagnosis (if onset is unknown). They should be reexamined at 3- to 6-month intervals until effusion is no longer present, significant hearing loss is identified, or structural abnormalities of the TM or middle ear are suspected.

   b. Hearing testing is recommended when OME persists for 3 months or longer or at any time that language delay, learning problems, or a significant hearing loss is suspected in a child with OME; language testing should be conducted for children with hearing loss.

   c. A child becomes a surgical candidate when OME lasts more than 4 months with hearing loss. Tympanostomy tube insertion is the preferred initial procedure. Adenoidectomy, myringotomy, or tonsillectomy may be performed as alternative procedures.

   d. Antihistamines and decongestants are ineffective for OME and are not recommended for treatment.

    e. Antimicrobials (e.g., amoxicillin for 14 days) and corticosteroids (e.g., prednisone 1 mg/kg/d for 7 days) have been used in the past with varying success. However, they do not have long-term efficacy and are not recommended for routine management.

4. Complications (Fig. 19-4)

OTITIS EXTERNA

1. Pathophysiology and etiology: Retention of water in the external canal, generally from swimming (thus called *swimmer's ear*) or excessive bathing, provides a moist environment for inflammation and infection by organisms that colonize the skin and canal (e.g., *S. aureus*, *P. aeruginosa*, *Proteus vulgaris*, and *S. pyogenes*).

2. Clinical features

    a. Pruritus of external canal

    b. Otalgia: Especially pain on movement (tugging) of the helix (this helps differentiate a draining purulent otitis externa [OE] from a perforated TM in AOM, which usually is *not* associated with pain on tugging)

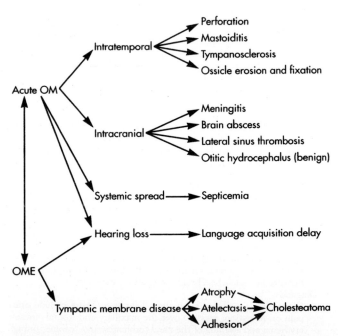

Figure 19-4   Complications of acute otitis media (AOM) and otitis media with effusion (OME). (Adapted from Balkary T, Pashley N: *Clinical Pediatric Otolaryngology.* St. Louis, 1986, Mosby.)

c. Purulent, foul-smelling discharge, erythema and swelling of ear

d. Cellulitis of tragus and helix, with adenopathy and fever

3. Differential diagnoses: Includes AOM, parotitis, preauricular adenitis, dental abscess, temporomandibular joint dysfunction, and foreign body

4. Management

   a. After external auditory canal has been cleansed, instill 2% acetic acid otic solution with or without steroids (VoSoL or VoSoL HC) 3 to 4 drops into the canal four times daily for 5 to 7 days for prophylaxis and mild cases; for severe infections, use for 10 to 14 days.

   b. Topical antibiotic otic solutions with or without steroids (Cortisporin, Floxin Otic, Cipro HC Otic) are available but are probably no more effective than the preceding approach.

   c. Progressive unresponsive infections: Systemic antimicrobials (may be given either orally or parenterally), using a combination of an aminoglycoside and antipseudomonal penicillin (ticarcillin, piperacillin)

   d. Avoid prolonged exposure to moisture and self-inflicted trauma to the canal.

   e. After bathing or swimming, gently dry the external ear with a cotton towel, and hold a hair dryer at arm's length on low/cool setting for 2 to 3 minutes to dry out canal further.

SINUSITIS

1. Pathophysiology and etiology: Inflammation of the paranasal sinus. Organisms are usually similar to those causing otitis media: *S. pneumoniae* (30%), *H. influenzae* (20%), *M. catarrhalis* (20%), and sterile/viral (30%). Note that *H. influenzae* or *M. catarrhalis* may produce beta-lactamase, rendering penicillin ineffective. A dental abscess may be the origin in older children.

2. Clinical features

   a. Sinusitis is generally rare in children younger than 24 months of age.

   b. The vast majority of infections primarily involve the maxillary sinuses.

   c. Acute (1 to 4 days): High fever; congestion, periorbital/facial swelling and pain, headache, and nasal discharge can be severe; daytime cough, halitosis

   d. Subacute (>10 days, <30 days)

      (1) Usually follows an upper respiratory infection (URI)

      (2) Symptoms less severe than with acute: Slight periorbital edema, purulent nasal discharge, and halitosis are most common.

      (3) Preauricular lymph nodes that drain the maxillary sinuses may be palpable.

   e. Chronic (>30 days): Symptoms may be vague: Cough that is worse at night or the morning on rising, nasal obstruction, postnasal drip, nonspecific headache, chronic congestion, and halitosis.

3. Diagnosis

   a. Diagnosis is usually made on clinical findings: These include sinus pain on palpation; pressure over the maxillary and frontal sinuses; erythema and swelling of the nasal turbinates; and "cobblestoning" of the posterior pharynx.

   b. CT scan is the study of choice and is particularly helpful in the evaluation of complications such as recurrent sinusitis, persistent

infection (especially unilateral), complicated infection (i.e., with suspected orbital or CNS involvement), and consideration of another diagnosis (e.g., tumor, foreign body).
c. Plain radiographs of sinuses (anteroposterior, lateral, and especially occipitomental view) may demonstrate complete or partial opacification of one or more sinuses, air–fluid levels, and mucosal thickening (≥4 mm). In children younger than 1 year, thick mucosa may indicate normal opacity of small, noninfected sinuses.
d. Sinus aspiration should be considered for the following indications:
    (1) Complicated infection(s)
    (2) Failure to obtain a clinical cure
    (3) Immunocompromised patients (i.e., to rule out a fungal etiology)
e. Laboratory studies such as CBC, ESR, and blood cultures may help define the severity of the infection and monitor resolution.
4. Management
    a. Antimicrobials given orally often produce clinical improvement within 48 to 72 hours and include
        (1) Amoxicillin (45 mg/kg/day)
        (2) Alternative regimens: High-dose amoxicillin (80 to 90 mg/kg/day) or amoxicillin-clavulanate, cefuroxime axetil, cefdinir, azithromycin, TMP/SMX, or clarithromycin
        (3) Treatment should be continued for a minimum of 14 to 21 days (except azithromycin); longer courses may be needed.
    b. Nasal decongestants, inhaled and oral β_2-adrenergic agonists, antihistamines, inhaled steroids, and saline nasal washes have shown no evidence for effectiveness in pediatric acute sinusitis.
    c. Consultation with an otolaryngologist may be needed for complicated infections.
5. Complications
    a. Orbital complications: Signs include proptosis, loss of extraocular movement (loss of upward gaze), diplopia, and exophthalmos. These findings may suggest
        (1) Subperiosteal abscess
        (2) Orbital abscess
        (3) Orbital cellulitis
        (4) Cavernous sinus thrombosis
    b. CNS complications: Signs such as increased ICP and focal neurologic findings may suggest
        (1) Subdural abscess
        (2) Epidural abscess
        (3) Brain abscess
    c. Bony complications present as osteomyelitis of the fontal bone (i.e., Pott's puffy tumor).
6. Risk factors for recurrent infection
    a. Recurrent viral URI (attendance at day care or school-age sibling)
    b. Allergic/atopic problems
    c. Immunodeficiency (e.g., HIV)
    d. Cystic fibrosis
    e. Anatomic problems (e.g., Down syndrome)
    f. Dysmotile cilia syndrome

PHARYNGITIS, TONSILLITIS, AND TONSILLOPHARYNGITIS

1. Etiology: Most cases are viral, but 15% to 20% are caused by GABHS.
    a. Viral: Adenovirus, Epstein-Barr virus (EBV), influenza, parainfluenza, enteroviruses
    b. Bacterial: GABHS, group C and G streptococci, *Arcanobacterium haemolyticum*, *Neisseria gonorrhoeae*, *Corynebacterium diphtheria*, *Mycoplasma pneumoniae*
2. Clinical features: Occurs generally in children older than 3 years of age, with seasonal peaks in late winter and early spring
    a. Table 19-10 helps differentiate the most common causes of febrile, exudative tonsillitis.
    b. The hallmarks of GABHS pharyngitis are tender, cervical adenopathy, foul breath, exudative tonsillitis, and soft palatal petechiae in a child *without* URI symptoms. Headache and abdominal pain are common.
    c. In infants, streptococcal infection is more likely to present with URI symptoms (streptococcosis): Persistent nasopharyngeal discharge with fever and cough.
3. Laboratory findings
    a. Throat culture detects GABHS in 85% or more of cases if done properly (vigorous swabbing of both tonsillar areas as well as the posterior pharynx, causing the patient to gag).
    b. Rising antistreptolysin O titers (≥500 Todd units as an absolute value on a single specimen, or a two-tube rise in serial specimens analyzed simultaneously) can be used for confirmation in uncertain or complicated cases. Rapid antigen detection tests are useful if performed in a standardized laboratory with experienced technicians.
    c. "Monospot" (heterophile antibody) test: EBV diagnosis is not reliable in children younger than 5 years.
    d. Atypical lymphocytosis with mild thrombocytopenia is often associated with EBV. It is important to note any history in the patient or family of recent or past streptococcal pharyngitis, scarlet fever, rheumatic fever, or penicillin allergy because management will be altered.
4. Management
    a. The major goal of antimicrobial therapy is to eradicate GABHS and prevent acute rheumatic fever (ARF).
    b. Penicillin remains the drug of choice in the nonallergic patient, shortening the duration of symptoms by 24 to 48 hours. Other options include clindamycin, cephalosporins, and macrolides.
        (1) IM penicillin (benzathine): Children can be given a single injection of 600,000 to 1,200,000 U, with the larger dose generally for children over 60 pounds.
        (2) Oral penicillin V: Children can be given 250 mg (i.e., 25 to 50 mg/kg/day) every 8 to 12 hours for 10 days. Adolescents and adults can be given 250 mg every 6 to 8 hours *or* 500 mg every 12 hours for 10 days. The entire 10-day course must be completed, even though the temperature returns to normal and the patient is better.

Table 19-10 Clinical Manifestations of Pharyngitis

	GABHS	Viral (Other than EBV)	EBV
Age	Generally ≥3 yr	Any age	>5 yr (especially late school age/adolescent)
Season	Fall to spring	Any	Any
Clinical	Tender cervical adenopathy, foul breath, tonsillar exudates, petechiae on soft palate, abdominal pain (mesenteric adenitis), headache, rash ("sandpaper" feel = scarlet fever), no rhinorrhea, cough, conjunctivitis (i.e., no URI symptoms)	Papulovesicular lesions or tonsillar ulcers common (e.g., herpangina-coxsackievirus A), URI symptoms common; if associated with conjunctivitis, adenovirus; rash often papulosquamous	Indolent onset, tonsillar exudates, lymphadenopathy, fatigue, hepatosplenomegaly, atypical lymphocytes in peripheral smear; rash will occur with penicillin; illness lasts more than 7-10 days (i.e., GABHS infection usually resolves within 7 days)

EBV, Epstein-Barr virus; GABHS, group A β-hemolytic streptococci; URI, upper respiratory infection.

    c. Emerging resistance to penicillin by GABHS may alter initial antimicrobial choices.

    d. Note that penicillin prevents ARF even when started as long as 9 days after the onset of acute symptoms (i.e., the rise in anti–M protein antibody, possibly responsible for ARF, takes time to develop). Thus, the brief delay in processing the throat culture before therapy is begun is not problematic. Penicillin does not prevent GABHS-associated glomerulonephritis.

5. Special considerations:

    a. For patients with documented penicillin allergy, oral first-generation cephalosporins, clindamycin, or macrolides should be used, depending on reaction type.

    b. Sulfonamides, although effective in the prophylaxis of streptococcal infection, are not effective in treatment of illness.

    c. For prophylaxis of rheumatic fever in patients with a well-documented history for ARF, see Section 19.9.

    d. After 24 hours of antibiotics, children are no longer contagious and may return to school as soon as the symptoms subside.

    e. *Symptomatic* family members should receive throat cultures and appropriate treatment. (Recurrent streptococcal pharyngitis, occurring in a family, may require antibiotic treatment of the entire family.)

    f. *Asymptomatic* GABHS pharyngeal carriers as well as children younger than 2 years of age are at little risk for development of ARF or spreading the infection to others.

PERITONSILLAR, RETROPHARYNGEAL, AND PARAPHARYNGEAL ABSCESSES

1. Pathophysiology and etiology: These deep tissue abscesses almost always follow tonsillopharyngitis or URI. Organisms include GABHS or *S. pyogenes*, oral anaerobes, *S. aureus*.

2. Clinical features: The child appears ill and complains of severe throat pain and dysphagia. Table 19-11 distinguishes clinical features among the deep neck infections.

3. Diagnosis: Often confirmed by cultures of abscess obtained during surgical drainage.

4. Management

    a. Initial treatment: Before surgical drainage, the patient may receive several doses of a broad-spectrum antibiotic.

    b. Surgical drainage: Performed under general anesthesia using a cuffed endotracheal tube to minimize the chances of aspiration or mediastinitis

    c. Antibiotics: The patient should be treated with a 10-day course of penicillin, initially IV until acute manifestations have subsided, and then continued orally. Other antimicrobial choices include

        (1) Nafcillin 100 to 150 mg/kg/day IV every 6 hours, maximum 12 g/day, or

        (2) Clindamycin 30 to 40 mg/kg/day IV or IM every 6 to 8 hours, maximum 2.7 g/day, or

        (3) Ampicillin/sulbactam 100 to 200 mg/kg/day IV every 6 hours, maximum 8 g ampicillin/day

Table 19-1 Distinguishing Deep Neck Infections

	Age	Source	Symptoms	Complications
Peritonsillar abscess	>10 yr	Pharyngitis	Sore throat, trismus, "hot potato voice," uvula pointing toward unaffected side	Aspiration, airway obstruction
Retropharyngeal abscess	<10 yr	Pharyngitis, foreign body, trauma	Stridor, dysphagia, drooling, anterior pharyngeal wall displacement	Obstruction, posterior mediastinitis, extension to lateral space
Parapharyngeal abscess	Any age	Pharyngitis, dental infection, parotitis, mastoiditis, cervical adenitis	Cervical swelling, trismus, dysphagia, medial displacement of pharyngeal wall	Carotid artery erosion, cord paralysis, Horner's syndrome, jugular vein thrombosis

d. Analgesic: Drugs may be needed for pain. Narcotics should be used cautiously because of risk of airway obstruction.

EPIGLOTTITIS

1. Pathophysiology and etiology
   a. A bacterial cellulitis of the supraglottic tissues (epiglottis and aryepiglottic folds) that is rapidly progressive, leading to narrowing of the airway inlet and eventual acute upper airway obstruction—a true medical/surgical emergency
   b. Almost always secondary to *H. influenzae* type b infection, although other organisms (e.g., staphylococci, streptococci) and toxins (e.g., gasoline inhalation) cause similar clinical manifestations. Immunization against type b *H. influenzae* has markedly reduced the incidence.
2. Clinical features (Table 19-12): Children with epiglottitis are 3 to 7 years of age and present with an abrupt onset of fever, severe sore throat, and dysphagia. Because of refusal to swallow, they often drool uncontrollably, and if they speak, they do so quietly and in a hoarse voice. Progressive respiratory distress (sitting in tripod posture with neck extended to keep airway open) and resulting hypoxemia leads to apprehension and delirium. Impending airway obstruction is signaled by stridor (especially inspiratory).
3. Diagnosis
   a. Must be made rapidly and on clinical suspicion
   b. Radiographs (e.g., lateral neck characteristically showing "thumbprint" sign of swollen epiglottis obliterating the valleculae) are unnecessary and should be performed only in confusing cases, under controlled conditions.
4. Management
   a. Epiglottitis should ideally be managed according to protocol:
      (1) Immediately notify anesthesia and otolaryngologic services.
      (2) Provide humidified oxygen with a minimum of intervention to the child—do not put anything into mouth! (unless intubating, of course).
      (3) In the operating room, direct visualization and prophylactic nasotracheal/orotracheal intubation will be performed. Intubation is usually required for only 1 to 3 days.
   b. Blood cultures (90% positive) and tissue cultures are obtained in the operating room after the airway is secured.
   c. Antimicrobial therapy: Antimicrobial therapy should be continued IV for 5 to 7 days.
      (1) Cefotaxime 100 to 200 mg/kg/day IV every 6 hours, *or*
      (2) Ceftriaxone 50 to 75 mg/kg/day IV every 24 hours, *or*
      (3) Ampicillin/sulbactam 100 to 200 mg/kg/day IV every 6 hours
   d. The child should be carefully sedated and monitored in an intensive care unit.
   e. A search for complications of *H. influenzae* infection should be undertaken once the patient is stable, such as pneumonia, pericarditis, and meningitis.
   f. Prophylaxis for *H. influenzae* type b infection: Rifampin prophylaxis (20 mg/kg/day orally, maximum 600 mg, given once daily for 4 days) should be provided to:

Table 19-12	Differentiating Epiglottitis from Similar Clinical Entities		
	Epiglottitis	**Viral Laryngotracheitis**	**Bacterial Tracheitis**
Etiology	*H. influenzae*, staphylococci, streptococci	Parainfluenza, influenza, respiratory syncytial viruses	Virus plus staphylococci, streptococci, *H. influenzae*, or enterics
Age	2-7 yr	3 mo-3 yr	3 mo-3 yr
Clinical characteristics	High fever, dysphagia, drooling, "toxic" appearance, refusal to speak	Low-grade fever, coryza, barking cough, hoarse voice	Improving croup, then worsens: high fever, stridor, anterior neck tenderness; no drooling
Plain radiography	Unnecessary (thumbprint sign on lateral neck)	Unnecessary (steeple sign on anteroposterior view)	Detached pseudomembrane gives soft tissue shadow

(1) Household contacts (individuals residing with index case 4 or more hours per day for at least 5 of the 7 days preceding the day of hospital admission), unless all household contacts younger than 48 months of age have completed their immunizations

(2) Index case if younger than 2 years of age

(3) Child care/nursery school contacts regardless of age, when two or more cases of type b H. *influenzae* invasive disease have occurred within 60 days (see AAP *Red Book*)

5. Prognosis: Within 48 to 72 hours after initiation of treatment, and barring complications, the child is usually considerably better and recovery is complete.

CROUP (VIRAL LARYNGOTRACHEOBRONCHITIS)

1. Pathophysiology and etiology: Inflammation and edema of subglottic tissue in an already anatomically small airway create obstruction. Parainfluenza viruses, respiratory syncytial virus (RSV), adenoviruses, and influenza viruses are the most common causes. Bacterial infection is rare.

2. Clinical features
   a. Children between 3 months and 3 years of age are most commonly affected.
   b. Mild upper respiratory symptoms are commonly followed by the sudden onset of a barking cough and hoarseness, often at night, worse on the second and third nights and lasting 72 to 96 hours.
   c. High fever or toxicity is unusual.
   d. Most children are comfortable at rest, and have a "barky," seal-like cough only when stressed or crying.
   e. Severely affected patients may have inspiratory stridor, tachypnea, and retractions at rest.
   f. Diminished breath sounds indicate critical narrowing of the airway.
   g. Restlessness, tachycardia, altered mental status, and pallor or cyanosis suggest impending hypoxemia.

3. Diagnosis
   a. Diagnosis is made primarily on clinical findings and confirmed by anteroposterior neck radiographs showing subglottic narrowing—the "steeple sign."
   b. Assess hypoxemia with pulse oximetry.
   c. Spasmodic croup: This chronic recurrent form of croup is neither uncommon nor directly tied to an infectious etiology. It is probably related to an upper airway response to an allergic trigger. Children are often slightly older than those with viral croup and the episodes are recurrent in children who are otherwise well (i.e., without fever, URI); also there is often a positive family history for allergies (atopy) or asthma, and the condition responds well to steroids and occasionally bronchodilators.
   d. Differential diagnosis: Besides epiglottitis, acute croup must be differentiated from foreign bodies and allergic reactions that involve the upper airway.

4. Management
   a. Mild croup: Croupy cough occurs only with cry; the patient is comfortable and in no respiratory distress. Usually, home therapy includes

a cool-mist humidifier, steam heat from bathroom, and frequent exposure to cool outdoor air. Parents should be instructed to call a physician if the child's respiratory distress increases.

b. Moderate croup: Mild inspiratory stridor, agitation, mild/moderate retractions

(1) Evaluate in an acute care setting. Provide sedation in the form of a quiet room where a parent may stay with the child and avoid unnecessary procedures to reduce the associated anxiety. Cool, moist air with oxygen is provided by a mist tent.

(2) Aerosolized racemic epinephrine (2.25% solution, 0.5 mL in 4 mL normal saline) may produce transient relief of symptoms. Frequent treatments are often necessary, and rebound may occur. Therefore these patients should be considered for admission.

(3) A single dose of corticosteroids (dexamethasone 0.15 to 0.6 mg/kg orally or 0.3 mg/kg IV) has been shown to lessen severity and duration of symptoms and hospitalization in patients with moderate to severe croup.

c. Severe croup: Inspiratory and expiratory stridor, retractions, and documented hypoxemia

(1) Hospital admission is warranted for observation, monitoring, racemic epinephrine, and treatment with mist tent or corticosteroids, depending on clinical preference.

(2) Intubation is indicated for impending respiratory failure (increasing work of breathing, accompanied by a falling respiratory rate in the face of worsening hypoxemia).

(3) Helium-oxygen therapy (usually 70% He:30% O2) can avoid or improve severe respiratory compromise.

19.7 Lymphadenitis

1. Pathophysiology and etiology

a. Lymphadenopathy often occurs as a host response to localized or systemic infection.

b. S. aureus and GABHS are the most likely organisms (see Table 19-13 for additional sources).

2. Clinical features: Progressive infection and inflammation within the node (i.e., adenitis) is accompanied by marked lymph node enlargement (often 3 cm or more) and is associated with warmth, tenderness, and erythema.

3. Diagnosis

a. A complete history (e.g., for trauma, skin infection, cat scratches, travel, TB exposure) and thorough examination of the area(s) drained by affected lymph nodes will often confirm the diagnosis and suggest a possible source.

b. Laboratory tests: Throat culture, EBV, cytomegalovirus (CMV), toxoplasmosis titers, CBC and differential, ESR, and PPD. Second-line tests include blood cultures, chest radiograph (CXR), and Venereal Disease Research Laboratory test (VDRL). If suspected, titers to the cat scratch bacillus (Bartonella henselae) should be obtained.

Location of Node(s)	Possible Etiologic Sources
Posterior auricular, posterior/suboccipital, occipital	Scalp infections (e.g., tinea capitis, pediculosis, impetigo)
Submandibular, anterior cervical	Oropharyngeal or facial infections (subacute, "cold" submandibular nodes suggest atypical or tuberculous mycobacteria)
Preauricular	Sinusitis, tularemia, cat scratch disease
Posterior cervical	Adjacent skin infection
Bilateral cervical of marked degree	Infectious mononucleosis, acute toxoplasmosis, secondary syphilis
Supraclavicular or scalene, lower cervical	Infiltrative process (e.g., malignancy), especially if firm, matted, immobile
Axillary	Cat scratch disease, sporotrichosis, hidradenitis suppurativa
Generalized adenopathy	Generalized viral infection (e.g., mononucleosis, viral hepatitis, human immunodeficiency virus), sarcoidosis, autoimmune diseases (e.g., systemic lupus erythematosus), neoplasms (e.g., lymphoma)
Inguinal adenopathy	Sexually transmitted diseases (e.g., syphilis, herpes simplex, chancroid, chlamydial infection) or nonvenereal (e.g., *S. aureus*, group A streptococci)

c. Needle aspiration of lymph node: After saline infusion, needle aspiration is useful for Gram and acid-fast bacillus (AFB) stains and culture for aerobes, anaerobes, and mycobacteria.

4. Management
   a. Antimicrobials: Because the vast majority of acutely infected nodes will be due to *S. aureus* and GABHS, a first-generation cephalosporin or penicillinase-resistant penicillin (e.g., cephalexin 25 to 50 mg/kg/day orally every 6 hours, or nafcillin IV 100 to 200 mg/kg/day every 4 hours) should be given as initial therapy. Clindamycin is an alternative agent.
      (1) The duration of treatment is determined by the patient's response; usually a 10- to 14-day course of antimicrobials suffices.
      (2) Improvement (decrease in fever, tenderness, and swelling) should occur within 48 to 72 hours in uncomplicated cases.
   b. Hot compresses and antipyretics are also helpful.
   c. Surgical consultation for potential drainage or excisional biopsy is appropriate for infected nodes that are fluctuant ("pitting edema") or refractory to 5 to 7 days of antimicrobial therapy. Fluctuant nodes indicating abscess usually require incision and drainage.

   d. Progressive adenopathy (especially in older children or in unusual locations) not responsive to aggressive medical management or adenopathy that persists beyond 4 to 6 weeks are indications for diagnostic excisional biopsy. In some cases, ultrasound-guided fine-needle aspiration may suffice as an alternative to excisional biopsy.

   e. Nontuberculous mycobacterial adenitis

     (1) Observation is the preferred initial management because nontuberculous mycobacterial strains respond poorly to the usual antituberculosis drugs and the adenopathy sometimes resolves spontaneously.

     (2) Complete surgical excision of the involved nodes is reserved for progressive or persistent adenopathy and is almost always curative. Antituberculosis chemotherapy offers no benefit. However, if surgical excision is incomplete or recurrence of adenopathy is noted, therapy with clarithromycin combined with ethambutol or rifabutin may be beneficial.

     (3) Infection is not communicable, so the child presents no risk to siblings or classmates.

19.8 Lower Respiratory Tract Infections

BRONCHIOLITIS

1. Definition: Bronchiolitis is a disease of infancy, characterized by signs and symptoms of airway obstruction.
2. Pathophysiology and etiology
   a. Primarily caused by RSV, a paramyxovirus. Other viral causes include parainfluenza (types 1 and 3) and adenoviruses.
   b. RSV has a predilection for the respiratory epithelium (especially of the terminal airway) and is associated with an intense inflammatory response by the host. This response may be immunoglobulin E (IgE) mediated with the resultant release of histamine and leukotriene-C4, producing bronchoconstriction, mucus secretion, and submucosal edema. This produces small-airway obstruction with variable degrees of hyperinflation and atelectasis.
3. Epidemiology
   a. Peak incidence is in the first 2 years of life (?.? cases/100 children/year).
   b. Most hospitalizations and deaths from bronchiolitis occur in infants younger than 6 months of age; especially affected are infants with chronic pulmonary disease (i.e., prematurity, bronchopulmonary dysplasia) or heart disease, and those who are immunocompromised.
   c. Most cases occur during cold weather months or during the rainy season in tropical climates and in infants who live in crowded home environments exposed to passive cigarette smoke.
   d. It is a significant cause of respiratory morbidity and mortality worldwide.
4. Clinical features
   a. General: Most children usually have a 3- to 5-day history of rhinorrhea, cough, and congestion due to thick secretions. Low-grade fever, tachypnea, tachycardia, restlessness/irritability, retractions of the

chest wall, and flaring of the ala nasi may be seen. Cyanosis of the oral mucosa can be present in severe cases.

b. Respiratory

(1) Cough worsens over time and audible wheezing and respiratory distress can become more evident, depending on the severity of the illness.

(2) Auscultation: Most infants will be wheezing or have diminished air exchange. Severe airway obstruction may be associated with inaudible wheeze. Fine crackles may be heard on inspiration and most likely represent small alveoli opening up.

(3) A severe episode is also suggested by paradoxical abdominal wall motion with respiration (i.e., the abdomen collapses with each inspiration).

5. Diagnosis: Based on clinical criteria

a. The infant who has had several days of URI symptoms and is wheezing during the cold weather months can reliably be assumed to have bronchiolitis.

b. CXR typically demonstrates hyperinflation, flattened diaphragms, or patchy atelectasis.

c. Pulse oximetry

(1) Helpful in determining the severity of illness. An *initial* SaO_2 under 95% may suggest the need for admission (i.e., impending hypoxemia and respiratory failure).

(2) Subsequent SaO_2 readings after bronchodilator therapy may *not* correlate well with the clinical examination; the patient may respond well clinically, but SaO_2 may decrease because of ventilation–perfusion mismatch (i.e., poorly ventilated lung units receiving enhanced blood flow secondary to therapy).

d. Enzyme-linked immunoassay (ELISA) or fluorescent antibody techniques are available for the rapid diagnosis of RSV, influenza virus, parainfluenza viruses and adenoviruses from respiratory secretions. Etiologic diagnosis is more important for epidemiologic and infectious control concerns than for pathogen-specific management.

6. Differential diagnosis

a. Foreign body aspiration

b. Cardiac disease with pulmonary edema

c. Structural defects: Laryngeal webs, vascular rings and slings (usually associated with chronic stridor), mediastinal masses

d. Aspiration syndromes (gastroesophageal reflux disease, tracheoesophageal fistulae)

e. Other causes of wheezing

f. Pneumonia

7. Management

a. This is often a self-limiting condition with 3 to 7 days of acute illness and full recovery in about 2 weeks, but longer in children with underlying pulmonary disease.

b. General: Most infants require only supportive care, hydration, O_2, nasal, or deep suctioning.

c. β_2 agonists: Infants with wheezing have been shown to respond to nebulized β_2 agonists (e.g., albuterol, salbutamol). However, the quality of the response is variable.

d. Steroids: Systemic steroid therapy has *not* been shown significantly to shorten the course of bronchiolitis. Nebulized/inhaled corticosteroids may shorten the course and especially benefit those with previous wheezing or severe illness, as well as those treated early in the course.

e. Hospitalization: Factors suggesting the need for hospitalization include the following:
   (1) "Toxic" or ill-appearing infants
   (2) History of prematurity (<34 weeks) or significant chronic cardiopulmonary disease or multiple congenital anatomic anomalies
   (3) Age less than 3 months
   (4) SaO_2 below 95%
   (5) Respiratory rate over 70 breaths/min, with signs of distress
   (6) Dehydration or poor feeding secondary to respiratory distress
   (7) Inability of parents to care for child

f. Other therapies: Severely ill patients may be treated in the pediatric intensive care unit with high-flow oxygen. Antivirals (e.g., ribavirin) are expensive and best reserved for severely ill patients. Empirical antibiotic therapy is not indicated.

g. Discharge: The decision to discharge the patient should be based on clinical improvement, *not* on SaO_2 measurements.

8. Prevention
   a. Patients are contagious during the 24 to 48 hours before the onset of symptoms and for several days thereafter. RSV-positive infants should probably be excluded from day care for 3 to 5 days after diagnosis.
   b. Contact precautions for hospitalized patients: Eye and nose goggles, gowns, gloves, and hand washing will restrict the spread of nosocomial infection.
   c. Immunization: Globulin preparations (RSV intravenous immune globulin [IVIG], palivizumab) with a high concentration of neutralizing antibody against RSV prevent severe illness due to RSV. The use of this agent has been recommended for the prevention of severe RSV illness in high-risk infants such as those with chronic lung disease and preterm birth (<35 weeks' gestation). This agent is administered once a month through the RSV season (see *Red Book* 2006, 27th edition).

9. Prognosis
   a. Short-term prognosis is excellent for infants and children with no underlying predisposing condition.
   b. Prognosis is more guarded for infants with moderate to severe bronchopulmonary dysplasia or cyanotic congenital heart disease. Early recognition of impending respiratory compromise is the key to avoiding morbidity and mortality.
   c. Long-term prognosis for subsequent or recurrent wheezing episodes or asthma is unclear.
      (1) As much as 40% to 50% of infants ill enough to be hospitalized with RSV infection will have recurrent episodes of wheezing.
      (2) The risk of recurrence may decrease markedly by 2 to 3 years of age in most infants; others will develop asthma.
      (3) Family history of atopy and exposure to environmental allergens, air pollution, and cigarette smoke may be contributing factors in the development of asthma for these infants.

PNEUMONIA/PNEUMONITIS SYNDROMES

1. Etiology and clinical features (Table 19-14)
   a. Neonates: Most neonatal bacterial pneumonias are caused by gram-positive cocci, particularly group B streptococci and occasionally S. aureus and gram-negative enteric bacilli.
   b. Children 1 month to 5 years of age: Respiratory *viruses* cause the majority of pediatric pneumonias in this age group.
      (1) The major *bacterial* pathogens in this age group are S. *pneumoniae* and type b H. *influenzae*. Pneumococci and type b H. *influenzae* are often associated with lobar or segmental consolidation, but bronchopneumonia can also be seen.
      (2) *Chlamydia trachomatis* produces an afebrile pneumonia syndrome in infants younger than 16 weeks of age, in which conjunctivitis is present in 50% of infants, eosinophilia is common, crackles are heard on chest examination, and the CXR shows hyperinflation and diffuse interstitial or patchy infiltrates.
      (3) S. *aureus* is usually seen in the very young (≤3 years), and severe pneumonia can lead to rapidly evolving respiratory distress, hypoxemia, empyema, and the characteristic radiologic features of rapid progression, lobular ectasia, and pneumatoceles.
   c. Children 5 years of age and older: S. *pneumoniae* and GABHS are the major causes of bacterial pneumonia in this age group.

Age Group	Etiologic Agents
Neonate	Group B streptococci
	Gram-negative enteric bacilli
	Listeria monocytogenes
	Cytomegalovirus
	Herpes simplex virus
Up to 3 mo	*Chlamydia trachomatis*
	RSV
	PIV type 3
	Bordetella pertussis
	Streptococcus pneumoniae
	Staphylococcus aureus
3 mo-5 yr	RSV, PIVs, influenza virus, rhinovirus, adenovirus
	S. *pneumoniae*
	Haemophilus influenzae
	Mycoplasma pneumoniae
	Mycobacterium tuberculosis
5-18 yr	M. *pneumoniae*
	S. *pneumoniae*
	Chlamydophila pneumoniae
	Mycobacterium pneumoniae

PIV, parainfluenza virus; RSV, respiratory syncytial virus.

(1) Illness is generally manifest by the sudden onset of a high fever and ill appearance and is associated with pallor, cough, tachypnea, pleuritic pain, and localized pulmonary findings (crackles and diminished breath sounds).

(2) An elevated WBC count (>15,000/mm^3) is common.

(3) Only 5% to 10% have positive blood cultures.

(4) The CXR may show local lobar or segmental infiltrates.

(5) Serosanguineous pleural effusion can occur.

(6) In patients with sickle cell disease, immunodeficiencies, and chronic pulmonary disease, pneumonia of any etiology can be severe.

d. M. pneumoniae is one of the most common causes of pneumonia in school-age children, adolescents, and young adults.

e. Bordetella pertussis, the etiologic agent of whooping cough, causes primarily a bronchitis but may be complicated by pneumonia in severe cases. It begins with mild upper respiratory tract symptoms (catarrhal stage) and progresses to cough and then usually with paroxysms of cough (paroxysmal stage), often with characteristic inspiratory whoop, followed by vomiting. Disease in infants may be atypical and apnea is a common manifestation.

f. In immunocompromised patients, pneumonia is commonly caused by the usual organisms, but gram-negatives, Pneumocystis carinii, and fungi are causes of primary or secondary infections also.

g. In children who aspirate, anaerobic bacteria, especially penicillin-sensitive oral anaerobes, can be associated with pneumonia and lung abscess.

h. TB should always be considered as a possible cause of pneumonia, especially in endemic areas or in the child who responds slowly or not at all to antibiotic therapy.

2. Laboratory findings

a. CXR (posteroanterior and lateral) utility is limited in nonseverely ill children with *clinically* documented pneumonia.

b. Tuberculin skin test (PPD), especially in endemic areas

c. Sputum or deep tracheal aspirate for Gram stain and culture

d. Cultures and fluorescent antibody techniques for respiratory viruses (which are rarely found in asymptomatic persons) are available but not generally necessary.

e. Blood culture(s) in patients who appear toxic or are immunocompromised

f. Serologic titers (acute and convalescent) can be helpful to diagnose mycoplasma (cold agglutinin titers of 1:64 or more), GABHS (antistreptolysin O titer), Chlamydia, Legionella, and Rickettsia (Q fever)

g. Thoracentesis can be helpful (for diagnosis and relief of Bordetella symptoms) if substantial pleural fluid is present.

h. Lung puncture or open lung biopsy is reserved for critically ill children to determine the etiologic agent and to guide antimicrobial therapy.

3. Management

a. Antimicrobials

(1) Mildly ill children with features suggestive of viral disease (e.g., coryza, conjunctivitis) can be managed without antibiotics, provided the patient can be closely followed.

(2) For patients with suspected bacterial illness, the choice of specific antibiotics is based on epidemiologic, clinical, and laboratory features (e.g., age, season).

(3) Specific recommendations for antimicrobial therapy *before* etiologic diagnosis:

    (a) Neonates (require hospitalization)

        (i) Ampicillin (<1 week of age): 100 mg/kg/day IV or IM every 12 hours; (≥1 week): 150 mg/kg/day IV or IM every 6 hours, *and*

        (ii) Cefotaxime (<1 week): 100 mg/kg/day IV every 12 hours; (≥1 week): 150 mg/kg/day IV every 8 hours, *or*

        (iii) Gentamicin (<1 week): 2.5 mg/kg/dose IV every 12 hours (≥1 week): 2.5 mg/kg/dose IV every 8 hours *or* 3.5 to 5 mg/kg/dose every 24 hours

        (iv) Add vancomycin or oxacillin if clinically toxic or with alveolar infiltrate

    (b) Hospitalized child 1 month to 5 years of age

        (i) Ampicillin/sulbactam 100 to 200 mg/kg/day in four divided doses, *or*

        (ii) Cefuroxime 75 to 100 mg/kg/day IV every 8 hours, *or*

        (iii) Cefotaxime 100 to 200 mg/kg/day IV every 8 hours, *or*

        (iv) Ceftriaxone 50 to 75 mg/kg/day IV or IM every 24 hours, *or*

        (v) Nafcillin *or* oxacillin 100 to 150 mg/kg/day IV every 6 hours, *and*

        (vi) Gentamicin 7.5 mg/kg/day IV or IM every 8 hours

        (vii) Continue IV therapy until afebrile for 72 to 96 hours before changing to an oral antimicrobial.

    (c) Nontoxic child 1 month to 5 years of age

        (i) Amoxicillin 80 to 90 mg/kg/day twice daily, for 7 to 10 days

        (ii) Amoxicillin-clavulanate (Augmentin) 80 to 90 mg/kg/day of amoxicillin orally twice daily, for 7 to 10 days

        (iii) Cefuroxime axetil (30 mg/kg/day every 12 hours for 7 to 10 days) is an alternative and also provides staphylococcal and amoxicillin-resistant *H. influenzae* coverage. If the clinical syndrome clearly suggests *Chlamydia*, clarithromycin or erythromycin should be administered for 14 days *or* azithromycin 10 mg/kg day 1 and 5 mg/kg days 2 to 5.

    (d) Older child with suspected M. *pneumoniae* infection

        (i) Erythromycin (30 to 50 mg/kg/day every 6 hours) or clarithromycin (15 mg/kg/day) for 14 to 21 days or azithromycin (10 mg/kg day 1 and 5 mg/kg days 2 to 5)

        (ii) *Note:* Failure to respond to one of the preceding regimens requires clinical reevaluation and adjustment of the choice of antimicrobials. For all pediatric age groups, empirical treatment for severe pneumonia normally includes vancomycin and one or two other agents.

b. Indications for hospitalization
   (1) Significant or worsening respiratory distress (e.g., SaO_2 <95%), cyanosis
   (2) Neonates or infants younger than 6 months of age if clinically unstable
   (3) Empyema or pleural effusion on CXR
   (4) Possible staphylococcal pneumonia
   (5) Anticipated inadequate home care or poor ability for follow-up
   (6) Persistent fever in a patient undergoing seemingly adequate outpatient antibiotic therapy (may be caused by loculated pleural fluid).

c. Symptomatic care
   (1) Oxygen if needed
   (2) Adequate hydration
   (3) High humidity
   (4) Bronchodilators if bronchospasm is present
   (5) Deep tracheal suctioning (especially for patients without adequate cough)
   (6) Postural drainage and physiotherapy (particularly with underlying bronchiectasis)

d. Outpatient management should include daily visits until definite clinical improvement can be documented.

e. Radiologic resolution generally lags behind clinical improvement, and abnormalities may remain on CXR for 4 to 6 weeks. Repeat CXR to document resolution is *not* necessary if clinical resolution occurs. However, persistent or recrudescent symptoms should alert the physician to possible underlying pulmonary processes (e.g., TB, foreign body, cystic fibrosis, immunodeficiency).

19.9 Cardiovascular System Infections

INFECTIVE ENDOCARDITIS

1. Pathophysiology and etiology
   a. Endocarditis is infection of the endocardial surface of the heart, including the heart valves. Infection of the endothelial surface of the blood vessels may also present as endocarditis.
   b. Organisms causing pediatric endocarditis primarily include *S. viridans* (other streptococci), *S. aureus*, *S. epidermidis*, and others.
   c. Risk factors for infective endocarditis
      (1) Congenital heart disease: especially Tetralogy of Fallot and ventricular septal defect
      (2) Surgically repaired congenital heart disease with patches, grafts, or artificial valves
      (3) Others
         (a) Indwelling central vascular catheters
         (b) IV drug use
         (c) Dental procedures

(d) Invasive GI or genitourinary surgery
(e) Rheumatic heart disease
2. Clinical features
a. Many symptoms are nonspecific; therefore, a high index of suspicion is required to diagnose endocarditis in a high-risk child.
b. Symptoms of infective endocarditis in children
(1) Fever of unknown origin, chronic, unrelenting fever (90%)
(2) Malaise/fatigue/arthralgias (50%)
(3) Anorexia/weight loss/arthralgias (25%)
(4) Abdominal pain/congestive heart failure (30%)
c. Signs of infective endocarditis in children
(1) Cutaneous manifestations: Petechiae (immune complex phenomena) are common. Janeway lesions, Osler's nodes, and splinter hemorrhages are more unusual.
(2) Splenomegaly (common)
(3) New or changing murmurs (especially regurgitant murmurs)
(4) Roth spots (white retinal patches with surrounding hemorrhage; rare)
(5) Neurologic abnormality (seizures, stroke; sudden and secondary to thromboemboli)
(6) Acute-fulminant sepsis
3. Diagnosis and laboratory studies
a. CBC (leukocytosis with left shift)
b. C-reactive protein (CRP), and ESR (increased in 90% to 95%)
c. CXR, electrocardiogram (ECG)
d. Blood cultures (bacteremia may be persistent and cultures will be positive in 70% to 98%). A positive blood culture in the right clinical setting confirms diagnosis. If the blood culture is negative, presumptive diagnosis can also be made based on typical clinical syndrome.
e. Urinalysis and culture (immune-complex nephritis leads to hematuria, proteinuria, casts)
f. BUN/creatinine (to assess renal function)
g. Rheumatoid factor (positive in 25%)
h. Complement (can be *low* if circulating immune complexes are present)
i. Cultures of potential sources of infection (lines, tips, etc.)
j. Echocardiography (for diagnosis and follow-up)
(1) Approximately 66% to 80% of children have valvular or endocardial vegetations demonstrated by two-dimensional technique.
(2) Vegetations smaller than 2 to 3 mm cannot be visualized (the longer the duration of symptoms, the larger the vegetations).
(3) Paravalvular abscesses and valvular insufficiency may be identified by echocardiography.
(4) The size of the vegetation may be a risk factor for embolization.
4. Management
a. Blood cultures recommendations for children with suspected endocarditis
(1) Acute endocarditis: Obtain two to three blood cultures separated by 15 minutes at *separate* venipuncture sites before initiating antibiotic therapy. Bacteremia is continuous in endocarditis; there is no need to wait for fever spikes.

            (2) Subacute endocarditis
                (a) Obtain three blood cultures at least 15 minutes apart on the
                    first day (in over 90% of patients, the first blood culture
                    drawn will be positive).
                (b) If all initial cultures are negative within 24 hours, obtain
                    two additional cultures.
                (c) If patient received prior antibiotic therapy, repeat two more
                    cultures on the third day.
        b. Antimicrobials
            (1) Initiation of antibiotics is critical and should not be delayed
                while blood culture results are pending.
            (2) Recommendations based on an identified pathogen appear in
                Box 19-4.
        c. Follow CBC, ESR, urinalysis, and complements as markers for
            improvement.
        d. Surgical intervention: Indications for surgery or replacement of
            infected valves
            (1) Worsening valvular function
            (2) Congestive heart failure (CHF) unresponsive to medical therapy
            (3) Multiple, major embolic events
            (4) Mycotic aneurysms
            (5) Fungal endocarditis not responsive to therapy
            (6) Removal of infected prosthetic valves
    5. Prevention of endocarditis
        a. Cardiac conditions and recommendations for endocarditis
            prophylaxis
            (1) Prosthetic cardiac valves, including bioprosthetic and homograft
                valves
            (2) Previous bacterial endocarditis, even in the absence of heart
                disease
            (3) Most congenital cardiac malformations
            (4) Rheumatic and other acquired valvular dysfunction, even after
                valvular surgery
            (5) Hypertrophic cardiomyopathy
            (6) Mitral valve prolapse with valvular regurgitation
            (7) Surgically constructed systemic pulmonary shunts or conduits
        b. Endocarditis prophylaxis not recommended
            (1) Isolated secundum atrial septal defect
            (2) Surgical repair without residua beyond 6 months of secundum
                atrial septal defect, ventricular septal defect, or patent ductus
                arteriosus
            (3) Physiologic, functional, or innocent heart murmurs
            (4) Previous Kawasaki's Disease (KD) without valvular dysfunction
            (5) Previous rheumatic fever without valvular dysfunction
            (6) Cardiac pacemakers and implanted defibrillators
        c. Endocarditis prophylaxis for at-risk individuals is recommended for
            the following procedures:
            (1) Dental procedures known to induce gingival or mucosal bleed-
                ing (includes professional cleaning)
            (2) Tonsillectomy and adenoidectomy

Box 19-4   Antimicrobial Therapy of Infective Endocarditis*

Viridans Streptococci and Enterococci

HIGHLY PENICILLIN SUSCEPTIBLE (MIC <0.1 μg/mL)
Penicillin G (150,000–200,000 U/kg/day) IV in six divided doses (every 4 hours) for 4 weeks
plus
Gentamicin (2-2.5 mg/kg/dose) IV every 8 hours for 2 weeks (peak level of 3.0 μg/mL desirable) for synergy
Penicillin-allergic child: vancomycin or cefazolin (two other regimens also recommended)
Ceftriaxone as alternative

MODERATELY PENICILLIN SUSCEPTIBLE (MIC >0.1 μg/mL BUT <0.5 μg/ml FOR PENICILLIN OR NUTRITIONALLY DEFICIENT VARIANTS)
Penicillin G (200,000-300,000 U/kg/day) IV every 4 hours *or* ampicillin (300 mg/kg/day) IV every 6 hours for 4 weeks
plus
Gentamicin (2-2.5 mg/kg/dose) IV every 8 hours for 2 weeks

LESS SUSCEPTIBLE (MIC = 0.5 μg/mL) OR ENTEROCOCCI
Same as for moderate penicillin susceptibility, but continue gentamicin for 4 weeks

Staphylococci[†]

METHICILLIN SUSCEPTIBLE
Nafcillin or oxacillin (150-200 mg/kg/day) IV in six divided doses for 4 to 6 weeks
plus
Gentamicin (2-2.5 mg/kg/dose) IV every 8 hours for 3 to 5 days
Penicillin-allergic child: cefazolin (100 mg/kg/day, maximum 6 g every 24 hours) IV every 8 hours, 4 to 6 weeks, and gentamicin for 3 to 5 days

METHICILLIN RESISTANT
Vancomycin (40-60 mg/kg/day) IV every 6 hours for 4 to 6 weeks

Staphylococci with Prosthetic Devices

Nafcillin, oxacillin, or cefazolin plus rifampin plus gentamicin

*Choices of antimicrobial therapy may need to be individualized and adjusted depending on organism (e.g., fungal infection) and host responses.
[†]Remove prosthetic material.
MIC, minimal inhibitory concentration.

      (3) Surgery involving intestinal or respiratory mucosa

      (4) Bronchoscopy with a rigid bronchoscope

      (5) Sclerotherapy for esophageal varices

      (6) Esophageal dilatation

      (7) Gallbladder surgery

      (8) Cystoscopy

      (9) Prostatic surgery

      (10) Urinary tract dilatation, catheterization, or surgery

      (11) Incision and drainage of infected tissue

      (12) Vaginal delivery in the presence of infection

      (13) Prophylaxis is *not* necessary for adjustment of orthodontic appliances, shedding of primary teeth, or tympanostomy tube insertion.

  d. *Standard* prophylactic antimicrobial regimens for dental, oral, or upper respiratory tract procedures in children at risk

      (1) Amoxicillin (50 mg/kg, maximum 3 g) orally, 1 hour before procedure

      (2) Penicillin-allergic patient

        (a) Clindamycin (20 mg/kg, maximum 600 mg) orally, 1 hour before procedure *or*

        (b) Azithromycin/clarithromycin (15 mg/kg, maximum 500 mg) orally, 1 hour before procedure

  e. *Alternative* prophylactic regimens if patient unable to take oral medication

      (1) Ampicillin (50 mg/kg, maximum 2 g) IV or IM, 30 minutes before procedure

      (2) If penicillin-allergic, clindamycin (20 mg/kg, maximum 600 mg) IV or IM, 30 minutes before procedure

ACUTE RHEUMATIC FEVER

1. Etiology: ARF generally follows symptomatic or asymptomatic GABHS pharyngitis by 2 to 3 weeks. The pathogenesis is unclear but may involve abnormal cell-mediated and humoral immune response to "rheumatic" strains of GABHS. Circulating immune complexes directed against M-proteins of GABHS cross-react with myosin/sarcolemma antigens shared by cardiac muscle.

2. Clinical features (Box 19-5). The Jones criteria help establish the diagnosis of ARF.

  a. Carditis may present as new or unexplained systolic murmurs signifying mitral or aortic insufficiency. Other evidence of carditis includes CHF, friction rub, muffled heart sounds, and ST-T wave change on ECG.

  b. Chorea (irregular, spasmodic, involuntary limb or facial movement) is a late, isolated finding and unusual in childhood.

3. Differential diagnosis

  a. Juvenile rheumatoid arthritis (JRA; migrating arthritis pattern is unusual in JRA)

  b. Systemic lupus erythematosus (SLE)

  c. Henoch-Schönlein purpura (HSP; purpuric, raised rash of HSP is much different than erythema marginatum)

  d. Serum sickness

Box 19-5   Jones Criteria for Diagnosis of Rheumatic Fever*

Major Criteria

Arthritis
Migratory, large joints
± Emotional lability
Chorea
Erythema marginatum (10%)
Subcutaneous nodules

Minor Criteria

Fever
Arthralgia (migration)
Elevated C-reactive protein or erythrocyte sedimentation rate
Prolonged PR interval

*Two major or one major with two minor criteria with recent evidence of streptococcal infection (positive throat culture or rapid antigen test, elevated or rising streptococcal antibody titers) are required for the diagnosis of acute rheumatic fever.

  e. Septic arthritis/osteomyelitis
  f. Postinfectious reactive arthritis (can follow GABHS infection, but Jones criteria not met)
4. Laboratory evaluation
  a. Elevated ESR and CRP with acute carditis and polyarthritis, but nonspecific
  b. CXR (cardiomegaly, signs of CHF)
  c. ECG (prolonged PR interval, ST-T changes)
  d. Echocardiography (evidence of pericarditis and valvular, especially aortic and mitral dysfunction). Mild valvular regurgitation by echocardiography alone without a clinical murmur is *not* a criterion.
  e. Documented streptococcal infection—throat culture or antigen test: antistreptolysin O titer increase (60% of cases ≥500 Todd units); follow titers serially to confirm previous infection. Also, anti-DNAase B and antihyaluronidase titers may be increased.
  f. Other: CBC, urinalysis, antinuclear antibody, bone scan, and cultures to help rule out other conditions
5. Management
  a. Eradication of streptococci should be undertaken (see section on Streptococcal Pharyngitis).
  b. Anti-inflammatory therapy may relieve symptoms.
    (1) Aspirin (acetylsalicylic acid [ASA]) is given for arthritis without carditis and also for children with mild cardiac involvement (75 to 100 mg/kg/day in four to six divided doses for a minimum of 4 to 6 weeks). Optimal serum concentration is 20 to 25 mg/100 mL.

      (a) Naproxen sodium (25 to 30 mg/kg/day in three divided doses) can also be used.

      (b) Although anti-inflammatory medications provide symptomatic relief (fever, arthralgias), they may not alter the course of myocardial injury.

      (c) These medications should be slowly tapered over a minimum of 4 to 6 weeks after *all* signs, symptoms, and laboratory test results (ESR) have returned to normal. Abruptly discontinuing the medication can lead to fulminant pancarditis.

    (2) Corticosteroid therapy for ARF remains controversial. In patients with severe carditis and CHF, corticosteroids are often needed.

      (a) Prednisone is usually given at a dose of 2 mg/kg/day, twice a day, for 4 to 6 weeks and then tapered over the next 2 to 4 weeks, depending on clinical response and laboratory tests.

      (b) As with other medications, corticosteroids will control inflammation but may not prevent residual valvular damage.

    (3) Digitalis and diuretics should be used with caution in patients with ARF complicated by CHF because of increased sensitivity of an inflamed myocardium to those agents.

    (4) Bed rest during the acute phase, especially if CHF is present, is necessary. Activity should be minimal until the ESR returns to normal.

    (5) Children with significant chorea are managed with psychiatric intervention and occasionally with medications (phenobarbital, chlorpromazine, diazepam, or haloperidol).

6. Prevention of ARF

  a. Prevention is indicated for individuals with one or more attacks of rheumatic fever because they have an increased risk of recurrence after GABHS pharyngitis.

  b. Risk of recurrence is highest in first 5 years after ARF, with multiple episodes, and with rheumatic heart disease.

  c. Secondary prophylactic regimens include

    (1) Benzathine penicillin G 1.2 million U IM every 3 to 4 weeks

    (2) Penicillin V 250 mg orally twice a day

    (3) Sulfisoxazole 1 g orally once daily if more than 60 pounds (27 kg) or 0.5 g once daily if less than 60 pounds, *or*

    (4) Erythromycin 250 mg orally twice a day

  d. Prophylaxis should begin soon after the diagnosis of ARF is made and initial therapy begun. It should be continuous and long term, perhaps for life in patients with carditis.

  e. Patients without rheumatic heart disease are at lower risk for recurrence. In these mild cases, it should be continued 5 or more years or at least until the patient is 21 years of age.

PERICARDITIS

1. Etiology and pathophysiology: Inflammation of the pericardial sac, possibly associated with effusion. Similar to endocarditis, pericarditis is often associated with acute bacterial infections such as *S. aureus*, *H. influenzae*, *S. pneumoniae*, and *N. meningitidis*. However, other etiologies to be considered, especially with recurrent pericarditis, include

ARF, SLE, systemic-onset JRA, uremia, postpericardiotomy, TB, multiple viruses (EBV, coxsackievirus), mycoplasmas, or parasites.
2. Clinical features
   a. Patients typically present with the following:
      (1) Chest pain (pericardial, referred to shoulder and back, better sitting up)
      (2) Dyspnea and tachypnea (shallow, rapid respirations)
      (3) Fever, malaise, fatigue
      (4) "Toxic" appearance (especially infants with sepsis)
   b. Physical examination may show the following:
      (1) Tachycardia
      (2) Decreased heart sounds
      (3) Pericardial friction rub (scratchy heart sounds)
      (4) Kussmaul's sign: distended neck veins with inspiration
3. Diagnosis and laboratory findings
   a. CXR: Early, left heart border straightened; later, enlarged "water-bottle" heart shape. Pneumonia may also be present.
   b. ECG: Low voltages, ST-T changes (ST segment elevation, T-wave inversion)
   c. Echocardiography: Diagnostic test of choice; qualifies and quantifies pericardial effusion
   d. Laboratory studies
      (1) Elevated WBC count (left shift)
      (2) Very elevated ESR
      (3) Obtain blood cultures, antinuclear antibody, complements, antistreptolysin O titers, BUN, creatinine, urinalysis
      (4) Place PPD
      (5) Viral serology and cultures, cold agglutinins, EBV titers
      (6) Cardiac enzymes
      (7) Total protein, albumin
      (8) Pericardial tap, if performed, may show the following:
         (a) If bacterial: Exudative protein (>3 g/l00 mL), low glucose, organisms on Gram stain, and highly elevated PMNs
         (b) If viral or collagen vascular: Transudative protein (<2 g/100 mL), normal glucose, and lymphocytosis
4. Management
   a. Bed rest is needed until symptoms resolve.
   b. Pericardiocentesis (or tube drainage) is required for bacterial infection (i.e., diagnosis and treatment).
   c. Antimicrobials (for bacterial pericarditis)
      (1) Nafcillin or oxacillin 150 mg/kg IV every 6 hours (maximum 12 g/day) *and either*
      (2) Gentamicin or tobramycin (normal renal function)
         (a) Younger than 5 years (except neonates): 2.5 mg/kg/dose IV every 8 hours
         (b) Older than 5 years: 2 to 2.5 mg/kg IV every 8 hours, *or*
      (3) Ceftriaxone 75 to 100 mg/kg/day IV every 12 hours (maximum 4 g/day), *or*
      (4) Cefotaxime 100 to 200 mg/kg/day IV every 6 to 8 hours (maximum 12 g/day)

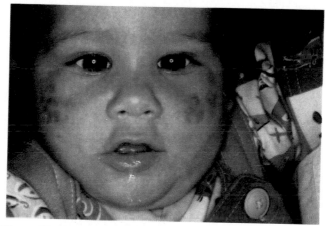

Figure 13-1 Infantile acne. (From Bolognia JL, Jorizzo JJ, Rapini RP [eds]: Dermatology. Philadelphia, Elsevier-Mosby, 2003.)

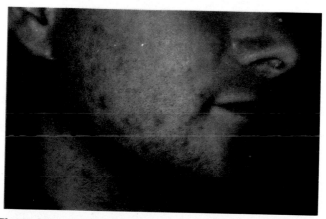

Figure 13-2 Papules, pustules, and scattered small cysts. (From Bolognia JL, Jorizzo JJ, Rapini RP [eds]: Dermatology. Philadelphia, Elsevier-Mosby, 2003.)

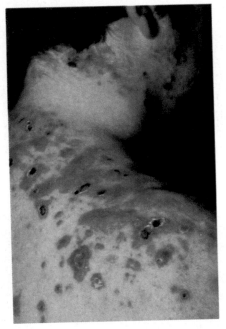

Figure 13-3 Severe cystic acne vulgaris. (From Bolognia JL, Jorizzo JJ, Rapini RP [eds]: Dermatology. Philadelphia, Elsevier-Mosby, 2003.)

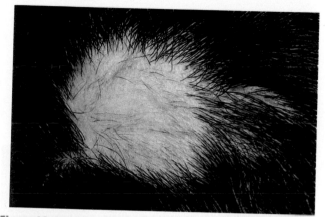

Figure 13-4 Localized alopecia areata. (From Weston WL, Lare AT, Morelli JG: *Color Textbook of Pediatric Dermatology,* 3rd ed. St. Louis, Mosby, 2002.)

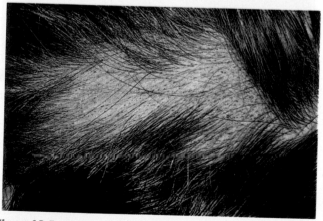

Figure 13-5 Circumscribed area of hair loss without scalp change and with hairs broken off at the follicular orifice. This is the black-dot pattern of *Trichophyton tonsurans* infection. (From Weston WL, Lane AT, Morelli JG: *Color Textbook of Pediatric Dermatology,* 3rd ed. St. Louis, Mosby, 2002.)

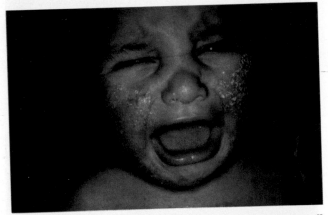

Figure 13-6 Atopic dermatitis on the face of an infant. (From Bolognia JL, Jorizzo JJ, Rapini RP [eds]: Dermatology. Philadelphia, Elsevier-Mosby, 2003.)

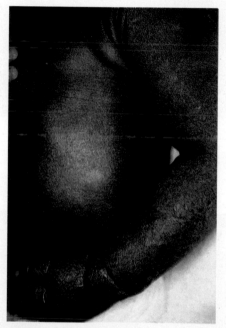

Figure 13-7 Atopic dermatitis on the extensor surface of an infant's arm. (From Bolognia JL, Jorizzo JJ, Rapini RP [eds]: Dermatology. Philadelphia, Elsevier-Mosby, 2003.)

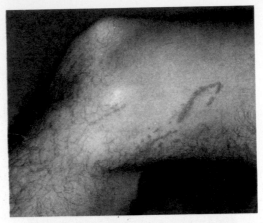

Figure 13-8 Allergic contact dermatitis on the legs secondary to poison oak; note the linear pattern where the leaf has brushed against the leg. (From Weston WL, Lane AT, Morelli JG: Color Textbook of Pediatric Dermatology, 3rd ed. St. Louis, Mosby, 2002.)

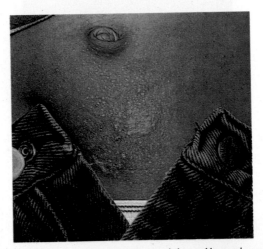

Figure 13-9 Allergic contact dermatitis to nickel caused by metal snap on blue jeans. (From Weston WL, Lane AT, Morelli JG: Color Textbook of Pediatric Dermatology. 3rd ed. St. Louis, Mosby, 2002.)

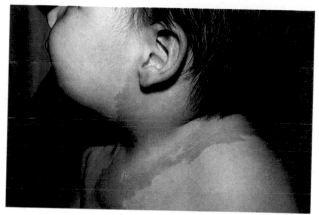

Figure 13-10 Large café au lait macule on a child's, neck. (From Weston WL, Lane AT, Morelli JG: Color Textbook of Pediatric Dermatology, 3rd ed. St. Louis, Mosby, 2002.)

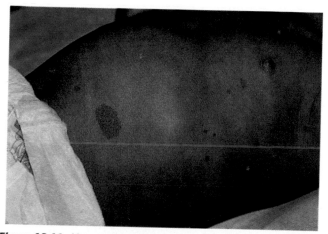

Figure 13-11 Numerous café au lait macules in a patient with neurofibromatosis type 1. (From Weston WL, Lane AT, Morelli JG: Color Textbook of Pediatric Dermatology. 3rd ed. St. Louis, Mosby, 2002.)

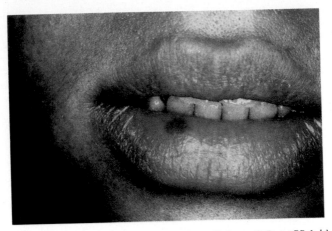

Figure 13-12 Junctional nevus. (From Bolognia JL, Jorizzo JJ, Rapini RP [eds]: Dermatology. Philadelphia, Elsevier-Mosby, 2003.)

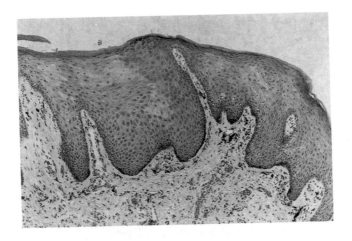

Figure 13-13 Compound melanocytic nevus. (From Bolognia JL, Jorizzo JJ, Rapini RP [eds]: Dermatology. Philadelphia, Elsevier-Mosby, 2003.)

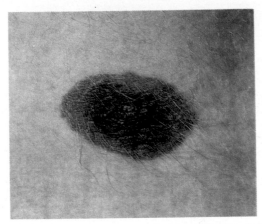

Figure 13-14   Dermal nevus. (From Weston WL, Lane AT , Morelli JG: Color Textbook of Pediatric Dermatology, 3rd ed. St. Louis, Mosby, 2002.)

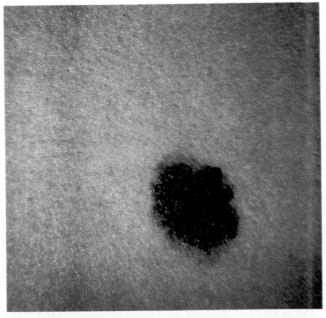

Figure 13-15   Small congenital nevus. (From Bolognia JL, Jorizzo JJ, Rapini RP [eds]: Dermatology. Philadelphia, Elsevier-Mosby, 2003.)

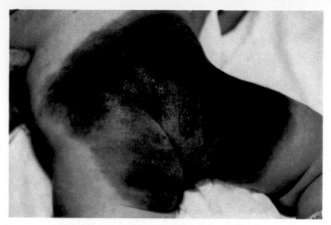

Figure 13-16 Giant congenital nevus. (From Bolognia JL, Jorizzo JJ, Rapini RP [eds]: Dermatology. Philadelphia, Elsevier-Mosby, 2003,)

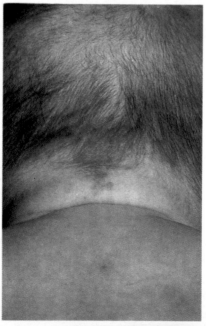

Figure 13-17 Salmon patch. (From Weston WL, Lane AT, Morelli JG: Color Textbook of Pediatric Dermatology, 3rd ed. St.Louis, Mosby, 2002)

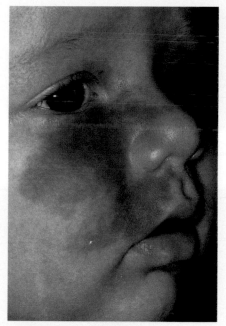

Figure 13-18 Port-wine stain in a cranial nerve V-2 distribution in an infant. (From Bolognia JL, Jorizzo JJ, Rapini RP [eds]: Dermatology. Philadelphia, Elsevier-Mosby, 2003.)

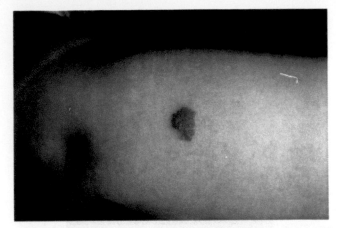

Figure 13-19 Superficial hemangioma. (From Bolognia JL, Jorizzo JJ, Rapini RP [eds]: Dermatology. Philadelphia, Elsevier-Mosby, 2003.)

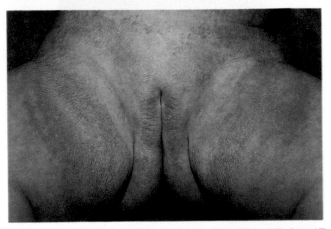

Figure 13-20 Chafing type of diaper dermatitis. (From Weston WL, Lane AT, Morelli JG: Color Textbook of Pediatric Dermatology, 3rd ed. St. Louis, Mosby, 2002.)

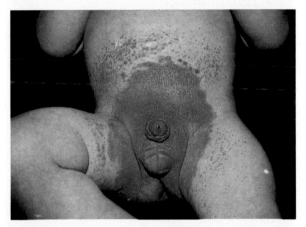

Figure 13-21 Candidiasis of diaper region. (From Weston WL, Lane AT, Morelli JG: Color Textbook of Pediatric Dermatology, 3rd ed. St. Louis, Mosby, 2002.)

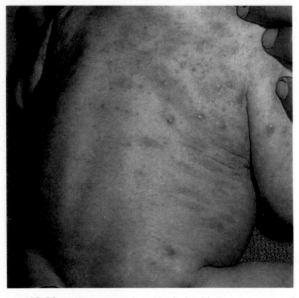

Figure 13-22 Scabies in an infant. Hundreds of lesions are present. (From Weston WL, Lane AT, Morelli JG: Color Textbook of Pediatric Dermatology, 3rd ed. St. Louis, Mosby, 2002.)

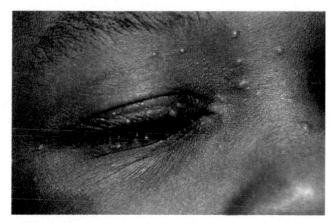

Figure 13-23 Multiple molluscum papules on a child's face. (From Weston WL, Lane AT, Morelli JG: Color Textbook of Pediatric Dermatology, 3rd ed. St. Louis, Mosby, 2002.)

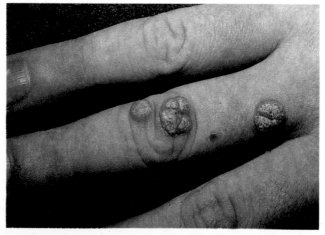

Figure 13-24 Multiple verrucae on a child's fingers. (From Weston WL, Lane AT, Morelli JG: Color Textbook of Pediatric Dermatology, 3rd ed. St. Louis, Mosby, 2002.)

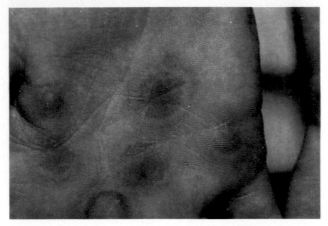

Figure 13-25 Classic target lesions on the palms. (From Bolognia JL, Jorizzo JJ, Rapini RP [eds]: Dermatology. Philadelphia, Elsevier-Mosby, 2003.)

Figure 13-26 Pityriasis rosea. (From Weston WL, Lane AT, Morelli JG: Color Textbook of Pediatric Dermatology, 3rd ed. St. Louis, Mosby, 2002.)

  d. Anti-inflammatory medications to control the inflammatory response
   (1) ASA 10 to 15 mg/kg/dose orally every 4 to 6 hours (maximum 2 to 3 g/day; warn family about Reye's syndrome) *or*
   (2) Ibuprofen 5 to 10 mg/kg/dose orally three or four times a day *and/or*
   (3) Prednisone 1 to 2 mg/kg/day orally twice a day, every day
   (4) Anti-inflammatory drugs may need to be continued at least until ESR returns to normal, or longer, depending on etiology.
  e. Pain/sedating medications
   (1) Morphine 0.1 mg/kg/dose every 2 to 3 hours IM or IV, *or*
   (2) Meperidine (Demerol) 1 to 2 mg/kg/dose every 2 to 3 hours as needed for pain
  f. Cardiovascular monitoring; check for pulsus paradoxus (>15 mm Hg suggests early tamponade).
5. Prognosis: Generally, most patients recover if infection is stabilized early with antibiotics or drainage; tamponade or constrictive pericarditis does not occur; and underlying etiologies (e.g., SLE, vasculitis) are controlled.

MYOCARDITIS

1. Etiology
  a. The most common cause of myocarditis is viral: coxsackievirus, echoviruses, influenza virus, adenovirus, mumps, rubella, HIV.
  b. Bacterial and other etiologies
   (1) *S. aureus, N. meningitidis*
   (2) *Rickettsia* (Rocky Mountain spotted fever [RMSF])
   (3) ARF (pancarditis)
   (4) KD
   (5) Toxic (lead)
   (6) Connective tissue disorders (JRA, SLE)
   (7) Systemic metabolic diseases (Pompe's disease, Hurler's syndrome)
   (8) Neoplasia (rhabdomyosarcoma, chemotherapy with doxorubicin)
2. Clinical features
  a. The presentation is associated with either an acute, fulminant course (as seen in young infants with sepsis) or a subacute/chronic yet unrelenting course (as sometimes seen in adolescents).
  b. Fever (especially in acute illness) followed by
   (1) Dyspnea (even with minor exertion)
   (2) Fatigue (may be indolent and occur over many months with subacute course)
   (3) Pallor
   (4) Dysrhythmias (especially with acute, fulminant course)
   (5) Tachypnea and tachycardia consistent with CHF
3. Diagnosis and laboratory evaluation
  a. CXR: Signs of CHF (increased vascular markings, pulmonary edema), enlarged heart (especially left atrium and ventricle)
  b. ECG: Nonspecific ST-T wave changes, low voltages, left ventricular hypertrophy and strain pattern

   c. Echocardiography: Poor contractibility, enlarged left atrium and ventricle
   d. Laboratory studies: CBC, ESR, CRP, viral cultures/serology, connective tissue work-up—most studies will be nonspecific.
   e. If performed, an endomyocardial biopsy will help differentiate viral from other etiologies.
4. Management
   a. Bed rest and supportive care (oxygen)
   b. Digitalis (low dose used because of myocardial sensitivity)
   c. Diuretics for CHF
   d. Afterload-reducing and adrenergic agents
   e. Careful cardiac monitoring
   f. Intubation and sedation to decrease work of breathing and myocardial strain
   g. Immunosuppressive agents and steroids *if* biopsy suggests fulminant inflammation or connective tissue disorder
5. Prognosis: The course and prognosis of myocarditis is variable; patients may experience spontaneous and complete recovery or may develop a progressive cardiomyopathy with chronic CHF, ultimately requiring transplantation.

19.10 Gastrointestinal Infections

ACUTE GASTROENTERITIS/DIARRHEA

1. Epidemiology
   a. GI infections are second only to acute respiratory infections as a cause of infectious morbidity in children worldwide.
   b. Enteropathogens are acquired through the fecal-oral route from person-to-person transfer or through contaminated food or water.
   c. In the United States, 9% of all hospitalizations of children younger than 5 years of age are due to diarrhea.
   d. Worldwide, diarrhea and dehydration cause 4 to 5 million deaths per year, mostly in developing countries.
2. Definition and pathophysiology of acute GI processes
   a. Diarrhea: Passage of unformed bowel movements at a daily rate twice that of the patient's usual rate; physiologically defined as a daily stool weight of more than 200 g/24 hours. Diarrhea may also be classified as follows:
      (1) Secretory: Very loose, watery stool due to an increased intestinal secretion of fluid and electrolytes (stool volume over 10 mL/kg/hr; fecal sodium over 85 mEq/L)
      (2) Osmotic: Due to nonabsorbable intraluminal molecules (stool osmolality is greater than the fecal sodium plus twice the fecal potassium concentration)
      (3) Exudative: Outpouring of inflammatory cells and mucosal sloughing
      (4) Anatomic bypass: Decreased surface absorptive area leading to diarrheal stool
   b. Acute dysentery: A syndrome of abdominal pain associated with stools containing gross blood and mucus and frequent small, loose

bowel movements. Characterized by microbial invasion of the colon causing inflammation.

c. Food poisoning: An illness of short incubation (<24 hours) presenting as pernicious vomiting, resulting from ingestion of a preformed toxin or from a toxin produced shortly after ingestion (most common causative agents are *S. aureus*, *Bacillus cereus*, and *Clostridium perfringens*)

d. Gastroenteritis: A misnomer because many enteric infections have minimal inflammation and very rarely directly affect the stomach

e. Vomiting alone, without diarrhea, should make one consider noninfectious etiologies: Head trauma or CNS infection (from increased ICP), gastric/peptic ulcer disease, toxins/poisons (e.g., lead), child abuse, metabolic disturbances (e.g., diabetes), or other causes

3. Etiology and clinical features

a. Viral diarrhea—rotavirus (most common)

   (1) Highest rate of illness in children 3 to 24 months of age

   (2) Peak incidence in winter months

   (3) Transmitted person-to-person by fecal-oral route

   (4) Selective infection and destruction of absorptive intestinal villus cells of jejunum and ileum leads to decreased absorption of sodium and water, resulting in net fluid secretion, poor glucose transport, carbohydrate malabsorption, and an osmotic diarrhea.

   (5) Illness begins 1 to 4 days after exposure and lasts from 3 to 7 days.

   (6) Viral gastroenteritis manifests as loose, watery stools that can be normal in color or acholic, odorless or foul smelling. Mucus and gross blood are absent. Up to 20 episodes of diarrhea or vomiting can occur per day.

   (7) Other, less common causes of viral gastroenteritis include enteric adenoviruses, caliciviruses, and astroviruses.

b. Bacterial diarrhea

   (1) Much less common than viral causes of diarrhea

   (2) Most bacterial enteric pathogens cause an inflammatory enteritis.

   (3) Principal agents in the United States include *Salmonella* species, *Shigella* species, *Campylobacter* species, *Yersinia enterocolitica*, *Vibrio parahaemolyticus*, enteroinvasive *E. coli*, enterohemorrhagic *E. coli*, and *Aeromonas hydrophilia*.

   (4) Clinically associated with

      (a) Abrupt onset of diarrhea with little or no vomiting before onset of diarrhea

      (b) Stool containing mucus (i.e., fecal leukocytes) or blood

      (c) Fever and possibly toxic or ill appearance if infection is severe

c. Traveler's diarrhea—enterotoxigenic *E. coli* (ETEC; most common cause)

   (1) A self-limited illness lasting several days

   (2) Affects 40% of travelers to developing countries

   (3) *Shigella* and *Salmonella* or other bacteria, viruses, and *Giardia* have also been associated.

d. Pseudomembranous colitis (antibiotic-associated colitis): Caused by *C. difficile* toxin (detected in the stool), produced as the organism overgrows the weakened gut flora of patients receiving antibiotics

e. Food poisoning
   (1) Caused by several bacteria (usually toxin producing), including staphylococci, C. perfringens, Clostridium botulinum (botulism), V. parahaemolyticus, and B. cereus
   (2) It may be possible to predict the offending organism from the incubation period (time from ingestion to onset of symptoms); for S. aureus, symptoms usually occur at 3 to 6 hours, but as early as 30 minutes; for C. perfringens, 1 to 25 hours, usually 8 to 12 hours. Food poisoning due to B. cereus may be characterized by short incubation, with onset of symptoms within 6 hours, or longer incubation (within 16 hours).
f. Parasitic enteritis
   (1) Intestinal parasites are most common among children with history of travel or immigration from endemic areas.
   (2) Immunocompromised hosts (eg., HIV, T-cell deficiencies) are at risk for intestinal parasites causing chronic diarrhea (Cryptosporidium, Microsporidium, Isospora)
   (3) Giardia lamblia is a common cause of abdominal pain, bloating, and nonbloody diarrhea in children.
   (4) In children with recent travel to a developing country presenting with fever and grossly bloody stool (dysentery), suspect Entamoeba histolytica (amebic dysentery).
4. Diagnosis
   a. History
      (1) It is important to consider the character, duration, quantity of stools, presence or absence of vomiting, bloody or mucusy stools, and a history of travel, outbreaks, ill contacts, antibiotic use, seafood ingestion, day care attendance, chronic illness, and sexual exposure.
      (2) The amount of fluid intake should be noted, and an assessment of hydration status should be made.
   b. Laboratory findings
      (1) Gram stain of stool (for suspected bacterial enteritis)
         (a) Obtain stool specimen by reversing diaper so that nonabsorptive side faces skin, which allows mucus-containing WBCs not to be absorbed into diaper.
         (b) The presence of sheets of fecal WBCs correlates with inflammatory (i.e., bacterial) disease.
      (2) Stool culture: The following are indications for obtaining a stool culture to assist in diagnosis and management:
         (a) Bloody stool, especially with abrupt onset of diarrhea (note: always perform a guaiac test on stool to be certain that blood is present)
         (b) Toxic appearance in patients with loose stools
         (c) Severe diarrhea (more than 10 stools/day in non-rotavirus season)
         (d) Chronic diarrheal disease
         (e) Impaired host defenses (e.g., HIV infection, T-cell immunodeficiencies)
         (f) During specific epidemics or with nosocomial infections

(3) Blood cultures in ill, hospitalized patients should be obtained.

(4) Assay for rotavirus is an enzyme immunoassay (EIA) test (usually results available same day).

(5) Stool test for C. *difficile* toxin

(6) Serologic titers for *Yersinia* (fourfold rise is diagnostic)

(7) Stool for ova and parasites (when *Giardia*, *Cryptosporidium*, amebae, or other parasites suspected)

(8) Culture for sexually transmitted diseases (STDs) if indicated (e.g., sexually active adolescents with proctitis).

5. Management and prevention
   a. Antimicrobial therapy
      (1) *Salmonella* gastroenteritis: Most mildly ill patients with *Salmonella* gastroenteritis are not treated because antimicrobials may prolong the carrier state (fecal excretion of organisms). Treatment is given only to children at increased risk for invasive disease.
         (a) Indications for antimicrobial treatment
            (i) Infection in young infants ($\leq$3 months)
            (ii) Immunocompromised patients
            (iii) Hemoglobinopathies (e.g., sickle cell disease)
            (iv) Malignant neoplasm
            (v) Chronic inflammatory bowel disease
            (vi) Severe toxicity
            (vii) Enteritis with bacteremia, especially if fever and toxicity are present at the time the results of a positive blood culture are obtained
         (b) *Salmonella* infections may be treated with ampicillin (200 mg/kg/day) or TMP/SMX (TMP 50 mg/kg/ day) in susceptible strains.
         (c) For resistant organisms, cefotaxime (150 to 200 mg/kg/day) or ceftriaxone (100 mg/kg/day) are usually effective.
      (2) *Shigella* enteritis: These organisms are likely to be highly resistant to ampicillin and TMP/SMX. Therefore, ceftriaxone (50 mg/kg/day) should be provided when *Shigella* is isolated before susceptibility is known.
         (a) Susceptible strains may be treated with ampicillin (100 mg/kg/day every 6 hours for 5 days).
         (b) Amoxicillin is too rapidly absorbed from the GI tract to be effective.
         (c) Antidiarrheal drugs should not be used because of risk of prolonging the course of the infection.
      (3) *Campylobacter* enteritis: May be successfully treated with erythromycin (40 mg/kg/day orally every 6 hours for 5 to 7 days) *or* azithromycin (10 mg/kg day 1, 5 mg/kg days 2 to 5 orally) *or* doxycycline (if older than 8 years of age; 2 to 4 mg/kg/day orally every 12 to 24 hours) if symptoms have not resolved by the time the culture result is known.
      (4) Traveler's diarrhea (ETEC)
         (a) Infection may be prevented by drinking only boiled or pre-bottled water or other processed beverages (e.g., soft drinks). Avoid unpeeled fruits, salads, and ice of questionable source.

(b) No specific prophylactic antibiotic therapy is recommended because the disease is generally self-limited.

(c) Treatment may be appropriate in cases where diarrhea is intractable or severe. Optimal therapy is not established and antibiotic resistance is common. Treatment may be considered with TMP/SMX or ciprofloxacin (however, this agent is not licensed for use in children younger than the age of 18 years).

(5) Pseudomembranous colitis (*C. difficile*): This condition is treated by withholding or withdrawing the offending antibiotic. In addition, treatment can be undertaken with metronidazole (30 mg/kg/day orally or IV) *or* vancomycin (40 mg/kg/day orally) for 7 to 10 days or until follow-up stools are negative for toxins.

(6) Other pathogens

    (a) *Yersinia*

        (i) No antibiotic treatment is needed for routine gastroenteritis.

        (ii) Severely ill or septic patients are treated with aminoglycoside plus a third-generation cephalosporin IV, *or* TMP/SMX orally.

    (b) *G. lamblia*

        (i) Metronidazole (Flagyl) 15 mg/kg/day orally three times a day, for 5 to 7 days, *or*

        (ii) Albendazole 15 mg/kg/day orally twice daily for 5 to 7 days, *or*

        (iii) Furazolidone 6 mg/kg/day orally four times a day, for 10 days

    (c) *E. histolytica* causing symptomatic disease (dysentery—pain, fever, tenderness, bloody, mucusy diarrhea) can be treated with metronidazole 30 to 50 mg/kg/day orally every 8 hours for 10 days (maximum 500 to 750 mg/dose), plus iodoquinol 30 to 40 mg/kg/day orally every 8 hours for 20 days.

    (d) *Vibrio cholerae*

        (i) TMP/SMX 10 to 50 mg/kg/day orally every 8 hours for 3 days

        (ii) Doxycycline 6 mg/kg as single dose (maximum 300 mg) in children older than 8 years of age

b. Fluid rehabilitation and maintenance therapy

(1) Oral rehydration (see also Chapter 9)

    (a) The mainstay of therapy for gastroenteritis is the proper restoration of normal baseline fluid and electrolyte status.

    (b) The presence of glucose (in oral rehydration therapy solution) in the small bowel lumen improves sodium absorption by means of coupled active transport across the mucosa, resulting in enhanced water absorption.

(2) Early feeding

    (a) Feeding should be reintroduced in the first 24 hours of the episode, if possible.

    (b) The advantages to early feeding include

        (i) Decreased intestinal permeability

(ii) Prevention of mucosal hypoplasia, which results in decreased absorption

(iii) Promotion of good weight gain and early cessation of diarrhea

(c) Initial foods include the following:

(i) Infants: Breast milk, diluted or full-strength formula, or milk

(ii) Older infants and children: Lean meats, yogurt, fruits, vegetables, rice, wheat, cereal, breads, potatoes, other complex carbohydrate foods

(d) Infants should be observed closely to detect and treat dehydration with IV fluids.

(3) Antidiarrheal therapy

(a) Because of the self-limited nature of gastroenteritis and potential side effects, antidiarrheal medications are generally not recommended for children.

(b) Described here are several regimens that should be used with caution if one chooses to treat complicated or prolonged infections.

(i) Kaolin with pectin (Kaopectate): 3 to 6 years: 15 to 30 mL/dose orally; 6 to 12 years: 30 to 60 mL/dose; over 12 years, 60 to 120 mL/dose after each loose bowel movement or every 3 to 4 hours as needed; or

(ii) Loperamide (Imodium): Initial doses for 2 to 5 years: 1 mg three times daily; 6 to 8 years: 2 mg twice daily; 8 to 12 years: 2 mg three times daily. After initial dosing, 0.1 mg/kg/dose after each loose stool but not to exceed initial dosage (1 mg/5 mL; capsules 2 mg); or

(iii) Diphenoxylate with atropine (Lomotil): Over 2 years, 0.3 to 0.4 mg/kg/day (maximum 15 mg diphenoxylate) orally 3 to 4 times a day (2.5 mg diphenoxylate/5 mL); or

(iv) Bismuth subsalicylate (Pepto Bismol): 3 to 6 years, 5 mL orally every 30 to 60 minutes as needed; 6 to 9 years, 10 mL orally every 30 to 60 minutes as needed; 9 to 12 years, 15 mL orally every 30 to 60 minutes as needed; over 12 years, 30 mL every 30 to 60 minutes as needed; up to eight doses per 24 hours

(4) Probiotics: For bacterial diarrhea, the effects of probiotics have been variable.

PERITONITIS

1. Etiology and pathophysiology: An acute infection of the peritoneal cavity; more than 250 polymorphonuclear cells/mm^3 of peritoneal fluid and evidence of infection by stain or culture. The types of peritonitis, associated risk factors, and etiologies are shown in Table 19-15.

2. Clinical features

a. Fever, anorexia, vomiting, lethargy, toxicity

b. Abdominal pain, tenderness (striking the heel with a fist produces pain in the abdomen) and rigidity

Table 19-15	Types of Peritonitis	
Type	Underlying Risk Factors	Etiology
Primary (blood or lymph borne; 3%-5% of all cases)	Ascites: nephrotic syndrome, cirrhosis, peritoneal dialysis	*E. coli* (most common), *S. pneumoniae*, *S. pyogenes*, *S. aureus*, *S. epidermidis*
Secondary (>80% of cases)	Perforated bowel, appendicitis	Enteric gram-negative rods: anaerobes, enterococci

    c. Abdominal wall cellulitis
    d. Decreased bowel sounds and fluid wave in abdomen
3. Diagnosis and laboratory findings
    a. Peritoneal lavage (for diagnosis and treatment); peritoneal fluid will have elevated protein and WBC count over 250/mm^3.
    b. Gram stain (to guide therapy)
    c. Aerobic/anaerobic, fungal, AFB cultures
    d. Plain abdominal film may show intestinal dilation, edema, fluid, obliteration of psoas shadow, and free air.
    e. Abdominal ultrasonography and CT scan can help identify the cause.
4. Management
    a. Early and initial antimicrobial therapy is empirical, often using three antimicrobial agents to cover multiple organisms (Table 19-16).
    b. Secondary *medical* management
       (1) Correction of hypovolemia and electrolyte stabilization to reestablish adequate urine output
       (2) Correction of hypoxemia with supplemental oxygen and mechanical ventilation, if necessary
       (3) Decompression of GI tract using nasogastric suction
    c. *Surgical* intervention often includes one or more of the following:
       (1) Closure or resection of perforated viscus
       (2) Irrigation of peritoneal cavity with or without antibiotics
       (3) Debridement of the peritoneum
       (4) Placement of drains into peritoneum for drainage and lavage

19.11 Joint and Bone Infections

SEPTIC ARTHRITIS (BACTERIAL INFECTIONS, EXCLUSIVE OF LYME ARTHRITIS)

1. Epidemiology: Septic arthritis (SA), an acute bacterial infection of a joint, can occur in children of all ages but is most common between the ages of 1 and 2 years. An associated osteomyelitis is found in 10% of cases of septic arthritis.
2. Pathophysiology

Table 19-16 Choices of Antimicrobials in Peritonitis

Intestinal Flora	Antimicrobials
Enteric gram-negative rods	Aminoglycosides: gentamicin or tobramycin (normal renal function): <5 yr (except neonates), 7.5 mg/kg/day IV every 8 hr; 5-10 yr, 6 mg/kg/day IV every 8 hr *plus*
Anaerobic	Clindamycin 20-40 mg/kg/day IV or IM every 6 hr (*or* metronidazole) *plus*
Enterococci	Ampicillin 100 mg/kg/day IV every 6 hr (*or* vancomycin)

a. SA is most commonly due to hematogenous spread of organisms; the primary source is often not apparent. Blood-borne bacterial invasion of synovial membranes results in synovial fluid exudate and subsequent signs of inflammation (warmth, redness, swelling, decreased range of motion).

b. Infection can occur by direct extension from a soft tissue site of infection or an iatrogenic inoculation (rare).

c. SA can result from complications of preexisting joint disease (e.g., rheumatoid arthritis) or from foreign bodies (e.g., prosthetic joint infections).

d. Penetrating injuries (or open lacerations) that involve joints should be considered at high risk for SA.

3. Etiology

 a. *S. aureus*: Most common organism causing SA in all ages (>50% of cases)

 b. *S. pneumoniae*: Uncommon in neonates; occasionally seen in infants and children

 c. *S. pyogenes*: Unlikely for neonates; common in children older than 5 years

 d. Group B streptococci: Common in neonates; uncommon in other children

 e. *N. gonorrhoeae*: Common in neonates and adolescents; uncommon in other age groups

 f. Gram-negative enteric bacteria (e.g., *E. coli*): Common in neonates; uncommon in other children

 g. *H. influenzae* type B: Unlikely for children who have been immunized

 h. *Salmonella*: Common in children with sickle cell anemia

 i. *Mycobacterium tuberculosis*: Common in children with epidemiologic risks of TB exposure

4. Clinical features

 a. Acute onset of fever, limp, joint pain, or refusal to walk are common features.

 b. Large weight-bearing joints (knee, hip, ankle) are most commonly involved. Usually infection is monarticular.

c. On examination, there is swelling, warmth, and erythema of the joint with decreased mobility. Range of motion can be so limited because of pain that the joint appears "frozen" (i.e., no mobility). A careful examination of all joints should be performed. Evaluate the patient for other foci of infection. Serial examinations may be required to determine whether any true limitation to range of motion exists.

d. When the hip is involved, the resting position may be a clue to infection: the child usually lies with hip flexed and leg abducted and externally rotated, refusing to change position.

e. In neonates, systemic symptoms may be minimal, but multiple joint involvement and contiguous osteomyelitis are common.

f. Gonococcal infection tends to be associated with a rash (vesicular or petechial) over the involved joint, migratory involvement of the small joints, and tenosynovitis.

5. Differential diagnosis
   a. Nonbacterial infection: Rarely associated with hepatitis and/or other viruses or fungi. Lyme infection (see section on Lyme Disease, later) is a very common cause of a "septic" arthritis–like presentation in endemic areas.
   b. JRA, other collagen vascular disease (less toxicity and fever): JRA is more often indolent and chronic; rarely is the joint motion "frozen."
   c. ARF (migratory arthritis/arthralgias common)
   d. Inflammatory bowel disease (chronic arthralgias/arthritis common)
   e. Leukemia (intense bone pain with range of motion relatively well preserved)
   f. When the patient is unable to bear weight and SA of the hip has been ruled out, toxic synovitis, psoas abscess, and pelvic osteomyelitis should all be considered as potential causes of hip pain.
   g. Reactive arthritis (*Shigella, Yersinia, Salmonella*; endocarditis)
   h. Trauma (hemarthrosis)
   i. Cellulitis (mimics SA when it occurs over a joint, but range of motion may be almost normal)

6. Laboratory evaluation/findings
   a. Plain radiographs and ultrasonography of joints may show joint space distention. Early in infection radiographs can be negative. CT or MRI may help define extent of infection or lead to another diagnosis.
   b. Arthrocentesis should be performed on all suspected cases of bacterial arthritis. Fluid is sent for cell count, Gram stain, glucose, character of mucin clot, and cultures.
      (1) The synovial fluid findings in three common causes of arthritis are shown in Table 19-17.
      (2) The presence of bacteria on a Gram stain specimen of synovial fluid, associated with a positive culture, confirms the diagnosis. However, synovial fluid culture may be negative in up to one third of cases, even when the child received no prior antibiotics.
   c. Bone-joint scans (gallium, technetium): If positive, the study is helpful, but it is not specific in ruling out infection if negative.
   d. Blood culture will be positive in approximately 40% to 60% of cases (depending on age and etiology).

Table 19-17 Synovial Fluid Findings in Various Types of Arthritis

	White Blood Cell Count (cells/mm³)	PMNs	Joint Fluid–Blood Glucose Ratio
Septic arthritis	>50,000	≥90%	Decreased
Juvenile rheumatoid arthritis	<15,000-100,000	60%	Normal to decreased
Lyme arthritis	15,000-100,000	50%+	Normal

PMNs, polymorphonuclear leukocytes.

    e. Other appropriate laboratory tests depending on differential diagnosis (e.g., Lyme titers for Lyme arthritis, and antistreptolysin O titers for ARF)
7. Management
    a. Drainage: Prompt aspiration of the involved joint is both diagnostic and therapeutic and can be crucial to the prevention of sequelae. Joint drainage prevents loculation, removes lysosomal proteolytic enzymes, and prevents increased intra-articular pressure, thus protecting articular cartilage.
    b. Antimicrobials: Empirical therapy (before Gram stain or culture results) is based on the patient's age and the presumptive etiology (Table 19-18).
        (1) Once the pathogen is identified, therapy may require modification to provide the most effective drug with the least toxicity.
        (2) Local instillation of antibiotics is not necessary because antimicrobials diffuse well into synovial fluid.
        (3) Other therapeutic measures include early immobilization of the joint and physical therapy when the inflammation subsides.
    c. Indications for surgery beyond initial aspiration
        (1) Joint swelling that persists or remains after repeat needle aspiration is an indication for surgical drainage.
        (2) Surgery is required for removal of foreign material secondary to penetrating injury.
        (3) SA of the hips or shoulder requires prompt open surgical drainage and irrigation of the joint space to prevent joint damage.
8. Prognosis and complications
    a. Outcome and complications depend on early diagnosis and initiation of therapy. Young age (<6 to 12 months) also increases the risk of sequelae.
    b. Prognosis is the worst for hip, followed by knee, then shoulder SA.
    c. Gram-negative bacillary infection has the worst prognosis.
    d. Complications include cartilage damage, stiff joint with poor mobility, abnormal bone growth if epiphysis involved, unstable joint, deformities, and chronic dislocation.

Table 19-18 **Antimicrobials for Septic Arthritis Based on Age***

Age	Agent	Duration
Neonate	Ampicillin *or* vancomycin *plus* aminoglycoside *or* ceftriaxone	4 wk
Infant or child	Nafcillin *or* clindamycin: add ceftriaxone *or* cefotaxime if not vaccinated against type b *H. influenzae*	3 wk
Adolescent	Nafcillin or clindamycin, add ceftriaxone if suspect gonococci	3 wk (7 days for gonococci)
Immunocompromised child	Vancomycin *plus* aminoglycoside and/or ceftriaxone	4 wk

*Criteria for oral therapy are the same as for osteomyelitis. If suspect methicillin-resistant *S. aureus*, replace beta-lactamase with vancomycin.

OSTEOMYELITIS

1. Epidemiology, etiology, and pathophysiology
   a. Acute osteomyelitis is a common infectious disease of childhood. The majority of infections occur in children younger than 5 years of age. Incidence is 2.5 times greater in boys than girls.
   b. The pathogenesis of acute osteomyelitis is related to three common mechanisms:
      (1) Hematogenous spread (especially in infants and young children)
      (2) Secondary to a contiguous focus or direct inoculation (e.g., trauma)
      (3) Associated with peripheral vascular disease (e.g., diabetes mellitus)
   c. Microbial etiology (Box 19-6)
   d. Predisposing factors related to osteomyelitis
      (1) Bacteremia in the setting of recent local trauma.
      (2) Penetrating trauma (e.g., nail puncture through sneaker can lead to *P. aeruginosa* osteochondritis; see later)
      (3) Hemoglobinopathies (especially sickle cell disease) associated with *Salmonella* or *E. coli* osteomyelitis
      (4) *Brucella* infection can lead to sacroiliitis.
      (5) IV drug abuse (*P. aeruginosa*)
      (6) Fractures, surgery, and prosthetic devices can lead to chronic osteomyelitis.
      (7) Dog or cat bite (*P. multocida*)
      (8) Contiguous infection (e.g., decubitus or diabetic ulcers, chronic sinusitis, mastoiditis)
      (9) Exposure to tuberculosis (e.g., vertebral osteomyelitis, or Pott's disease)

Box 19-6   Common Organisms Associated with
Osteomyelitis by Age Group

Neonate

Group B streptococci
S. aureus
Candida species
Enterobacter species
Other streptococci

Infant

S. aureus*
S. pyogenes
S. pneumoniae
H. influenzae

Older Child

S. aureus*
S. pyogenes
Salmonella (in sickle cell anemia)

*Responsible for 75% to 80% of cases.

      (10) Immunodeficiency (e.g., chronic granulomatous diseases associated with S. aureus, Candida, Nocardia)
2. Clinical features (Table 19-19)
  a. The child usually presents with a relatively acute onset of fever with limitation of the use of the involved extremity; refusal to use the extremity or bear weight is common.
  b. Point tenderness is an important diagnostic feature in older children, often associated with localized swelling, warmth, erythema, and pain.
  c. Most common sites involve long bones (femur, tibia, humerus).
  d. Hip pain or abdominal pain, difficulty walking, and rectal mass can be signs of pelvic osteomyelitis.
  e. Back pain and tenderness over spinous processes with few other symptoms may herald vertebral osteomyelitis.
  f. Neonates
    (1) Osteomyelitis is frequently accompanied by SA because, unlike for older children, blood vessels of metaphysis and epiphysis are freely connected, allowing infection to damage the epiphysis and rupture into the joint.
    (2) Pseudoparalysis of the joint is common. Erythema and swelling can be significant over the involved bone.
  g. Pseudomonas osteochondritis
    (1) A foot puncture wound is followed by local findings (swelling, warmth, redness, tenderness of soft tissue) 48 to 96 hours after injury.

Table 19-19 **Signs and Symptoms of Osteomyelitis According to Age**

Newborn	Children 2 wk to 4 yr	Children 4 to 16 yr
Symptoms		
Clinical sepsis	Pain	Local pain
Irritability	Limp	Mild limp
Pseudoparalysis	Refusal to use limb	Fever, malaise
Signs		
Redness	Point tenderness	Point tenderness
Massive swelling		
Progression		
Rapid	Subperiosteal abscess	Rare
Secondary septic arthritis		

(2) Fever is not prominent, and symptoms can occur as late as 2 to 3 weeks after injury.

3. Diagnosis and laboratory findings
   a. Clinical suspicion is important, especially with a history of the acute onset of bone pain, fever, tenderness, disuse of the extremity (especially after penetrating or blunt trauma or soft tissue infection).
   b. Laboratory tests: CBC (elevated WBC count), ESR (often high, above 50), CRP (markedly elevated)
   c. Radiographs: Early in the course of infection, plain films may be negative. Soft tissue edema initially is nonspecific; specific findings of new bone formation and gross bone destruction take 10 to 21 days to become apparent by radiographs.
   d. MRI is a sensitive test for osteomyelitis that detects changes in bone marrow signal. CT scan of bone is less sensitive.
   e. Technetium bone scintigram ("nuclear scan") is helpful in early detection and localization. In general, the study has a high sensitivity (over 90%) but relatively low specificity (60% to 70%), and false-positive and false-negative results can occur.
   f. Blood culture: Positive in 60% of cases
   g. Bone culture: Subperiosteal needle or surgical aspirate can be performed to increase diagnostic yield.
   h. Differential diagnosis
      (1) Cellulitis (because of skin tenderness)
      (2) Skeletal or blood neoplasia (Ewing's sarcoma, leukemia)
      (3) Bone infarction in patient with a hemoglobinopathy
      (4) Hemophilia with bleeding into soft tissue
      (5) Thrombophlebitis
      (6) Child abuse/trauma
      (7) Toxic synovitis
      (8) Abdominal processes (appendicitis, UTI, psoas abscess)
4. Management
   a. Antimicrobials: Penetration of antimicrobials into a relatively avascular "abscess" is poor (in contrast to the joint space) and thus

necessitates high doses and prolonged courses with parenteral antimicrobials (Table 19-20).

b. In certain cases, given good clinical response to initial IV antibiotics, and adequate medication compliance and regular follow-up, high-dose oral antibiotics may be given as "follow-through" treatment (usually after minimum of several days of IV treatment).

c. Surgical debridement and drainage is necessary in some cases (especially chronic osteomyelitis and *Pseudomonas* osteochondritis). Also, *Pseudomonas* osteochondritis requires tetanus prophylaxis.

5. Prognosis
   a. The goal of therapy is to prevent sequelae and chronic osteomyelitis.
   b. A major therapeutic problem arises when there is bone necrosis, producing a possible nidus for chronic infection.
   c. Prognosis is worse in the neonate, in an immunocompromised child, or with a residual nidus for infection.

DISKITIS

1. Pathophysiology and etiology

   Diskitis may be related to trauma and, secondarily, poor blood flow. It is unclear whether this condition represents a noninfectious necrosis of the disk or bacteremic seeding of the disk space. Staphylococcal species are the most common cause of infectious diskitis.

2. Clinical features are age dependent:
   (1) Infant: Refusal to sit, pain when changing diaper
   (2) Young child: Hip/leg complaints and refusal to walk or walks with a limp; often irritable
   (3) Older children: Back pain and stiffness, occasionally abdominal pain

   a. Other symptoms/signs include tenderness on palpation over vertebral processes (most common in lumbar area, L3-4), low-grade fever,

Table 19-20	**Antimicrobials for Osteomyelitis**	
Organism	**Agent**	**Duration (Minimum)**
S. aureus*	Nafcillin/oxacillin or cefazolin; alternative, clindamycin	4 wk
Streptococci*	Penicillin	4 wk
P. aeruginosa osteochondritis	Piperacillin or ceftazidime (±aminoglycoside)	7-10 days if adequate debridement
Salmonella	Cefotaxime or ceftriaxone (TMP/SMX or ampicillin if susceptible)	4-6 wk

*Therapy can be completed with oral antibiotics in an older infant or child if (1) the organism is recovered and susceptible to an appropriate agent, (2) the patient is afebrile for 3 days and improving on intravenous antibiotic, (3) the child can tolerate an oral drug, and (4) the parents are reliable. Try to achieve a peak serum bactericidal concentration of more than 1:8. For chronic osteomyelitis, oral therapy is continued for 6 to 12 months.

and paraspinal muscle spasm. Symptoms are indolent and chronic (median duration of 10 to 12 weeks).

b. Differential diagnosis includes trauma, toxic synovitis, JRA, vertebral osteomyelitis, epidural abscess, pelvic osteomyelitis, sacroiliitis (from brucellosis).

3. Laboratory findings
   a. ESR usually is elevated; WBC count may be normal.
   b. Plain radiographs: Disk space narrows (earliest sign) by 2 to 4 weeks; later, destruction of adjacent vertebral edges occurs, but vertebral body compression is rare.
   c. Bone scan demonstrates abnormal uptake at disk space and adjacent vertebral bodies.
   d. MRI or CT may be useful if clinical and initial radiographic findings are not typical.

4. Management/prognosis/complications
   a. Bed rest
   b. If severe, begin IV antistaphylococcal antibiotic, followed by oral doses for 4 to 6 weeks or until ESR is below 20 mm/hr.
   c. Risk of dissemination of infection is low.
   d. Young children reconstitute disk space well; older patients may have spontaneous spinal fusion.

MYOSITIS

1. This represents an inflammatory response within muscle, after an infection, usually viral or mycoplasma.
2. There is generalized muscle tenderness (prominent in distal muscle group such as the calves).
3. Strength is normal.
4. Creatinine phosphokinase and aldolase may be elevated.
5. Management includes rest, moist heat, and anti-inflammatory medications.

19.12 Infections Associated with Rashes (Exanthems and Enanthems), Swellings, and Other Manifestations

There is a broad spectrum of diseases in children associated with fever and rash. The fever pattern and characteristics of the rash aid clinical diagnosis.

MAJOR CHILDHOOD VIRAL EXANTHEMS

1. Introduction/definition
   a. Exanthems: Blanching macular or papular lesions (usually <1 cm in diameter)
   b. Scarlatiniform: Lesions with sandpaper feel on palpation (e.g., scarlet fever)
   c. Morbilliform: Lesions that coalesce, typically maculopapular

2. Diagnosis
   a. In well-appearing children with fever and exanthema, a careful history and physical examination may yield a diagnosis without the need for laboratory evaluation.
   b. Specific tests that may be useful include the following:

(1) Enterovirus: Culture of stool or oropharyngeal secretions, polymerase chain reaction (PCR) blood, urine, CSF
(2) Measles: Serology, measles-specific IgM
(3) Rubella: Serology, rubella-specific IgM; culture from nasal secretions
(4) Parvovirus B19: Serology, parvovirus-specific IgM, or PCR in immunocompromised subjects
(5) EBV: Serology, EBV-specific antibody panel, PCR in immunocompromised subjects
(6) Adenovirus: Culture and rapid antigen detection on secretions, PCR blood/urine

3. Rubella
  a. Congenital rubella
    (1) Etiology: Rubella virus, a rubivirus
    (2) Timing
      (a) Infection in first or early second trimester potentially leads to a spectrum of defects, with an overall 20% chance of birth defects if maternal infection occurs in first or early second trimester.
      (b) Long-term prognosis is often poor (retardation, congenital heart disease, deafness).
      (c) Pathogenesis is unknown, but the virus is suspected to cause mitotic arrest.
    (3) Congenital defects
      (a) Ophthalmologic: Cataracts, microphthalmia, glaucoma, chorioretinitis
      (b) Cardiac: Patent ductus arteriosus, atrial septal defect, ventricular septal defect, peripheral pulmonary artery stenosis
      (c) Auditory: Sensorineural deafness
      (d) CNS: Microcephaly, meningoencephalitis, mental retardation
      (e) Skin: "Blueberry muffin" purple skin lesions
      (f) Thrombocytopenia, hepatosplenomegaly, growth retardation
  b. Postnatal rubella
    (1) Epidemiology: Although less contagious than measles, transmission is by respiratory droplets (even from asymptomatic persons); congenitally infected infants shed the virus for months.
    (2) Clinical features
      (a) A mild rash on face, trunk (faint, rose-pink, maculopapular) begins in hairline and spreads down into a "kaleidoscope" rash with changing color. A pink to red exanthema can occur (punctate red spots on soft palate).
      (b) Hemorrhagic complications (low platelets, vascular damage) are common.
      (c) Asymptomatic infections are frequent.
      (d) History of disease is not useful for judging immunity.
      (e) Symptoms are more pronounced in adults than in children (arthralgia, arthritis, especially in adult women).
      (f) The disease is not more severe in immunocompromised patients.

(3) Diagnosis
    (a) Culture virus (expensive, limited availability)
    (b) Acute and convalescent antibody titers. A rise in rubella-specific IgM is diagnostic.

(4) Management and prevention
    (a) Supportive and individualized, according to number and type of congenital defects
    (b) Infants are contagious until 1 year of age.
    (c) Children are excluded from school for 7 days after the onset of rash.
    (d) Immune globulin (IG) is not recommended for postexposure prophylaxis.
    (e) Immunization: measles, mumps, and rubella (MMR) vaccine: In postpubertal female patient, check rubella susceptibility. If susceptible, check pregnancy test before giving vaccine. Counsel patient not to get pregnant for at least 3 months after vaccination, although vaccine-associated rubella infection is very rare.

4. Measles (rubeola)
  a. Etiology: Paramyxovirus (RNA virus)
  b. Epidemiology
    (1) Peak incidence: Preschool, early school age
    (2) Epidemic: Every 2 to 3 or more years; late winter, early spring
    (3) Transmission: Highly contagious by droplets or airborne transmission; contagious for approximately 4 days until just after the onset of the rash
    (4) Vaccine has led to a more than 95% reduction in cases.
  c. Clinical features
    (1) Generalized infection with prodrome of
      (a) Fever (to 104° F), chills, malaise, headache
      (b) Conjunctivitis
      (c) Coryza
      (d) Cough (dry, hacking, refractory)
    (2) Koplik spots (enanthema): These can appear 2 days before rash and consist of fine, blue-white, "sandpaper" lesions on buccal mucosa around second molars and Stensen's duct.
    (3) Maculopapular (i.e., morbilliform) rash starts on the face/scalp as discrete, purple-red macules; it becomes confluent as it moves down the body, like a bucket of paint was dropped on the patient's head. Rash fades in order of appearance and may be associated with desquamation.
    (4) Clinical variants
      (a) Modified: Usually seen in previously vaccinated individuals; mild illness and immunity follow a modified infection.
      (b) Atypical: Atypical measles is seen with incomplete immunity with hypersensitivity to measles exposure. In contrast to typical measles, the atypical variant has the following features:
        (i) The rash is mostly centripetal with a peripheral vasculitis-like rash that begins on the hands, feet, palms, and

soles and spreads centrally; it resembles RMSF and can be purpuric.
- (ii) The illness is often associated with an interstitial pneumonitis.
- (c) Severe
    - (i) Illness presents with a hemorrhagic rash, associated with giant cell (Hecht) pneumonia or chronic encephalitis.
    - (ii) It can be seen in immunocompromised or malnourished patients with poor cell-mediated immunity.
- (d) Subacute sclerosing panencephalitis
    - (i) A rare degenerative CNS syndrome. Intellectual deterioration, seizures, dementia, coma, and death can occur over a 6-month course.
    - (ii) Persistent infection occurs with a defective measles virus.
    - (iii) Most infected are boys who have had measles before 2 years of age. Neurologic deterioration begins, on the average, 7 years later.
    - (iv) It is associated with high serum and CSF antibody titers.
- d. Differential diagnosis: Rubella, scarlet fever, RMSF, drug eruption, other viral infection (note: rash of measles is purple-red, rubella is pink-red, and scarlet fever is yellow-red)
- e. Laboratory findings
    - (1) Virus isolation or antigen detection (blood, nasopharynx, conjunctiva, urine) can be made during the diagnostic febrile phase.
    - (2) A fourfold or greater increase in antibody titer occurs. The clinician may miss this rise because the positive titer occurs at the onset of the rash. IgM may be present immediately after rash onset, but is gone 30 to 60 days later.
    - (3) Assess immune status by measuring antibodies by ELISA; very low titers may indicate lack of protection.
- f. Complications
    - (1) Otitis media (10%)
    - (2) Pneumonia/croup (5%)
    - (3) Diarrhea (5%)
    - (4) Encephalitis (0.1%)
    - (5) Increased severity in children in developing countries (mortality 5% to 15%) because of malnutrition and other causes
        - (a) Hemorrhagic rash, diarrhea, bacterial superinfection
        - (b) Especially in first 4 years of life
    - (6) Increased severity in adults and immunocompromised (e.g., leukemia, HIV positive)
- g. Management and prevention
    - (1) Supportive
    - (2) IV ribavirin has been given in severely affected immunocompromised patients, but there are no controlled data.
    - (3) Vitamin A has been shown to reduce morbidity and mortality in patients with measles from developing countries. Vitamin A

(50,000 IU/mL) is given at 100,000 to 200,000 IU orally for children 6 months of age or older in two doses separated by 24 hours for hospitalized, immunocompromised, or malnourished children. This treatment is repeated once 4 weeks later.

    (4) Postexposure control

        (a) Vaccine, if given within 72 hours of measles exposure, may prevent clinical infection.

        (b) IG needs to be given within 6 days of exposure.

           (i) 0.25 mL/kg IM, once

           (ii) 0.50 mL/kg IM, once, for immunocompromised patients (maximum 15 mL)

           (iii) Need to wait 5 months before giving MMR vaccine

        (c) IVIG may offer some protection; it can be given as late as 3 weeks after exposure, 100 to 400 mg/kg, once.

        (d) Vaccine recommendations are presented in Chapter 2.

5. Mumps

  a. Etiology/epidemiology

    (1) Paramyxovirus—spread by respiratory route

    (2) Most common in late winter, spring

    (3) Outbreaks can occur in highly vaccinated populations.

    (4) Peak incidence at 10 to 14 years of age

  b. Clinical features

    (1) It is not usually associated with an exanthem (skin rash).

    (2) An "exanthem" in the case of mumps is not in the form of a rash but swelling of the salivary glands (especially parotids) and erythema around Stensen's duct.

    (3) Parotid swelling may begin spontaneously and unilaterally, then becomes bilateral in 50% of cases.

    (4) Jaw movement (i.e., chewing) can be painful.

    (5) Systemic illness involves a prodrome of high fever, headache, and myalgias followed by painful swelling of the parotid gland.

    (6) Differential diagnosis includes cervical adenitis (the parotitis obliterates the prominence of the ramus of the mandible, whereas cervical adenitis should not) and parotitis from other causes (bacterial, viral [parainfluenza virus, echoviruses, coxsackievirus], and parotid stones).

    (7) Clinical variants and complications of mumps

        (a) Pancreatitis (increase in lipase and alpha amylase)

        (b) Aseptic meningitis (common: 10% to 30% of mumps cases can have meningeal signs, CSF pleocytosis, and low CSF glucose)

        (c) Encephalitis (1 in 6000 cases)

        (d) Orchitis (10% to 20%), usually unilateral, occurs at the end of the first week and lasts 4 to 7 days; atrophy can occur in 10% to 50% of orchitis cases.

        (e) Oophoritis (5% of women)

        (f) Hearing loss (major sequela; most acute loss is temporary)

        (g) Congenital infection (rare)

  c. Diagnosis and laboratory findings

    (1) Tissue culture (saliva, CSF)

    (2) Fourfold rise in antibody titer (ELISA)

d. Management: Supportive (fluids, bland diet; avoid sour foods)
e. Prevention
   (1) Active immunity: Live, attenuated vaccine (see Chapter 2, section on Immunizations). The vaccine is not effective in preventing infection after exposure.
   (2) Passive immunity: Mumps IG is usually not effective.
6. Roseola, human herpes virus 6 (HHV6) (exanthem subitum, or sixth disease)
   a. Etiology
      (1) HHV6 (humans are the only natural host for HHV6)
      (2) Disease of young children (6 months to 3 years; peak at 6 to 12 months)
   b. Clinical features
      (1) High fever without a focus (30%)
      (2) Fever with URI, otitis media, vomiting, and diarrhea (50%)
      (3) Signs of classic illness of roseola (20%)
         (a) Fever (39° C to 40° C) lasts 3 to 7 days.
         (b) Erythematous, maculopapular, rose-pink rash that resembles rubella and appears as defervescence occurs (i.e., usually on day 3) and is short-lived, lasting hours to days
         (c) Rash begins on trunk and spreads to neck and extremities.
         (d) Few other symptoms occur; children are usually well between temperature elevations.
   c. Diagnosis is made by clinical findings.
   d. Management
      (1) Supportive (antipyretics, fluids, reassurance)
      (2) If immunocompromised patient with severe disease, may consider using ganciclovir
   e. Complications include febrile seizures (common association with HHV6 infection). HHV6 infection can be a problem in immunocompromised patients, causing pneumonitis, encephalitis, and bone marrow suppression.
7. Parvovirus B-19 (erythema infectiosum, or fifth disease)
   a. Etiology and epidemiology
      (1) DNA virus; B-19 only parvovirus to affect humans
      (2) Primarily infection in school-age children (5 to 15 years of age)
      (3) Late winter, spring
      (4) Immunity in 50% of adults
   b. Clinical features
      (1) Mild systemic symptoms include fever in 15% to 30% of patients and an intense red rash on face with circumoral pallor, giving a "slapped cheek" appearance.
      (2) A maculopapular, reticular, lacelike rash then appears on the trunk, arms, and buttocks. The rash can become more intense with sunlight, heat, baths, and the like, and can last from days to weeks, usually causing no discomfort. The condition is often confused with buccal cellulitis if the rash is unilateral, but the rash from parvovirus is *not* tender.
      (3) Other clinical syndromes

(a) Arthritis/arthralgias: Most commonly seen in older children and adult women. Usually presents with symmetric involvement of small joints (wrists, hands, feet) and may last weeks or months, or may develop into chronic arthritis.

(b) Transient aplastic crisis

    (i) Develops during primary infection in patients with chronic hemolytic anemias (e.g., sickle cell disease)

    (ii) Prodromal illness with fever, malaise, myalgias, usually no rash

    (iii) Lasts 7 to 10 days, then reticulocytosis occurs

(c) Chronic marrow suppression

    (i) Chronic parvovirus B-19 infection in immunocompromised patients leads to chronic red blood cell aplasia.

    (ii) May resolve with IVIG therapy

(d) Fetal infection (infection in first half of pregnancy)

    (i) Usually asymptomatic (majority)

    (ii) Fetal death (occurs in <10%)

    (iii) Hydrops fetalis (severe anemia, CHF) unusual but can occur

    (iv) Not associated with congenital malformations

c. Diagnosis and laboratory findings

  (1) Made by typical clinical picture

  (2) Parvovirus B-19–specific IgG or IgM antibody (present in 90%); not detected in immunocompromised patients because they cannot mount an antibody response

d. Management

  (1) Supportive

  (2) Patients with red blood cell aplasia may require transfusion.

  (3) IVIG in immunocompromised patients with chronic infection

e. Prevention

  (1) Routine exclusion from a workplace of pregnant women with children who may contract erythema infectiosum (e.g., day care, schools) is not needed. If necessary, susceptibility of adults may be determined by antibody testing.

  (2) Children may attend child care or school because they are not contagious.

  (3) Patients with aplastic crisis are the most highly contagious; therefore, pregnant women should avoid close contact with these patients.

8. Enteroviruses (coxsackievirus, echoviruses, enteroviruses)

a. Etiology, pathophysiology, and epidemiology: RNA nonpolio enteroviruses are spread by oral-oral or fecal-oral routes, with attack rates highest under conditions of poor hygiene and overcrowding. In temperate climates, the disease is most common in summer and fall.

b. Clinical features: A wide variety of clinical manifestations, including

  (1) Hemorrhagic conjunctivitis (severe, can least several weeks)

  (2) Mucocutaneous lesions that are characteristically associated with coxsackievirus infection (i.e., papulovesicular rash on hands, feet, and buttocks), and similar enanthem (vesicles and white patches) on the posterior pharynx (the so-called "hand, foot, and mouth" syndrome; commonly occurs in endemics in summer)

      (3) Pneumonia/pleurodynia, "devil's grip" (severe chest wall pain on inspiration from intercostal myositis, pleuritis)

      (4) Gastroenteritis

      (5) Myopericarditis

      (6) Nonspecific exanthems (nonspecific, viral rashes)

      (7) Aseptic meningitis and encephalitis (common in summer; photophobia, headache, neck stiffness)

  c. Diagnosis is usually made by clinical findings, but cultures of the throat, rectum, or CSF may yield the virus.

  d. Management

      (1) Supportive care (e.g., antipyretics/analgesics, rest)

      (2) IVIG in immunocompromised patients and severe neonatal infection

9. Herpes viruses

  a. Etiology and epidemiology

      (1) Two types of HSV

         (a) Type 1 (HSV-1) causes predominantly oral, skin and cerebral disease.

         (b) Type 2 (HSV-2) is responsible for most genital and congenital infections.

      (2) After infection, latency is established in the sensory neural ganglia and often serves as the reservoir for recurrent disease.

      (3) Transmission is by direct contact with infected secretions.

      (4) The source of primary infection is often an asymptomatic excreter. Most previously infected individuals shed HSV at irregular intervals in saliva for HSV-1 or genital secretions for HSV-2.

  b. Clinical features and management

      (1) Gingivostomatitis

         (a) Characterized by high fever, irritability and drooling in infants

         (b) Multiple oral ulcers on the tongue, buccal, and gingival mucosae

         (c) Pharyngeal ulcers (in older children and adolescents); may coalesce and result in diffuse swelling of the gums and cervical lymphadenopathy

         (d) Management is generally with supportive care. Occasionally helpful is "magic mouthwash" (combination of diphenhydramine, lidocaine, and Maalox; swish and spit).

      (2) Cutaneous infections

         (a) Direct inoculation onto cuts or abrasions may produce localized vesicles or ulcers.

         (b) Deep infections on the fingers (herpetic whitlow) should be differentiated from bacterial infection. HSV infection of eczematous skin may result in extensive areas of vesicles (eczema herpeticum) and may be mistaken for impetigo.

      (3) Recurrent mucocutaneous infection

         (a) After primary infection, recurrent oral shedding is usually asymptomatic.

         (b) Perioral recurrences characteristically begin with a prodrome of tingling or burning sensation in the perioral region followed by eruption of vesicles, which crust and scab over 3 to 5 days.

(c) Recurrent genital infection is common after initial infection with HSV-2.

(d) Additional management for gingivostomatitis and other mucocutaneous HSV infection includes oral acyclovir, valacyclovir or famciclovir. Treatment beneficial for gingivostomatitis and other mucocutaneous manifestations only if begun early. IV treatment is recommended for severe disease or extensive disease in immunocompromised.

(4) Keratoconjuctivitis

(a) Involvement of the eyes may be part of the primary infection or spread from oral infection or reactivation of latent virus in the ciliary ganglion.

(b) Typically presents with photophobia, pain, and conjunctival irritation and may be associated with dendritic ulcers on the cornea.

(c) Management includes topical antivirals: 1% trifluridine, 5% acyclovir, and 3% vidarabine (use with guidance from an ophthalmologist).

(d) The use of steroids is contraindicated, and expert ophthalmic consultation must be obtained.

(5) Encephalitis

(a) CNS involvement is unusual in infants outside the neonatal period; encephalitis may occur at any other age.

(b) Presents without cutaneous manifestation

(c) HSV is the most common cause of sporadic severe encephalitis.

(d) Typically associated with headache, behavioral changes, neurologic deficits, and focal seizures

(e) CSF pleocytosis is typically mononuclear leukocyte predominant with elevated protein.

(f) MRI is more sensitive and positive early in the course of infection.

(g) Culture of CSF is rarely positive and etiologic diagnosis is most readily achieved by PCR for the detection of HSV DNA.

(h) Management includes IV acyclovir 500 mg/m^2 every 8 hours for 21 days or 20 mg/kg IV every 8 hours for neonatal disease (minimum 21 days for CNS disease or 14 days for skin, eye, or mouth).

(i) Prognosis is poor without antiviral therapy.

(6) Neonatal infections

(a) Neonatal infection is acquired by transmission of infection from the genital tract.

(b) A history of genital infection in the mother is usually absent.

(c) The infant presents within a few days up to 4 weeks of delivery with skin vesicles (especially at trauma sites, such as scalp electrode sites).

(d) Infection may be limited to skin, eye, and mouth, whereas others may be acutely ill, with systemic symptoms such as hepatitis, shock, sepsis, and respiratory distress.

(e) Management of neonatal HSV infection includes parenteral acyclovir. Acyclovir should be administered to all neonates with HSV infection, regardless of manifestations and clinical findings. The dosage of acyclovir is 60 mg/kg/day IV in three divided doses for 14 days if disease is limited to the skin, eye, and mouth, and for 21 days if disease is disseminated or involves the CNS.

(f) Prognosis: The best outcome in terms of morbidity and mortality is seen in infants with disease limited to the skin, eyes, and mouth. Although most neonates treated for CNS HSV survive, substantial neurologic sequelae is the rule. Despite antiviral therapy, approximately 25% of neonates with disseminated disease die.

10. Varicella-zoster (chickenpox)
   a. Primary infection with varicella-zoster virus results in varicella, the most distinctive of all childhood exanthems.
   b. The incubation period is 10 to 21 days. Contact may have been unrecognized because the index case is infectious 1 to 2 days before the appearance of the rash.
   c. The usual case consists of mild systemic symptoms followed by crops of red macular rash that rapidly become small vesicles with surrounding erythema (often described as a "dew drop on a rose petal"), these progress to pustules, become crusted, and then scab over.
   d. The rash is typically on the trunk and face. Lesions may also occur in the scalp, nose, and mucosal surfaces such as the mouth, conjunctiva, and vagina.
   e. Once crusting occurs the patient is no longer contagious.
   f. Management: Supportive care, avoid prolonged courses of acetaminophen or ibuprofen—may lead to hepatotoxicity
   g. Complications
      (1) Secondary bacterial infection with staphylococci or GABHS is most common (impetigo or in severe cases as necrotizing fasciitis or sepsis).
      (2) Encephalitis occurs in 0.1% of cases.
      (3) Fetal infection (first or second trimester) can present in varicella embryopathy.
   h. Prognosis: Chickenpox generally has a very favorable prognosis; prevention is with varicella vaccine (see Chapter 2).
11. Herpes zoster
   a. Reactivation of latent varicella-zoster virus in dorsal root ganglia can lead to shingles (herpes zoster). Vesicles appear in groups along one to three sensory dermatomes, often associated with pain and tingling. Other unusual complications include optic neuritis, myocarditis, transverse myelitis, and arthritis.
   b. Management includes limiting progression by starting treatment at first signs of illness with oral acyclovir 80 mg/kg/day in three divided doses, maximum 1000 mg/day for 5 to 10 days. Medication that treats neuropathic pain (i.e., gabapentin [Neurontin]) can also be helpful.

c. Infection with varicella-zoster virus usually confers lifelong immunity. The virus remains latent in sensory nerves and this forms the reservoir for herpes zoster in later life.

SCARLET FEVER ("SCARLATINA")

See also section on pharyngitis.

1. Etiology, pathophysiology, and epidemiology: A systemic erythrogenic exotoxin is produced by GABHS strains that leads to the classic cutaneous findings. It is seen late in fall, winter, and early spring.
2. Clinical features
   a. Usually the child is older than 2 to 3 years.
   b. Scarlet fever is associated with GABHS pharyngitis or less often with pyoderma or an infected wound.
   c. The hallmark of infection is the typical rash.
      (1) The rash appears within 24 to 48 hours of sore throat, fever, headache, and abdominal pain—all symptoms typical of GABHS pharyngitis.
      (2) The exanthem begins around the neck and then spreads to the trunk and extremities.
      (3) The rash is best appreciated if felt; it consists of diffuse, fine, "gooseflesh" erythematous papules, feeling much like sandpaper.
      (4) It is more prominent in skin creases (axillae, groin, antecubital areas), and is termed *Pastia's lines*.
      (5) Circumoral pallor may also be seen.
      (6) The enanthema of mucous membranes includes soft palatal petechiae, with the tongue (days 1 to 2) coated white; on days 2 to 3, the red, edematous papillae project through, creating a white "strawberry tongue"; on days 4 to 5, denuded tissue produces the red "strawberry tongue."
      (7) The rash lasts 4 to 5 days, leaving a brawny edema associated with desquamation of the fingers and toes.
3. Diagnosis and laboratory findings
   a. The characteristic rash with history of fever and exudative pharyngitis suggest the diagnosis.
   b. Laboratory and throat cultures indicate rising antistreptolysin O and other GABHS antibodies.
   c. Differential diagnosis includes KD, rubeola, viral exanthems (e.g., EBV), and staphylococcal scarlet fever. (In staphylococcal illness, the rash is tender, the throat culture is negative, and there is no desquamation.)
4. Management: Antimicrobials as for GABHS pharyngitis
5. Complications: ARF, glomerulonephritis

KAWASAKI'S DISEASE

1. Etiology: Unknown, but likely caused by an infection in a susceptible host. The condition is associated with protean systemic manifestations secondary to a vasculitis mostly involving small and medium vessels.
2. Epidemiology: KD most commonly affects children under 2 years old (50% of cases); 80% are younger than 5 years. Epidemics occur in winter and spring at 2 to 3 year intervals.

3. Diagnosis and clinical features
   a. The following clinical criteria have been suggested to make a diagnosis:
      (1) Fever of no other known cause, lasting 5 days or more (it is imperative for fever to be present to make the diagnosis). Fever usually is not accompanied by prodromal symptoms of cough, rhinorrhea, vomiting, and so forth. However, with the fever the child may be extremely irritable and agitated.
      (2) Four of the following *other* criteria should be present:
         (a) Bilateral conjunctival congestion (dilated blood vessels without purulent discharge and with limbic sparing), that is, conjunctival suffusion. Occurs 2 to 4 days after onset of fever.
         (b) Changes in the mucous membranes of the upper respiratory tract: Redness, dryness or fissuring of lips, strawberry tongue, diffuse injection of oral and pharyngeal mucosa. Occurs within 2 to 4 days; subsides within 7 days.
         (c) Changes in the extremities: Edema, erythema of the hands and feet so they become warm, red, and swollen, causing irritability and refusal to grasp objects or bear weight, usually 2 to 5 days after fever onset. Desquamation of the fingers or toes 10 to 15 days after onset may begin, usually around nails and spreading over palms and soles. Transverse furrows (Bow's lines) develop in the nails 30 to 60 days after onset.
         (d) Rash(es): Diffuse polymorphous rash (ranging from macules to bullae to an erythematous exanthem) of the trunk. Most commonly a morbilliform or scarlatiniform rash; usually not crusting or vesicular, which occurs over days 1 to 5 and disappears within 7 days.
         (e) Cervical lymphadenopathy: Begins at onset of fever with an acute, nonpurulent, firm swelling of the nodes which measure 1.5 to 5 cm. It is the least commonly seen criterion.
      (3) In addition to the preceding criteria, the illness cannot be explained by another disease process.
      (4) Extreme irritability is so common in KD that its absence should lead to a reconsideration of the diagnosis.
   b. Additional clinical features
      (1) Cardiovascular (Box 19-7): Heart murmur, gallop rhythm, distant heart sounds, ECG changes (prolonged PR, QT intervals, abnormal Q wave, low voltage, ST-T changes, arrhythmias), CXR findings (cardiomegaly), two-dimensional echocardiography findings (pericardial effusion, coronary aneurysms, aneurysm of peripheral arteries other than coronary), angina pectoris, or myocardial infarction
      (2) GI tract: Diarrhea, vomiting, abdominal pain, hydrops of gallbladder, paralytic ileus, mild jaundice, slight increase of serum aminotransferases, hypoalbuminemia
      (3) Blood: Leukocytosis with shift to the left, thrombocytosis, increased ESR and CRP, hypoalbuminemia, increased α_2-globulin, slight decrease in erythrocyte and hemoglobin levels

Box 19-7   Specific Features of Cardiac Involvement in Kawasaki's Disease

When coronary artery disease is detected, Kawasaki's disease may be diagnosed even with fewer than four of the previously listed criteria.

Major cause of morbidity and mortality (0.5% in the United States)

Related to small and medium vessel arteritis during inflammatory stages of Kawasaki's disease, with weakening of vessel walls and subsequent thrombosis or aneurysm formation

Clinical manifestations

   Carditis, pericarditis, CHF, dysrhythmias (can occur early in acute stages)

   Aneurysmal dilatation of coronary vessels, sometimes accompanied by thrombosis (occurs as early as 3 days but most commonly 2 to 4 weeks after onset)

Patients at increased risk include boys, infants younger than 12 months of age, those with fever lasting more than 10 days, and those with early cardiac involvement.

Mild and simple coronary dilatation can resolve within 6 to 8 weeks. Coronary aneurysms (<4 mm in diameter) may regress within 1 year; saccular and diffuse lesions (>8 mm) are more concerning.

---

    (4) Genitourinary tract: Proteinuria, increase of leukocytes in urine sediment (i.e., sterile pyuria)

    (5) Joints: Arthritis/arthralgias

    (6) Neurologic: Pleocytosis of mononuclear cells in CSF, seizures, facial palsy, paralysis of the extremities

    (7) Eyes: Uveitis

4. Laboratory findings: No specific confirmatory tests are currently available. Baseline work-up:

    a. CBC with differential

    b. Serial platelet count (platelet counts rising to over 1 million are common findings in KD)

    c. Electrolytes

    d. Urinalysis

    e. Liver enzymes

    f. ESR/CRP

    g. Blood culture

    h. Two-dimensional echocardiogram

5. The differential diagnosis includes the following:

    a. Scarlet fever (patients older than typical patient with KD; no hand, foot, or conjunctival involvement)

    b. Stevens-Johnson syndrome (mouth sores and cutaneous bullae and crusts are characteristic)

    c. Measles (rash occurs after fever peaks and begins in head/scalp)

    d. Other viral infection (EBV, adenovirus, hepatitis B)

    e. JRA (usually a longer duration of fever at presentation)
    f. Drug reaction
    g. Toxic shock syndrome (older patients, fever of shorter duration)
    h. Leptospirosis
    i. Acrodynia (mercury poisoning)
    j. Bacterial endocarditis (unusual in early childhood)
    k. Rheumatic fever (older patients)

6. Management
    a. Exclusion and treatment of other similar conditions are imperative.
    b. Early evaluation by a pediatric cardiologist for detection of early cardiac involvement is critical. Close follow-up with pediatric cardiologists is mandatory.
    c. Therapy should be instituted when the diagnosis is established.
    d. IVIG should be initiated within 10 days of onset of fever (in conjunction with ASA), which will decrease the prevalence of coronary artery dilatation and lead to early resolution of fever and other symptoms. A dosage of 2 g/kg IVIG as a single infusion over 10 to 12 hours is currently recommended. For the 10% who may not respond (i.e., persistent or recurrent fever, other symptoms), a second infusion at 1 to 2 g/kg may be helpful.
    e. ASA
        (1) Initial *anti-inflammatory dose* during acute stage (first 7 to 10 days): 80 to 100 mg/kg/day in four divided doses (serum salicylate levels kept at 20 to 30 mg/dL).
        (2) As fever subsides and symptoms abate, use a dose to prevent platelet aggregation: 3 to 5 mg/kg/day (e.g., one baby aspirin per day for at least 6 to 8 weeks or until platelet count and ESR return to normal).
        (3) Explain risk of ASA therapy (i.e., Reye's syndrome) to parents.
        (4) If no coronary abnormalities are detected by 6 to 8 weeks after onset of illness, ASA can be discontinued.
        (5) If coronary abnormalities persist, dipyridamole (4 mg/kg/day, divided in three doses) may be added to the ASA regimen.
    f. Corticosteroids are generally not used except under certain conditions (e.g., carditis); they may increase the frequency of a coronary aneurysm.
    g. Subsequent immunizations
        (1) Delay MMR and varicella immunizations for 11 months after IVIG therapy, unless exposure to measles occurs.
        (2) Other immunizations should not be interrupted.
        (3) Influenza vaccine should be given yearly to patients on long-term ASA therapy.

7. Prognosis
    a. Relates to whether the cardiovascular system (or other major organ system) is involved, which has decreased with IVIG and ASA therapy. Without significant vasculitis/arteritis, the prognosis is excellent and recovery is complete. Parents should be reassured.
    b. The larger and more extensive coronary aneurysms that do not respond to therapy may thrombose or fail to regress, leading eventually to myocardial ischemia.

19.13 Tick-Borne Infections

LYME DISEASE

1. Etiology/epidemiology
   a. Lyme disease is a tick-borne spirochetal infection with rash and influenza-like initial symptoms, sometimes followed by joint, CNS, and cardiac sequelae weeks to years later.
   b. The occurrence of Lyme disease is directly dependent on the distribution of vectors that carry B. burgdorferi, the causative organism.
   c. Tick vectors (B. burgdorferi resides in the GI tract and saliva)
      (1) Ixodes scapularis (deer tick) in the northeastern and upper midwestern United States
      (2) Ixodes pacificus (western black-legged tick) in the Pacific states
   d. Host reservoirs for the organism in the northeastern and upper midwestern United States include white-footed mice (most common) and other small mammals and birds. Deer are not competent hosts because they do not maintain the growth cycle of the spirochete. In the Pacific coastal United States, lizards are reservoirs.
   e. Transmission
      (1) Risk of transmission to humans depends on the likelihood that a tick is infected (varies by geography, stage of tick life cycle, and species). Most disease transmission to humans in the United States occurs between May and December; in most cases, before August.
      (2) Risk of transmission is related to the duration of feeding. The disease is unlikely if the tick is removed within 24 to 48 hours of attachment (use forceps with counterclockwise twist). Note: a nonengorged tick is the size of a pencil point.
2. Clinical features
   a. Early localized disease (3 to 30 days after tick bite)
      (1) The major sign of early localized Lyme disease is the characteristic erythema migrans (EM) rash, which is diagnostic (no need for serologic confirmation).
         (a) There may be a single lesion that begins as a pimple or vesicle(s) at site of the tick bite, (which may occur anywhere on the body).
         (b) A primary lesion develops and expands to form a large (15 cm), annular, erythematous macule with partial central clearing. Rash is occasionally uniformly erythematous and may have a vesicular or necrotic center. Secondary lesions of early disseminated disease are smaller.
         (c) EM presents 3 to 30 days after the bite (average, 10 days) and can last up to 30 days.
      (2) Differential diagnosis of EM primarily includes tinea corporis (ringworm), granuloma annulare, erythema multiforme, and spider bite.
   b. Early disseminated disease
      (1) Manifestations
         (a) Multiple secondary EMs, evanescent red blotches, malar rash, urticaria

    (b) Flulike illness may accompany secondary rash (fever, headache, myalgias, conjunctivitis, fatigue, arthralgias)

    (c) Meningitis

      (i) Presents as an aseptic meningitis (stiff neck, photophobia)

      (ii) Diagnosis is usually based on CSF findings that are consistent with aseptic meningitis (low-grade lymphatic pleocytosis, normal glucose, protein, negative Gram stain).

      (iii) Serologic confirmation of Lyme disease is essential for diagnosis of Lyme meningitis.

    (d) Seventh-nerve palsy (Bell's palsy) is most common, usually lasts 2 to 8 weeks, and resolves completely.

      (i) May present with few other symptoms; occasionally associated with headache and fatigue.

      (ii) Treatment may not affect resolution; antimicrobial treatment is instituted to prevent late Lyme disease. Corticosteroids are not recommended.

    (e) Carditis: Varying degrees of heart block (first- or second-degree) occur in less than 1% of cases, and these usually resolve without intervention, although in rare cases a temporary pacemaker may be required.

  c. Late disease

    (1) Can occur months and occasionally years after infection

    (2) Major manifestations

    (a) Arthritis is the major manifestation of late disseminated Lyme disease in children.

      (i) Knees are involved over 90% of the time.

      (ii) Arthritis is monoarticular or pauciarticular (i.e., fewer than four joints) and nonsymmetric; swelling may be impressive, but the range of motion is better than expected from the degree of swelling (in contrast to bacterial arthritis).

      (iii) Duration of arthritis is variable, usually resolving completely with treatment, although it recurs in 5% to 10% of treated children and usually resolves with retreatment.

    (b) Encephalopathy (chronic headache; change in behavior, school performance; may rarely occur in children)

    (c) Polyneuropathies are rare in children

    (d) Uveitis (similar to that seen in JRA) has been reported.

3. Diagnosis

  a. Clinical suspicion should be high in endemic areas.

  b. Centers for Disease Control and Prevention (CDC) criteria for diagnosis

    (1) Physician-diagnosed EM (≥5 cm) *or*

    (2) One or more clinical manifestations of early disseminated or late Lyme disease (aseptic meningitis, arthritis, or Bell's palsy) *and* positive serology

  c. Serologic tests (EIA test as a screen, Western immunoblot as confirmatory)

(1) Specific IgM: Often not found but detectable 3 to 4 weeks after infection. IgM peaks between 3 and 6 weeks after infection, then declines.

(2) Specific IgG: More likely to be positive with significant symptoms: meningitis, arthritis, multiple EM rash. It is detectable 4 to 12 weeks after infection, peaks 4 to 6 months after infection, and may remain elevated indefinitely. Early antimicrobial treatment may abate antibody response.

(3) False-positive EIA test results are *common* because of cross-reactive antibodies from other infections, including viral, bacterial, and spirochetal.

d. Caveats on obtaining serologic tests in specific clinical situations

(1) Do not obtain titers in patients with vague, nonspecific symptoms (not likely related to Lyme disease).

(2) Patient recently bitten by deer tick: Antibody tests will be negative at the time of the bite.

(3) Patient with EM: Antibody tests are negative at the time EM is seen.

(4) Patient with late Lyme disease (e.g., monoarticular arthritis): Get antibody tests to confirm diagnosis, but repeat titers are not helpful because IgG may remain elevated.

(5) Patient with seventh-nerve palsy: Antibody test is useful; most patients will have detectable antibody.

4. Management: There are few comparative studies on the management of Lyme disease in childhood. Most recommendations are extrapolated from adult studies. Rarely, in less than 5% of patients, a Jarisch-Herxheimer reaction (fever, chills, flulike symptoms) may occur after antimicrobial treatment as spirochetes are killed and toxins are released.

a. Antimicrobial treatment of Lyme disease (Table 19-21)

b. Nonsteroidal anti-inflammatory agents may help to control arthritis symptoms. The majority of patients recover after antimicrobial therapy.

c. Prevention of tick infestation

(1) Avoidance of tick-infested areas and protective clothing (keep pants tucked in socks; wear boots)

(2) Skin repellents

(a) Insect repellents: diethyltoluamide (DEET)—very effective. Do not put on face; toxicity rarely leads to seizures.

(b) Less active: Dimethylphthalate (DMP); citronella-based products

(c) Clothing repellents: Permethrin (0.5%) placed directly on clothing (avoid spraying onto skin)

(3) Tick removal (grasp tick with a fine tweezers close to the skin and gently pull straight out or twist counter clockwise)

(4) Chemoprophylaxis once a tick bite has occurred may not be helpful in preventing Lyme disease; not routinely recommended.

ROCKY MOUNTAIN SPOTTED FEVER

1. Etiology/epidemiology

a. *Rickettsia rickettsii* is the causative organism.

Table 19-21 Recommended Treatment of Lyme Disease in Children	
Disease Category	**Drug(s) and Dose***
Early Localized Disease*	
>8 yr of age	Doxycycline 100 mg orally twice a day for 14-21 days
All ages	Amoxicillin 25-50 mg/kg per day orally, divided into two doses (maximum 2 g/day), for 14-21 days
Early Disseminated and Late Disease	
Multiple erythema migrans	Same oral regimen as for early disease but for 21 days
Isolated facial palsy	Same oral regimen as for early disease but for 21-28 days†‡
Arthritis	Same oral regimen as for early disease but for 28 days
Persistent or recurrent arthritis§	Ceftriaxone sodium 75-100 mg/kg IV or IM once a day (maximum 2 g/day) for 14-21 days; *or* penicillin 300,000 U/kg/day IV, given in divided doses every 4 hr (maximum 20 MU/day) for 14-28 days; *or* same oral regimen as for early disease
Carditis	Ceftriaxone or penicillin: see persistent or recurrent arthritis
Meningitis or encephalitis	Ceftriaxone or penicillin: see persistent or recurrent arthritis, but for 30-60 days

*For patients who are allergic to penicillin, cefuroxime axetil and erythromycin are alternative drugs.

†Corticosteroids should not be given.

‡Treatment has no effect on the resolution of facial nerve palsy; its purpose is to prevent late disease.

§Arthritis is not considered persistent or recurrent unless objective evidence of synovitis exists at least 2 months after treatment is initiated. Some experts administer a second course of an oral agent before using an IV-administered antimicrobial agent.

    b. Tick vector: *Dermacentor variabilis* (most common) in spring–summer; south Atlantic, southeastern, and southern regions

    c. Most patients younger than 15 years of age; highest incidence in 5- to 9-year-old age range

2. Pathophysiology and clinical features

    a. *R. rickettsii* multiply within the endothelial cells lining small blood vessels, resulting in cell damage. Perivascular mononuclear cell infiltration (vasculitis), thrombosis, and leakage of blood into tissue ensue.

    b. Vasculitis and inflammation can occur in any organ system. Clinically, presents early with flulike symptoms associated with a maculopapular or petechial skin rash (often on the wrists). CNS disturbance (severe headache, mental confusion), or large vessel involvement of an extremity (gangrene) can also occur.

   c. Hyponatremia is a very common finding and results from the leakage of water (intracellular to extracellular) and the loss of renal sodium. This characteristic hyponatremia is almost pathognomonic for RMSF.

3. Diagnosis and laboratory findings
   a. A high index of clinical suspicion is crucial because a definitive diagnosis often cannot be made until the second week of illness.
   b. Laboratory parameters
     (1) Leukopenia, thrombocytopenia, anemia
     (2) Hyponatremia (very consistent finding)
     (3) Elevated aminotransferases, bilirubin, BUN
   c. Serology
     (1) Indirect hemagglutination (fastest increase in titers), latex agglutination (easiest)
     (2) Diagnosis is probable with titer of 1:128 or greater.
   d. Skin biopsy: Fluorescent or peroxidase-tagged antibody test (only in patients with rash; best lesions for test are petechial). Specificity is 100% and sensitivity is 70%. Skin biopsy may be falsely negative if the patient has had treatment for more than 48 hours.

4. Differential diagnosis: The differential includes enteroviruses, measles (especially atypical), rubella, infectious mononucleosis, HSP, and drug hypersensitivity. Also in the differential are scarlet fever, leptospirosis, *N. meningitides*, type b *H. influenzae*, ehrlichiosis, and tularemia (typhoidal).

5. Management
   a. Presumptive therapy and diligent fluid management are critical to avoid shock. Monitor blood pressure and fluid status.
   b. Children (fever without rash) may be observed for 2 to 4 days after onset of illness; studies show mortality is rare if antibiotics are begun before day 6.
   c. Doxycycline is the drug of choice for any age, given as 4 to 5 mg/kg/day orally or IV twice a day for 7 to 10 days (or until afebrile for at least 3 days and demonstrated clinical improvement).

6. Prognosis: Predictors of poor outcome include a delay in diagnosis (i.e., prognosis is worse if diagnosed after 6 days), glucose-6-phosphate dehydrogenase deficiency, male sex, nonwhite race, age older than 30 years.

CAT SCRATCH DISEASE

1. Etiology/epidemiology
   a. *Bartonella henselae* (a rickettsial bacterium) is the causative organism.
   b. It is transmitted by the scratch of healthy kittens, cats, and occasionally dogs (possible flea-borne disease).

2. Clinical features
   a. Usually a mild, self-limited infection begins as a skin papule at the site of inoculation; then, 1 to 2 weeks later, it may become associated with regional lymphadenopathy and occasionally fever.
   b. Cervical lymphadenitis (painful swelling, warmth) or nontender lymph enlargement are the most common presentations.
   c. Parinaud's syndrome (involvement of face/eyes with intense conjunctivitis, regional adenopathy) is possible.

3. Diagnosis
   a. Serology (indirect fluorescent antibody)
   b. Warthin-Starry silver stain on tissue can identify the organism.
   c. PCR for confirmation
4. Management
   a. Usually self-limited; resolution of adenopathy can be prolonged but usually occurs within 2 to 4 months.
   b. Antimicrobial choices for acutely or severely ill patients include azithromycin, TMP/SMX, gentamicin, and rifampin.

BABESIOSIS

1. Babesiosis is caused by *Babesia microti*, an intraerythrocytic protozoon.
2. In the United States, the primary reservoir host for *B. microti* is the white-footed mouse, and the primary vector is the *I. scapularis* tick (also the vector for Lyme disease and ehrlichiosis). Babesiosis can also be acquired through blood transfusions.
3. Babesiosis generally causes transient symptoms. More severe disease is associated with malaise, anorexia, and fatigue, followed by spiking temperatures, myalgias, arthralgias, and nausea and vomiting. Physical examination may reveal hepatomegaly, splenomegaly, jaundice, or pallor. Laboratory features can include anemia, elevated bilirubin, positive direct Coombs' test, and thrombocytopenia. The cornerstone of diagnosis is identification of intraerythrocytic parasites on Giemsa- or Wright-stained thick and thin blood smears. Because *B. microti* infection is usually self-limited, treatment is reserved for children with more severe illness.
4. Clindamycin (20 to 40 mg/kg/day in children) plus quinine (25 mg/kg/day) is given for 7 days. Alternatively, atovaquone (20 mg/kg twice daily in children) plus azithromycin (12 mg/kg daily) for 7 to 10 days appears to be equally efficacious.

TULAREMIA

1. Tularemia is a zoonotic disease caused by *Francisella tularensis*, a gram-negative pleomorphic coccobacillus.
2. In the United States, transmission to humans by ticks is most common. Less commonly, transmission occurs through direct contact with non-domesticated rabbits and other infected animals.
3. Clinical manifestations include constitutional symptoms of fever, chills, malaise, and fatigue. Several tularemic syndromes are recognized and include glandular tularemia with adenitis, oculoglandular disease, oropharyngeal disease, and typhoidal tularemia that results from ingestion of contaminated food (high and prolonged fever is typical). Diagnosis is made by serum agglutination testing (a fourfold increase in titer between two sera obtained at least 2 weeks apart) is diagnostic. Management includes a 7-day course of an aminoglycoside antibiotic (streptomycin, gentamicin, or amikacin). Alternative treatments include either ciprofloxacin or imipenem-cilastatin.

19.14 TUBERCULOSIS

1. Etiology and pathophysiology (see also section on Screening in Chapter 2)
   a. TB is caused by *M. tuberculosis*, an AFB. It is very important to distinguish TB *infection* from TB *disease*.

    (1) Infection: Patients who are *infected* have a positive tuberculin skin test (PPD) but a negative CXR and *no* signs or symptoms consistent with TB.

    (2) Disease: Patients with *disease* have manifestations of pulmonary or extrapulmonary infection, manifested by radiographic findings *and/or* clinical signs and symptoms.

  b. TB is transmitted by inhalation of droplet nuclei produced by an adult or adolescent with infectious pulmonary TB. Most patients are noninfectious within a few weeks of starting effective therapy.

  c. Children are usually noncontagious because their lesions are small, discharge of bacilli is minimal, and cough is minimal or nonexistent.

  d. The incubation period from the infection to the development of a positive PPD is between 2 and 10 weeks.

  e. The risk for development of TB is highest in the first 2 years after infection.

  f. Usually an untreated infection becomes dormant and never progresses to clinical disease in the healthy host.

2. Epidemiology

  a. Infants and children are at high risk for disease from recent infection.

  b. Rates of TB are highest among urban, low-income populations, the homeless, residents of correctional facilities, Hispanics, blacks, Native Americans, Alaskan natives, and Asians, and first-generation immigrants from high-risk countries.

3. Clinical features

  a. Latent TB infection is defined as M. *tuberculosis* infection in a person who has a positive tuberculin skin test result, no physical findings of disease, and chest radiograph findings that are normal or reveal evidence of healed infection such as granulomas or calcification in the lung, hilar lymph nodes, or both.

  b. Most infected children are asymptomatic. The primary complex is usually not seen on CXR.

  c. Early disease (occurring from 1 to 6 months after the initial infection) includes

    (1) Lymphadenopathy (hilar, mediastinal, cervical, or other nodes)

    (2) Pulmonary involvement of a segment or lobe

    (3) Atelectasis

    (4) Pleural effusion

    (5) Miliary TB

    (6) Tuberculous meningitis

  d. Late disease (occurring months to years after the initial infection) includes

    (1) Pulmonary involvement (reactivation of primary infection)

    (2) Extrapulmonary disease (middle ear, mastoid, bones, joints, skin, renal, meningeal, and miliary).

    (3) Late disease affects 25% of children younger than 15 years of age with TB.

4. Diagnosis and laboratory findings

  a. Isolation of the bacillus establishes the diagnosis. The best culture material for the diagnosis of pulmonary TB in young children is an early morning gastric aspirate to obtain swallowed sputum. The organism is isolated from less than 40% of children with pulmonary TB.

b. Histologic examination of lymph nodes, pleura, liver, bone marrow biopsies, or other tissues can be very valuable for the diagnosis when AFBs are demonstrated.

c. Identification of a source case should be actively pursued to obtain a specimen for culture that will determine possible drug resistance in the source case, select the appropriate drugs to be used, and identify all infected or diseased contacts.

d. A CXR showing hilar node enlargement with or without segmental atelectasis suggests the possibility of TB.

e. Culture materials should always be obtained when no source case is isolated, the source case isolated is drug resistant, the child is immunocompromised (HIV in particular), and extrapulmonary disease is present.

f. Tuberculin skin testing (see also Chapter 2): The PPD is the best tool for diagnosing TB infection in asymptomatic individuals. A positive reaction means that the person is infected with M. *tuberculosis*. Tuberculin reactivity usually appears 3 to 6 weeks and up to 3 months after the initial infection. Tuberculin reactivity is usually present for life, even after chemotherapy is given.

g. PCR can be used for diagnosis in children with significant pulmonary disease but without firm clinical diagnosis or epidemiologic link with known disease.

5. Management
   a. Recommended treatment regimens for drug-susceptible TB in infants, children, and adolescents are described in Table 19-22.
      (1) Treatment for HIV-infected patients should include at least three drugs initially and continue for 9 months.
      (2) Preventive isoniazid (INH) therapy should be started in exposed contacts with impaired immunity (e.g., HIV infection) and all household contacts younger than 4 years of age.
         (a) Individuals with a negative skin test should be retested 12 weeks after last contact; if their PPD is negative, INH can be discontinued. If it is positive, INH should be continued for a total of 9 months.
   b. Commonly used drugs for the treatment of TB in infants, children, and adolescents are described in Table 19-23. Note: If the reliability of self-administration of medications is doubtful, a health care worker or other responsible individual should be present when the patient takes medications.
   c. Drug-resistant TB is most common in immigrants from high-risk areas (Russia and the former Soviet Union, Asia, Africa, and Latin America), in people previously treated for TB, and children with TB whose adult source case is in one of the preceding groups.
   d. Children with drug-resistant TB should be treated for 12 to 18 months and in consultation with an expert on infectious diseases.
   e. Testing for HIV should be performed on all children with TB.
   f. Children who are being treated for TB can receive any of the recommended childhood immunizations, unless they are severely ill, receiving corticosteroids, or have specific vaccine contraindications.

Table 19-22 Recommended Treatment Regimens for Drug-Susceptible Tuberculosis in Infants, Children, and Adolescents

Infection or Disease Category	Regimen*	Remarks
Asymptomatic infection (positive skin test, no disease): INH-susceptible INH-resistant	9 mo of INH daily 9 mo of R daily	If daily therapy is not possible, twice-weekly therapy may be used for 9 mo. If daily therapy is not possible, twice-weekly therapy may be used for 6 mo.
Pulmonary and extrapulmonary (including hilar adenopathy)	6-mo regimen (standard): 2 mo of INH, R, and Z daily, followed by 4 mo of INH and R daily *or* 2 mo of INH, R, and Z daily, followed by 4 mo of INH and R twice weekly	If possible drug resistance is a concern, another drug (ethambutol or streptomycin†) should be added to the initial three-drug therapy until drug susceptibility is determined. Drugs can be given two or three times per week under direct observation in the initial phase if nonadherence is likely. For hilar adenopathy, a regimen consisting of 6 mo of INH and R daily is sufficient.
Meningitis, disseminated (miliary), and bone/joint	2 mo of INH, R, Z, and S* daily, followed by 7-10 mo of INH and R daily	S* is given in initial therapy until drug susceptibility is known. For patients who may have acquired tuberculosis in geographic areas where resistance to S is common, capreomycin (15-30 mg/kg/day) or kanamycin (15-30 mg/kg/day) may be used instead of S.

*Duration of therapy is longer in HIV-infected persons.
†Available from Pfizer Streptomycin Program, Pfizer Pharmaceuticals, New York, NY (800/254-4445).
INH, isoniazid; R, rifampin; Z, pyrazinamide; S, streptomycin.
Adapted from American Academy of Pediatrics; Pickering LK, Baker CJ, Long SS, McMillan JA (eds): Red Book: 2006 Report of the Committee on Infectious Diseases, 27th ed. Elk Grove, Ill, American Academy of Pediatrics, 2006.

Table 19.23 Commonly Used Drugs for the Treatment of Tuberculosis in Infants, Children, and Adolescents

Drugs	Dosage Forms	Daily Dose (mg/kg/day)	Twice Weekly Dose (mg/kg per dose)	Maximum Dose	Adverse Reactions
Ethambutol	Tablets: 100, 400 mg	15-25	50	2.5 g	Optic neuritis (reversible), decreased red-green color discrimination, gastrointestinal disturbance, hypersensitivity
Isoniazid*	Scored tablets: 100, 300 mg Syrup: 10 mg/mL	10-15	20-30	Daily: 300 mg Twice weekly: 900 mg	Mild hepatic enzyme elevation, hepatitis,† peripheral neuritis,† hypersensitivity
Pyrazinamide*	Scored tablets: 500 mg	20-40	50	2 g	Hepatotoxicity, hyperuricemia
Rifampin*	Capsules: 150, 300 mg Syrup: formulated in syrup from capsules	10-20	10-20	600 mg	Orange discoloration of secretions/urine, staining of contact enses, vomiting, hepatitis, flu-like reaction, and thrombocytopenia; may rende· birth control pills ineffective
Streptomycin† (IM administration)	Vials: 1, 4 g	20-40	20-40	1 g	Ototoxicity, nephrotoxicity, skin rash

*Rifamate is a capsule containing 150 mg of isoniazid and 300 mg of rifampin. Two capsules provide the usual adult (>50 kg body weight) daily doses of each drug. Rifater is a capsule containing 50 mg of isoniazid, 120 mg rifampin, and 300 mg pyrazinamide.
†When isoniazid is used in combination with rifampin, the incidence of hepatotoxicity increases if the isoniazid dose exceeds 10 mg/kg/day.
‡Available from Pfizer Streptomycin Program, Pfizer Pharmaceuticals, New York, NY (800/254-4445).
Adapted from American Academy of Pediatrics; Pickering LK, Baker CJ, Long SS, McMillan JA (eds): Red Book: 2006 Report of the Committee on Infectious Diseases, 27th ed. Elk Grove, Ill, American Academy of Pediatrics, 2006.

g. Isolation: Most children do not need to be isolated. Only those whose sputum smears have shown AFB and are coughing or have cavitary pulmonary TB or suspected congenital TB should be isolated. Patients can reside in an open ward once effective chemotherapy has been started, their sputum smears are negative, and their cough is resolving.

6. Prevention
   a. Bacillus Calmette-Guerin (BCG) vaccine is a live attenuated strain of *Mycobacterium bovis*. Its efficacy is unknown, and it is not currently indicated for immunization of all children in the United States. However, its administration should be considered for patients with a negative skin test result who are not infected with HIV in the following circumstances:
      (1) A child who is exposed continually to a person or people with contagious pulmonary TB resistant to isoniazid and rifampin and cannot be removed from exposure
      (2) A child who is exposed continually to a person or people with untreated or ineffectively treated contagious pulmonary TB and cannot be removed from such exposure or given antituberculous therapy

19.15 Sexually Transmitted Diseases

INTRODUCTION

See also Chapter 6.
1. Epidemiology
   a. STDs represent an epidemic among teenagers; adolescents account for one third of the reported cases in the United States.
   b. *Asymptomatic* infections occur frequently.
   c. Gonorrhea and chlamydial infection are the most common bacterial STDs.
   d. Human papillomavirus (HPV), the most common viral STD, affecting 20% to 50% of adolescent girls.
   e. HSV-2 is common; up to 20% of youth acquire genital herpes in adolescence.
   f. The prevalence of HIV infection is increasing in the teenage population.
2. Serious sequelae of STDs
   a. Pelvic inflammatory disease (PID)
   b. Gonorrhea and chlamydial infection are linked to ectopic pregnancy and infertility.
   c. HPV is associated with cervical cancer.

CHLAMYDIAL INFECTION

1. Epidemiology
   a. Sexually active adolescent boys have a prevalence of asymptomatic chlamydial infection of 8% to 12%.
   b. The prevalence of chlamydial infection among asymptomatic sexually active inner-city adolescent girls is 11% to 23%, among college students, 5%.

   c. Recurrent infection within 14 months occurs in nearly 40% of previously infected adolescent girls; therefore, reassessment is indicated.
2. Clinical features
   a. Many infections are asymptomatic (approximately one third in adolescent girls, and even higher among adolescent boys).
   b. Urethral syndrome/urethritis is probably the most common symptomatic presentation for chlamydial infection, responsible for one half of symptomatic cases in male patients
   c. Cervicitis
      (1) Mucopurulent cervicitis is often caused by chlamydial infection.
      (2) It is diagnosed by mucopurulent discharge from cervical os, with edema, erythema, and friability of cervix, and 10 to 30 PMNs on a Gram stain or wet preparation.
   d. Epididymitis
      (1) In heterosexual men younger than 35 years of age, C. *trachomatis* is the most common cause of epididymitis, which occurs in 1% to 3% of untreated cases of chlamydial infection.
      (2) The onset is often gradual (abrupt in one third); the involved scrotum is red and edematous, with swelling beginning in tail and spreading to head of epididymis.
   e. PID (see PID section, later)
   f. Perihepatitis (Fitz-Hugh-Curtis syndrome): This type of low-grade PID is characterized by upper right quadrant pleuritic-type pain and liver tenderness on percussion.
   g. Proctitis
      (1) This is often asymptomatic, except when caused by lymphogranuloma venereum, which is often an aggressive, invasive disease.
      (2) Non–lymphogranuloma venereum infection is characterized by rectal discharge, tenesmus, and rectal pain; suspect in women and gay men who present with proctitis and have anal intercourse.
3. Diagnosis and laboratory findings
   a. Urine screening: Routinely screen asymptomatic adolescent boys using a urine dipstick, looking for urine leukocyte esterase activity on unspun urine.
      (1) Sensitivity is 72% to 100%, specificity 83% to 93%.
      (2) *Note*: A positive result cannot distinguish gonorrhea from chlamydial infection.
   b. Cell culture: Gold standard, but may miss 20% of infections
   c. ELISA: Lower sensitivities in asymptomatic subjects
   d. Direct fluorescent antibody: Used directly on clinical samples; provides greater clinical accuracy than other methods
   e. Nonamplified DNA probes: Easy to use, can combine gonorrhea and chlamydial infection
   f. Nucleic acid amplification tests (i.e., PCR and ligase chain reaction techniques): Swab and urine tests available for both chlamydial infection and gonorrhea; recommended screening test for chlamydial infection
4. Management (Box 19-8)

> ### Box 19-8   Treatment of Uncomplicated Chlamydial and Gonococcal Infections
>
> *For Uncomplicated Chlamydial Infection*
>
> Doxycycline 100 mg orally twice daily for 7 days
>
> *or*
>
> Azithromycin 1 g orally for one dose*
>
> *For Uncomplicated Gonococcal Infection*
>
> Ceftriaxone 125 mg IM for one dose
>
> *or*
>
> Cefixime 400 mg orally for one dose*
>
> *or*
>
> Ofloxacin 400 mg orally for one dose*
>
> *or*
>
> Ciprofloxacin 500 mg orally for one dose*
>
>   *plus* (always treat for possible chlamydial coinfection)
>
> Doxycycline 100 mg orally twice daily for 7 days
>
> *or*
>
> Azithromycin 1 g orally for one dose*
>
> It is now possible to treat both uncomplicated chlamydial and gonococcal infections with one-dose oral regimens. Cost factors must be evaluated locally. The effect of such regimens on incubating syphilis is not known.
>
> Although azithromycin and ofloxacin have been approved by the U.S. Food and Drug Administration for those 16 years of age or older and 18 years of age or older, respectively, recent studies have shown them to be safe in younger adolescents also.

Adapted from Centers for Disease Control and Prevention: Sexually transmitted diseases treatment guidelines 2002. MMWR Morb Mortal Wkly Rep 51(RR-6):1-80, 2002.

GONORRHEA

1. Epidemiology
   a. The prevalence rate among 15- to 19-year-old girls is 24/1000 among sexually experienced individuals.
   b. Of sexually active adolescent boys, 1% to 3% have asymptomatic gonorrhea.
   c. Antimicrobial resistance is rising.
2. Clinical features
   a. Many infections are asymptomatic, especially in teens.
   b. The most common presentation in male patients is urethritis, which occurs approximately 1 week after exposure.
   c. Rectal infection in women is usually asymptomatic and accompanies 10% to 30% of *urogenital* infections (autoinoculation).
   d. Rectal infection is the only site in 40% of gay men infected with gonorrhea; infected gay men are more likely to have symptomatic

infection (pruritus, mucopurulent rectal discharge or coating of stools, rectal pain, tenesmus).
   e. Other presentations, similar to chlamydial infection, include PID, Fitz-Hugh-Curtis syndrome, and mucopurulent cervicitis.
   f. Bartholin's or Skene's gland abscesses present with pain and swelling of labia minora in the former and periurethrally in the latter.
   g. Pharyngitis is usually asymptomatic (up to 90%).
   h. Disseminated gonococcal infection occurs in 1% to 3% of untreated cases of gonorrhea.
3. Diagnosis and laboratory findings
   a. As with chlamydial infection, screen asymptomatic male patients for gonorrhea with unspun urine using leukocyte esterase activity.
   b. In symptomatic male patients, urethral Gram stain has excellent sensitivity (90% to 98%) and specificity (95% to 100%).
   c. Culture with selective media has been the standard of diagnosis for gonorrhea.
   d. Other diagnostic methodologies include DNA probes, PCR, ligase chain reaction, and ELISA.
4. Treatment: see Box 19-8

GENITAL ULCER DISEASE

Table 19-24 categorizes the various infections associated with genital ulcers.

GYNECOLOGIC CLINICAL SYNDROMES

1. Vaginitis
   a. Inflammatory response of vaginal mucosa after exposure to chemical irritant or STD
   b. Common causes: *Candida albicans*, *Trichomonas vaginalis*, and *Gardnerella vaginalis* (Table 19-25)
2. Cervicitis
   a. Hallmark of endocervicitis is "mucopurulent cervicitis": Yellow-green discharge, edema and erythema, friability of cervix, and 30 or more PMNs on Gram stain smear
   b. Mainly caused by *C. trachomatis* and *N. gonorrhoeae*
3. PID
   a. Epidemiology
      (1) Ascending infection that can involve the uterus, fallopian tubes, ovaries, and surrounding structure
      (2) Incidence
         (a) Ten to 15% of women of reproductive age have one or more episodes of PID.
         (b) Each year 750,000 to 1,000,000 new cases arise.
      (3) Impact
         (a) Recurrent disease common
         (b) Chronic abdominal pain (18% after resolution of acute PID)
         (c) Causes half of all ectopic pregnancies (risk increased sixfold)
         (d) Infertility (8% after one episode, 45% after three or more)—causes 15% to 30% of cases of involuntary infertility in the United States

Table 19-24 Genital Ulcer Syndromes

	Herpes Simplex	Syphilis (Primary, Secondary)	Chancroid	Lymphogranuloma Venereum
Agent	Herpes simplex virus	Treponema pallidum	Haemophilus ducreyi	Chlamydia trachomatis
New cases*	~250-500,000	35,147	4998	303
Incubation (days)	2-7	12-40	3-40	20-40
Primary lesions	Vesicle	Papule	Papule-pustule	Papule-vesicle
Size (mm)	1-2	5-15	2-20	2-10
Number	Multiple, clusters (coalesce ±)	Single	Multiple (coalesce ±)	Single
Depth	Superficial	Superficial or deep	Deep	Superficial or deep
Base	Erythematous, nonpurulent	Sharp, indurated, nonpurulent	Ragged border, purulent, friable	Varies
Pain	Yes.	No	Yes	Yes
Lymphadenopathy	Tender, bilateral	Nontender, bilateral	Tender, unilateral, may suppurate, unilocular fluctuance	Tender, unilateral, may suppurate, multilocular fluctuance

Laboratory diagnosis	Smear (Pap) Tzanck preparation: multinucleated cells (low sensitivity) Cell culture (sensitivity varies with stage of disease) Direct immunofluorescence stain	Dark-field microscopy; serology: RPR, VDRL; FTA-ABS, MHA-TP	Culture	Complement fixation, immunofluorescent antibody serologic tests
Treatment[†]	Primary genital: acyclovir 200 mg orally five times daily for 7-10 days or to resolution. Recurrent: most do not benefit	Benzathine penicillin G 2.4 million U IM, or if penicillin allergy, tetracycline 500 mg orally four times daily for 15 days, if not pregnant	Erythromycin base 500 mg orally four times daily for 7 days, or ceftriaxone 250 mg IM	Doxycycline 100 mg orally twice daily for 21 days

*New cases in United States in 1987.

†Centers for Disease Control and Prevention: STD Treatment Guidelines. Washington, DC, U.S. Department of Health and Human Services, Public Health Service, 1989. Screen and treat all partners and encourage use of condoms.

FTA-ABS, fluorescent treponemal antibody absorption; MHA-TP, microhemagglutination—T. pallidum; RPR, rapid plasma reagin; VDRL, Venereal Disease Research Laboratory.

Adapted from Hook EW: Syphilis and HIV infection. J Infect Dis 160:530, 1990.

Table 19-25 Diagnosis and Treatment of Vaginitis*

Vaginal pH	<4.5	≥5.0	≥5.0
Discharge	Nonhomogeneous	Yellow-green, frothy, malodorous	Watery gray
Potassium hydroxide (KOH) preparation	Yeast mycelia pseudohyphae buds on microscopy	Negative on KOH microscopy	Fishy odor when 10% KOH added to slide preparation
Sodium chloride (NaCl) preparation (microscopy)	Few PMNs	Many PMNs, motile trichomonads	Few PMNs, clue cells
Diagnosis	Candidiasis (yeast)	Trichomoniasis	Bacterial vaginosis†
Treatment (first rule out pregnancy)	Intravaginal clotrimazole 100 mg at bedtime for 3 or 7 days‡ (treat partners)	Metronidazole 2 g orally, once	Metronidazole 500 mg orally twice a day for 7 days§

*Symptoms (any/all): discharge, pruritus, dysuria; rule out urethritis, cystitis by clean-catch urinalysis; look for motile trichomonads in *fresh* urine sediment. Clinicians should be aware that trichomoniasis and bacterial vaginosis can coexist and that sexually transmitted cervicitis can coexist with vaginitis.

†Bacterial vaginosis was formerly called nonspecific, *Gardnerella*, or *Haemophilus* vaginitis.

‡Other comparable medications include butoconazole, miconazole, tioconazole, and terconazole.

§Alternative regimens include clindamycin cream (2%) intravaginally at bedtime for 7 days; or metronidazole gel (0.75%) intravaginally once a day for 5 days.

PMNs, polymorphonuclear leukocytes.

Adapted from Centers for Disease Control and Prevention: Sexually transmitted diseases treatment guidelines 2002. MMWR Morb Mortal Wkly Rep 51 (RR-6):1–80, 2002.

(4) Risk factors
  (a) Teenage years: A sexually active 10- to 14-year-old is three times as likely to get PID compared with a 20- to 29-year-old.
  (b) Partners (multiple partners, high rate acquiring new partners)
  (c) Contraceptive practices: Gonococci and *Chlamydia* can attach to sperm; therefore, preventing sperm from entering the uterus will lower the risk of PID.
b. Microbiology and pathogenesis
  (1) In the first episode, gonorrhea (in half of all cases) and chlamydial infection (in one third of all cases) are the most likely causes; approximately one third of untreated cases of gonorrhea or chlamydial infection will evolve into acute PID.
  (2) *Bacteroides, Peptostreptococcus, Peptococcus,* and *E. coli* may play a role because PID is a polymicrobial disease.
  (3) There is an association between vaginal bacterial colonization/low-grade infection and PID.
c. Clinical features and diagnosis
  (1) The most common presenting symptom of PID is lower abdominal pain; gonorrheal PID is more abrupt and dramatic in its presentation. Therefore, suspect PID in *all* adolescents with abdominal pain.
  (2) Diagnostic criteria appear in Box 19-9.
d. Treatment and management
  (1) Treat partners. In PID, 53% of partners will have chlamydial infection, 41%, gonorrhea.
  (2) Indications for hospitalization include fever, toxicity, vomiting, severe abdominal pain, and overt peritonitis.
  (3) Outpatient recommendations
    (a) Regimen A: Ofloxacin 400 mg orally twice a day for 14 days, *or* levofloxacin 500 mg orally once daily for 14 days, with or without metronidazole 500 mg orally two times a day for 14 days
    (b) Regimen B: Cefoxitin 2 g IM, plus probenecid 1 g orally, in a single dose, or ceftriaxone 250 mg IM, *or* another third-generation cephalosporin (e.g., ceftizoxime or cefotaxime), *plus* doxycycline 100 mg orally twice a day for 14 days, with or without metronidazole 500 mg twice daily for 14 days
  (4) Inpatient protocols
    (a) Regimen A: Cefoxitin 2 g IV four times a day, *or* cefotetan 2 g IV twice a day, *plus* doxycycline 100 mg IV or orally twice a day, to continue 24 hours after improvement, then doxycycline 100 mg orally twice a day for a total of 14 days
    (b) Regimen B: Clindamycin 900 mg IV three times a day, *plus* gentamicin loading dose 2 mg/kg, followed by maintenance 1.5 mg/kg every 8 hours,* to continue 24 hours after

---

*Single daily dosing may be substituted.

Box 19-9   Diagnostic Criteria for Pelvic Inflammatory Disease

Major Diagnostic Criteria

Treat empirically for PID if all are present and no other causes are plausible:
- Lower abdominal tenderness
- Adnexal tenderness
- Cervical motion tenderness

Additional Criteria

If severe clinical signs are present, these criteria help in differential diagnosis and increase the specificity of the diagnosis:
- Oral temperature above 38.3° C
- Abnormal cervical or vaginal discharge
- Elevated erythrocyte sedimentation rate
- Elevated C-reactive protein
- Laboratory-documented *N. gonorrhoeae* or *C. trachomatis* cervical infection

Other Criteria

These criteria are based on findings consistent with PID delineated during additional testing when appropriate and available:
- Evidence of endometritis on biopsy
- Tubo-ovarian mass on ultrasonography
- Laparoscopic evidence of inflammation/infection

PID, pelvic inflammatory disease.
From Shafer MAB: Sexually transmitted diseases in adolescents: Prevention, diagnosis, and treatment in pediatric practice. Adolesc Health Update 6(2):6, 1994.

        improvement, then doxycycline 100 mg orally twice a day, or clindamycin 450 mg orally four times a day for a total of 14 days
4. Urethritis
   a. Nongonococcal
      (1) C. trachomatis (30% to 50% of cases), Ureaplasma urealyticum (10% to 40%).
      (2) Twenty to 30% of cases associated with T. vaginalis, yeasts, viruses, and possibly mycoplasmas
   b. Gonococcal: The most common presentation of gonorrhea in a male patient is urethritis with copious, green-yellow penile discharge.
   c. Diagnosis and treatment (see Table 19-25)

GENITAL WARTS: HUMAN PAPILLOMAVIRUS

1. Etiology and significance
   a. HPV is a DNA virus; it cannot be cultured, and, to date, no antibody test is available.

b. This is a highly prevalent STD (13% to more than 50% depending on the population and diagnostic method).

c. HPV is responsible for the majority of Papanicolaou (Pap) smear abnormalities and is linked to cervical cancer.

d. It is a possible indicator of child sexual abuse.

2. Diagnosis

a. Differential diagnosis includes molluscum contagiosum, condyloma lata, and "pearly penile papules" (benign).

b. Routine diagnostic modalities include

(1) Visual inspection/identification (condylomata acuminata) will identify only the "tip of the iceberg" in terms of the extent of infection.

(2) Colposcopy poses problems with access and cost.

(3) Cytology (Pap smear) has low sensitivity/specificity but is the most practical.

(4) Molecular hybridization, using dot-blot (ViraPap/ViraType), is commercially available for HPV detection and typing.

3. Management (Table 19-26). A new vaccine to prevent the spread of HPV (and subsequent cancer) is available and will be given to girls (aged 13 years) and young women.

ASSESSMENT FOR SEXUALLY TRANSMITTED DISEASES IN THE WELL ADOLESCENT

The evaluation of the sexually active adolescent for possible *asymptomatic* infection is outlined in Table 19-27 (screening girls) and Figure 19-5 (screening boys).

HUMAN IMMUNODEFICIENCY VIRUS

1. Epidemiology, etiology and risk factors

a. HIV-1 infection is caused by an enveloped RNA retrovirus.

b. Worldwide, 1500 children are infected daily.

c. In the United States, there are fewer than 500 new infections per year in infants.

d. Risk factors for mother-to-child transmission (MTCT) include

(1) High maternal viral load

(2) Low CD4 count

(3) Preterm delivery

(4) Chorioamnionitis

(5) Breast-feeding

(6) Prolonged rupture of membranes

e. General risk factors for transmission are in Table 19-28.

2. Pathogenesis and transmission

a. HIV is transmitted by exposure to HIV-infected blood or body fluids (see previously).

b. Ninety-five percent of cases in young children occur through MTCT.

c. After infection, there is a variable and often long period of clinical latency (up to 10 years in adolescents, but shorter in infected children).

d. Active viral replication in CD4+ T cells gradually overwhelms the immune system, and opportunistic infections occur.

Finding	Regimen	Comments
Visible warts	Podophyllin (10%-25%) *or*	Systemic toxicity; unsafe in pregnancy
	Trichloroacetic acid or bichloracetic acid (80%-90%) *or*	Safe on mucosa and with pregnancy; local sensitivity
	Cryotherapy/surgical removal	
Pap smear: signs of human papillomavirus virus infection, squamous intraepithelial neoplasia	Colposcopy with biopsy	Refer for colposcopy

Adapted from Centers for Disease Control and Prevention: Sexually transmitted diseases treatment guidelines 2002. MMWR Morb Mortal Wkly Rep 51(RR-6):1-80, 2002.

Site	Test
Vagina	pH
	Potassium hydroxide (KOH) odor test
	Sodium chloride (NaCl; "wet") and KOH preparations for microscopic examination
Cervix	Pap smear
	Gonococcal and *Chlamydia* culture (or nonculture tests, e.g., ELISA or DFA tests)
Skin, mucosa	Inspect vulva for warts, ulcers, discharge
	RPR or VDRL
	Urine human chorionic gonadotropin to rule out pregnancy
	Hepatitis B panel
	Human immunodeficiency virus antibody
	Clean-catch urinalysis (to rule out urinary tract infection)
	Serology as indicated

DFA, direct fluorescent antibody; ELISA, enzyme-linked immunosorbent assay; RPR, rapid plasma reagin; VDRL, Venereal Disease Research Laboratory.
Adapted from Shafer MAB: Sexually transmitted diseases in adolescents. Adolesc Health Update 6(2):2, 1994.

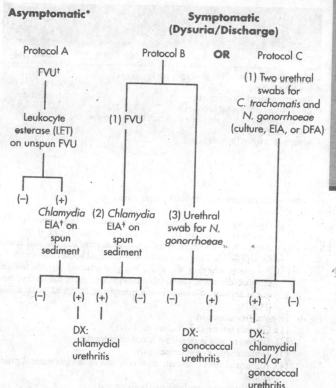

Figure 19-5 Screening for urethritis in male patients. DFA, direct fluorescent antibody test. (Adapted from Shafer MAB: Sexually transmitted diseases in adolescents: Prevention, diagnosis, and treatment in pediatric practice. Adolesc Health Update 6[2]:5, 1994.)

Exposure	Risk (%)
Mother-to-infant, if no therapy, no breast-feeding	20-30
Breast-feeding	10-15
Receptive anal intercourse	0.5-3.2
Receptive vaginal intercourse	0.05-0.15
Occupational exposure; needle-stick from known HIV-positive patient	0.3
Insertive vaginal intercourse	0.03-0.09

3. Diagnosis: History and physical examination
   a. History
      (1) Ascertain history of risk factors in parents (e.g., known HIV infection or risks for HIV such as IV drug use or STDs).
      (2) Ascertain risk factors in the child/adolescent (e.g., sexual activity and STDs, drug use, transfusions, sexual abuse).
      (3) Ascertain whether the child has unexplained growth failure, chronic diarrhea, unexplained hepatitis, encephalopathy, frequent serious or unusual infections (e.g., *P. carinii* pneumonia [PCP]).
   b. Physical examination
      (1) Growth failure (i.e., failure to thrive)
      (2) Persistent and generalized lymphadenopathy
      (3) Hepatomegaly or splenomegaly
      (4) Abnormal development, especially loss of developmental milestones
      (5) Oral thrush beyond the newborn period
      (6) Unexplained chronic lung disease (lymphoid interstitial pneumonia, pulmonary nodular hyperplasia, chronic hypoxemia)
      (7) Unexplained parotid gland swelling/parotitis
4. Diagnosis: Laboratory tests
   a. HIV antibody testing should be encouraged for
      (1) All pregnant women
      (2) Sexually active adolescents
      (3) All children who have one or more HIV-positive parent
      (4) *Note:* Children with any of the aforementioned physical examination findings or risk factors reviewed on history taking should also be screened for HIV.
   b. HIV antibody testing
      (1) HIV ELISA is the usual screening test
         (a) Tests for HIV-1 IgG antibodies
         (b) This test is highly sensitive and specific, but occasional false-positive results occur. It is a good screening test for HIV infection in children and adolescents.

(c) HIV-exposed newborns will have antibodies detected at birth owing to transplacental transfer of maternal IgG. Maternal antibodies will disappear by 18 months of age.

(2) HIV Western blot

(a) Tests for HIV-1 IgG antibodies; more specific than the ELISA test

(b) Used as the confirmatory test, when HIV ELISA test is positive

(c) For children older than 18 months of age, a positive HIV ELISA and positive Western blot confirms the child as HIV infected.

c. PCR tests

(1) These are used to detect presence of HIV genomic material, thus they are "direct tests" for the virus.

(2) HIV DNA PCR test is a qualitative (detected vs. not) test for HIV, and is the preferred test for early diagnosis in HIV exposed newborns. The test is highly sensitive and specific when performed at 1 month of age or older.

(3) HIV RNA PCR test is a quantitative test for the patient's "viral load." The usual use for this test is to monitor the viral load in HIV-infected patients.

d. Diagnostic evaluation of HIV-exposed infants (born to HIV-positive mothers)

(1) HIV DNA PCR test should be obtained at birth, 1 month, and 3 to 6 months of age. A positive test should be immediately repeated. Two positive PCR tests confirm HIV infection in an infant.

(2) An HIV-exposed infant with a positive HIV antibody test at 18 or more months of age is considered to be HIV infected; however, if negative, then HIV can be excluded.

(3) If two PCR tests are negative (one of the tests must be when the infant is older than 3 months), then HIV infection is highly doubtful.

(4) Note that standard recommended HIV PCR tests lack sensitivity for detecting HIV strains that originate from outside the United States (e.g., West Africa). In such cases, consult with a pediatric HIV expert.

e. Laboratory findings in children with HIV infection

(1) Anemia of chronic disease, with or without iron deficiency

(2) Neutropenia/leukopenia (often secondary to therapy), lymphopenia

(3) Thrombocytopenia (immune-mediated)

(4) Low CD4/CD8 ratio

(5) Elevated hepatic aminotransferases (even without a documented infectious cause)

(6) Elevated amylase/lipase (secondary to HIV or therapy)

(7) Hypergammaglobulinemia (IgG, IgA, IgM two to three times normal), especially in infants. Paradoxically, these immunoglobulins are dysfunctional.

(8) Hypoproteinemia/albuminemia (from malnutrition or renal loss)

(9) Renal functional abnormalities (proteinuria) from HIV nephropathy

5. Management
   a. Management of *HIV-exposed* infants
      (1) Start newborn on oral zidovudine (ZDV) for the first 6 weeks of life, then discontinue prophylaxis (antiretroviral drugs continue only if the infant has proven infection).
      (2) At 6 weeks, begin TMP/SMX, given 3 days/week, for PCP prophylaxis.
      (3) Test infant by HIV-1 DNA PCR assay at birth, 1 month, and 3 to 6 months of age. If the 1-month and 3- to 6-month PCR tests are negative, discontinue TMP/SMX.
      (4) Give routine immunizations to HIV-exposed infants who are without signs/symptoms of HIV.
   b. Management of *HIV-infected* infants
      (1) Basic monitoring includes history, physical examination, CBC, CD4 percentage, and viral load at least every 3 months
      (2) TMP/SMX should be given through the first year of life, and then depending on CD4 measures.
      (3) Combination antiretroviral treatment should be given to
         (a) All HIV-infected infants identified before 12 months of age
         (b) All children with HIV-related signs and symptoms
         (c) Children with moderate or severe suppression of CD4 percentage
   c. Antiretroviral agents: There are five classes of antiretroviral agents, each with its own mechanism of action and short- and long-term toxicity profile. See the *Red Book*, 27th edition (2006) for more information on specific HIV therapy in children. All HIV-infected children require care and management by a pediatric HIV treatment specialist.

6. Complications and definition of acquired immunodeficiency syndrome (AIDS): Late-stage complications of HIV infection are considered to be AIDS-defining conditions by the CDC (Box 19-10).

7. Prevention of HIV infection
   a. Postexposure prophylaxis
      (1) Risk of transmission of HIV based on mechanism of exposure (Table 19-28)
      (2) Prevention of MTCT
         (a) MTCT can occur in utero, intrapartum, or through breast-feeding (which is contraindicated for HIV-exposed newborns in developed countries).
         (b) Zidovudine prophylaxis, when given to mother and infant, results in a 67% reduction in MTCT. Further decreases in risk may be achieved when mothers receive additional antiretroviral agents or planned cesarean section delivery.
      (3) Postexposure prophylaxis for occupational exposure: Retrospective studies suggest a greater than 80% decrease in transmission rate if postexposure prophylaxis given.

Box 19-10   Diagnoses Indicative of Acquired Immunodeficiency Syndrome (AIDS) in Children, Adolescents, and Adults: CDC Surveillance Case Definition for AIDS

Criteria for All Ages

Candidiasis of the esophagus*†
Candidiasis of the trachea, bronchi, or lungs†
Coccidioidomycosis, disseminated or extrapulmonary‡
Cryptococcosis, extrapulmonary*
Cryptosporidiosis, chronic intestinal*
Cytomegalovirus disease (other than liver, spleen, nodes), onset after 1 month of age*
Cytomegalovirus retinitis (with loss of vision)*†
Herpes simplex ulcer, chronic (>1 month's duration) or pneumonitis or esophagitis, onset after 1 month of age†
HIV encephalopathy‡
Histoplasmosis, disseminated or extrapulmonary‡
Isosporiasis, chronic intestinal (>1 month's duration)‡
Kaposi's sarcoma*†
Lymphoma, primary brain†
Lymphoma (Burkitt's or immunoblastic sarcoma)‡
Mycobacterium avium-intracellulare complex or Mycobacterium kansasii, disseminated or extrapulmonary†
Mycobacterium tuberculosis, disseminated or extrapulmonary‡
Other Mycobacterium species, or unidentified species, disseminated or extrapulmonary†

*If indicator disease is diagnosed definitively (e.g., by biopsy or culture) and no other cause of immunodeficiency is present, laboratory documentation of HIV infection is not required.
†Presumptive diagnosis of indicator disease is accepted if laboratory evidence of HIV infection is present.
‡Laboratory evidence of HIV infection is required.

Continued

Box 19-10   Diagnoses Indicative of Acquired Immunodeficiency Syndrome (AIDS) in Children, Adolescents, and Adults: CDC Surveillance Case Definition for AIDS—cont'd

Criteria for All Ages—Cont'd

Pneumocystis carinii pneumonia[*†]
Progressive multifocal leukoencephalopathy[†]
Toxoplasmosis of brain, onset at 1 month of age[*†]
Wasting syndrome due to HIV[‡]

Additional Diagnoses Applicable for Children Younger than 13 Years of Age

Lymphoid interstitial pneumonitis[*†]
Multiple or recurrent serious bacterial infections[‡]

Additional Diagnoses for Adolescents (≥13 Years of Age) and Adults

Cervical cancer, invasive[‡]
M. tuberculosis, pulmonary[‡]
Pneumonia, recurrent[‡]
Salmonella septicemia, recurrent[‡]
CD4+ T-lymphocyte count of 200 cells/mm^3 or fewer, or a CD4 percentage of 14[‡]

HIV, human immunodeficiency virus.
Adapted from Centers for Disease Control and Prevention: Revised classification system for HIV infection and expanded surveillance case definition for AIDS among adolescents and adults. MMWR Morb Mortal Wkly Rep 41(RR-17):1-19, 1992.

(4) For high-risk occupational exposure from known HIV-positive patient, offer postexposure prophylaxis.

    (a) If high risk, start combination therapy for 4 weeks. Generally use three drugs, most frequently ZDV+3TC (available as one tablet, to be taken twice daily) plus nelfinavir (five tablets, twice daily). Drug regimen is adjusted for index patient's antiretroviral treatment history, resistance, and viral load, as well as profile of exposed patient (pregnant, other medical issues).

    (b) For low/medium risk, consider two-drug prophylaxis (fewer side effects) or no drugs.

(5) Exposures to saliva and body fluid contact with intact skin are considered *low risk*, with no postexposure prophylaxis indicated.

(6) For percutaneous exposure to discarded "needles on the street," consider offering postexposure prophylaxis on a case-by-case basis, depending on local HIV prevalence among IV drug users.

(7) For sexual contact, consider exposure and risk of treatment. Postexposure prophylaxis for ongoing sexual relationship not appropriate except in instances of failure of barrier contraceptive method. Postexposure prophylaxis may be indicated in cases of sexual abuse. Consider HIV risks involved (e.g., anal or vaginal penetration, trauma, and risk profile of perpetrator).

(8) Postexposure prophylaxis is unlikely to have benefit if initiated more than 72 hours after exposure.

(9) Studies

    (a) Obtain baseline HIV ELISA/Western blot, CBC, liver function tests before starting postexposure prophylaxis.

    (b) Treat for 1 month (if indicated) with repeat HIV ELISA/Western blot at 6, 12, and 24 weeks after exposure.

(10) Consultation with an HIV treatment specialist for individualized approach to postexposure prophylaxis

REFERENCES

1. McCarthy PL, Sharpe MR, Spiesel SZ, et al: Observation scales to identify serious illness in febrile children. Pediatrics 70:802-809, 1982.

2. Whitney CO, Farley MM, Hadler J, et al: Decline in invasive pneumococcal disease after the introduction of protein-polysaccharide conjugate vaccine. N Engl J Med 348:1737-1746, 2003.

SUGGESTED READING

American Academy of Pediatrics; Pickering LK, Baker CJ, Long SS, McMillan JA (eds): Red Book: 2006 Report of the Committee on Infectious Diseases, 27th ed. Elk Grove Village, Ill, American Academy of Pediatrics, 2006.

American Academy of Pediatrics Subcommittee on Management of Acute Otitis Media: Diagnosis and management of acute otitis media. Pediatrics 113:1451-1465, 2004.

American Academy of Pediatrics Subcommittee on Management of Sinusitis and Committee on Quality Improvement: Clinical practice guideline: Management of sinusitis. Pediatrics 108:798-808, 2001.

American Academy of Family Physicians; American Academy of Otolaryngology–Head and Neck Surgery; American Academy of Pediatrics Subcommittee on Otitis Media With Effusion: Otitis media with effusion. Pediatrics 113:1412-1429, 2004.

Baker CJ, Nadelman RB, Dattwyler RJ, et al: Change in management of skin/soft tissue infections needed. AAP News 25(3):105-112, 2004.

Baltimore RS, Shapiro ED: Lyme disease. Pediatr Rev 15:167-173, 1994.

Baraff LJ, Brass JW, Fleisher GR, et al: Practice guideline for the management of infants and children 0 to 36 months of age with fever without source. Ann Emerg Med 36:602-614, 2000.

Bisno AL, Gerber MA, Gwaltney JM Jr, et al: Practice guidelines for diagnosis and management of group A streptococcal pharyngitis. Clin Infect Dis 35:113-125, 2002.

Carillo JA, Fields AI, Task Force Committee Members: Clinical practice parameters for hemodynamic support or pediatric and neonatal patients in septic shock. Crit Care Med 30:1365-1378, 2002.

Centers for Disease Control and Prevention: Sexually transmitted diseases treatment guidelines 2002. MMWR Morb Mortal Wkly Rep 51(RR-6):1-80, 2002.

Christy C, Siegel DM: Lyme disease—what it is, what it isn't. Contemp Pediatr 12:64-86, 1995.

Feign RD, Cherry JD (eds): Textbook of Pediatric Infectious Diseases, 4th ed. Philadelphia, WB Saunders, 1998.

Gilbert DN, Moellering RC Jr, Eiopoulos GM, Sande MA (eds): The Sanford Guide to Antimicrobial Therapy, 34th ed. Hyde Park, Vt, Antimicrobial Therapy, 2004.

Horsburgh CR Jr, Feldman S, Ridzon R: Infectious Diseases Society of America practice guidelines for the treatment of tuberculosis. Clin Infect Dis 31:633-639, 2000.

Hsiao AL, Baker MD: Fever in the new millennium: A review of recent studies of markers of serious bacterial infection in febrile children. Curr Opin Pediatr 17:56-61, 2005.

Jensen HB, Baltimore RS (eds): Pediatric Infectious Diseases: Principles and Practice. Norwalk, Conn, Appleton & Lange; 1995.

Kaplan SL: Treatment of community-associated methicillin-resistant Staphylococcus aureus infections. Pediatr Infect Dis J 24:457-460, 2005.

King CK, Glass R, Bresee JS, Duggan C, Centers for Disease Control and Prevention: Managing acute gastroenteritis among children: Oral rehydration, maintenance, and nutritional therapy. MMWR Morb Mortal Wkly Rep 52(RR-16):1-16, 2003.

Long SS, Pickering LK, Prober CG (eds): Principles and Practices of Pediatric Infectious Diseases, 2nd ed. New York, Churchill Livingstone, 2003.

La Via WV: Parasitic gastroenteritis: Infectious diarrhea. Pediatr Ann 23:556-560, 1994.

McCarthy PL: Fever without apparent source on clinical examination. Curr Opin Pediatr 16:94-106, 2004.

Pizzo PA, Wilfert CM (eds): Pediatric AIDS: The Challenge of HIV Infection in Infants, Children, and Adolescents, 2nd ed. Baltimore, Williams & Wilkins, 1993.

Sander R: Otitis externa: A practical guide to treatment and prevention. Am Fam Physician 63:927-936, 941-942, 2001.

Shafer MAB: Sexually transmitted disease in adolescents: Prevention, diagnosis, and treatment in pediatric practice. Adolesc Health Update 6(2):1-7, 1994.

Teitelbaum JE: Probiotics and the treatment of infectious diarrhea. Pediatr Infect Dis J 24:267-268, 2005.

Tunkel AR, Hartman BJ, Kaplan SL, et al: Practice guidelines for the management of bacterial meningitis. Clin Infect Dis 39:1267-1284, 2004.

Wormser GP, Nadelman RB, Dattwyler RJ, et al: Practice guidelines for the treatment of Lyme disease: The Infectious Diseases Society of America. Clin Infect Dis 31(Suppl 1):1-14, 2000.

WEBSITES

American Academy of Pediatrics: www.aap.org
Centers for Disease Control and Prevention: www.cdc.gov
Infectious Diseases Society of America: www.idsociety.org
National Guideline Clearinghouse: www.guideline.gov

Neurologic Disorders 20

Sonia Partap and Randal C. Richardson

20.1 Seizures and Epilepsy: Overview of Diagnosis and Treatment

1. Definitions
   a. A seizure is a sudden change in motor, sensory, or cognitive behavior due to abnormal electrical discharges from the brain.
   b. Epilepsy is defined as more than one unprovoked seizure.
2. Diagnosis
   a. The first step in diagnosis: *Is the event a seizure or not?* Table 20-1 lists paroxysmal events that are not seizures.
   b. Next, describe onset and presentation of the seizure, which is useful in guiding anticonvulsant therapy and classification. Is the seizure focal or generalized? Is consciousness lost or preserved? The following terms help describe seizure presentation (Fig. 20-1):
      (1) Preictal: Is there a subjective sensation not detected by the observer (prodrome or aura), such as abnormal sensations or smells, indicating an impending event?
      (2) Ictal
         (a) Onset of seizure: Is it focal (e.g., hand jerking, facial twitching) or generalized (e.g., starts with bilateral involvement)?
         (b) Progression: What is the sequence of phenomena after onset? This progression correlates with the path of propagation of abnormal electrical discharges along brain networks, also known as "Jacksonian march."
      (3) Postictal
         (a) Nonspecific symptoms: Headache, confusion, lethargy, vomiting, amnesia
         (b) Lateralizing symptoms: *Hemiplegia* (Todd's paralysis) indicates that ictal focus is in contralateral hemisphere; aphasia (word-finding and naming difficulty) indicates left hemisphere focus in the majority of right- and left-handed people.
   c. The third step: *Is the event provoked?* (e.g., fever, central nervous system bleed, medications, etc.)
   d. The final step is the attempt to classify the epilepsy syndrome. Note that the majority of epileptic seizures do not fall into well-defined

Syncope	Sleep Disorder	Movement Disorder	Migraine
Vasovagal	Night terrors	Tics (as in Gilles de la Tourette's syndrome)	Acute confusional migraine (vs. complex partial seizures)
Breath-holding spells	Nightmares	Myoclonus (vs. myoclonic seizure)	Basilar migraine
Reflex syncope (stimuli: needles, blood, bad news, unexpected trauma)	Restless legs syndrome	Pseudoseizures (psychogenic)	Visual auras (vs. occipital epilepsy)
Long Q-T syndrome	Somniloquism (vs. complex partial seizures)	Periodic paralysis: hyperkalemic or hypokalemic	Abdominal migraine
Acute life-threatening event (ALTE or near-sudden infant death syndrome)	Somnambulism	Clonus	Benign paroxysmal vertigo
Gastroesophageal reflux	Normal sleep phenomena: hypnic jerks; phasic movements of REM sleep	Chorea (e.g., Sydenham's)	Hemiplegic migraine (vs. postictal Todd's paralysis)

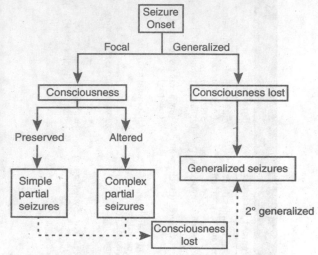

Figure 20-1 Classification of seizure based on presentation. (With permission from Jonathan Birnkrant, MD.)

seizure syndromes (see Section 20.4). If there is any evidence of focality on history or examination, or if the patient has had two unprovoked seizures, then electroencephalography (EEG) and magnetic resonance imaging (MRI) should be considered.

20.2 Seizure Types

Classification of seizures is important because partial-onset seizures frequently indicate an epileptogenic brain lesion. Seizure classification is the first step toward the diagnosis of an epilepsy syndrome, which leads to possible etiologies, specific medical treatment, and prognosis. Described here are the two categories of seizure, generalized and partial. *Note:* Neonatal seizures can present as either of these two (see Section 20.4); febrile seizures are described in Section 20.3.

1. Generalized seizures
   a. Pathophysiology: Primary generalized seizures (in contrast to secondarily generalized seizures; see Fig. 20-1) are bilaterally simultaneous in onset, clinically and electrically.
   b. Etiology: Often idiopathic or genetic, involving thalamocortical networks
   c. EEG: Bilaterally synchronous spike-wave or polyspike-wave complexes
   d. Age: Onset is usually in childhood and adolescence.
   e. Subtypes: Based on motor activity:
      (1) Tonic: Sustained appendicular or axial posture (i.e., stiff)

    (2) Clonic: Repetitive rhythmic and synchronous jerking, usually of extremities

    (3) Myoclonic: Single or multiple jerks, which may be confused with clonic seizures, but are usually arrhythmic

    (4) Atonic: Sudden loss of muscle tone, affecting posture (head drop, head nodding if repetitive, falls or drop spells)

    (5) Absence: Sudden staring, often with eye blinking, lasting seconds in primary generalized absences ("petit mal"), or longer in atypical absences

2. Partial seizures

  a. Pathophysiology: Partial seizures begin with focal or unilateral symptoms and indicate activation of neurons in a specific part of a cerebral hemisphere. Subtypes are determined by level of consciousness during seizure presentation.

    (1) Simple partial seizure: Consciousness is *intact*.

    (2) Complex partial seizure: Consciousness is *impaired*.

  b. Clinical features: Presentation depends on where in the brain the discharges originate and propagate. Clinical manifestations of partial seizures may be localized on the basis of the site of origin. For example, if the discharges are located in the right motor arm cortex, the left arm will begin to jerk. Wherever they originate, discharges may spread to both hemispheres, thus becoming secondarily generalized seizures.

  c. Subtypes

    (1) Simple partial seizures: Preservation of consciousness

      (a) Simple partial motor (focal motor): focal repetitive jerking of hand, face, or leg

      (b) Simple partial sensory (focal sensory)

        (i) Hemisensory paresthesiae

        (ii) Visual hallucinations, often in a half-visual field distribution

        (iii) Auditory hallucinations, usually sounds rather than voices

        (iv) Uncinate auras (unpleasant smells)

    (2) Complex partial seizures: Accompanied by impairment of consciousness

      (a) Temporal lobe origin: Often an aura (déjà vu, feeling of fear), speech arrest if from left temporal lobe, and motor automatisms (semipurposeful movements such as lip smacking, grooming, picking at clothes)

      (b) Frontal lobe origin: Usually no auras, present with bizarre automatisms (bicycling, swimming, other well-performed complex movements) that can be mistaken for pseudoseizures, often nocturnal and brief in duration with minimal to absent postictal state

20.3 Febrile Seizure

1. Definition and epidemiology: Most common seizure syndrome in pediatrics, occurring in 3% to 5% of children 6 months to 5 years of age. Simple febrile seizures are always generalized and may present before

there is awareness that the child is febrile. To be classified as complex febrile seizures, one of the following criteria must be met: duration greater than 10 to 15 minutes, two or more seizures in a 24-hour period, partial seizures, or focal examination findings (including a transient Todd's paresis).

2. Diagnosis and management

   a. If the child presents to an emergency department with the seizure already lasting 10 minutes (*febrile status epilepticus*), suppressive treatment is indicated.

   b. When seizures occur with fever, determine whether the cause of the fever is an acute systemic infection or an acute central nervous system infection (Table 20-2). Do a lumbar puncture if meningitis is suspected or if younger than 12 months of age.

   c. Pharmacologic treatment: only for febrile seizures greater than 5 minutes and actively seizing

      (1) Immediate suppression of seizures

	Febrile Seizures	Acute CNS Infection
Seizure type	Generalized	Partial or generalized
Mental status	Rapidly improves to baseline with fever control and hydration	Persistently altered
Physical examination	Identifiable source of infection or UTI	May or may not have identifiable source, nonblanching rash
Neurologic examination	Nonfocal	Meningismus, encephalopathy, focal signs
Cerebrospinal fluid	Normal	Significant leukocytosis, protein may be increased and glucose low in bacterial meningitis
Brain computed tomography	Normal	If brain swelling, small ventricles; often normal
Brain magnetic resonance imaging	Normal	Focal or diffuse brain edema; increased uptake on T1-weighted imaging with contrast in meninges; if encephalitis, T2-weighted/FLAIR signal changes

CNS, central nervous system; FLAIR, fluid-attenuated inversion-recovery.

(a) Lorazepam: 0.05 mg to 0.1 mg/kg intravenously (IV), maximum 8 mg; may repeat in 5 minutes as needed for continuous seizures

(b) Diazepam: 0.1 to 0.3 mg/kg IV (0.5 mg/kg rectally), maximum 10 mg; may repeat in 5 minutes as needed for continued seizures

(c) If status is not stopped, phenobarbital 20 mg/kg IV (see Section 20.10, Management of Status Epilepticus in Children)

(2) Intermittent therapy: Rectal diazepam, 5 to 20 mg suppository, can be given by parents at home, for any febrile seizure lasting greater than 5 minutes. May be repeated once, 10 minutes after initial dose, as needed.

(3) Prophylactic therapy: There is no effective prophylactic therapy for febrile seizures other than aggressive temperature control *after* onset of a febrile illness.

20.4 Epileptic Syndromes and Antiepileptic Drugs

1. Definition: An epileptic syndrome is a combination of specific seizure types, EEG findings, and neurodevelopmental/neurologic examination findings, with a typical age of onset, natural history, and prognosis.
2. Epilepsy syndromes of infancy (Table 20-3): Neonatal seizures
   a. Seizures that appear to be focal may actually be generalized, but because of immature/incomplete myelination, fail to spread globally.
   b. Clinical features: Presentation is subtle; progression movements (pedaling, rowing, swimming); roving eye movements; sucking, chewing, tongue protrusions; sudden arousal with transient, increased random motor activity.
   c. Neonatal seizures are usually provoked or due to underlying brain abnormalities; rarely, the diagnosis is primary epilepsy syndrome.
3. Epilepsy syndromes of childhood (Table 20-4)
4. Epilepsy syndromes of adolescence and adulthood (Table 20-5)
5. Figure 20-2 shows drugs of choice for different *seizure types*. Note that for children, these antiepileptic drugs may not be U.S. Food and Drug Administration labeled.
6. Table 20-6 gives antiepileptic drug dosages.

20.5 Headaches

1. Acute headaches: See Table 20-7 for cause, presentation, work-up, and treatment of acute headaches.
2. Chronic recurrent nonmigrainous headaches: These are uncommon in children younger than 10 years of age, more common in adolescence (Table 20-8).
3. Migraine
   a. Definition and clinical features: episodic headache characterized by recurrent episodes of throbbing head pain of variable intensity,

Text continued on page 627

Table 20-3 Epilepsy Syndromes in Infancy (0-12 Months)

Syndromes	Clinical	EEG	Management	Prognosis
Ohtahara's*	Before 3 mo, tonic spasms in clusters and sporadically, etiology usually brain dysgenesis	Suppression-burst pattern in wake and sleep	ACTH; clonazepam, sodium valproate usually ineffective	Early death or severe retardation, intractable seizures; may evolve to infantile spasms
Infantile spasms†	Peak onset at 4-6 mo of massive myoclonus (flexion spasms), causing developmental arrest	Hypsarrhythmia	ACTH for 3 wk, then rapid taper; vigabatrin if etiology is tuberous sclerosis	Developmental delay, other seizures; idiopathic > prior delay > overt cause (worst prognosis)
Benign myoclonic epilepsy of infancy	4 mo-3 yr; brief bouts of generalized myoclonus, normal development/ examination, positive family history	Generalized SW often only in early sleep	Valproic acid/sodium valproate	Seizures easily controlled if treated early; then, normal development
Severe myoclonic epilepsy of infancy	Onset with generalized or unilateral febrile clonic seizures, family history of epilepsy/febrile seizures, later—myoclonic jerks at 1-4 yr	Generalized SW, polyspike waves, early photosensitivity	Phenobarbital, sodium valproate, clonazepam, zonisamide, pulse IV methylprednisolone, intravenous immune globulin, ketogenic diet, VNS‡	Neurodevelopmental deterioration, followed by static encephalopathy, intractable seizures

*Also called early-infantile epileptic encephalopathy with suppression-bursts (EIEE).
†Also called West's syndrome if triad of spasms, hypsarrhythmic EEG, and mental retardation seen.
‡Vagus nerve stimulation treatment by a surgically implantable prosthesis.
ACTH, adrenocorticotropic hormone; EEG, electroencephalogram; SW, spike-and-wave discharge.

Table 20-4 Epilepsy Syndromes in Childhood (1-12 Years)

Syndromes	Clinical	EEG	Management	Prognosis
Lennox-Gastaut	Multiple seizure types, including drop attacks and nocturnal tonic seizures Often with prior delay or seizures, including infantile spasms	Poor background, multifocal slow SW pattern	Polytherapy: valproate, benzodiazepines, lamotrigine, topiramate Felbamate and corpus callosotomy stop drop attacks Ketogenic diet, VNS*	Intractable seizures, mental retardation
Childhood absence epilepsy†	Onset 3-12 yr; peak 6-7 yr; normal children, genetic predisposition	Bilateral, synchronous 3-Hz SW discharges activated by hyperventilation	Ethosuximide, valproic acid, zonisamide	65%-80% remission, usually by puberty; 15% will evolve into juvenile myoclonic epilepsy
Benign rolandic epilepsy‡	Common; onset most at 5-10 yr; often nocturnal and brief with perioral sensory aura leading to motor manifestations	Slow, diphasic, high-voltage, centrotemporal spikes, activated by sleep	No treatment recommended; however, may opt for gabapentin	Seizures stop and EEG normalizes in most patients, usually by second decade

*Vagus nerve stimulation by surgically implanted neuroprosthesis.
†Not to be mistaken for juvenile absence epilepsy, differing by age of onset and prevalence of other seizures.
‡Also called benign centrotemporal epilepsy or benign rolandic epilepsy with centrotemporal spikes.
EEG, electroencephalogram; SW, spike-and-wave discharge.

Table 20-5 Epilepsy Syndromes of Adolescence and Adulthood (>12 Years)

Syndromes	Clinical	EEG	Management	Prognosis
Generalized epilepsy, febrile seizures plus	Febrile convulsions, absences, nonfebrile convulsions, strongly positive family history of same, normal neurologically	Bilaterally synchronous spikes or SW discharges	Valproic acid	Good; seizures usually easily controlled; normal neurologically as adults
Juvenile myoclonic epilepsy	Onset prepuberty or postpuberty; early morning myoclonic jerks, absences, and generalized convulsions	Bilaterally synchronous, fast, irregular, polyspike and SW, activated by photic stimulation	Valproic acid, lamotrigine, clonazepam	Good for seizure suppression, but relapse frequent after drug withdrawal; normal neurologically
Temporal lobe epilepsy, due to mesial temporal sclerosis	Aura (fear), psychomotor automatisms, may secondarily generalize	Spikes in anterior, mesial temporal, or zygomatic leads	Carbamazepine, oxcarbazepine, lamotrigine, topiramate, anterior temporal lobectomy	Medically refractory by adolescence, 80% seizure-free after temporal lobectomy

EEG, electroencephalogram; SW, spike-and-wave discharge.

Anticonvulsant Selection Guide

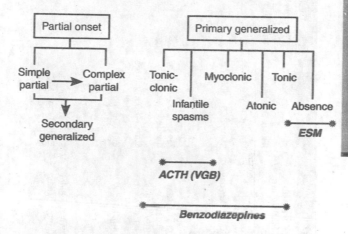

Figure 20-2 Anticonvulsant selection guide. (Courtesy of John Kuratani, MD, Seattle, WA.)

Table 20-6 Antiepileptic Drugs and Dosing Recommendations

Medication	Pediatric Start	Dosing Regimen	Pediatric Escalation Rate and Maintenance/Maximum	Adult Dosing	Therapeutic Goal (µg/mL)
Carbamazepine (Tegretol, Carbatrol, Teg XR, CBZ)	<6 yr: 5-10 mg/kg/day 6-12 yr: 100 mg twice daily	Three times daily—Tegretol Twice daily—TegXR/Carbatrol	E: 5 mg/kg/d every 3-7 days Max: 20-30 mg/kg/day	Start: 200 mg twice daily Max: 800-1600 mg/day	8-12
Ethosuximide (Zarontin, ESM)	<6 yr: 7.5-15 mg/kg/day >6 yr: 250 mg twice daily	Twice daily	E: <6 yr: 7.5 mg/kg/day every 4-7 days >6 yr: 7.5mg/kg/day every 4-7 days M: 15-50 mg/kg/day	Start: 250 mg twice daily Max: 1500-2000 mg divided twice daily	*
Felbamate (Felbatol, FBM)	15 mg/kg/day	Three times daily	E: 15 mg/kg/day every week M: 45-60 mg/kg/day	Start: 400 mg three times daily E: 1200 mg every week M: 32-56 mg/day two or three times daily	
Gabapentin (Neurontin, CBP)	10 mg/kg/day twice daily	Three times daily	E: 10 mg/kg/day daily M: 60-100 mg/kg/day	Start: 300 mg/day E: 300 mg daily M: 900-3600 mg/day	*

Lamotrigine without valproic acid (Lamictal, LTG)	0.3 mg/kg/day for 2 wk (>12 yr, see adult)	Twice daily	E: 0.6 mg/kg/day for 2 wk, then 1.2 mg/kg/day for 1-2 wk M: 5-18 mg/kg/day	Start: 50 mg/day for 2 wk E: 50 mg twice daily for 2 wk, then 100 mg/day every 1-2 wk M: 300-500 mg/day	*
Lamotrigine with valproic acid (Lamictal, LTG)	<12 yr and >17 kg: 0.15 mg/kg/day for 2 wk (>12 yr, see adult)	Twice daily	E: 0.3 mg/kg/day for 2 wk >12 yr: 25 mg every day for 2 wk Continue increase every 2 wk M: 5 mg/kg/day	Start: 25 mg four times a day for 2 wk E: 25-50 mg/day every 1-2 wk M: 100-400 mg/day	*
Levetiracetam (Keppra, LTA)	10-20 mg/kg/day	Twice daily	E: 20 mg/kg/day every week M: 40-60 mg/kg/day	Start: 250 mg twice daily E: 1000 mg/day every week M: 500-1500 mg twice daily	*
Oxcarbazepine (Trileptal, OXC)	8-10 mg/kg/day (to convert meds, OXC:CBZ ratio is 1.5:1)	Twice daily	E: 10 mg/kg/day every week M: 20-45 mg/kg/day	Start: 300 mg twice daily E: 600 mg/day every week Max: 1200 mg twice daily	10-35

Continued

Table 20-6 Antiepileptic Drugs and Dosing Recommendations—cont'd

Medication	Pediatric Start	Dosing Regimen	Pediatric Escalation Rate and Maintenance/ Maximum	Adult Dosing	Therapeutic Goal (μg/mL)
Phenobarbital (Luminal, PB, and PB-IV)	<2 mo: 3-5 mg/kg/day <2 yr: 6-8 mg/kg/day Loading: 20 mg/kg once	Once or twice daily	M: 3-6 mg/kg/day	1-3 mg/kg/day	15-40
Phenytoin (Fosphenytoin-IV, Dilantin, PHT)	3-5 mg/kg/day (can orally load 20 mg/kg divided three times daily or 20 mg/kg IV once)	Once or twice daily	E: 1-2 mg/kg/day every week M: 5-8 mg/kg/day (higher in infants)	Start/M: 300 mg/day	10-20 Free level: 1-2
Primidone (Mysoline, PRM)	Neonates: 10-20 mg/kg/day <8 yr: 50-125 mg every bedtime (>8 yr, see adult)	Two or three times daily	E: <8 yr: 50-125 mg every 3-7 days M: <8 yr: 10-25 mg/kg/day	Start: 125 mg/day E: 125-250 mg every 3-7 days M: 500-1500 mg/day	8-12 (or check PB level and aim for 15-40)

Topiramate (Topomax, TPM)	1-3 mg/kg/day	Twice daily	E: 0.5-1 mg/kg/day every 1-2 wk M: 5-9 mg/kg/day	Start: 50-100 mg/day E: 100 mg/day every 1-2 wks M: 200-800 mg/day	*
Valproic acid (Depacote, Depacon-IV, Depakene, VPA)	10-15 mg/kg/day	Two or three times daily	E: 5-10 mg/kg/day every 3 days Max: 30-60 mg/kg/day	Start: 1000 mg twice daily (60 mg/kg/day)	50-120
Zonisamide (ZNS)	2-5 mg/kg/day	Once or twice daily	E: 2-5 mg/kg/day every 1-2 wk M: 5-12 mg/kg/day	Start: 100 mg/day E: 100 mg/day every 1-2 wk M: 200-600 mg/day	*

All menstruating female patients on antiepileptic drugs should be on folate supplementation (4 mg/day).

Therapeutic serum levels for some antiepileptic drugs are widely accepted, such as CBZ, OXC, PB, PHT, and VPA. Which are useful for compliance, titration, and toxicity issues.

Note: Many antiepileptic drug pediatric doses are not FDA approved, and usage of these drugs should be discussed with an experienced neurologist

E, escalation rate; M, maintenance; Max, maximum.

*, no consensus on acceptable Therapeutic goal.

Table 20-7 Acute Headaches: Presentation, Work-up, and Management

Etiology	Clinical	Investigations	Management
Systemic illness	Location diffuse, constant, usually systemic viral infection, fever, neurologic examination negative	Determine etiology of systemic illness	Nonsteroidal anti-inflammatory drugs Treat systemic illness
Meningitis	Resistance to passive neck flexion, Kernig's and Brudzinski's signs, fever	Complete blood count; CSF cells, Gram stain, culture	Antibiotics for bacterial, antifungals for mycotic, supportive for viral
Encephalitis	Seizures, altered mental status, neurologic examination signs	Electroencephalogram, CSF to rule out meningoencephalitis, brain MRI	Acyclovir for herpes simplex, otherwise supportive
Increased intracranial pressure from mass/tumor	Headache wakes patient from sleep, vomiting; papilledema	CT/MRI brain	Dexamethasone load 0.5-1 mg/kg IV, then 0.25-0.5 mg/kg/24 hr, divided into every 6 hours Neurosurgical intervention
Decreased intracranial pressure	Headache on assuming upright posture, steady, most commonly post-lumbar puncture	None necessary	Prone position, increase fluid intake, PO/IV caffeine, if severe—blood patch
Subarachnoid hemorrhage	Sudden onset, severe, stiff neck	CT brain acutely; brain MRI/MRA	Intensive care unit admission, neurosurgical emergency
Intracerebral hemorrhage	Headache may be unilateral, focal neurologic signs, hypertension	CT brain acutely; brain MRI/MRA	Lower blood pressure, neurosurgical consultation

CT, computed tomography; CSF, cerebrospinal fluid; MRA, magnetic resonance angiography; MRI, magnetic resonance imaging.

Table 20-8 Recurrent Nonmigrainous Headaches in Children

Etiology	Clinical	Management
Chronic daily headache syndrome	Dull, bilateral; response to ordinary analgesics variable; often no obvious stressors	Prophylactic: Amitriptyline 0.1-2 mg/kg every bedtime; psychosocial support; see tension headache
Pseudotumor cerebri	Dull, bilateral, nonspecific; papilledema, often normal neuro exam; may be associated with steroid or antibiotic use and obesity	Acetazolamide 25 mg/kg/day divided every 6-8 hr, repeated lumbar punctures, serial ophthalmologic examinations to monitor visual fields.
Muscular contraction (tension)	Dull, constant, frontal or occipital, worse at end of day, related to stress; pain from isometric contraction of frontalis/occipitalis muscles	Acetaminophen, ibuprofen, stress management, relaxation therapy, biofeedback muscle relaxation therapy, psychological evaluation, behavioral contingency management
Other	Consider analgesic rebound, caffeine withdrawal; sleep deprivation; psychogenic (conversion reaction, malignancy)	As per each condition

duration, and frequency with associated nausea and vomiting, as well as photophobia or phonophobia. Most highly associated items with childhood migraine:

b. Family history of migraine: 70% to 75%

c. Motion sickness: 60% to 75%

(1) Common migraine (80%): These headaches have no warning/aura (initial neurologic symptoms, such as visual scotomata, scintillations).

(2) Classic migraine (15%): Preceded by an aura

(3) Complicated migraine (5%): The neurologic symptoms associated with the initial intracranial vasoconstrictive phase of the

migraine attack predominate, and the headache may be minimal or absent. This is a diagnosis of exclusion. Characteristic (and rare) variants include the following:

(a) Basilar artery migraine: Symptoms like those of vertebral-basilar transient ischemic attack in adults—vertigo, ataxia, diplopia, dysarthria, hemianopsia and usually associated with an occipital headache.

(b) Acute confusional migraine: The patient presents with an acute confusional state, with impaired memory after the event that may last hours. It may be a single event or repetitive. Need to rule out toxic encephalopathy if not resolved at time of presentation.

(c) Hemiplegic migraine: Hemiparesis may precede, accompany, or follow the headache and it may last hours after the resolution of the headache.

(d) Ophthalmoplegic migraine: Presents with orbital pain and extraocular muscle paralysis. The pain is unilateral, severe, and located behind the eye. Ophthalmoplegia may persist for days to weeks after the pain has resolved.

(4) Migraine variants: Several syndromes occurring in childhood are considered precursors to migraine.

(a) Cyclic vomiting and abdominal migraine; diagnoses of exclusion, usually do not present with headache and may treat with antiemetics

(b) Alternating hemiplegia of childhood

(c) Benign paroxysmal vertigo of childhood

(d) Paroxysmal torticollis; rare disorder usually occurring in infants, consisting of paroxysmal recurrent episodes of head tilt associated with sudden distress and vomiting

d. Diagnosis—inquire about:

(1) Headache characteristics, including location, severity, and duration. Duration of migraine headache in children can be shorter than in adults.

(2) Precipitants: Parents may note an association with certain foods (cheese, chocolates, MSG, caffeine), sunlight, or excessive television. Variable sleep schedules, poor sleep hygiene, and changes in stress levels are also precipitants. Obstructive sleep apnea should be excluded as well. Girls may experience exacerbations temporally related to menses.

(3) The child's grades, depressive symptoms, and number of school days missed.

(4) Red flags: These include positional nature, awakened from sleep or present when awake, change in headache pattern, or increasing severity. These can indicate masses causing increased intracranial pressure. Papilledema without a mass can indicate pseudotumor cerebri.

(5) Have the parents keep a headache calendar to track the frequency and severity of headaches. It is also helpful to know when medications are implemented (including doses and frequency), and if they were effective.

e. Laboratory findings
  (1) Usually no studies are necessary because migraine is purely a clinical diagnosis made by a well-taken history and normal results on the neurologic examination.
  (2) The following red flags may necessitate studies:
    (a) Acute confusional migraine warrants an EEG to rule out nonconvulsive status epilepticus and a lumbar puncture to exclude encephalitis.
    (b) Consistently unilateral headache, especially if a bruit is heard over the head or eyes, warrants neuroimaging to rule out arteriovenous malformation or aneurysm (computed tomography [CT], angiography, or magnetic resonance angiography).
    (c) Abnormal results on neurologic examination merit MRI and consideration of mitochondrial encephalopathies.
f. Management
  (1) *Abortive treatment for migraine*: Taking medication at the time of the attack to stop it; works best if there is an aura or warning, as in classic migraine. To help prevent rebound withdrawal headaches, these medications should not be used more than twice a week. If abortive therapy is needed more frequently, prophylactic therapy may be warranted.
    (a) First line: Nonsteroidal anti-inflammatory drugs, over-the-counter medications
      (i) Acetaminophen 15 mg/kg/dose every 4 hours
      (ii) Ibuprofen 10 mg/kg/dose every 6 hours
    (b) Second line: Triptans, along with an antiemetic such as metoclopramide, prochlorperazine, or promethazine (Phenergan), should be given at the onset of an aura or headache. The dose can be repeated after 30 minutes. Triptans and vasoconstrictors are contraindicated in complicated migraine because of increased risk of stroke.
    (c) Third line: Ergotamine derivatives can be useful; however, the risk of nausea and rebound withdrawal headaches can limit their effectiveness.
  (2) Treatment for unrelenting migraine: The following are indicated when a migraine headache is refractory to the preceding treatment, or the child is unable to take oral medications.
    (a) Prochlorperazine 0.15 mg/kg PO/PR (maximum 10 mg) or metoclopramide 0.5 mg/kg (maximum 10 mg), fluid bolus 20 mL/kg; may be followed by ketorolac IV.
    (b) Sumatriptan 0.06 mg/kg subcutaneously, maximum dose 6 mg. A prescription can be given for abortive self-treatment at home.
    (c) Dihydroergotamine 0.5 mg IV, wait 1 hour, then 1 mg IV every 8 hours. For children 6 to 9 years of age, use 0.1 mg as final dose, 9 to 12 years of age 0.15 mg, and 12 to 16 years 0.2 mg. Give with an antiemetic, such as metoclopramide 0.2 mg/kg IV. Watch for extrapyramidal reactions, which can be countered with diphenhydramine. Do not use for more than 24 to 48 hours because of rebound effect.

    (3) Prophylactic treatment of migraine
       (a) Tricyclic antidepressants: Amitriptyline 0.1 to 2 mg/kg at bedtime
       (b) Beta blockers: Propranolol 0.6 to 1.5 mg/kg/day divided three times daily
       (c) Calcium channel blockers: Verapamil 4 to 8 mg/kg divided three times daily
       (d) Antiepileptic drugs: Valproic acid (VPA), initial dose 10 to 15 mg/kg/day divided three times daily; maintenance 30 to 60 mg/kg/day divided three times daily
       (e) Cyproheptadine: 0.25 mg/kg/day daily or divided twice daily
4. Chronic nonprogressive headaches: These are tension or muscular contraction headaches, usually in adolescents. They may coexist with migraine (mixed headache syndromes) and may need to be managed by multiple disciplines (see Table 20-8).

20.6 Hypotonia and Weakness

1. Hypotonia: Reduction in postural tone with or without alteration in deep tendon reflexes (DTRs)
   a. Central (cerebral)
   b. Peripheral: Categorized as a lesion in the anterior horn cells of the spinal cord, peripheral nerve, neuromuscular junction, or muscle fiber
   c. Myopathy: Generalized weakness but proximal muscles are weaker than distal and DTRs are preserved
   d. Neuropathy: Generalized weakness but distal muscles are weaker than proximal and absent/reduced DTRs
   e. Combination central and peripheral (e.g., mitochondrial disorders)
   f. Table 20-9 shows causes of hypotonia.
2. Weakness: Defined as the loss of muscle strength, it can be divided into acute and chronic onsets. Etiology, presentation, and management of acute weakness are given in Table 20-10, and chronic weakness in Table 20-11.
3. Electromyography and muscle biopsy: Electromyography and nerve conduction times are necessary if it is unclear whether loss of muscle tone or strength is due to a myopathy versus a neuropathy. Muscle biopsy is still helpful in nondystrophic cases of muscle disease, such as in polymyositis or mitochondrial diseases. Molecular genetic testing for diagnosis is replacing invasive studies for many diseases.

20.7 Childhood Ataxias

1. Ataxia: Disruption of fine control in posture and movements
2. Midline cerebellar lesions can be manifested by truncal or gait ataxias.
   a. Truncal ataxia is an irregular swaying forward, backward, or sideways while in a sitting or standing position.
   b. Gait ataxia is walking off balance, particularly when walking a straight line (tandem gait) or on turning.
3. Lateral cerebellar lesions can be described as appendicular ataxia. This is indicated by dysdiadochokinesis, past-pointing, end-intention tremor with the upper extremities or poor heel-to-shin testing with the lower extremities.

Table 20-9 **Etiology of Hypotonia**		
Category	**Disease**	**Laboratory Tests**
Chromosomal abnormalities (central)	Prader-Willi syndrome Fragile X syndrome Trisomies	PWS genetic testing Fragile X screen High-resolution chromosomes
Cerebral palsy (central)	Hypoxic ischemic encephalopathy Perinatal factors	Neuroimaging
Peroxisomal disorders (central)	Zellweger's syndrome Neonatal adrenoleukodystrophy	Very–long-chain fatty acid screen
Spinal muscular atrophies*	Spinal muscular atrophy types 1, 2, or 3	Spinal muscular atrophy testing
Polyneuropathies	Demyelinating types* Axonal types	EMG/NCV, lumbar puncture, nerve biopsy
Disorders of neuromuscular junction*	Myasthenic syndromes Botulism	EMG/NCV, acetylcholine receptor antibody, edrophonium testing Serologies
Myopathies	Fiber-type disproportion myopathy Metabolic myopathy Inflammatory	Muscle biopsy, erythrocyte sedimentation rate
Muscular dystrophies*	Duchenne's Becker's Congenital myotonic dystrophy	Elevated creatine kinase, genetic testing, EMG/NCV, muscle biopsy

*Discussed in Tables 20-10 and 20-11.
EMG, electromyography; NCV, nerve conduction velocity.

4. Diagnosis and etiology of the ataxias are chiefly determined by the presentation and course (Table 20-12).

20.8 Stroke

1. Etiology and pathophysiology: Focal and persistent neurologic deficits due to a loss of blood supply or hypoxia. Stroke is rarely seen in childhood.
2. Prenatal: Usually occur in the third trimester and are asymptomatic in the child. Usually noticed as hemiplegia around sixth postnatal month; hand dominance should never be evident before 1 year of age. CT and MRI show old infarct or porencephalic cyst. Physical and occupational therapy are required.
3. Perinatal: Strokes can be secondary to birth trauma, placental insufficiencies, congenital malformations, or other idiopathic causes.
4. Postnatal/childhood: Strokes usually occur as a complicating factor from meningitis, coagulopathies, sickle cell anemia, cyanotic congenital

Table 20-10 Acute Weakness: Etiology and Treatment

Etiology	Clinical	Laboratory Tests	Management
Guillain-Barré syndrome	Pain and dysesthesia in legs, ascending weakness, complete in hours to days May have cranial nerve palsies Viral infection 2-4 wk prior Absent deep tendon reflexes	CSF for increased protein, normal cell count Nerve conduction, electromyographic studies	Check inspiratory function; intravenous immune globulin 2 g/kg given over 2-5 days; consider plasmapheresis if bulbar involvement, or respiratory failure
Transverse myelitis	Flaccid paralysis, spinal cord motor/sensory level Back pain, bladder/bowel dysfunction	MRI with contrast of spinal cord CSF can have increased protein and cell count	Methylprednisolone 15 mg/kg/day for 3 days
Acute demyelinating encephalomyelitis	Hemiparesis, ataxia, encephalopathy, seizures; can be present in spinal cord; preceding viral infection or vaccines.	MRI, CSF for elevated protein and cell count to rule out infection	Steroids—as for transverse myelitis, then oral prednisone 2 mg/kg/day Treat with acyclovir until herpes simplex virus negative

Stroke	Increased risk in cyanotic congenital heart disease, sickle cell disease	Computed tomography acutely to rule out hemorrhage Brain MRI with diffusion-weighted imaging Coagulation work-up	Exchange transfusion in sickle cell disease Contact neurologist for stroke <3 hr of onset Consider aspirin treatment
Myasthenic crisis	Generalized weakness, respiratory failure; if cholinergic crisis, excess bronchial secretions	Edrophonium test: improves if myasthenia gravis, worsens if cholinergic crisis Repetitive nerve stimulation test	Neostigmine 0.01 to 0.04 mg/kg every 3 hr
Bell's palsy	Weakness of upper and lower face, pain behind ear, hyperacusis, loss of taste	Lyme titers in endemic area	Prednisone 2 mg/kg/day for 5 days, if patient seen in first 3 days after onset Acyclovir may be given orally three times daily Eye protection

CSF, cerebrospinal fluid; MRI, magnetic resonance imaging.

Etiology	Clinical	Laboratory Tests	Management
Spinal muscular atrophy	Hypotonia, "frog-leg" posture, absent deep tendon reflexes	DNA testing for SMN1 gene exon 7 deletions, other mutations If negative, muscle biopsy	Supportive treatment Inevitably fatal if SMA types 1 or 2
Duchenne's/Becker's* muscular dystrophy	Toddler-age onset, boys, large calves, Gower's sign, waddling gait	DNA testing for dystrophin gene mutations, electrocencephalography, respiratory function tests, muscle biopsy	Prednisone may delay need for wheelchair for about 18 months.
Juvenile myasthenia gravis/transient neonatal myasthenia	1. Juvenile—fatigability, mild hip, neck extensor weakness 2. Neonatal—hypotonia, poor suck within first hours to days of life; mother with history of myasthenia gravis	Edrophonium test Repetitive nerve stimulation test with EMG Acetylcholine receptor antibodies	Juvenile: pulsed gamma globulin IV, pulsed methylprednisolone IV, thymectomy, pyridostigmine Neonatal: neostigmine NG
Inherited neuropathies	Distal atrophy, weakness, sensory ataxia, stork legs, claw hands, stocking-glove sensory loss	EMG, sensorimotor nerve conduction times DNA mutation analysis for CMT1, CMT2 (autosomal dominant), CMT4 (recessive)	Supportive, genetic counseling, very slowly progressive, compatible with long life

*Becker type has a more benign course with longer survival.
CMT, Charcot-Marie-Tooth disease; EMG, electromyography.

Etiology	Disorders	Clinical	Laboratory Findings	Management
Vertiginous	Labyrinthitis, vestibular neuritis, benign paroxysmal vertigo, perilymphatic fistula	Vertigo, nystagmus, nausea/vomiting, truncal ataxia; Dix-Hallpike maneuver	Pneumato-otoscopy	Antivertigo drugs (meclizine, diazepam)
Postinfectious	1. AC 2. ADEM	AC: 2-7 yr, gait ataxia. ADEM: any age, multifocal neurologic signs	Brain MRI, toxicology. Cerebrospinal fluid to rule out infection	AC: self-limited. ADEM: steroids, see Table 20-11
Toxic	Drugs: phenytoin, sedatives, psychiatric drugs. Alcohol	Gait and lateralized ataxia, dysarthria	Toxic screen, serum drug levels	Supportive, antidote or reversant if available
Vascular	Cerebellar or brain stem stroke from dissection of vertebral artery	Preceding fall, trauma to head or neck; lateral medullary neurologic signs. See Table 20-13	MRI/MRA of brain/neck	Interventional radiology consult
Paraneoplastic	Opsoclonus-myoclonus syndrome			

AC, acute cerebellitis; ADEM, acute disseminated encephalomyelitis; MRA, magnetic resonance angiography; MRI, magnetic resonance imaging.

heart disease, vascular malformations, or trauma/dissection of the neck vessels. Rarely, a progressive occlusion of the main cerebral vessels, also known as moyamoya, can occur. Venous strokes are less common. MRI and CT scanning are recommended.

20.9 Movement Disorders

1. Etiology and pathophysiology: Movement disorders (MDs) can be described as nonepileptic abnormal involuntary movements. They are usually associated with disorders of the basal ganglia and its connections (Table 20-13).
2. Clinical features: MDs are often difficult to describe and are rarely constant. If not directly observed, have the caregiver videotape the events. Initial assessment should be directed toward excluding seizures (see Differential diagnosis, later):
   a. Choreoathetosis: A combination of chorea (quick muscle jerks that spread randomly to different muscle groups) and athetosis (continuous writhing movements of muscle groups that tend to spread in a predictable manner to adjacent muscle groups). All have a similar differential diagnosis.
   b. Ballismus: Violent, large-amplitude, irregular flinging movements of the extremities.
   c. Myoclonus: Extremely rapid, jerklike contraction that may cluster and even appear rhythmic. Secondary causes of myoclonus need to be excluded (toxic, hypoxic, infectious, vascular, demyelinating, neoplastic, or traumatic).
   d. Tremor: Prolonged or continuous rhythmic movement of a body part resulting from alternating contractions of antagonist muscles. May be subdivided into resting (extremity is relaxed) or action (extremity in fixed position or during movement).
   e. Dystonia: Sustained contractions of both agonist and antagonist muscles that results in maintained abnormal postures. One muscle group may have more power, resulting in sustained movement or even spasms.
   f. Tics: Stereotyped, arrhythmic, rapid movements of the muscles. Although complex motor and vocal tics are easily recognized, simple tics in isolation (eye blinking, grimacing, shoulder shrugs, arm and leg jerks) may be subtle.
3. Differential diagnosis: Always exclude the possibility of seizures first.
   a. Seizures are usually rhythmic, unlike MDs. EEG may be necessary to differentiate the two.
   b. Bilateral spread of abnormal movements, with consciousness preserved, is not seen in seizures.
   c. MDs rarely occur during sleep (except some dystonias and nocturnal myoclonus). Seizures occur at any time.

20.10 Management of Status Epilepticus in Children

1. Convulsive and non convulsive status epilepticus (continous or cluster of seizures without returning to base line lasting greater than 15 min): general principles

Disease	Clinical	Etiology	Investigatory
Sydenham's chorea	Choreoathetosis, often of distal extremities Triad: chorea, hypotonia, and emotional lability; other Jones' criteria	Possible poststreptococcal; related to rheumatic fever	Review Jones' criteria (antistreptolysin O titer may be insensitive) Need to rule out lupus chorea and hyperthyroidism
Juvenile Huntington's disease	Rigidity and dystonia more common than proximal choreoathetosis in juvenile form	AD inheritance pattern with progressive dementia and seizures	MRI; number of CAG trinucleotide repeats in *huntingtin* gene (4p16.3)
Wilson's disease (hepatolenticular degeneration)	Dystonia, rigidity, and resting tremor	Autosomal recessive inherited liver disease with variable course Neurologic signs seen after age of 5 yr Psychiatric involvement common	MRI; slit-lamp examination (Kayser-Fleischer rings); serum ceruloplasmin; 24-hour urine copper; liver biopsy
Essential tremor	Tremor (postural or intentional), maximal in arms and head, distal > proximal	AD trait with complete penetrance but variable age of onset	Family history of essential tremor in >95% of patients
Gilles de la Tourette's syndrome	More than one motor and at least one vocal tic lasting longer than 1 yr	Largely AD inheritance with onset between 2-18 yr Attention deficit hyperactivity disorder, obsessive-compulsive disorder are common	Tics must occur outside of the effects of medicines (e.g., stimulants) or illness

Continued

Disease	Clinical	Etiology	Investigatory
Myoclonic encephalopathy of infancy (opsoclonus-myoclonus syndrome)	Acute simultaneous onset of chaotic myoclonic jerks and rapid dancing eye movements (opsoclonus)	Associated with occult neuroblastoma, viral illness, aseptic meningitis, or idiopathic causes	Serial urine catecholamine levels and computed tomography of chest, abdomen, and pelvis to exclude neuroblastoma
Physiologic myoclonus	Myoclonus occurring in special circumstances only, such as initiation or maintenance of sleep	1. Sleep-associated (hypnic jerks, nocturnal myoclonus) 2. Exercise-induced myoclonus	Isolated finding with absence of other clinical clues

AD, autosomal dominant; MRI, magnetic resonance imaging.

a. Perform the ABCs (airway, breathing, circulation) of general emergency care.
b. After drawing blood for baseline electrolytes, venous blood gases, glucose, liver and renal chemistry profiles, and toxic screen, treat with IV/PR anticonvulsants.
  (1) *Diazepam* 1 to 2.5 mg IV in young infants, 5 mg IV in older infants/young children; may be repeated once, 10 minutes later, as needed (PR preparation available).
  (2) *Lorazepam*, 0.1 mg/kg IV.
  (3) Immediately after (1) and (2), load with long-acting antiepileptic drugs to prevent recurrence:
    (a) *Phenobarbital* 20 mg/kg IV over 10 to 15 minutes. The risk of respiratory suppression is minimal, but is increased if there have been repeated doses of diazepam or its derivatives previously.
    (b) *Phenytoin* 20 mg/kg IV in normal saline solution, or *fosphenytoin* at same phenytoin-equivalent dose, IM or IV in any IV solution. IV solutions drip in over 20 to 30 minutes.
    (c) *Sodium valproate (Depacon)* 20 to 25 mg/kg, load IV, obtain a serum VPA level about 6 hours later, then adjust for maintenance dose. Desired therapeutic level is between 80 and 100 µg/dL.
  (4) If status is still not controlled, intubate and transfer to the intensive care unit, and proceed with several possible general anesthesia approaches with continous EEG monitoring to ensure burst suppression patterns:
    (a) *Pentobarbital coma*
    (b) *IV midazolam drip*
    (c) *IV propofol drip* (may cause sudden death in children)

SUGGESTED READING

Fenichel GM: Clinical Pediatric Neurology: A Signs and Symptoms Approach, 5th ed. Philadelphia, Elsevier Saunders, 2005
Lewis D, Ashwal S, Hershey A, et al: Practice parameter: Pharmacological treatment of migraine headaches in children and adolescents. Neurology 63:2215-2224, 2004.
Maizels M: The patient with daily headaches. Am Fam Physician 70:2299-2306, 2004.
Pellock JM, Dodson WE, Bourgeois BF: Pediatric Epilepsy: Diagnosis and Therapy, 2nd ed. New York, Demos, 2001.
Rothner D (ed): Pediatric Headaches. Semin Pediatr Neurol 8(1), 2001.
Silberstein S, Lipton R, Dalessio D: Wolff's Headache and Other Head Pain, 7th ed. New York, Oxford University Press, 2001.
Wheless JW, Bourgeois BF: Choosing antiepileptic drugs for developmentally normal children with specific epilepsy syndromes and behavioral disorders. J Child Neurol 19(Suppl 1):539-548, 2004.

WEBSITES

Child Neurology Society (practice parameter resources): www.childneurologysociety.org
Epilepsy Foundation (for patients and families): www.epilepsyfoundation.org
Family Village (good resource for parents, families): www.familyvillage.wisc.edu
Migraine Awareness Group (for patients and families): www.migraines.org
National Institute of Neurological Disorders and Stroke, Ataxias and Cerebellar or Spinocerebellar Degeneration Information Page: www.ninds.nih.gov/disorders/ataxia/ataxia.htm

National Institute of Neurological Disorders and Stroke, Epilepsy Information Page: www.ninds.nih.gov/disorders/epilepsy/epilepsy.htm

National Institute of Neurological Disorders and Stroke, Headache Information Page: www.ninds.nih.gov/disorders/headache/headache.htm

Spencer S. Eccles Health Science Library, University of Utah (good outline of the pediatric neurologic exam): http://library.med.utah.edu/pedineurologicexam/html/home_exam.html

Developmental Disabilities

21

Maya Liza C. Lopez and Jo-Ann Blaymore Bier

21.1 Developmental Evaluation

1. Introduction: This section discusses an approach to the evaluation and differential diagnosis of children with suspected or known abnormalities in development.
2. General principles and definitions
   a. Developmental domains
      (1) Cognition: Intellectual ability
      (2) Gross motor: The use of large muscle groups of the body
      (3) Fine motor: The use of the smaller muscle groups of the hands
      (4) Adaptive: Practical and self care skills
      (5) Socioemotional: Self-awareness and social interaction skills
      (6) Language: Ability to communicate ideas and understand others
   b. Developmental evaluation: An assessment of a child's level of functioning in each of the six developmental domains
   c. Developmental variation: Achievement of a milestone occurs at an age range and not at a precise age. *For example*, the mean age for walking may be 12 months, but some children may walk as early as 8 months or as late as 15 months.
   d. Developmental delay: A lag in the acquisition of developmental milestones with skills *significantly* below that which is expected by an individual's chronologic age. Statistically significant delay means the child's developmental level is 2 standard deviations below the mean.
   e. Developmental quotient (DQ): A measure that can be determined for each domain of development. DQ can be calculated by dividing the child's skills age by his or her chronologic age, then multiply by 100. A DQ of 70 and below signifies significant developmental delay.
3. Etiology: Developmental delays may occur in otherwise healthy children or may be manifestations of medical conditions, such as genetic syndromes, metabolic derangements, or neurologic diseases.
4. Clinical features
   a. Parental concern: Suspicion of developmental delay usually arises with parental observations.

641

b. Symptoms and signs (these should raise suspicion of possible abnormality)
   (1) Abnormal muscle tone
   (2) Asymmetry of muscle tone
   (3) Inability to receive or convey communication
   (4) Regression or loss of milestones
c. Screening: Pediatricians periodically screen (using tools such as the Denver Developmental Screening Tool; see Appendix VII-C) for developmental delay during well child visits. The purpose of screening is to identify children who require more formal diagnostic testing by a trained professional, such as a psychologist or a speech and language pathologist.
d. Specific developmental domains
   (1) Motor: In the first year of life, motor delay is the most common presenting concern. Significant motor delays sometimes lead to a diagnosis such as cerebral palsy, whereas milder delays may be the presenting feature of a wide range of developmental diagnoses.
   (2) Language: By 2 to 4 years of age, delayed language is the most common presenting complaint. Language is the developmental domain most closely correlated to cognitive development. Many children identified with mental retardation initially present with delayed language development. See Appendix VII-D for the CLAMS language assessment tool.
e. History: A comprehensive history provides information that is vital in the diagnosis and management of children with developmental delay. Focus on the historical factors in Table 21-1.
f. Physical examination: A careful physical examination should be performed, with special attention to neurologic findings and dysmorphology.
   (1) Neurologic: One of the key areas, extensive neurologic evaluation should include
      (a) "Hard neurologic signs": These include deep tendon reflexes (DTRs), abnormal muscle tone, asymmetry, weakness, spasticity, and ataxia.
      (b) "Soft neurologic signs": These include difficulty with gross motor coordination skills.
      (c) Motor symptoms: In younger children, gait pattern and stooping and recovering may be observed for any abnormalities; older children may be asked to perform hopping, tandem gait, and rapid alternating movements.
   (2) Screening developmental skills: Observe the performance of developmental skills in gross motor, fine motor, social interaction, language (be aware of a possible hearing deficit), and adaptive skill domains.
   (3) Examination for developmental disorders should include
      (a) Length/height, weight, head circumference
      (b) Skin examination for neurocutaneous stigmata (e.g., café au lait macules and axillary/inguinal freckling of neurofibromatosis; ultraviolet lamp examination for hypopigmented "ash leaf" macules of tuberous sclerosis)

History	Factors
Birth and maternal	Maternal factors (e.g., alcohol/illicit drug use, medications, maternal illness)
	Complications of pregnancy (e.g., preterm labor and bleeding, multiple pregnancy, polyhydramnios or oligohydramnios, abnormal α-fetoprotein level, abnormal findings on ultrasonography and amniocentesis, intrauterine growth retardation)
	Perinatal complications (e.g., meconium aspiration, placenta previa, difficult delivery and labor)
	Immediate neonatal course (e.g., birth length, weight, and head circumference, hyperbilirubinemia, feeding issues, respiratory difficulties, seizures, sepsis)
Past medical	Head trauma
	Elevated lead level
	Prolonged hospitalizations or illnesses
	History of surgeries
	Human immunodeficiency virus infection
	Growth concerns
	Seizures
	Chronic middle ear effusions
	Vision or hearing concerns
	Immunization status
	Behavior problems
Developmental	Age at acquisition of developmental milestones
	Any regression or loss of developmental skills
	Current developmental functioning
	Participation in early intervention program, Head Start, or special education programs
Family	First- and second-degree relatives with similar problems
	History of miscarriages, stillbirths, consanguinity, ancestry, parental intellectual ability
	Parental learning difficulties and education level
Social	Parental substance abuse
	History of physical or sexual abuse
	Deprived social environment
	Parental mental illness
	Parental employment
	Child care arrangements

(c) Scalp hair whorl direction/pattern

(d) Abdominal examination: liver, spleen

(e) Dysmorphic features: hand and foot position deformities, scoliosis

g. Table 21-2 provides an easy-to-reference practical guide to developmental screening.

21.2 Mental Retardation

1. Introduction

    a. Definition: Mental retardation (MR) is a disability characterized by significant limitations both in intellectual functioning and in adaptive behavior. This disability originates before 18 years of age (American Association on Mental Retardation, 2002). Examples of adaptive behavior include

       (1) Conceptual skills—money concepts, reading, language

       (2) Social skills—interpersonal, gullibility, responsibility

       (3) Practical skills—dressing, toileting, feeding

    b. Levels of MR: Current classification of MR is largely based on the types and intensities of supports and services needed by the individual (Box 21-1).

2. Etiology: Aside from the idiopathic cases, causes of MR may be organized according to the timing of insult: prenatal, perinatal, and postnatal (Box 21-2). The majority of cases of MR are attributed to prenatal causes. Cases of severe MR are more likely to have an identified etiology than cases of mild MR. Genetic technology is advancing rapidly, leading to more specific and more reliable methods of identification of the etiologies of MR.

3. Clinical presentation: The most common presenting complaint is global language delays. Parents may note that their child is slow in learning self-help skills (toileting, dressing, feeding), especially when there is a younger sibling who "passes" the child in question. The younger the child when he or she presents, often the more severe the degree of MR.

4. Diagnosis

    a. Standardized tests: Performance on standardized tools that measure intelligence quotient (IQ) and adaptive behavior that is 2 standard deviations below the mean (a score of approximately 70 or below) and presence of disability before 18 years of age

    b. Diagnostic work-up: It is essential to have a comprehensive medical and developmental history, including a three-generation family history and a complete physical examination. Supplemental information may be gathered through an audiologic evaluation, vision examination, autism screen, and a speech and language evaluation. Further testing, such as genetic testing, brain imaging, and other laboratory work-up, should be guided by specific clinical features.

5. Management: Interventions

    a. Medical: Specific medical surveillance and treatment depending on etiology and associated medical conditions

    b. Education

       (1) Overall educational goal should be to maximize functional independence in preparation for independent living (e.g., using a Life Skills curriculum).

Developmental Concern	Signs and Symptoms	Associated Condition
Abnormal motor milestones	Spastic, pathologic reflexes, increased deep tendon reflexes, decreased range of motion, asymmetry	Cerebral palsy
Delayed motor milestones	Proximal muscles weaker than distal muscles, hypertrophied calves, Gower's sign	Muscular dystrophy
	Dysmorphic features, short stature, complex congenital heart disease, hypotonia	Down syndrome
Delayed language milestones	Lack of interest in peers, impaired social skills, stereotypical repetitive behaviors	Autism spectrum disorder
	Intact nonverbal communication skills, clumsiness, garbled speech	Apraxia
	Visual responsiveness, poor response to sounds	Hearing impairment
Delayed socioemotional skills	Lack of eye contact, limited tracking, no social smile	Visual impairment, autism spectrum disorder
Delayed development in two or more domains	No significant dysmorphism, no focal neurologic deficits	Mental retardation of unspecified etiology, social deprivation
	Syndromic dysmorphologic features	Genetic syndrome with mental retardation (fragile X, Angelman's)
Developmental regression	Staring spells, normal results on physical examination	Seizures
	Staring spells, hypomelanotic macules, confetti lesions	Tuberous sclerosis
Failure to thrive with delayed development	Hypotonia, seizures, vomiting	Inborn errors of metabolism
Poor school performance	Poor concentration, disruptive behaviors, low frustration tolerance	Learning disability, attention deficit hyperactivity disorder

Box 21-1　Level of Support for Mental Retardation

Intermittent/mild (IQ 50-69): Support on an as-needed basis (e.g., help finding a job)

Limited/moderate (IQ 35-49): Certain supports over a period of time (e.g., help handling finances or job training for a few months)

Extensive/severe (IQ 20-34): Constant support but not in all environments (e.g., daily support needed in some aspects of living)

Pervasive/profound (IQ <20): Constant support in all environments (e.g., continual intensive supports in all aspects of life)

Box 21-2　Representative Etiologies of Mental Retardation

Prenatal

Chromosomal abnormalities: Down syndrome, Prader-Willi syndrome, fragile X syndrome, Angelman's syndrome, Rett's syndrome, trisomy 18

Neurocutaneous syndromes: tuberous sclerosis, neurofibromatosis

Metabolic disorders: phenylketonuria, Lesch-Nyhan syndrome

Endocrine disorder: Congenital hypothyroidism

Central nervous system malformation: anencephaly, severe hydrocephalus

Fetal conditions: TORCH infections (toxoplasmosis, other agents, rubella, cytomegalovirus, herpes simplex virus), intrauterine growth retardation

Teratogen exposure: Fetal alcohol syndrome

Perinatal

Prematurity
Kernicterus
Hypoxic encephalopathy

Postnatal

Traumatic brain injury
Near-drowning
Meningitis
Brain tumor
Severe malnutrition
Severe psychosocial deprivation

(2) Special education services available up to 21 years of age, including a transition plan into adulthood (e.g., job training and placement).

   c. Behavior management: Functional analysis of problem behaviors (recognizing the antecedent and consequent circumstances) in order to devise appropriate coping strategies

   d. Pharmacologic adjuncts: Consider treatment to target certain behaviors such as severe aggression, depression, self-injurious behaviors, and poor concentration.

   e. Family services: Family support groups, respite programs, alternative funding sources (e.g., supplemental security income), and sibling support

   f. Legal: At age 18 years, a guardian must be legally appointed.

6. National resources and websites

   a. American Association on Intellectual and Developmental Disabilities (formerly the American Association on Mental Retardation; www.aamr.org)

   b. The Arc (www.theArc.org)

21.3 Down Syndrome

1. Etiology: Three copies of chromosome 21 (trisomy 21, translocation, mosaicism, or partial trisomy 21)

2. Clinical features

   a. Head/skull

      (1) Brachycephaly (shortened anteroposterior diameter of the skull)

      (2) Delayed closure of fontanelles

      (3) Hypoplasia of mid-facial bones

   b. Eyes

      (1) Epicanthal folds, obliquely placed palpebral fissures

      (2) Brushfield spots (white/gray areas on the surface of the iris)

   c. Nose: depressed nasal bridge

   d. Ears: Auricles may be small with abnormal structure—overlapping and folding of the helices, prominent antihelix, absent or attached earlobes, narrow auditory canals.

   e. Mouth

      (1) As the child grows, lips may become more prominent, thickened, and fissured.

      (2) Protrusion of the tongue may be present, as well as a broad alveolar ridge ("pseudo high palate"); as the child gets older, papillary hypertrophy and fissuring of the tongue may be present.

   f. Neck: Short, sometimes with abundant skin and subcutaneous tissue at birth. With growth, the increased tissue may become less apparent.

   g. Musculoskeletal

      (1) Extremities may appear short.

      (2) Hand may have a single palmar transverse crease and there may be a short, incurved fifth finger (brachyclinodactyly).

      (3) Foot may have a gap between the first and second toes.

(4) Muscular hypotonia with increased extremity range of motion and delayed postural controls are common.

3. Diagnosis: May initially be suspected based on clinical features; chromosomal analysis is used to make a definitive diagnosis.

4. Medical problems
   a. Cardiovascular: Congenital heart disease (arteriovenous canal defects); an echocardiogram should be done shortly after birth.
   b. Gastrointestinal: Duodenal atresia, Hirschsprung's disease, celiac disease
   c. Visual: Congenital cataracts occur in 3% to 4% of newborns with Down syndrome. A higher incidence of myopia and strabismus has also been reported. An ophthalmologic examination at birth is indicated.
   d. Endocrine: Hypothyroidism is common, and clinical symptoms may not be obvious; thyroid function studies should be obtained at regular intervals.
   e. Musculoskeletal: Atlantoaxial instability can result in spinal cord damage, so cervical spine radiographs should be obtained at regular intervals to avoid a delay in recognizing this condition.
   f. Hearing: Children with Down syndrome have an increased incidence of sensorineural hearing loss. They also have an increased incidence of otitis media (eustachian tube dysfunction), which may result in conductive hearing loss. Formal assessment of audiologic function is required.
   g. Other: Other conditions occurring fairly frequently in children with Down syndrome include seizure disorders, hematologic diseases, and sleep apnea.

21.4 Cerebral Palsy

1. Etiology and pathophysiology: Cerebral palsy (CP) is a disorder of posture or movement secondary to a static lesion of the developing brain. With CP, there is a disconnection of lower motor neurons from cerebral control (occurring before or during birth, or postnatally during early childhood). This leads to alterations in muscle tone, persistent primitive reflexes, and postural reactions.

2. Prevalence: 2 to 3 cases per 1000 live births

3. Clinical features
   a. Age of presentation: During the first few months of life, much of the motor repertoire is reflex based. Consequently, CP may not present until 4 to 5 months of age, at which time motor delay and fixed asymmetry may be demonstrated.
   b. Motor function: The following are common presenting symptoms and signs in infants and toddlers:
      (1) Sucking/swallowing problems
      (2) Increased or decreased muscle tone
      (3) Abnormal extensor posturing (e.g., scissoring of the legs)
      (4) Abnormal reflexes (e.g., increased DTRs, persistent ankle clonus, obligatory tonic neck reflex)
      (5) Persistence of primitive reflexes

(6) Delayed or abnormal motor milestones (asymmetric creeping or "bunny hop" creep)

(7) Early hand preference, asymmetric fisting

c. Important clinical points

(1) A child with CP who sits up without assistance by 12 months of age will likely be able to walk. If not sitting up by 12 months, motor disability is more likely to be significant.

(2) Motor delay with *normal* results on neuromuscular examination should not be diagnosed as CP.

4. Diagnosis: Classification is based on the clinical description of the neuromotor dysfunction:

a. Spastic (60% to 78%): Increased tone, clonus, decreased range of motion, and hyperreflexia

(1) Monoplegia: One extremity involved

(2) Hemiplegia: Involvement of one side of the body (upper more than lower)

(a) Asymmetric use of extremities at 4 to 6 months of age (reaching with only one hand or protective reflexes on only one side, e.g., one-sided parachute reflex)

(b) Asymmetry presenting earlier than 4 months of age suggests lower motor neuron injury (e.g., brachial plexus injury).

(c) With vertical suspension and the soles of the feet touching the examining table, the involved ankle will assume the equinovarus position (i.e., on tip-toes).

(3) Diplegia: Primarily lower extremities

(a) A brief period of hypotonia in infancy that progresses to hypertonia between 1 and 2 years of age

(b) Increased tone is more marked in lower extremities and is associated with hyperreflexia, ankle clonus, and decreased range of motion.

(c) With vertical suspension, lower extremities tend to rotate internally and adduct (scissoring). When the soles of the feet touch the examining table, an exaggerated positive support reaction will be present with feet in the plantar flexed position.

(4) Quadriplegia: Involvement of all four extremities

(a) Affected infants may be hypotonic or hypertonic in the first 6 months of life.

(b) Infants with hypotonia and increased DTRs typically become hypertonic near the end of the first year of life.

(c) Findings commonly include decreased abduction of hips and bilateral fisting.

(d) Typically presents as a neurologically involved child with delayed gross motor milestones and significantly aberrant motor patterns.

b. Athetoid (20% to 25%)

(1) First year of life: Tone is mixed—hypertonia, hypotonia, or normal.

(2) After 12 months: Uncontrolled, writhing movements in extremities and face are seen.

   c. Ataxic (5%)

     (1) May initially present as hypotonia and normal reflexes.

     (2) Characterized by a poor sense of balance, impaired depth perception, and tremors

     (3) Intention tremor or truncal ataxia is usually seen after the first year of life.

     (4) Posterior fossa processes must be ruled out.

   d. Mixed type (10% to 20%): Combination of 2 types (e.g., spastic and ataxic)

5. Differential diagnosis (i.e., CP vs. other conditions associated with para-neurologic findings)

   a. Rule out progressive disorders. The following findings are less likely to be found in CP and would increase suspicion of a progressive disorder:

     (1) Signs of increased intracranial pressure: papilledema and Cushing's triad (hypertension, bradycardia, and irregular respirations)

     (2) Ophthalmologic findings, such as cataracts, pigmentary degeneration of the retina, cherry red spot, or optic atrophy

     (3) Skin abnormalities, such as vitiligo, café au lait spots, hypopigmented macules, nevus flammeus

     (4) Hepatomegaly or splenomegaly: Possible storage disease

     (5) Markedly decreased or absent DTRs: Possible lower motor neuron disease

     (6) Progressive decrease in DTRs and degeneration of neurologic status: Possible leukodystrophy

   b. Endocrine disorders (e.g., hypothyroidism): may present with delayed motor development or hypotonia

6. Management

   a. Physical and occupational therapy: enhance functional mobility and self-care skill

   b. Bracing: Control abnormal joint postures and permit better mechanical alignment to prevent contractures of the joints

   c. Orthopedic surgery: Prevent or correct fixed deformities (e.g., tendotomy, hamstring release, Achilles tendon lengthening)

   d. Neurologic: Selective dorsal rhizotomy (cutting of spinal nerve rootlets, which leads to decreased spasticity) may be done as part of an intensive treatment program.

   e. Medications: Baclofen (gamma-aminobutyric acid agonist; oral, intrathecal) and botulinum toxin decrease spasticity but do not directly act on function.

   f. Early intervention program: Infants and toddlers should be referred to an early intervention program to improve muscle tone and muscle control.

   g. Psychologic/psychiatric intervention: Significant disabilities occur in impaired peer interactions and poor self-image. Young adults may experience sexual dysfunction and social isolation.

   h. Chronic problems associated with CP

     (1) Neurologic: Seizures, ophthalmologic diagnoses (e.g. nystagmus, strabismus), hearing deficits

     (2) Developmental/behavioral deficits: MR, learning disabilities, speech disabilities, impaired gross motor and fine motor skills,

attention deficit hyperactivity disorder (ADHD), behavior problems

(3) Orthopedic: Leg length discrepancies (hemiparesis), skeletal deformities (scoliosis, hip subluxation or dislocation), joint contractures

(4) Feeding and growth: Oral-motor dysfunction, swallowing dysfunction/dysphagia, gastroesophageal reflux disease

(5) Other: Failure to thrive, recurrent emesis, constipation, impaired saliva management

  i. Family supports: United Cerebral Palsy (www.ucp.org), We Move (www.wemove.org)

21.5 Muscular Dystrophy

1. Etiology and pathophysiology
   a. Muscular dystrophy (MD) refers to a group of genetic disorders with progressive degeneration of skeletal muscle and no associated structural abnormality in the central nervous system or peripheral nerves. Examples of specific diagnoses in this group include
      (1) Duchenne's MD
      (2) Becker's MD
      (3) Congenital MD
      (4) Limb girdle MD
      (5) Fascioscapulohumeral MD
   b. These conditions differ on the basis of body distribution of affected areas, severity of muscle weakness, pattern of inheritance, and localization of the defective gene. Of all the MDs, Duchenne's MD is the best clinically described condition.
   c. Both Duchenne's and Becker's MD are X-linked recessive conditions that are associated with mutations in the DMD gene. The DMD gene encodes for the protein dystrophin, which is a component of the cell membrane cytoskeleton. In classic Duchenne's MD, the complete dystrophin molecule is absent or nearly absent. In Becker's MD, dystrophin is present in reduced amounts or normal amounts but with aberrant molecular configuration.
2. Diagnosis: Duchenne's MD and Becker's MD
   a. Duchenne's MD (1 in 3500 live male births)
      (1) Genetics: The Duchenne's MD gene has been localized to the Xp21 region of the X chromosome. DNA analysis (polymerase chain reaction or Southern blot analysis) can provide a definitive diagnosis. Restriction fragment length polymorphisms (RFLPs) may be useful for carrier detection or prenatal diagnosis in families without known deletion.
      (2) Clinical features
         (a) Developmental milestones: Delayed between 3 and 6 years of age (e.g., difficulty running, climbing stairs, or rising from floor)
         (b) Speech problems (3%), learning disabilities (5%)
         (c) Motor: Waddling gait may be seen, with progressive weakness in the proximal muscles noted before involvement of distal muscles.

(d) Physical findings
(i) "Pseudohypertrophied" gastrocnemii that feel firm/"rubbery" on palpation
(ii) Positive Gower's sign (use of hands for support to counteract weakness of pelvic girdle muscles when rising from a supine position)
(e) Cognitive: Static cognitive deficits, verbal IQ often lower than performance IQ
(f) Clinical course: Rapid progression, often wheelchair dependent by early adolescence
(g) Prognosis: Few survive beyond third decade of life, with death commonly due to cardiorespiratory complications.
(h) Laboratory findings (in addition to genetic testing described previously)
(i) Markedly elevated serum creatinine phosphokinase level
(ii) Electromyogram indicates a myopathic process.
(iii) Muscle biopsy shows degeneration, regeneration and fibrosis, peripheral nuclei, and variable fiber size.
(3) Management
(a) Cardiac: Cardiac muscle involvement (50% to 80% of cases) can be seen as early as 5 to 6 years of age. Periodic electrocardiograms and echocardiograms are recommended to follow cardiac status.
(b) Respiratory: Periodic pulmonary function testing is done once child reaches adolescence and repeated more often as the child becomes wheelchair dependent. Risk of respiratory infection increases at the end-stage of disease.
(c) Infectious disease: Influenza and pneumococcal vaccine are recommended.
(d) Orthopedic deformities: Physical therapy is recommended to prevent contractures; monitor for scoliosis.
b. Becker's MD
(1) Clinical features: Clinical presentation, diagnosis, and management are similar to those for Duchenne's MD, with the following exceptions:
(a) Clinical course: Later onset, slower rate of progression, and less severe symptoms
(b) Physical findings
(i) Weakness of quadriceps femoris may be the only sign.
(ii) Preservation of neck flexor muscle strength (not seen in Duchenne's MD)
(c) Motor: Activity-induced cramping in some individuals, wheelchair dependency after 16 years of age
(d) Other: These patients have normal intelligence and little cardiac involvement.

21.6 Spina Bifida

1. Etiology and pathophysiology
a. *Myelodysplasia* (commonly known as *spina bifida*) is a neural tube defect (NTD) that occurs when the fetal neural tube fails to close in

the first month of gestation (neural folds form on day 20 postconception and normally fuse by day 28). The result is incomplete development of the brain, spinal cord, and meninges.

b. NTDs have a multifactorial etiology, including genetic (e.g., family history) and environmental (e.g., heat, folate antagonists, maternal nutrition).

c. Incidence in the United States is 0.6 to 0.8 per 1000 live births. Among mothers who have already given birth to a child with spina bifida, the risk of having a second similarly affected child is between 3% and 5%.

d. Three common types

   (1) *Spina bifida occulta*: A bony defect results from failure of the vertebrae to fuse. The spinal cord is normal and is covered only by skin. Usually asymptomatic.

   (2) *Meningocele*: Meninges of the spinal cord bulge through the bony defect. Usually the spinal cord is normal, but some nerve rootlets may be affected and relatively minor neurologic symptoms are possible.

   (3) *Meningomyelocele/myelomeningocele*: The most severe form, in which the spinal cord itself protrudes through the bony defect along with its meninges. In most cases, the meningomyelocele does not have a skin covering and may leak cerebrospinal fluid. Symptoms include flaccid paralysis, sensory loss below the level of the defect, hydrocephalus (70% to 90% of cases), and neurogenic bowel and bladder.

e. Decreased incidence of neural tube defects occurs with daily maternal intake of folic acid (400 μg).

2. Diagnosis: Elevated maternal serum α-fetoprotein (AFP) at 16 weeks' gestation may indicate presence of NTD. Fetal liver produces AFP, which leaks through the spinal defect and enters the maternal circulation. If an elevated AFP is found, level II ultrasonography is indicated.

3. Management

a. Surgical: Closure of the spinal defect in the first 24 to 48 hours after birth is done to prevent infection and physical injury to the exposed neural tissue.

b. Hydrocephalus: Occurs either prenatally or as a consequence of the spinal closure. Symptoms of increased intracranial pressure (e.g., bulging fontanelle, irritability, lethargy, high-pitched cry, seizures, poor feeding) must be monitored for at least 2 months after surgical closure of spinal defect.

c. Genitourinary: Neurogenic bladder is frequently present, unless the lesion is very low on the spinal cord. There is also an increased risk of other genitourinary defects or kidney malformations (e.g., horseshoe kidney). A voiding cystourethrogram (rule out vesicoureteral reflux) and renal ultrasonography should be performed before discharge from nursery. Later, cystometric studies are completed to evaluate bladder capacity.

d. Chronic medical issues (by system)

   (1) Neurologic

      (a) Shunt malfunction: Symptoms include vomiting, poor feeding, swelling along the shunt, irritability, drowsiness, headaches, downward deviation of the eyes, bulging fontanelle in infants, and personality change and deterioration in school performance in older children.

(b) Shunt infection: Fever, together with the symptoms and signs listed in (a)

(c) Tethering of spinal cord: Scarring from spinal surgery may cause tethering of spinal cord with symptoms such as worsening gait and scoliosis, marked incontinence, pain, and new onset of spasticity.

(d) Seizures: Occur in 5% to 25% of children with meningomyelocele

(e) Arnold-Chiari malformations: Nearly 100% of individuals with meningomyelocele have type II Arnold-Chiari malformation, which is the downward displacement of the cerebellum, lower pons, and medulla oblongata through the foramen magnum. However, only a minority of patients are symptomatic (e.g., stridor, apnea, dysphagia, and facial palsy) and require posterior fossa decompression.

(f) Syrinx (fluid within the spinal cord): Common level is cervical and may present as "tingling" and numbness in the upper extremities

(2) Genitourinary

(a) Neurogenic bladder: Urinary retention is common because of dyssynergy of the bladder wall muscle and sphincter. Recurrent symptomatic urinary tract infections or postvoiding residual urine of 20 mL or greater need to be relieved by clean intermittent catheterization (CIC) before starting preschool; CIC is used to achieve continence in the majority of patients. Medications that decrease bladder contractions (oxybutynin [Ditropan]) and enhance storage of urine (imipramine [Tofranil]) may also need to be used in concert with catheterization to improve continence.

(b) Vesicoureteral reflux: This is a common problem requiring treatment with prophylactic antibiotics to protect the kidneys from infection. Multiple genitourinary surgeries are common.

(c) Urinary tract infections: Increased risk secondary to urinary retention. Colonization is not uncommon, so antibiotics are typically used to treat positive cultures only if the patient is symptomatic (unless vesicoureteral reflux has been diagnosed). Prophylactic antibiotics are recommended if patient has vesicoureteral reflux or recurrent symptomatic urinary tract infections.

(3) Gastrointestinal: Attention to stool consistency to avoid problems with constipation should begin in infancy. Between 2.5 and 4 years of age, bowel training can begin with routine toilet visits after meals to encourage the gastrocolic reflex. Bowel emptying may be facilitated by a stool softener (docusate [Colace]), laxative (Senokot; polyethylene glycol [MiraLax]), fiber supplement (Perdium, Metamucil), or rectal suppositories (bisacodyl [Dulcolax]). Water enemas or colonic irrigation are additional treatments.

(4) Musculoskeletal: Decreased mobility and muscle imbalance around the joint area lead to deformities and dislocations (e.g., club foot, hips, scoliosis, kyphosis) that interfere with sitting and ambulation and may compromise pulmonary function. Physical therapy is begun shortly after birth and occupational therapy soon follows with age and activity level. Proper positioning (bracing or casting) to correct and prevent deformities begins during infancy. Older children may need corrective surgery (e.g., scoliosis surgery). Fractures are common because of poor bone mineralization and decreased weight bearing.

(5) Skin: Children are predisposed to decubitus ulcers in the weight-bearing areas (e.g., buttocks, legs). Prevention is by frequent inspection and providing properly fitted shoes, braces, and pads.

(6) Allergies: Latex allergies can occur owing to repeated exposure to latex.

(7) Cognitive: Although most children with meningomyelocele have average to low average intelligence, they are at increased risk for MR and learning disabilities.

21.7 Neurocutaneous Disorders

1. Etiology and pathophysiology: A group of hereditary disorders that manifest as widespread abnormalities in structures of ectodermal origin (skin, eye, and nervous system). These disorders are associated with a variety of developmental conditions and present with cutaneous findings very early in life, often before the onset of neurologic symptoms.

2. Neurofibromatosis type 1 (NF1)
   a. Etiology and pathophysiology
      (1) NF1 is an autosomal dominant disorder. The gene for NF1 is located on chromosome 17. Genetic linkage studies using linked polymorphic markers can be used for prenatal or presymptomatic diagnosis, provided two or more generations of affected individuals are available for study. Fifty percent of affected individuals have de novo mutation.
      (2) Severity of the condition in offspring cannot be based on the severity in other family members; however, the severity tends to increase with each generation.
      (3) Incidence: 1 in 3000 to 4000 births
   b. Clinical features
      (1) Seizures and headaches may occur.
      (2) Visual-spatial deficits and ADHD are often seen.
      (3) Learning disabilities occur in about 50% of cases.
   c. Diagnosis: Clinically diagnosed by the presence of two or more of the following findings:
      (1) Multiple café au lait macules (nearly 100%)
         (a) If prepubertal: At least six café au lait macules over 5 mm in greatest diameter
         (b) If postpubertal: One or more café au lait macule greater than 15 mm in diameter

(2) Axillary or inguinal freckling (found in 90%)

(3) Distinctive osseous lesion (e.g., sphenoid dysplasia or thinned long bone cortex with or without pseudoarthrosis)

(4) Optic glioma

(5) Two or more iris Lisch nodules on slit-lamp examination

(6) First-degree relative with NF1 by the preceding criteria

(7) Two or more neurofibromas of any type, or one plexiform neurofibroma

d. Management: Medical surveillance with annual physical examination, annual ophthalmologic examination, regular blood pressure checks, scoliosis screening, and regular developmental assessment. Baseline and follow up neuroimaging are obtained.

3. Neurofibromatosis type 2 (NF2): Bilateral acoustic neurofibromatosis

a. Etiology and pathophysiology: NF2 is inherited as an autosomal dominant disorder. The NF2 gene has been localized on chromosome 19. Incidence is 1 in 40,000.

b. Diagnosis

(1) Computed tomography (CT) or magnetic resonance imaging (MRI) evidence of bilateral internal auditory canal masses consistent with acoustic neuroma, or

(2) A first-degree relative with NF2 and either a unilateral eighth nerve mass or two of the following:

(a) Neurofibroma

(b) Meningioma

(c) Glioma

(d) Schwannoma

(e) Juvenile posterior subcapsular lenticular opacity

(3) All individuals at genetic risk for NF2 should be examined periodically for vestibular schwannoma by brain stem auditory evoked potentials or MRI. It is recommended that MRI be done even in the absence of signs or symptoms of vestibular schwannoma in adolescence and again after age 30 years.

4. Tuberous sclerosis

a. Etiology and pathophysiology: A disorder of the CNS with multiple tubers in the cerebral cortex and associated cutaneous symptoms. Incidence is 1 per 5800 live births. It is an autosomal dominant disorder.

b. Clinical features

(1) MR and seizures are common.

(2) Behavioral: Associated conditions include ADHD, autism, and aggression.

c. Diagnosis: Clinically diagnosed with two major features or with one major and two minor features (Box 21-3)

d. Management: Medical surveillance

(1) Genitourinary: Renal ultrasonography every 1 to 3 years

(2) Neurologic

(a) Cranial CT/MRI every 1 to 3 years

(b) Electroencephalogram for seizure management

(3) Echocardiography/chest CT with follow-up for cardiopulmonary symptoms

Box 21-3   Diagnosis of Tuberous Sclerosis

Major Features

Facial angiofibromas
Ungual or periungual fibromas
Hypomelanotic ("ash leaf") macules (three or more)
Shagreen patch
Multiple retinal hamartomas
Cortical tubers
Subependymal nodule or astrocytoma
Cardiac rhabdomyoma
Lymphangiomyomatosis
Renal angiomyolipoma

Minor Features

Multiple pits in dental enamel
Hamartomatous rectal polyps
Bone cysts
Cerebral white matter radial migration
Gingival fibromas
Nonrenal hamartoma
Retinal achromic spot
"Confetti" skin lesions
Multiple renal cysts

(4) Developmental and behavioral evaluations: at school entry and as needed
(5) Information resources: National Neurofibromatosis Foundation (www.nf.org), Tuberous Sclerosis Alliance (www.tsalliance.org)

21.8 Public Policy

1. The Education for All Handicapped Children Act (PL 94-142)
   a. PL 94-142 was enacted by Congress in 1975 and has been reauthorized four times. It is currently known as the Individuals with Disabilities Act (IDEA). Part B of the IDEA pertains to children with disabilities (3 to 21 years), whereas Part C cover services for infants and toddlers with disabilities (from birth until they turn 3 years of age).
   b. Children and youth with disabilities (Part B): Based on IDEA, children and youth with disabilities are provided with the following:
      (1) Free and appropriate education with emphasis on special education and all related services to meet each child's unique needs (3 to 21 years)
      (2) Placement in the "least restrictive environment" (e.g., children with disabilities are integrated with typical peers as much as possible)
      (3) An Individualized Education Plan (IEP)

(4) The right to be involved in decisions about their special education

(5) The right to have an impartial hearing if there is conflict over the special education services

(6) Transition plan from high school to adult living (planning should start at 14 years of age)

(7) Assistive technology devices and services needed to achieve potential

c. Infants and toddlers with disabilities (Part C): Part C of IDEA provides for a statewide program that offers identification and therapy services for children 0 to 2 years of age with developmental delays. Through early intervention, infants and toddlers with disabilities are provided with family-centered, culturally sensitive, individualized developmental services in their natural environments. This program also facilitates transition of these children into special education of the local school department, if necessary.

d. Basic special education process under IDEA

(1) Child Find: Each state conducts activities that would identify and evaluate all children with disabilities. A parent or a professional may ask to have the child evaluated for a possible disability.

(2) Evaluation: Child undergoes evaluation in all areas related to suspected disability. Qualified professionals and parents comprise a multidisciplinary team.

(3) Eligibility: Multidisciplinary team reviews evaluation results and determines if child is eligible for services.

(4) IEP: Once eligible, the child's educational goals and services required to achieve these goals are written in the IEP by the team of professionals and parents.

(5) The IEP then guides the delivery of special education services to the child.

(6) Monitoring: Progress reports are provided to parents on a regular basis.

(7) Review: The IEP is reviewed on a yearly basis or more often if parents and school personnel request it.

(8) Reevaluation: The child is reevaluated at least once every 3 years or more often at the request of parents or school personnel.

2. Section 504 of the Rehabilitation Act of 1973

a. Section 504 is a federal law designed to protect the rights of individuals with disabilities in programs and activities that receive federal funds from the U.S. Department of Education. This regulation requires a school district to provide free appropriate public education to students with disabilities in a manner that meets their individual needs. All individuals who are deemed disabled under IDEA are handicapped and thus are protected under Section 504, but not vice versa. Under IDEA, eligible students must have certain specified types of disabilities and must need special education because of their disability. Section 504, however, has a more generalized definition of disability.

b. Examples of potential Section 504 handicapping conditions *not* typically covered under IDEA are communicable diseases such as human immunodeficiency virus infection and tuberculosis, medical conditions such as asthma, temporary conditions due to illness or accident, ADHD, behavioral difficulties, and a history of drug/alcohol addiction. Section 504 does not require a written IEP, but does require a formal plan.

SUGGESTED READING

American Academy of Pediatrics: AAP Policy Statement on The Medical Home. Pediatrics 110:184-186, 2002. Also available at http://aappolicy.aappublications.org/cgi/content/full/pediatrics;110/1/184.

American Academy of Pediatrics, Section on Genetics: Health supervision for children with Down syndrome. Pediatrics 107:442-449, 2001.

American Association on Mental Retardation: Mental Retardation: Definition, Classification and Systems of Support, 10th ed. Washington, DC, AAMR Publications, 2002.

Batshaw ML, Perret YM (eds): Children with Disabilities. Baltimore, Brookes Publishing, 1997.

Capute AJ, Accardo PJ (eds): Developmental Disabilities in Infancy and Childhood, 2nd ed. Baltimore, Brookes Publishing, 1996.

Friedman JM: Neurofibromatosis 1. GeneReviews, updated January 7, 2007. Available at www.ncbi.nlm.nih.gov/books/bv.fcgi?rid=gene.chapter.nf1.

Johnson CP: Early clinical characteristics of children with autism spectrum disorder. In Gupta V (ed): Autism Spectrum Disorders in Children. New York, Marcel Dekker, 2004, pp 85-125.

Korf BR, Darras BT, Urion DK: Dystrophinopathies. GeneReviews, updated August 25, 2005. Available at www.ncbi.nlm.nih.gov/books/bv.fcgi?indexed=google&rid=gene.chapter.dbmd.

Menkes JH, Sarnat HB (eds): Child Neurology, 6th ed. Philadelphia, Lippincott Williams & Wilkins, 2000.

Northrup H, Au K-S: Tuberous sclerosis complex. GeneReviews, updated December 5, 2005. Available at www.ncbi.nlm.nih.gov/books/bv.fcgi?indexed=google&rid=gene.chapter.tuberous-sclerosis.

U.S. Department of Education: Policy Article: History of IDEA. U.S. Department of Education, March 2003. Available at www.ed.gov.

U.S. Department of Education: Policy Guidance: The Civil Rights of Students with Hidden Disabilities under Section 504 of the Rehabilitation Act of 1973. U.S. Department of Education, Office for Civil Rights, December 2000. Available at www.ed.gov.

Behavioral and Psychiatric Disorders of Childhood

22

Andrea R. Carlsen, Jonathan D. Birnkrant,
Judith A. Owens, Randy Rockney,
Natalia Golova, Horacio B. Hojman,
and Barry M. Lester

22.1 The Psychiatric Interview of the Infant, Child, and Adolescent

1. Goals
   a. Understand a child's behavior, thoughts and feelings in relation to past and present stressors in the home, school, and interpersonal setting. Gather psychiatric history, both individual and family. Assess strengths in the individual, family, academic, and interpersonal realm.
   b. Define psychopathology, if present, in a child and family. Treat a child based on that psychopathology using medical as well as behavioral and psychosocial interventions.
2. Clinical interview
   a. History of the problem: Onset, type, and severity of symptoms and associated symptoms, especially across different settings (school, home). Important: Probe for stressors (life events, separations and losses) in the child's life now and in the past.
   b. Psychiatric history: Previous diagnosis and comorbid conditions, therapist and medications, previous admissions for psychiatric reasons, previous suicide attempts, substance abuse (including alcohol, cigarettes, or recreational drugs), history of abuse (physical, sexual, emotional/psychological)
   c. Developmental history: Pregnancy and birth, major milestones, and results of previous developmental evaluations
   d. Social history: Who does the child live with? Family constellation, educational level of parents and siblings, marital history, history of domestic violence and sexual or physical abuse, recent or ongoing stressors in the home, and family response to the child's symptoms/behavior/academic problems. Assess the psychiatric state of each parent, their marriage, and significant family relationships. Assess relationship with family members and peers (e.g., best friends, social habits, sports, hobbies).

660

e. School history: Previous and current academic standing as well as behavioral difficulties, current educational program and setting (classroom size and child's placement in the classroom, e.g., self-contained?), special education services/resource help, Individualized Education Plan (IEP), recent report card results, academic strengths and weaknesses, homework management, peer relationships in school setting

f. Medical history: Significant/chronic illnesses, lead poisoning, significant head trauma, allergies, and medications

g. Family history: Attention deficit hyperactivity disorder (ADHD), academic problems/learning disabilities (LDs), mood/anxiety disorders, thought disorders, substance/alcohol abuse, and thyroid disease

h. Physical examination: Growth parameters, baseline vital signs, and brief neurologic examination.

i. Child interview: Observation of symptoms in the office setting (although their presence in that setting is not necessary to make the diagnosis), oppositional/defiant behavior, general cognitive and language level, child's understanding of behavioral concerns, and parent–child interactions

j. Biologic functions: Appetite, bladder and bowel control, growth, menstruation. Sleep history: Sleep onset difficulties, night waking, quality and duration of sleep (restlessness), early awakening, symptoms of obstructive sleep apnea (disruptive snoring, gasping), enuresis

k. Assessment for LDs: Review any previous educational/achievement test results and neuropsychological (e.g., intelligence quotient [IQ], language, cognitive, processing abilities) evaluation results. Any child in whom learning problems are suspected should have a neuropsychological assessment done by the school or a qualified neuropsychologist.

3. Mental status examination
   a. When performing a mental status examination in a child, always consider his or her age and developmental level.
   b. Physical appearance
      (1) Stature (age appropriateness, precocity) and head circumference
      (2) Dysmorphic features (e.g., Down syndrome, fragile X, fetal alcohol syndrome)
      (3) Focal neurologic signs
      (4) Tics, biting of lips, hair pulling (e.g., Tourette's syndrome, anxiety)
      (5) Momentary lapses of attention, staring, head nodding, eye blinking (e.g., epilepsy, hallucinations)
      (6) Dress, cleanliness, hygiene (e.g., level of caring)
      (7) Mannerisms (e.g., tics, thumb sucking, nail biting)
   c. Separation
      (1) Easy separation may denote superficial relationships.
      (2) Excessive difficulty in separation may denote ambivalent parent–child relationships.
   d. Orientation (may be impaired by organic factors, intelligence, anxiety, or a thought disorder)

(1) To person: Verbal children should know their names.
(2) To place: Young children will know whether they are at home.
(3) To time: A complete sense of time is formed by 8 or 9 years of age. Young children can tell whether it is day or night.
e. Central nervous system (CNS) function: soft signs (neurodevelopmental immaturities that persist) include
(1) Gross motor coordination
(2) Fine motor coordination: Child is asked to copy the following geometric designs—circle at 2 to 3 years of age, cross at 3 to 4 years, square at 5 years, rhomboid at 7 years.
(3) Laterality (right and left discrimination identified by 5 years of age)
(4) Rapid alternating movements (heel-to-toe walking, hopping on one foot by 7 years of age)
(5) Attention span (e.g., distractibility, hyperactivity in ADHD)
f. Reading or writing difficulties (e.g., dyslexia)
g. Speech and language difficulties (e.g., autism, mental retardation [MR], organic syndromes, deprivation, drug intoxication, and regression)
h. Intelligence (vocabulary, level of comprehension, ability to identify body parts by 5 years of age, drawing ability, mathematical ability)
i. Memory: Child can count five digits forward and two backward; poor performance may indicate poor attention span, brain damage, or MR.
j. Thought process
(1) Are thoughts logical and coherent?
(2) Is there any evidence of disorders of perception such as hallucinations?
(3) Is there any evidence of suicidal ideation, homicidal ideation, phobias, obsessions, delusions?
k. Fantasies and inferred conflicts (evaluated through dreams, naming three wishes, drawing, spontaneous play)
l. Affect: Anxiety, anger, depression, apathy—their level, intensity, range, appropriateness, and control
m. Defense organization (e.g., denial, projection, introversion, extroversion)
n. Judgment and insight (what the child believes caused the problem, how upset the child appears to be about the problem, and how the clinician can help)
o. Adaptive capacities (problem-solving capacities, resiliency)
4. Diagnosis
a. Assess categories of psychopathology. Ask the following questions:
(1) What degree of organic dysfunction is present, and to what extent does it affect perception, coordination, attention, learning, emotions, and impulse control?
(2) Is there any evidence of a thought disorder? Is there any evidence of depression, anxiety, or behavioral symptoms (e.g., phobias, obsessive-compulsive behaviors)?
(3) Is the child reacting to an unfavorable environment (e.g., family, school, community, society)?
b. Determine the patient's developmental level (cognitive, affective, interpersonal, moral, etc.).

c. Assess predisposing or causative factors.
  (1) Genetic (e.g., dyslexia, ADHD, MR, autism, schizophrenia)
  (2) Organic (e.g., malnutrition, intrauterine drug exposure, prematurity, head injury, CNS infections/tumors, metabolic conditions, toxins)
  (3) Developmental immaturity and attachment
  (4) Temperament of the child: "Difficult" and "slow-to-warm-up" temperaments are at risk for emotional and behavioral problems, whereas "easy" children are relatively protected from these problems.
  (5) Inadequate parenting (parental deprivation, separation, loss, abusive parents, psychiatric disorders in parents)
  (6) Stress factors (illness, injury, surgery, hospitalizations, school failure, poverty, racial discrimination)

22.2 Excessive Crying and Colic

1. Normal development
   a. Crying in normal infants increases during the first few weeks of life
   b. By 6 weeks, about 25% of infants normally cry more than 2.75 hours per day.
2. Definition of excessive crying
   a. Excessive crying occurs in 20% to 25% of infants and affects over 700,000 infants in the United States each year.
   b. Excessive crying is defined using the "rule of 3":
     (1) Crying for more than 3 hours a day
     (2) For at least 3 days a week
     (3) For 3 consecutive weeks in otherwise healthy infants during the first 3 to 4 months of life
   c. The amount of daily crying in these infants is above the 75th percentile of the distribution of crying in normal, healthy infants.
3. Colic
   a. Infants with colic are a subset of infants with excessive crying (one third to one half of infants with excessive crying have colic).
   b. Infants with colic meet the "rule of 3" criteria for excessive crying but also show an additional set of characteristics.
     (1) Episodic/paroxysmal crying
       (a) Rapid and abrupt onset
       (b) Little buildup but more of an "on/off" quality
       (c) Unpredictable extreme reaction with no warning and may have the quality of an attack, spell, or "fit"
       (d) Well-demarcated start and stop time, with the infant often described as frantic, out of control, or in pain
     (2) Cry quality (qualitative change in the sound of the cry during the colic episode)
       (a) Can be high-pitched, loud, painlike cry with a piercing, screeching, and annoying quality—more like a scream than a cry
       (b) Periods of elongated cry bursts followed by long periods of inspiration

      (3) Physical signs
         (a) Often associated with *hypertonia* (stomach tightened or hard, clenched fists or hands, legs and knees drawn up, breath holding, arched back, red face, cold feet, pale around the mouth)
         (b) Usually occurs in clusters
         (c) The number of characteristics, not the specific characteristic, is most important.
         (d) Inconsolability: Infant is difficult if not impossible to quiet, and often the episode needs to run its own course. Some infants are responsive to calming techniques; others actively resist being soothed and appear even more frantic when attempts are made to quiet them.

  c. Etiology of colic
      (1) Exact causes of colic are unknown.
      (2) *Biologic factors* are probably responsible: The infant's temperament coupled with a lower threshold of reactivity secondary to autonomic imbalance, hypertonia secondary to gastrointestinal contraction (gas), and immaturity of the gastrointestinal tract.
      (3) *Parenting factors* are associated with colic but are not the cause of colic. These may include maternal anxiety, depression, inappropriate handling, poor mother–infant interaction, breast-feeding, and overfeeding or underfeeding.
      (4) Parental characteristics will determine how parents behave toward their crying infant, which will in turn affect the infant's behavior. Colic is a violation of expectations that the parents have for their infant and can lead to difficulty in the parent–infant relationship. Thus, what begins as a biologically based condition may be mediated and perpetuated by social and emotional factors in the parents.

4. Management of colic and excessive crying
  a. Rule out other medical conditions, such as a cow's milk allergy to protein, in which it is best to change to a protein hydrolysate or soy-based formula.
  b. Pharmacologic treatments (chloral hydrate, phenobarbital, simethicone, homeopathic medicines) are not indicated because they are ineffective or may have adverse effects.
  c. Mechanical aids, such as swings, music, and vibration, may produce a brief reduction in crying in some infants but may not be effective in some cases of colic.
  d. The psychosocial intervention approach is to view colic as a perturbation or short-term disruption in the parent–child relationship that will resolve through a combination of successful management of the infant's behavior and the parent's ability to cope. This approach involves parent counseling to differentiate infant-based issues from parent-based issues. Counseling also focuses on helping parents manage the infant, describe their feelings as caregivers, and identify issues within the larger family system that may be affecting their ability to cope.

e. Suggestions
   (1) Get a thorough history of the infant's crying and other behavior, including formula changes and sleep patterns, by having the mother complete questionnaires and diaries.
   (2) Use this information to determine whether the infant has a milk allergy, the infant has excessive crying rather than colic, and there are associated behavior problems such as a sleep disturbance.
   (3) Acknowledge that colic can also affect the parents' relationship with the infant and emphasize how difficult and stressful colic can be for parents. Referral may be needed.

22.3 Sleep Disorders

NORMAL SLEEP: DEVELOPMENTAL CONSIDERATIONS

1. Infancy (0 to 1 year)
   a. Neonates spend approximately 70% of every 24 hours asleep (16 to 20 hours/day). Neonatal sleep periods last 3 to 4 hours, followed by 1 to 2 hours awake.
   b. At about 3 to 6 months, most infants start to "settle" (sleep through the night). During the first 6 months, total rapid eye movement (REM) sleep volume markedly decreases. By 6 to 8 months, sleep periods may last 6 hours, and the total sleep time decreases to an average of 13 to 14 hours.
   c. By 1 year, 60% to 70% of infants self-soothe.
2. Early childhood (2 to 5 years)
   a. By 3 to 5 years, sleep periods are gradually consolidated into a single 10-hour nocturnal period. Daytime nap periods decrease.
   b. Average sleep onset latency is 15 minutes in younger children (3 to 4 years of age) and 15 to 30 minutes for older children (5 to 6 years of age).
   c. Night wakings remain problematic in up to one third of preschoolers.
   d. Sleep becomes more dependent on environmental cues and family expectations and bedtime routines.
3. Middle childhood (6 to 12 years)
   a. Average sleep duration is 9 to 11 hours. The sleep pattern becomes more stable, with night-to-night consistency.
   b. The level of daytime sleepiness is low. Naps are rare.
4. Adolescence
   a. By mid-adolescence, total sleep time decreases to 8.5 hours.
   b. Sleep duration varies during school and nonschool nights. "Catch-up" sleep occurs on weekends secondary to relative sleep deprivation.
   c. Adolescents do not have less need for sleep as they mature. The increased need for sleep often leads to cumulative sleep deprivation that can produce lower daytime alertness and greater daytime sleepiness.

SLEEP PROBLEMS

1. Dyssomnias (insomnias, hypersomnias, and circadian rhythm sleep disorders)

a. Definition: Disorders of initiating and maintaining sleep (DIMS) in which there is difficulty in or resistance to falling asleep or frequent and disruptive night wakenings

b. Sleep onset association disorder
   (1) Clinical presentation
      (a) The child is unable to self-soothe and requires certain associations (e.g., parental presence, pacifier) to complete sleep transition, fall asleep at bedtime, and fall back asleep during night wakenings.
      (b) It is most common between 6 months and 3 years of age.
   (2) Management
      (a) Consistency: Parents develop and maintain consistent and persistent responses. Parents should briefly reassure child that everything is OK and that they are there for the child.
      (b) Parents may use the *cry it out* approach, allowing the child to cry until he or she falls asleep. Alternatively, parents may gradually increase the time intervals of the response to the night wakenings (*cry-wait-respond*).
      (c) Often the child's crying and protesting intensifies briefly once the treatment plan is started. Treatment is easier to accomplish *before* the child is developmentally able to climb out of the crib. Improvement is generally seen within 1 week if parents are consistent.

c. Limit-setting sleep disorder: The parents are unable to set consistent bedtime rules, which leads to prolonged bedtime struggles and refusal behavior (protests, requests, excuses).
   (1) Clinical presentation: Prolonged sleep onset latency (i.e., child cannot fall asleep). Night wakening is usually not problematic. It is most common in 2- to 6-year-olds.
   (2) Management: Provide education and support of parents regarding developmentally appropriate limit setting, including using a gate at the bedroom door, using sticker/star charts to reinforce appropriate bedtime behavior, temporarily establishing a later bedtime to increase the likelihood of sleep readiness, exploring the role of marital discord, and determining environmental constraints.

d. Stress- or anxiety-related DIMS
   (1) Types
      (a) Adjustment sleep disorder: Acute onset of difficulty in initiating/maintaining sleep, usually following a stressful life event
      (b) Nighttime fears: These include separation fears that often develop at 2 to 3 years of age, and are developmentally appropriate.
   (2) Management: Parental support and reassurance (including parental presence at bedtime), positive reinforcement (sticker/star chart), progressive relaxation at bedtime, avoidance of frightening stimuli (TV shows, stories), pet fish tank, transitional objects, and night lights

e. DIMS can also be related to medical conditions (e.g., colic, otitis media, medication effects).

2. Disorders of excessive somnolence include inappropriate daytime sleepiness (excessive daytime sleepiness), total daily sleep in excess of developmentally appropriate levels (hypersomnolence), and excessive napping.

   a. Etiologies
      (1) Obstructive sleep apnea
      (2) Narcolepsy
      (3) Medications/drugs/toxins (lead)
      (4) CNS lesions (tumors)
      (5) Depression

   b. Clinical presentation: Daytime symptoms of decreased alertness with motor restlessness, inattention, distractibility, impulsivity/aggressiveness, day-dreaming

3. Parasomnias: A group of disorders occurring during sleep or sleep–wake transition state characterized by fairly dramatic symptoms, including confusion and disorientation of the child, as well as treatment resistance

   a. Somnambulism (sleepwalking)
      (1) Epidemiology: Incidence—overall, 1% to 15% of the population; equal male and female occurrence, with age at onset between 4 and 6 years; duration 5 years for 33%, 10 years for 12%
      (2) Clinical characteristics: Some children remain quiet, others agitated; automatic behaviors may be present.

   b. Confusional arousals
      (1) Epidemiology: Incidence—3% to 5% (brought to medical attention); equal male and female occurrence; age of onset—most common during first 3 years, usually before age 7; duration 6 months to 13 years
      (2) Clinical characteristics: Agitation, crying/moaning verbalizations; some automatic arousal; some displacement from bed; may develop quiet sleepwalking as adolescent

   c. Pavor nocturnus (sleep/night terrors)
      (1) Epidemiology: Incidence—1% to 3%, 10% of sleepwalkers; greater male than female occurrence; age at onset—4 to 12 years, peaks at 5 to 7 years; frequency—often highest at onset, often higher (greater than once a week) in younger onset; duration—usually disappears within 1 to 4 years, longer with positive family history; continuation into adolescence for 30%
      (2) Clinical characteristics: Occurs during first third of night; dramatic, sudden onset with scream; duration of 1 to 10 minutes; extreme autonomic arousal—tachycardia, tachypnea, diaphoresis, dilated pupil; child seems "out of control" and "out of it," usually does not remember event; may have displacement from bed; can be triggered by auditory stimuli during slow-wave sleep

   d. Nightmares (dream anxiety attacks)
      (1) Clinical characteristics: extremely common; occur during last third of night (with increased percentage of REM sleep); usually some to good recall for content; fully awake afterward; little motor behavior during dream; may be exacerbated by stress, anxiety, and medications that increase REM

PREVENTION OF SLEEP PROBLEMS: GENERAL PRINCIPLES

1. Prevention in infants (>4 months)
   a. Put the infant to bed drowsy but awake.
   b. Avoid rocking to sleep; avoid putting to bed with a bottle
   c. Make night waking contacts reassuring but brief and boring, 5 to 15 minutes.
   d. Avoid removing the infant from the crib or bringing the infant into the parents' bed in response to night waking.
   e. Establish transitional objects (e.g., mother's T-shirt).
   f. Avoid keeping the crib in the parents' room, or cover the side rails of the crib with a blanket.
   g. Eliminate long (>2 hours) daytime naps.
   h. Avoid changing diapers during the night.
   i. Discontinue middle-of-night feeding after 4 months.
2. Prevention in children (2 to 5 years)
   a. Establish a consistent bedtime and a regular bedtime routine or calm-down time.
   b. Allow child to self-soothe; encourage the use of transitional objects.
   c. Avoid reinforcing bedtime procrastination (e.g., offering extra drinks, food).
   d. Use positive reinforcement (sticker, stars) for staying in bed.
   e. Return child to bed gently but firmly if he or she is up after bedtime.
   f. Avoid using the bedroom for time-out.
3. Older children and adolescents: Development of good sleep hygiene
   a. Keep regular bed and wake-up times, with bedtime routine (e.g., quiet time before bed).
   b. Avoid daytime naps and activities in bed (e.g., watching TV and reading).
   c. Avoid caffeine and cigarettes.
   d. Get out of bed if having difficulty falling asleep.
   e. Avoid heavy meals late at night.
   f. Encourage physical exercise, but not just before bedtime.

22.4 Disorders Related to Incontinence

ENURESIS

1. Definitions
   a. *Enuresis:* Involuntary voiding of urine beyond the age at which control of voiding is normally attained, usually age 4 to 6 years or school age; most often presents as bed-wetting (nocturnal enuresis)
   b. *Primary enuresis:* Wetting by children who never had control
   c. *Secondary enuresis:* Wetting by children preceded by consistent period of dryness, 6 months to 1 year (20% to 25% of cases)
   d. *Diurnal enuresis:* Daytime wetting while awake (15% to 20% of cases; more common in girls)
2. Normal development of bladder control

a. Infancy: Void by reflex; bladder filling triggers bladder contraction (spinal reflex arc).

b. 1 to 2 years: Conscious sensation of bladder fullness

c. 2 to 3 years: Ability to void or inhibit voiding voluntarily

d. 4 years: Adult pattern of urinary control

3. Epidemiology

a. Incidence: Enuresis is seen in 10% to 20% of 5-year-olds, 5% of 10-year-olds, and 1% of 18- to 20-year olds.

b. The male-to-female ratio is about 3:2.

c. Spontaneous resolution occurs in about 15% per year after 5 years of age.

4. Etiology: This symptom has multiple etiologies, alone or in combination.

a. Genetic: Fifteen percent incidence in nonenuretic families; 44% and 77% of children are enuretic when one or both parents, respectively, are enuretic.

b. Sleep: Most parents ascribe etiology to the child being an extremely sound sleeper, which is an unproven theory.

c. Psychiatric morbidity: Enuretic children are little different emotionally and behaviorally from nonenuretic children, although their self-esteem may suffer as a result of enuresis. On the other hand, psychiatric issues can be associated with enuresis, especially trauma.

d. Urodynamic findings: Diminished functional bladder capacity and uninhibited bladder contractions are more common in enuretic patients and may be related to genetic/developmental aspects of the symptom.

e. Delayed attainment of central control of bladder function

f. Anatomic disorder of the urinary tract is unusual in the absence of persistent daytime incontinence, history of urinary tract infections (UTIs), abnormal voiding pattern, or family history of inherited anatomic abnormalities.

g. Constipation/encopresis may contribute through crowding of urinary tract structures.

h. Abnormal diurnal/nocturnal variation in antidiuretic hormone levels

i. Miscellaneous: Upper airway obstruction, sickle cell disease, diabetes insipidus and mellitus

5. Diagnosis

a. A baseline record of enuresis frequency can be helpful

b. History: To determine the extent of evaluation necessary and to initiate supportive aspects of therapy

(1) History of constipation or soiling (should be addressed first)

(2) Past medical history: Sickle cell anemia, diabetes mellitus, neurologic impairment, symptoms of upper airway obstruction (sleep apnea, snoring)

(3) Primary versus secondary

(4) Wetting incidence (at night only, day only, both day and night)

(5) Wetting frequency

(6) Changes or no changes in symptom over time

(7) Previous UTI or other symptoms such as urinary hesitancy that indicate a need to perform a more extensive work-up

        (8) Possible sexual abuse

        (9) Family history of enuresis

      (10) Parents' and child's attitude toward symptom

      (11) Previous efforts to treat: For example, fluid restrictions or previous medical evaluations and treatments (e.g., medication or alarm trials—age and duration of trial are important)

  c. Physical examination

      (1) Height, weight, growth percentiles, blood pressure

      (2) Mental status examination: Motivation to work toward cure, level of intellectual functioning, any comorbid psychopathology

      (3) Abdominal examination: Distended bladder or colon (result of fecal retention)

      (4) Genital examination: Urethral position and size, scarring or redness of vulva

      (5) Rectal examination: Anal sensation, sphincter tone, fecal impaction

      (6) Back: Scoliosis, dimple, or hairy patch

      (7) Neurologic examination: Peripheral reflexes, gait

  d. Laboratory evaluation

      (1) Urinalysis: Specific gravity above 1.020 rules out concentrating deficit and diabetes insipidus; check for glucosuria, white blood cells, protein, bacteria.

      (2) Urine for culture and sensitivity, especially in girls

  e. Radiologic work-up: Renal ultrasonography and voiding cystourethrogram if the patient has a history of previous UTIs or obstructive signs or symptoms

6. Management

  a. Basic principles: Determine whether treatment is actually necessary (rarely treat those younger than 5 years of age), and whether the child is motivated to work toward a cure (usually a function of age).

  b. Supportive measures (used alone or in conjunction with other modalities)

      (1) Educate the patient and family that

         (a) The symptom of bedwetting is not under conscious control.

         (b) Punishment is not helpful.

         (c) Bedwetting is very common (i.e., the child is not alone).

         (d) Children often get better on their own.

      (2) Suggest that the parents should

         (a) Engage the child in working toward a cure.

         (b) Offer praise for success, encouragement for lack of success.

         (c) Encourage responsibility for symptom (changing bed, putting bedclothes into the washing machine).

         (d) Encourage record keeping (calendar/stickers or star chart).

  c. Behavior modification approaches

      (1) Positive reinforcement therapy: Star chart alone or in combination with agreed-on rewards for attainment of goals (25% cure, 75% improved); requires longer treatment than medications but possibly has a lower relapse rate

(2) Bedwetting alarm: Conditioning therapy
   (a) Best overall success rate with lowest rate of relapse (65% to 100% cure after 4 to 6 months, 30% relapse)
   (b) The family and child must be extremely motivated and compliant because a long course of treatment (several weeks to months) is necessary for a positive outcome.
   (c) Poor choice if other siblings are in the room or the child is frightened by the alarm

d. Pharmacotherapy
   (1) Imipramine (tricyclic antidepressant [TCA])
      (a) Fifty percent have a positive response; 60% have a relapse when treatment is discontinued.
      (b) The dosage range is 0.9 to 1.5 mg/kg/dose given once at bedtime (25 mg every bedtime for children 5 to 8 years; 50 to 75 mg every bedtime for older children).
      (c) This approach works immediately and is helpful for sleepovers.
      (d) If successful, continue for 3 to 6 months, then taper.
      (e) Side effects: Anxiety, insomnia, dry mouth
      (f) Warn the family about overdose (cardiac toxicity); especially at risk are younger siblings and suicidal youth.
      (g) Initial success is 50%; long-term cure is 25% after discontinuation.
   (2) Desmopressin acetate (DDAVP)
      (a) Similar to vasopressin (antidiuretic hormone) in that it reduces urine output after dose is administered.
      (b) Available as a nasal spray (10 µg DDAVP per spray) or oral tablet 0.2 mg/tablet
      (c) Initial dose: 20 µg (one spray in each nostril) or 0.2 mg at bedtime
      (d) Increase to maximum dose of 40 µg (two sprays each nostril) or 0.6 mg
      (e) Up to 75% success rate; high relapse rate
      (f) Rare side effect of water intoxication
      (g) Relatively expensive
   (3) Oxybutynin (Ditropan)
      (a) Anticholinergic; acts by reducing uninhibited bladder contractions
      (b) Rarely beneficial for nocturnal enuresis
      (c) May help if patient has diurnal enuresis with frequency and urgency
      (d) Dose (>6 years of age): 5 mg two to three times a day
      (e) Side effects: Dry mouth, facial flushing

e. Complicated enuresis
   (1) Uninhibited contractions: Anticholinergics (oxybutynin, hyoscyamine [Levsin])
   (2) Infrequent voiders ("lazy" bladder): Timed voiding
   (3) Associated constipation/encopresis: Bowel regimen (enemas, fiber, etc.)

ENCOPRESIS

1. Definition (based on the *Diagnostic and Statistical Manual of Mental Disorders*, 4th edition, text revision [DSM-IV-TR]) and classification
   a. Repeated passage of feces into inappropriate places (e.g., clothing or floor), whether involuntary or intentional
   b. At least one such event a month for at least 3 months
   c. Chronologic age is at least 4 years (or equivalent developmental level).
   d. The behavior is not due exclusively to the direct physiologic effects of a substance (e.g., laxatives) or a general medical condition except through a mechanism involving constipation.
   e. Classification
      (1) Primary: Always a problem; possible organic cause
      (2) Secondary: Fecal continence for 6 months to 1 year before onset of encopresis
2. Prevalence
   a. Among 7- to 8-year old children, 2% for boys and 1% for girls; among 10- to 12-year-olds, 1% and 0.3%, respectively. Many researchers and clinicians believe that the problem is significantly underreported.
   b. Accounts for 3% of visits to a general pediatric outpatient clinic
   c. Male-to-female ratio is 3:1 to as great as 6:1.
3. Etiology
   a. Most often multifactorial; differs from child to child
   b. Critical stages in the potentiation of encopresis from infancy to early school years
      (1) Infancy: Constipation, congenital anorectal problems
      (2) Toddlerhood: Chaotic toilet training, hard or painful stools
      (3) School years: ADHD, school bathroom avoidance
   c. Fecal retention and consequent loss of sensation of rectal distention and overflow incontinence is the usual final common pathway.
   d. Sexual abuse is rarely of etiologic significance.
   e. Psychopathology is seldom related.
4. Diagnosis
   a. Identify common but not invariable historical points (large-caliber stools, hiding soiled underwear, soiling in late afternoon or early evening).
   b. Determine whether the child perceives an urge to defecate or is not bothered by the smell (sources of confusion).
   c. Assess stool withholding behaviors (source of confusion).
   d. Abdominal distention and lower left quadrant sausage-shaped mass are variable.
   e. A rectum full of stool or obvious soiling is common.
   f. Check anal tone, sensation, and position (anterior displacement).
   g. Laboratory tests are not routine, but consider thyroid studies and erythrocyte sedimentation rate.
   h. Order a plain abdominal radiograph to diagnose retention if the rectal examination is negative or contraindicated; may also be used as a teaching/demystification tool.
   i. Rectal manometry can be used in conjunction with biofeedback.

      j. A barium enema or rectal mucosal biopsy is required if Hirschsprung's disease is suspected.

      k. Psychological or psychiatric consultation may be useful when a psychiatric condition comorbid with encopresis is known or suspected.

5. Management

    a. There is no universal agreement on the best approach to management of encopresis.

    b. Most interventions combine education and demystification, bowel catharsis, and behavior modification.

    c. Approaches to bowel catharsis

      (1) Four consecutive 3-day cycles of treatment, each cycle consisting of an enema (day 1), a suppository (day 2), and a laxative tablet (day 3)

      (2) Daily enemas for 3 to 7 days, depending on the output of feces

      (3) High dose of mineral oil, up to 1 ounce per year of age twice a day (compliance can be problematic)

      (4) Balanced electrolyte solution (GoLYTELY); requires high volumes

    d. Components of behavior modification/maintenance therapy

      (1) Goals statement: No soiling, regular (every 1 to 2 days) or hyper-regular (one to two times per day) bowel movements

      (2) Stool softeners/laxatives alone or in combination: MiraLax, mineral oil, Agoral, lactulose, Senokot, milk of magnesia for 4 to 6 months or longer

      (3) Stool softener should be titrated to produce desired effect, at least one or two soft bowel movements per day; for example, begin with MiraLax 17 g (one capful) twice a day, increase or decrease dose as needed.

      (4) Toileting habit changes: Increased time on toilet to relax and complete defecation; regular toileting time; feet planted firmly on floor

      (5) Lots of fluids, especially water or juices that promote regularity

      (6) Increased exercise

      (7) High-fiber diet (25 to 35 g/day of fiber)

      (8) The parents and clinician may individualize the specific regimen for each child.

6. Prognosis: Generally good, with 63% to 94% improvement; tends to improve with time, although some patients do not improve for many years

    a. High-risk groups are those who are poorly compliant and have the nonretentive type.

    b. For those who do not succeed, parents must be persistent and should consider group therapy (peer and parent support) and biofeedback (helps short-term but not long-term).

7. Comorbid association with enuresis

    a. Eighteen to 20% of enuretic patients have encopresis.

    b. Thirty to 40% of encopretic patients have enuresis.

    c. Treat encopresis first because it is more bothersome and more curable; it may ameliorate enuresis.

22.5 Stuttering

1. Definition, etiology, and pathophysiology
   a. Stuttering is an involuntary repetition, prolongation, hesitance, or blockage in the production of a speech sound.
   b. Both motor and sensory etiologies for stuttering exist.
2. Epidemiology
   a. Five percent of all children stutter for several months or more at some point in their lives.
   b. Stuttering runs in families and is most prevalent among preschoolers.
   c. The prevalence of stuttering is 1% in children, with a male-to-female ratio of 3:1. The incidence is 7/1000 children.
   d. Most children who stutter start doing so before the age of 5 years.
   e. Children who stutter have no higher incidence of psychological problems, anxiety disorders, history of emotional trauma, or abnormal child-rearing practices than those who do not.
3. Clinical features
   a. Children who stutter have problems getting words started and have disruption in speech usually occurring at the beginning of a sentence.
   b. Parts of words (sound or syllables) are repeated rather than entire words or phrases.
   c. Stuttering begins gradually during a period of rapid language acquisition, usually once the child is speaking in short, meaningful phrases.
   d. If a speech-motor or sensory deficit is present, the speech difficulties are in excess of those usually associated with these problems.
4. Management
   a. Parents and home
      (1) Try to provide a calmer, less hurried lifestyle in the home.
      (2) Speak less hurriedly when talking to the child.
      (3) Allow the child to finish his or her thoughts without interrupting, filling, or speaking for the child.
      (4) Pause a second or so before responding, using some of the same words.
      (5) Do not expect the child to talk rapidly, precisely, and maturely at all times.
      (6) Do not force the child to give speeches, perform in plays, or read aloud to visiting friends, relatives, and neighbors.
   b. Referral: A child who stutters should be referred for evaluation and treatment to a speech therapist when the following conditions apply:
      (1) The stuttering has been present for more than 6 months and is becoming constant from day to day and more consistent from one situation to the next.
      (2) Tension (in the face or chest) is noticeable accompanying the stuttering.
      (3) Distress, fear of talking, or avoidance of speech is evident.
5. Prognosis: Stuttering resolves in as much as 80% of all children, with at least 50% stopping stuttering within a year. Persistent, consistent stuttering is unlikely to disappear without therapy.

22.6 Attention Deficit Hyperactivity Disorder

1. Etiology and risk factors
   a. Recent studies support a neurobiologic basis for this disorder. Multiple neurotransmitters are most likely involved, including dopamine, norepinephrine, and serotonin. Recent theories of the pathophysiology of ADHD have focused on dysfunction in the prefrontal cortex, which is involved in many executive functions. These functions (e.g., impulse control, planning, organization) are often impaired in people with ADHD.
   b. Biologic risk factors
      (1) Prenatal or perinatal: Prenatal alcohol or substance abuse, prematurity, birth asphyxia, and birth complications
      (2) Genetic syndromes: Increased incidence in fragile X syndrome, developmental delay, and MR
      (3) Postnatal: Significant head trauma, CNS infections, and neurotoxins (lead exposure)
      (4) Other medical conditions with secondary ADHD-like symptoms: Hyperthyroidism, medications (e.g., theophylline, phenobarbital), obstructive sleep apnea
   c. Psychosocial risk factors: Lower socioeconomic class, lack of parental education, maternal depression or mental illness, marital discord and domestic violence, and sexual and physical abuse
2. Epidemiology
   a. Estimated 3% to 5% of school-age children in the United States
   b. Much more common in boys (male-to-female ratio of 3:1 to 10:1), especially the hyperactive/impulsive subtype
   c. Positive family history in 30% to 50% of children with ADHD
   d. Comorbid conditions include oppositional defiant disorder, conduct disorder, generalized anxiety disorder, and major depressive disorder (MDD).
3. Clinical features
   a. The chronicity, persistence, pervasiveness, and developmental inappropriateness of symptoms help distinguish the child with ADHD from the behaviorally disordered child.
   b. Onset of symptoms usually occurs before 7 years of age; more severely affected children may be recognized in preschool.
   c. Symptoms frequently persist into adolescence and adulthood.
   d. Major features
      (1) Inattention: Difficulty in focusing, sustaining, and redirecting attention
      (2) Distractibility: Inability to screen out internal and external stimuli; difficulty in focusing on tasks
      (3) Impulsivity: "Acting without thinking"; can be verbal or physical; often results in a multitude of secondary behavioral concerns, such as aggressiveness with peers and disruptiveness in the classroom setting
      (4) Hyperactivity: Restlessness, fidgetiness, inability to sit still, excessive talking; more prominent in younger children
   e. ADHD in adolescence

    (1) Disorganized approach with variability in academic performance
    (2) Mental fatigue (often interpreted as "laziness" or "boredom")
    (3) Associated processing and memory problems
    (4) Inattention to detail
    (5) Difficulty in distinguishing between salient and irrelevant material ("the forest for the trees" phenomenon)
    (6) Behavioral impulsivity/risk-taking behaviors

4. Diagnosis
  a. Diagnostic categories
    (1) ADHD, hyperactive/impulsive type
    (2) ADHD, inattentive type
    (3) ADHD, combined type
  b. Evaluation: Consider the following issues in your interview, which are either directly related to the diagnosis of ADHD or to diagnoses you would not want to miss, but also present with symptoms similar to ADHD.
    (1) History of the problem: Onset, type, and severity of ADHD symptoms, behavior across different settings (school, home), current and previous attempts at behavioral management, and description of the child's typical behavior in situations that are likely to be problematic (mealtimes, chores, bedtime)
    (2) Developmental history: Major milestones, but especially results of previous developmental evaluations
    (3) School history: Previous and current academic and behavioral difficulties, history of grade retention, current educational program and setting (classroom size and child's placement in the classroom), special education services/resource help, IEP, recent report card results, academic strengths and weaknesses, homework management, peer relationships
    (4) Medical history: Lead poisoning, significant head trauma
    (5) Sleep history: Difficulty sleeping can lead to symptoms similar to ADHD, especially inattentive type.
    (6) Family history: ADHD, academic problems/LDs, mood/anxiety disorders, substance/alcohol abuse, thyroid disease
    (7) Social history: With whom does the child live? Assess family constellation, marital history, history of domestic violence and sexual or physical abuse, recent or ongoing stressors in the home, and family response to the child's behavior/academic problems.
    (8) Physical examination: Growth parameters, baseline vital signs, and brief neurologic examination. Although ADHD may be associated with neurologic "soft signs" (e.g., clumsiness, poor fine motor coordination), their significance is unclear. Unless specific signs or symptoms emerge, laboratory testing, neuroimaging, or electroencephalography is not indicated in the general evaluation of ADHD.
    (9) Child interview: Observation of ADHD target symptoms in the office setting (although their presence in that setting is not necessary to make the diagnosis), oppositional/defiant behavior, general cognitive and language level, child's understanding of behavioral concerns, and parent–child interactions

    (10) Standard ADHD questionnaires: Connor's Parent and Teacher's Questionnaires, the Achenbach Child Behavior Checklist

    (11) Assessment for LDs: Review of any previous educational/achievement test results and neuropsychological (IQ, language, cognitive, processing abilities, etc.) evaluation results. Any child in whom learning problems are suspected should have a neuropsychological assessment done by the school or a qualified neuropsychologist.

5. Management

  a. School: Educational intervention by the school involves both diagnosing and addressing any specific coexisting LDs as well as designing programs for classroom management. Parents should be strongly encouraged to become active participants in their child's educational plan. They need to be made aware of federally mandated special education services for children with ADHD-related significant academic impairment, under the 1990 Individuals with Disabilities Education Act, and provisions for classroom modification under Section 504 of the Rehabilitation Act of 1973. The IEP, which operationalizes the stated educational goals, should be part of the patient's medical record and reviewed with parents periodically by the primary care physician.

    (1) Classroom management consists of age- and child-specific modifications to improve attention and impulse control, enhance organizational skills and self-esteem, and increase productivity.

  b. Home behavioral management of the child with ADHD

    (1) Use sticker/star charts or token-reward systems for specific target behaviors.

    (2) Engage the child's attention before giving directions and avoiding multistep directions.

    (3) Anticipate and structure problematic situations in which the child is likely to be overstimulated.

    (4) Use time-out or "cool-off" periods.

    (5) Encourage activities that require selective attention.

  c. Psychotherapy: Individual psychotherapy referral may be necessary for children with significant self-esteem concerns and comorbid disorders. Family therapy may help deal with problematic family relationships. Parent support groups such as Children and Adults with Attention Deficit Disorder (CHADD) are often extremely helpful in providing emotional support, practical management techniques, and information to parents.

  d. The role of dietary factors (e.g., excessive sugar consumption, food additives and dyes, food allergies) in exacerbating ADHD is questionable.

  e. Psychopharmacology

    (1) General principles

      (a) Select medication on the basis of specific target symptoms. Target symptoms should be well defined and measurable whenever possible (e.g., percentage of schoolwork completed, number of times out of seat). Treatment success should be measured on the basis of remission of, or at least improvement in, these symptoms as evidenced by standardized questionnaires such as the Connor's or Vanderbilt. Even better is a written narrative by the teachers/parents.

(b) Before starting a stimulant medication, all children should have a routine physical examination, including baseline blood pressure, pulse, height, and weight.

(c) Consider age and developmental stage. Note that preschool-age children tend to metabolize psychostimulants faster and may need a more frequent dosing schedule. They also tend to have more unpredictable behavioral effects from these medications. Because of the risk for cardiac dysrhythmia, TCAs should be used with caution in prepubertal children.

(d) Start medication at the lower end of the dosage range and gradually titrate up. The shorter-acting medications such as methylphenidate may be increased more quickly.

(e) Titrate medication to maximize the cognitive and behavioral benefits, while minimizing the development of both short- and long-term side effects.

(f) Try different medications in the same class before moving on to another class; give each an adequate trial (dose and length of trial). Initiate medications one at a time. If this fails, you may need to consider alternative or additional diagnoses or combination of medications; a consult to a child psychiatrist may then be warranted.

(g) During initial titration and dose adjustments, there should be weekly phone contact, with follow-up appointments made on a monthly basis until the patient's symptoms have stabilized. Follow every child on medication for ADHD for continued medication efficacy and side effects at a minimum of every 4 months once a stable dose has been reached. Because stimulants are class II drugs, there can be no refills and prescriptions must be written on a monthly basis.

(2) Psychostimulants (see Table 22-1; abbreviations Box 22-1) such as methylphenidate (Ritalin) and amphetamines (Dexedrine, Dextrostat, Desoxyn, Adderall) are first-line medications for treatment of ADHD.

(a) A black box warning for stimulants has been issued by the FDA for cardiac risks based on questionable evidence of case reports of sudden death. Caregivers need to weigh the risks/benefits, especially in patients with cardiac history or family history of sudden death; an ECG to check for conduction abnormalities or cardiology consult prior to stimulant initiation may be considered.

(b) Doses should be given two to three times per day: after breakfast, after lunch and, if needed, in the afternoon to help with homework. The short half-life of most psychostimulants allows for rapid effect.

(c) There are advantages and disadvantages to "drug holidays" on weekends and school and summer vacations. This strategy may result in rapid return of symptoms. In general, drug holidays are not routinely recommended. To date, no long-term statistically significant delays have been found in the development of normal weight and height.

(d) Many adolescents and adults with ADHD continue to benefit substantially from ongoing pharmacotherapy; the class of drug used, dose, and dosing intervals may require modification over time.

(3) Antidepressants are also used in the pharmacotherapy for ADHD (see Tables 22-2 through 22-4). Most of the antidepressants may be used in combination with stimulants, especially for comorbid ADHD and mood/anxiety disorders, often allowing a reduction in the dose of both drugs.

 (a) Consider using antidepressants for the following conditions:
   (i) Failure to respond to adequate stimulant trial or intolerance of stimulant side effects
   (ii) High risk of stimulant abuse
   (iii) Patient or family history of tic disorder or Tourette's syndrome
   (iv) Comorbid conditions—depressive/anxiety disorder, enuresis
   (v) Strong family history of affective disorders/alcohol abuse
   (vi) Preference for once-daily dosing and/or avoidance of in-school medication administration

 (b) Atomoxetine (Stattera) is a selective norepinephrine reuptake inhibitor and the only FDA approved nonstimulant for the treatment of ADHD and is widely considered second line choice for treatment of ADHD (it may in fact be first line in those for whom stimulants are not appropriate or acceptable). The effects on ADHD treatment may take weeks before they are noticed.

 (c) Bupropion (Welbutrin) is a norepinephrine dopamine reuptake inhibitor which has data supporting its use in ADHD.

 (d) TCAs (see Table 22-2) such as imipramine (Tofranil), desipramine (Norpramin), nortriptyline (Pamelor), and amitriptyline (Elavil) have been used in the past as second-line pharmacotherapy for ADHD, but their side effect profile has led to decreased use by clinicians.

 (e) Selective serotonin reuptake inhibitors (SSRIs), such as fluoxetine (Prozac), sertraline (Zoloft), and paroxetine HCL (Paxil), can be used in children as young as 4 years, with generally fewer side effects than TCAs.

(4) α_2-Adrenergic agonists (see Table 22-5), such as clonidine (Catapres) and guanfacine (Tenex), appear to be particularly effective in decreasing arousal levels in ADHD, without significantly altering distractibility and attention.

 (a) Major effects
   (i) Clinically most useful in treating highly active, impulsive, and aggressive children with ADHD with an early onset of symptoms
   (ii) Also used in ADHD with comorbid oppositional and conduct disorders
   (iii) May be also particularly helpful in treating children with ADHD with a personal or family history of motor tics

(b) Drug interactions
  (i) A combination regimen of methylphenidate and cloni-
      dine can be useful in treating children with both severe
      hyperactivity/impulsivity and significant inattentive-
      ness, allowing for up to a 40% reduction in the methyl-
      phenidate dose used. This combination may particularly
      help reduce methylphenidate side effects, including
      rebound symptoms.
  (ii) Be aware of possible severe hypotensive/hypertensive
      episodes on this combination regimen, and never use in
      combination with beta blockers.
(c) Treatment strategies
  (i) Clonidine is usually initiated with a bedtime dose;
      daily dose is increased every 3 days (see Table 22-5).
  (ii) Clinical effects of clonidine may not be evident until
      2 to 4 weeks into treatment; maximum effect may not
      be reached until 2 to 3 months.
  (iii) Clonidine is available in transcutaneous patch form.
      Advantages of the patch include considerable conve-
      nience (replaced every 5 days) and less sedation. Switch
      to patch after the appropriate oral dose has been titrated.
  (iv) The longer half-life of guanfacine allows for a less
      frequent dosing schedule (once to three times a day).
      Tolerance to both clonidine and guanfacine may also
      develop, necessitating an increase in dose.

5. Prognosis
   a. About half of children with ADHD have no or minimal symptoms as
      older adolescents or adults.
   b. About 30% to 50% continue to have mild symptoms, including cog-
      nitive dysfunction, inattention, distractibility, impatience, and irri-
      tability/mood lability into adulthood.
   c. About 10% to 20% have significant functional impairment leading
      to difficulties in school achievement, job performance, and intimate
      relationships; drug and alcohol abuse; motor vehicle accidents; and
      low personal satisfaction/self-esteem.
   d. Poor prognosis is associated largely with comorbid disorders, espe-
      cially conduct disorders.

22.7 Pervasive Developmental Disorders: Autism and Asperger's Syndrome

1. Introduction
   a. Definition: Pervasive developmental disorders (PDD) is defined in
      DSM-IV-TR as severe, pervasive impairment in developmental areas
      (e.g., social interactions or communication) or the presence of ste-
      reotyped behaviors, interests, and activities.
   b. PDD includes autism, Asperger's syndrome, Rett's syndrome, child-
      hood disintegrative disorder, and PDD not otherwise specified
      (NOS). Only autism and Asperger's syndrome are covered in this
      section.

   c. Disease severity: Even within a particular diagnosis, the degree of functional impairment can vary widely.

   d. MR: Many children with PDD have comorbid MR. This too varies widely—for example, up to 75% of children with autism have some degree of MR, whereas most with Asperger's syndrome have average to above-average intelligence.

2. Etiology and pathophysiology

   a. The etiology for autism is unknown. There are many studies suggesting influence from many factors, including genetic, congenital, neuroanatomic, biochemical, and immunologic. No one factor has been consistently found in autistic patients.

   b. Parental role: Studies have disproved the hypothesis that parental interactions with children play a role in the development of PDD/autism.

   c. Immunizations: Concerns were raised that there is an association between the measles, mumps, rubella (MMR) vaccine or the mercury exposure associated with it and autism. However, major epidemiologic studies have found no evidence for this. See references at end of chapter.

3. Epidemiology

   a. All cultures, ethnic backgrounds, and socioeconomic levels are affected.

   b. Autism: Prevalence is approximately 4 per 10,000; male-to-female ratio is 5:1, but girls tend to have more severe forms of the disorder with lower IQs.

   c. Asperger's syndrome: Prevalence is approximately 20 to 25 per 10,000; male-to-female ratio is between 3.8 and 10.5:1.

4. Clinical features

   a. Autism

     (1) Onset: Autism is usually evident in the first year of life, although delays in case recognition are very common. Infants with autism often display the following behaviors:

       (a) Lack of reciprocity in their social interactions

       (b) Inappropriate gaze behaviors

       (c) Poor attachment (even with their parents)

       (d) Paucity of joint play

       (e) Poor communicative skills

     (2) Domains of impairment

       (a) Social interaction: Delays in social development including the lack of social engagement and reciprocity, often present from the first days of life (see earlier)

       (b) Communication/language delay: Many autistic children are nonverbal and have severely limited communication ability. In those children who are verbal, the speech tends to be monotonous and expressionless; echolalia is common.

       (c) Restrictive and repetitive activities: Rigid and inflexible thinking and pervasive need for sameness. The degree of impairment varies considerably from discomfort around changing routines to repetitive self-injurious behaviors or preoccupation with numbers, schedules, and the like.

(3) Comorbid disorders
    (a) Seizure disorders are relatively common in autistic patients.
    (b) Psychiatric disorders: ADHD, obsessive-compulsive disorder (OCD), and mood disorders
    (c) Aggression: Often a serious concern, especially as the child physically matures

b. Asperger's syndrome
    (1) Onset: Usually recognized later because language skills are normal to precocious; furthermore, although social skills are impaired, there is often a strong desire by the child with Asperger's syndrome to have friends and interact. These children tend to be described as strange or annoying by peers, often shunned and ridiculed.
    (2) Domains of impairment
        (a) Social interaction impaired
            (i) Failure to develop peer relationships
            (ii) Lack of social or emotional reciprocity: Clumsy, awkward, or forced social approach (e.g., overly focused on the handshake or rote greetings); unable to express pleasure in other people's happiness; difficulty identifying feelings and nonverbal expressions/cues of others
        (b) Restrictive and repetitive activities: rigid and inflexible thinking and pervasive need for sameness
            (i) Difficulty with changing routines or impulsive activities
            (ii) Focus on unique topic to the exclusion of most others: from dinosaurs to fire alarm boxes
    (3) Communication and language: Asperger's syndrome is distinguished from autism by no significant language delay (may even be precocious) and even an increased drive to talk. However, studies have consistently shown the following findings:
        (a) Poor prosody and frequent abnormalities in inflection (flat or monotone)
        (b) Conversations are described as stilted, thought disordered, or preoccupied with idiosyncratic interests, sometimes described as pseudoconversations: Patients can talk endlessly about specific and often strange topics without regard for the audience's level of interest (at times irritated or perplexed when others are not interested in the topic).
        (c) The speech of adolescents with Asperger's syndrome is often described as pedantic or odd.

5. Diagnosis (consult DSM-IV-TR for detailed diagnostic criteria)
    a. Domains of impairment
        (1) Autism: Social interaction; communication; restrictive and repetitive activities
        (2) Asperger's syndrome: Social interaction; restrictive and repetitive activities; no language delay
    b. Scales and measures (may require neuropsychiatric testing)
        (1) General/PDD: Vineland Adaptive Behavior Scale
        (2) Autism: Autism Behavior Checklist, Autism Screening Questionnaire, Autism Spectrum Disorder Screening Questionnaire, Checklist for Autism in Toddlers, Childhood Autism Rating Scales, Pre-Linguistic Autism Diagnostic Observation Schedule

(3) Asperger's syndrome: Gilliam Asperger's Scale, Asperger's Syndrome Diagnostic Scale

6. Differential diagnosis
   a. Language disorder
   b. Learning disorder with or without autistic features
   c. Rett's syndrome: Distinguish by progressive deterioration after period (approximately 2 years) of normal development (compare with no normal development period in autism); usually seen in girls
   d. Neurodegenerative and disintegrative disorders
   e. Early deprivation
   f. Fragile X syndrome
   g. Deafness

7. Management
   a. Treatment modalities include social skill training, parental counseling, behavioral modification, special education in highly structured environment, sensory integration training speech therapy, and certain medications.
   b. Pharmacologic: Medications are directed at problematic symptoms, such as aggression, mood disorders, and comorbid medical conditions. Medications such as mood stabilizers, antipsychotics, and stimulants are commonly prescribed. Of note, doses are often much different (usually lower) than in the general population.

8. Prognosis
   a. These are chronic disorders. For autism, only a third are able to achieve some degree of personal independence as adults. Patients with Asperger's syndrome are somewhat more successful, often achieving independence; however, they often lead lonely lives as they continue to relate awkwardly to other adults as well as be shy and uncomfortable socially.
   b. Goals of treatment are to increase socially acceptable behavior and to aid in the development of verbal and nonverbal communication.
   c. Predictors of function include IQ and acquisition of verbal language.

22.8 Disruptive Behavior: Conduct Disorder and Oppositional Defiant Disorder

INTRODUCTION

1. Characterized by willful disobedience
2. Two types
   a. Conduct disorder (see definition later)
   b. Oppositional defiant disorder (see definition later)
3. Differential diagnosis: Behavior problems can be the presenting symptom in a number of psychiatric illnesses; most of these diagnoses have specific treatments that, when initiated, can also reduce the behavioral problems.
   a. Learning disorders
   b. ADHD
   c. Mild MR
   d. Seizure disorders
   e. Schizophrenia

f. Mood disorders
g. Antisocial personality disorder: People with this disorder consistently lie and are often referred to as *sociopathic*. These individuals have lifelong patterns of behavior and thinking that are inflexible—exactly the antithesis of childhood and adolescence, where the personality is still developing.
h. Substance abuse
i. Post-traumatic stress disorder (PTSD)

CONDUCT DISORDER

1. Definition: A *conduct disorder* is a disturbance of behavior that lasts at least 12 months in which the basic rights of others or the major age-appropriate norms and rules of society are violated.
2. Epidemiology
   a. Conduct disorder affects boys more than girls.
   b. Most children come from lower socioeconomic backgrounds, have experienced punitive rearing methods, and are temperamentally difficult with a high activity level and intensity of response.
3. Clinical features
   a. Four basic categories recognized in DSM-IV-TR
      (1) Aggression to people or animals: Bullying, intimidating, physical cruelty, forcing sexual activity
      (2) Destruction of property: Fire setting, etc.
      (3) Deceitfulness or theft: Lying, nonconfrontive stealing
      (4) Serious violation of rules: Truancy, running away, substance abuse, disobedience
   b. Additional features
      (1) Substance abuse (drugs and alcohol)
      (2) Suicidal ideation and suicide attempts
      (3) Scores in the low-normal or borderline range in standard intelligence tests
      (4) Learning disorders
4. Diagnosis (consult DSM-IV-TR for detailed diagnostic criteria)
   a. Nature of the problematic behaviors: Circumstances and precipitants; amount of control and remorse/guilt the child exhibits
   b. Degree of parent involvement, attempts to control problem behaviors
   c. Past medical history focusing on serious accidents or injuries, physical or sexual abuse
   d. Presence of comorbid psychiatric disorders such as ADHD, LDs, mood disorder, substance abuse
   e. Neurologic examination, neuropsychological testing, and a psychoeducational evaluation
5. Management
   a. Parent management training, in which parents are trained in conflict resolution
   b. Functional family therapy, focusing on enhancing direct communication and supportive behaviors among family members
   c. Problem-solving skills training, teaching alternative ways of handling difficult situations

d. Community-based treatments, in which adults act as friends, advocates, and role models

e. The use of medications tailored to treating specific symptomatic behaviors and comorbid disorders (e.g., ADHD, mood disorder). Examples include ADHD medications and mood stabilizers/antidepressants. Aggression has been treated effectively with both mood stabilizers and antipsychotic medications. (See tables at end of chapter.)

6. Prognosis

a. Only those children with milder forms of the disorder tend to improve over time.

b. Nearly half of seriously antisocial children are antisocial as adults.

c. Aggressive behavior in school-age children, particularly when it is associated with school failure, is predictive of later delinquency.

OPPOSITIONAL DEFIANT DISORDER

1. Definition: Hostile, negative, defiant, and disobedient attitudes and behaviors, especially toward authority figures

2. Epidemiology: Prevalence ranges from 2% to 16%; twice as common in boys

3. Clinical features

a. Negativism (argue with adults)

b. Hostility (angry, vindictive, and sometimes aggressive behavior)

c. Defiance of adults' rules (refuse to comply with adult requests and rules more often than typically observed in those of comparable age and developmental level)

4. Diagnosis (Consult DSM-IV-TR for detailed diagnostic criteria)

a. This disturbance in behavior must be present for at least 12 months and impair the ability to function socially, academically, and at work.

b. The degree of behavioral disturbance falls short of the repetitive and serious violations associated with conduct disorder.

5. Management (see tables at end of chapter)

a. Management of comorbid diagnosis: ADHD, mood disorders, PTSD, etc.

b. Aggression: Antipsychotic medication has been used effectively in acute situations and mood stabilizers for chronic treatment.

22.9 Anxiety Disorders

INTRODUCTION

1. Anxiety disorders are one of the most prevalent categories of childhood and adolescent psychopathology. They include a heterogeneous group of disorders involving excessive worry that causes significant impairment in developmental functioning. They are not an isolated group of symptoms but instead belong within a broader context of traits that include timidity, hypersensitivity, social withdrawal, lack of self-confidence, and dysphoria.

2. Anxiety disorders include the following diagnoses: generalized anxiety disorder, separation anxiety disorder, OCD, social phobia, panic disorder, specific phobia, and selective mutism. Specific diagnostic criteria for each disorder can be found in the DSM-IV-TR.

3. Etiology and pathophysiology: The interaction of five main factors contributes to the development of anxiety disorders in childhood:

   a. Genetics and temperament: Behavioral inhibition (i.e., the tendency to approach unfamiliar situations with distress or avoidance) at a young age (9 to 31 months) is thought to have both a genetic component and to be an enduring temperamental trait. Behavioral inhibition has been linked to an increased risk of social phobia in adolescence.

   b. Attachment: Insecure attachment between mother and child contributes to the development of anxiety disorders.

   c. Parental anxiety: Children whose parents have anxiety disorders are at a greater risk for developing anxiety disorders. Parental anxiety may not be a direct cause but instead may be expressed through another mechanism (e.g., parenting style).

   d. Parenting style: Parents of children who develop anxiety disorders have been described as granting less autonomy and perceived by their children as less accepting.

   e. Life experiences: Certain negative conditioning experiences (loss of a grandparent, frightening events on the news, seeing a parent worry) have been described as contributing to anxiety in children. By themselves, stressful life events do not fully explain the development of anxiety disorders. They are instead a backdrop or contributing factor along with other important variables.

SEPARATION ANXIETY DISORDER

1. Definition: An overwhelming fear of losing a parent or caregiver that is inappropriate for the child's level of development and that interferes with the child's functioning

2. Epidemiology: Prevalence rate of approximately 4% (female, 4.3%; male, 2.7%). Rates of separation anxiety disorder (SAD) decrease with age.

3. Etiology: Level of ego development is strongest predictor of having SAD.

4. Clinical features

   a. Separation anxiety is a normal part of development, beginning around 6 months, peaking around 18 months, and then declining after 30 months of age. Subclinical separation anxiety (e.g., fear of harm to attachment figures or to self) is a reasonably common phenomenon through childhood and early adolescence.

   b. However, once the worry becomes persistent, excessive, and impairing, a diagnosis of SAD should be considered; at the time of separation, a child with SAD may literally be in a panic.

   c. Because of their fear of separation, children with SAD will procrastinate in numerous ways: they will be slow in their morning routine; they will refuse to attend school or to leave the side of their parent when its time for school. They will often describe multiple somatic complaints (stomachaches, headache). Over time, their anxiety may compromise their performance and may delay their maturation and development.

   d. Of note, the refusal to attend school is not specific for SAD and may also be seen in other disorders such as social phobia, specific school phobia, or depression.

5. Management
   a. Cognitive behavioral therapy (CBT): Includes recognizing anxious feelings and thoughts, identifying physical reactions to anxiety, developing a coping plan when symptoms arise, desensitization, prolonged exposure, modeling, role playing, relaxation training
   b. Medication: SSRIs, TCAs (second-line because of cardiac risks), benzodiazepines (short term and in conjunction with an SSRI), atypical antipsychotics. See Tables 22-2 to 22-9 for medications and dosing suggestions.
6. Prognosis: SAD has a good prognosis, especially if the patient's ego is strong.

GENERALIZED ANXIETY DISORDER

1. Definition: Generalized anxiety disorder (GAD) is characterized by excessive and uncontrollable worry about numerous things, or none at all, for at least 6 months.
2. Epidemiology: Prevalence of approximately 2% (female, ~2.4%; male, ~1%); more prevalent among older children and adolescents. Rates increase with age.
3. Clinical findings: Although anxiety is a normal part of development, children with GAD find their excessive worry difficult to control, and it often interferes with their ability to function.
4. Management
   a. CBT: Recognizing anxious feelings and thoughts, identifying physical reactions to anxiety, developing coping plans when these symptoms arise, desensitization, prolonged exposure, modeling, role playing, relaxation training
   b. Medication: SSRIs, TCAs (second-line because of cardiac risks), benzodiazepines (short term and in conjunction with an SSRI), atypical antipsychotics. See Tables 22-2 to 22-9 for medications and dosing suggestions.
5. Prognosis
   a. High rate of recovery (~80%).
   b. Children with GAD are at an increased risk for developing additional psychiatric disorders (e.g., social phobia, MDD, GAD, panic disorder).

OBSESSIVE-COMPULSIVE DISORDER

1. Definitions
   a. Obsessions are persistent thoughts, images, or impulses that are intrusive and pointless. Often, the child realizes that these thoughts are excessive and is distressed by them.
   b. Compulsions are repetitive behaviors that the child feels driven to perform in response to the obsessions.
2. Epidemiology: Incidence of childhood OCD is estimated to be between 0.8% to 1.2%; lifetime prevalence is 1.9% to 3.0%. OCD is significantly associated with both tics and ADHD.
3. Etiology
   a. Multiple factors are implicated in the development of OCD: these include genetic susceptibility, neurotransmitter dysregulation (serotonin and perhaps dopamine) and environmental triggers.

b. Frontal lobe-limbic-basal ganglia dysfunction may also contribute to OCD. Specifically, damage to the basal ganglia is associated with the onset of OCD (e.g., tumors, trauma, carbon monoxide poisoning, illnesses like postencephalitic Parkinson's).

c. Children with Sydenham's chorea and children with pediatric autoimmune neuropsychiatric disorders associated with streptococcal infections (PANDAS) have an increased incidence of OCD, suggesting a possible autoimmune response in OCD.

4. Clinical findings

a. The obsessions and compulsions cause significant distress or interfere in the patient's life.

b. Children with early-onset OCD are more likely to be male and to have a family member with either OCD or a tic disorder.

c. Young children often experience compulsions without obsessions.

d. The most common ritual seen in children is excessive cleaning (e.g., handwashing, toothbrushing, showering). Other common behaviors include repeating rituals (e.g., going in and out of doors, restating phrases, rereading) and checking rituals (checking the doors are locked, the appliances are turned off, the homework is perfect).

e. Most patients, over time, experience many different obsessions and compulsions with no clear pattern of progression.

f. Other behaviors that may indicate a child dealing with OCD: rigid rituals, an excessive need for reassurance, or long unproductive hours spent doing homework. A dramatic increase in laundry volume or an insistence on wearing clothes only once may indicate an obsession with germs.

5. Differential diagnosis

a. MDD: Ruminating and brooding preoccupations are often seen in MDD, but they tend to be content specific and are not followed by senseless compulsive acts.

b. Other anxiety disorders (GAD/social phobia/SAD): The focus of the worry is different and there are no accompanying compulsive rituals in these disorders.

c. Eating disorders: The obsessive and compulsive behaviors associated with bulimia and anorexia are all related to food, weight gain, and body image.

d. Tic disorder/Tourette's syndrome: It can be difficult to distinguish between complex motor tics (see section on Tic Disorders) and a compulsive ritual. In OCD, the ritual is typically preceded by a specific thought/cognition. On the other hand, tics are either spontaneous and involuntary, or they may be preceded by a persistent "urge" that is relieved by the tic. The treatments for OCD and tic disorders are different, so it is important to distinguish between them. Children with tic disorder may also have OCD.

6. Management

a. CBT has been shown to be effective in reducing symptoms in OCD and is considered to be first-line treatment. Treatment usually consists of information gathering, exposure with response prevention (E/RP), and homework assignments. For example, a child with a fear of germs will gradually be exposed to "germy" things and then must refrain from handwashing until his or her anxiety has substantially decreased. E/RP can also be combined with other therapy modalities, such as psychodynamic therapy and family therapy. Psychopharmacologic therapy in combination with CBT is especially helpful.

b. The SSRIs, including fluoxetine (Prozac), fluvoxamine (Luvox), and sertraline (Zoloft), have been approved by the U.S. Food and Drug Administration (FDA) in children and all have been shown to be superior to placebo in the treatment of OCD symptoms. Generally, patients experience a 30% to 40% reduction in OCD symptoms. A 12-week trial of an SSRI at an adequate or even high dose is considered necessary for a patient to experience a reduction in symptoms (see Table 22-2).

c. Other medications, including benzodiazepines (e.g., clonazepam [Klonopin]), atypical antipsychotics (e.g., risperidone [Risperdal]), and TCAs (particularly clomipramine [Anafranil]), have been shown to be effective for augmentation or monotherapy. However, their side effects, mortality in overdose, and need for monitoring (e.g., electrocardiogram for prolonged QTc and arrhythmia in TCAs) warrant consultation with a child and adolescent psychiatrist.

7. Prognosis: Follow-up studies indicate that 30% to 68% of children with OCD will remain symptomatic as adults. A small population continues with a chronic debilitating course. A potentially better outcome occurs if children have consistent access to SSRIs and behavioral therapy.

SOCIAL PHOBIA

1. Definition: A person with social phobia experiences fearful apprehension, distress, and somatic symptoms in social situations in which they are exposed to unfamiliar persons or to scrutiny by others.

2. Epidemiology: The prevalence rate is approximately 1% (likely underestimated) in children. Lifetime prevalence rates for adolescents are between 5% and 15%. Social phobia has an early age of onset and a bimodal distribution, with peaks before age 5 and again at about age 13 years.

3. Clinical findings
   a. Marked, persistent fear of social or performance situations, and worrying about acting in a way that is humiliating or embarrassing
   b. Social phobia affects all ages but can manifest itself differently depending on the age of the patient. For example, young children may cry or have a tantrum and school-age children may avoid classroom presentations. Adolescents and young adults will have difficulties with dating and may drop out of college classes in which a presentation is required.
   c. The most commonly feared situations include public speaking, social gatherings, interactions with authority figures, asking for directions, or speaking with strangers.
   d. Somatic symptoms are common (racing heart, sweating, blushing, tremulous hands or voice), as is the fear that others will notice these symptoms.
   e. People with social phobia have an increased incidence of alcohol abuse, more suicidal ideation and suicide attempts, more physical and mental health problems, and greater use of health care services than do people without social phobia.
   f. There is a high comorbidity with other anxiety disorders and with avoidant personality disorder.

4. Management
   a. CBT for individuals, groups, and families has been shown to be effective.
   b. SSRIs (fluvoxamine, fluoxetine) are considered the treatment of choice and can play an important role in the treatment plan.
5. Prognosis: Long-term outcome in children is unknown. Longitudinal studies with adults indicate it is often a chronic disorder.

PANIC DISORDER

1. Definition: Recurrent, spontaneous episodes of panic characterized by physical (e.g., tachycardia, diaphoresis) and psychological (fear) symptoms
2. Epidemiology: Studies indicate peak age of onset is between 15 and 20 years of age, although numerous cases have been described before puberty. One study of adolescents 14 to 17 years of age estimated the prevalence of panic disorder to be 0.6%. The incidence of panic attacks is much higher than the incidence of full-blown panic disorder and greatly increases with the onset of puberty. The prevalence of panic attacks/panic disorder before puberty is unknown.
3. Clinical findings
   a. Panic disorder involves recurrent, unexpected, discrete episodes of intense fear (panic attacks) accompanied by specific physical symptoms and associated with anticipatory anxiety of having another attack.
   b. A panic attack lasts about 10 minutes and is characterized by four or more of the following symptoms: Palpitations or pounding heart, sweating, trembling or shaking, shortness of breath, feeling of choking, chest pain, nausea, dizziness, surrealness, fear of losing control or "going crazy," fear of dying, paresthesias, and chills. Cognitive symptoms (fear of losing control or dying) are reported less frequently in adolescents.
   c. Panic disorder with or without agoraphobia usually begins in adolescence or early adulthood but can develop at any age.
   d. An important and common feature is the presence of comorbid SAD. Children who develop SAD at an early age are at an increased risk for later development of panic disorder.
   e. Offspring of parents with panic disorder have a more than threefold increased risk for development of SAD.
4. Management
   a. Adult studies have shown the efficacy of TCAs, MAOIs, SSRIs, and benzodiazepines. Although no systematic treatment trials of SSRIs in children have been done, SSRIs are emerging as the medication treatment of choice in clinical practice.
   b. Preliminary evidence suggests that CBT is effective for childhood and adolescent panic disorder.
5. Prognosis: Long-term outcome in children is unknown. Longitudinal studies with adults indicate it is often a chronic disorder.

ANXIETY DUE TO A GENERAL MEDICAL CONDITION

1. Generalized anxiety or panic attacks can be seen in certain medical conditions, including hypoglycemic episodes, cardiac arrhythmias, pheochromocytoma, hyperthyroidism, asthma or encephalitis, migraines, seizures, or medication reactions (e.g., antihistamines, antiasthmatics, sympathomimetics, steroids, SSRIs, antipsychotics [akathisia], and over-the-counter preparations).

2. PANDAS: Abrupt development of obsessions and compulsions defined by five clinical characteristics:
   a. The presence of OCD or a tic disorder (or both)
   b. Prepubertal symptom onset
   c. Dramatic onset and acute exacerbations with an episodic course of symptom severity
   d. Temporal association between symptom exacerbations and group A beta-hemolytic streptococcal infection
   e. Associated neurologic abnormalities (e.g., choreiform movements)

22.10 Tic Disorders

1. Definition
   a. Tics are repetitive, involuntary, sudden, rapid, brief, stereotyped movements or vocalizations.
   b. They are increased by anxiety, stress, excitement, and fatigue.
   c. They are less noticeable during sleep, periods of relaxation, and absorbing activities (e.g., studying).
   d. Tics are briefly suppressible, but this provokes the buildup of inner, emotional tension, which is relieved by reinitiating of tic activity.
   e. Patients often attempt to mask their tics by converting them into pseudovoluntary movements or noises.
2. Etiology and pathophysiology: Etiologic factors in tic disorder include genetic (monozygotic and dizygotic twin studies, family studies), neuroanatomic (abnormalities in the basal ganglia and in the dopaminergic system), perinatal, and autoimmune.
3. Epidemiology: Tics are common in childhood. The highest prevalence occurs between ages 7 and 11 years. As much as 18% of boys and 11% of girls have "tics." Most childhood tics remit by adolescence. Childhood tics may be a risk factor for the development of OCD and other anxiety symptoms in adolescence.
4. Clinical features
   a. Motor tics
      (1) *Simple*: Involving an individual muscle group (i.e., eye blinking, nose twitching, and shoulder shrugging)
      (2) *Complex*: Involving several muscle groups (i.e., facial grimacing, jumping, smelling, obscene gestures)
   b. Vocal tics
      (1) *Simple*: Grunting, coughing, throat clearing, barking, sniffing, snorting
      (2) *Complex*: Words, syllables, sentences, phrases, palilalia (repeat one's own words), echolalia (repeat other's words), coprolalia (obscene words)
      (3) Most vocal tics tend to occur at phrase junctions during speech, resulting in a blockage or hesitation.
   c. Sensory tics: Uncomfortable sensations (tickle, irritation, change in temperature, or unusual feelings) that cause the patient to produce voluntary movements or sounds
5. Diagnosis
   a. Transient tic disorder; mildest and most common tic disorder

(1) Tics last for more than 4 weeks but less than 1 year.
(2) Usually affects the face, neck, head, or arms and occurs in approximately 5% to 24% of school-age children
b. Chronic tic disorder
(1) Tics last for more than 1 year and during this period there is never a tic-free period of more than 3 consecutive months.
(2) Onset of tics before 18 years of age
(3) Single or multiple motor or vocal tics (but not both) have been present at some time during the illness.
(4) No other medical explanation for the tics
c. Tourette's syndrome: Diagnosis is similar to chronic tics, with the following unique features:
(1) Both multiple motor tics and one or more vocal tics
(2) A waxing and waning course
(3) Gradual replacement of old symptoms with new ones
d. Nonspecific tic disorder: The patient does not meet the criteria for a specific tic disorder (i.e., onset in adulthood, motor and vocal tics for less than 1 year).
6. Management: Therapy should be targeted to those symptoms that are functionally disabling for the patient; both tics and associated problems such as ADHD, OCD, and behavioral difficulties need to be identified and treated according to the individual's greatest disability.
a. Pharmacology
(1) For chronic tics, clonidine or guanfacine can be used as an initial medication for patients with mild symptoms and for those in whom behavioral problems predominate.
(2) The most potent medications for suppressing tics are the neuroleptics, including the newer atypicals such as risperidone, olanzapine, and ziprasidone. However, their side effects, although less severe than with the older neuroleptics, limit their use to more severe cases of chronic tic disorders or to those that are unresponsive to clonidine or guanfacine.
(3) Children with ADHD: Clonidine or guanfacine should be tried. Certain TCAs, including desipramine or nortriptyline, can also be useful, but electrocardiographic monitoring must be done because of the risk of cardiac arrhythmias and conduction disorders with these medications. If the foregoing medications are ineffective, a brief trial with a psychostimulant (e.g., methylphenidate) can be initiated and withdrawn if tics worsen.
(4) Children with tic disorder and OCD: The SSRIs (e.g., fluoxetine) are useful. Of note, tic-related OCD is less responsive to SSRIs, and the addition of a neuroleptic can be helpful in improving treatment response.

22.11 Mood Disorders: Depression and Bipolar Disorder

INTRODUCTION

1. Mood disorders have a common underlying abnormality: Alteration in mood. Two types discussed here are MDD and bipolar disorder.

2. Mood disorders are alterations in common feelings that are ongoing over extended periods and interfere with daily activities or normal development.

MAJOR DEPRESSIVE DISORDER

1. Etiology and pathophysiology
   a. The younger the age, the more environment influences mood. The older the child/adolescent, the more genetic factors come into play.
   b. Risk factors: Low self-esteem, poor interpersonal skills, aggressive (verbally or physically) coping skills, abuse or neglect, stress, loss of a parent or loved one, romantic relationship problems, trauma, chronic illnesses
   c. Depression in parents: When one of the parents has a mood disorder, the child has a 30% chance of also having one. When both parents are affected, the child has a 50% to 70% chance of having a mood disorder.
2. Epidemiology
   a. Depression is present in as much as 1% of preschoolers, 2% to 3% of school-age children, and 4% to 8% of adolescents.
   b. Incidence increases with age and is most prevalent and severe during adolescence.
   c. Depression affects both sexes almost equally before puberty but is more common in girls after puberty.
3. Clinical features
   a. Onset: Often acute in retrospect, symptoms may be compounded if the diagnosis is delayed. The common presentation is a severe disruption in daily activities (developmental, social, or academic).
   b. Some clinical manifestations occur at all developmental stages: Sadness; lack of enjoyment in usual activities; irritability or oppositional behavior; disturbances in eating, sleeping, and play.
   c. Age-specific features
      (1) Infants and toddlers: Failure to thrive; delays in speech and gross motor skills
      (2) Preschoolers: Disruptions in play activities; preoccupation with morbid, even suicidal, thoughts; enuresis or encopresis; frequent accidents or "accidental" ingestions
      (3) School-age, prepubertal children: Somatic complaints (head aches and recurrent abdominal pain); psychomotor-agitation; problems at school (poor academic performance, falling grades, school phobia); social isolation; poor self-esteem; antisocial behaviors (stealing or lying); mood-congruent hallucinations common
      (4) Adolescent and older children can express their feelings of sadness and may also present with restlessness, grouchiness, and mood swings; acting-out/antisocial behaviors (substance abuse, running away from home, stealing, lying); aggression and psychomotor agitation; withdrawal, isolation, and problems with family and school; feeling not understood; and suicidal thoughts or even attempts.
4. Diagnosis (consult DSM-IV-TR for detailed diagnostic criteria)

a. The major distinction between adults and children is the allowance of irritability in substitution for depressed mood.
b. Five or more of the following symptoms must be present for the same 2-week period:
  (1) Depressed or irritable mood
  (2) Loss of interest in previously enjoyed activities
  (3) Change in appetite or weight
  (4) Insomnia or hypersomnia
  (5) Psychomotor agitation or retardation
  (6) Fatigue or loss of energy
  (7) Feeling worthless or guilty
  (8) Decreased concentration
  (9) Thoughts of death
c. Rule out medical conditions causing depression (e.g., hypothyroidism, Lyme disease, chronic infections, acquired immunodeficiency syndrome) with a complete physical examination.
d. Identify substances that can cause depression: oral contraceptives, clonidine, alcohol, illicit drug use, and so forth.
e. The interview: Speak with the child/adolescent and parents separately; and identify the burden of suffering, degree of dysfunction, and duration and persistence of symptoms.
f. Identify common comorbid diagnoses: anxiety, OCD, PTSD, ADHD.
5. Management.
  a. Safety
    (1) Ask about suicidal thoughts or a plan and hospitalize if necessary.
    (2) Ask about weapons/guns in the home, access to prescription/over-the-counter drugs, and general safety in the home; have the parents/guardian remove all dangerous items from the home.
    (3) Determine who will keep the child/adolescent safe; if they cannot, consider hospitalization.
  b. Therapy: CBT has been shown to be effective in depression.
  c. Medication: See the section on Pediatric Psychopharmacology for specific recommendations and warnings.
    (1) Antidepressants: First line is the SSRIs. Note that fluoxetine (Prozac) is the only antidepressant approved for the treatment of MDD in children in the United States. Also note that in 2004, the FDA issued a "black box" warning about the safety of antidepressants in children and adolescents because of a presumed increased risk of suicidal thinking and behavior in children with MDD and other psychiatric disorders. In the study which the FDA based their black box warning, it is important to recognize that the relative risk of adverse events (suicidal thoughts or behavior) actually increased from 2% in the placebo group to just 4% in the SSRI group; especially important is the fact that no children completed suicide.
    (2) Mood stabilizers: Often used as an adjunct to antidepressants; some (e.g., lithium and lamotrigine [Lamictal]) augment the antidepressant.

BIPOLAR DISORDER

1. Etiology and pathophysiology
   a. Compared with the relatively vast body of knowledge and research on depression, there is little information about bipolar disorder in children; moreover, there continues to be significant debate about the diagnosis and management, especially because the presentation is often significantly different from that in adults.
   b. Genetic factors and environmental factors are thought to contribute. The impact of these factors, as well as other comorbid conditions such as ADHD, is a matter of debate.
   c. Mean age of onset for childhood bipolar disorder is 8.1 years.
2. Clinical features
   a. Presentation: The presentation in children/adolescents is often unique compared with adult standards.
      (1) Mania is seldom characterized by euphoric mood; more commonly prolonged irritability, with extended agitated or aggressive outbursts, frustration, moodiness, sleep disturbance, and impulsivity, are defining characteristics.
      (2) There is rarely a distinct separation between periods of mania and depression; in fact, depressive periods are often lacking.
      (3) Unlike in adults, the course of childhood-onset bipolar disorder tends to be chronic and continuous.
   b. Common symptoms include prolonged, aggressive outbursts lasting from an hour to a day or longer with extremely low frustration tolerance; moodiness with disruptive behavior; difficulty sleeping at night; impulsivity, hyperactivity, and explosive anger.
   c. Age differences
      (1) Younger than 9 years: Irritability and emotional lability are common (two very nonspecific symptoms).
      (2) Older than 9 years: Euphoria, elation, paranoia, and grandiosity may be seen.
3. Diagnosis (consult DSM-IV-TR for detailed diagnostic criteria)
   a. Manic episode: Distinct period of abnormally and persistently elevated, expansive, or irritable mood
   b. Symptoms present during the period of mood disturbance—at least three of the following (four if mood is irritable).
      (1) Inflated self-esteem or grandiosity
      (2) Decreased need for sleep
      (3) More talkative or pressured speech
      (4) Flight of ideas or racing thoughts
      (5) Distractibility
      (6) Increased goal-directed activity (e.g., cleaning) or psychomotor agitation
      (7) Increase in risk-taking behaviors
   c. Mixed episode: Rapidly alternating moods between symptoms associated with mania and those associated with depression
   d. Time factor: At least 1 week of mood disturbance is needed for the diagnosis.

4. Management
   a. Safety: As with major depression, ensuring the child's or adolescent's safety is of the utmost concern. Identify suicidal thoughts or plans; determine the safety of being in the home (e.g., presence of firearms). Hospitalize as necessary if there is any question of a child's or adolescent's safety.
   b. Therapy: Parent training, family therapy, and intensive community services have all been helpful.
   c. Medication: See the tables at the end of the chapter for specific recommendations and warnings.
      (1) Mood stabilizers: First line in treatment of bipolar disorder (e.g., lithium, valproic acid [Depakote], lamotrigine)
      (2) Antidepressants: Used for specific depressive symptoms if not effectively covered by the mood stabilizer. Care must be taken because SSRIs may cause manic episodes in bipolar patients who are stable on a mood stabilizer.
      (3) Antipsychotics: Atypical antipsychotics have been found to have mood-stabilizing properties; they are especially effective with the agitation commonly seen in bipolar disorder. They can be used as an adjunct to a mood stabilizer or as a monotherapy.
   d. Acute agitation: Classic (chlorpromazine [Thorazine]) and atypical antipsychotics (see Tables 22-8 and 22-9) have been used on an as-needed basis for severe agitation.
5. Differential diagnosis
   a. Dysthymia is present in children who do not meet the full criteria for major depression but have feelings of sadness, low self-esteem, and three to four neuronegative signs that persist for 2 years.
   b. Cyclothymia is characterized by recurrent episodes of hypomania and depression.
   c. Psychoses such as schizophrenia may be the primary disorder, with depression as the presenting symptom.
   d. PTSD: often presents with both mood disturbance and agitation
   e. ADHD: Mood symptoms are commonly associated with ADHD and agitation can be a central part of this diagnosis; ADHD is one of the most common and difficult differential diagnoses for bipolar disorder.
   f. Anxiety disorders: An anxiety disorder is often comorbid with depression; however, it can also be the presenting symptom of MDD.
   g. Conduct disorder: Again, often comorbid with bipolar disorder. However, it is commonly misdiagnosed in a child with primary bipolar disorder.

22.12 Childhood Schizophrenia

Schizophrenia is rare in children and seldom apparent before 9 years of age; the reader is referred to online web sources for more information about childhood schizophrenia.

22.13 Munchausen Syndrome by Proxy

1. Definition: Munchausen syndrome by proxy is a disorder in which a person persistently fabricates symptoms of illness on behalf of another,

so causing that person to be regarded as ill. When children are involved, mothers almost exclusively fabricate the illness.

2. Clinical features
   a. The illness appears to be multisystemic, and the children appear to have different types of illness at different times.
   b. Bleeding is the most common presentation. The apparent bleeding may be from the gastrointestinal tract or the genitourinary or respiratory systems. Presenting symptoms also include diarrhea, vomiting, fever, seizures, CNS depression, and apnea.
   c. Actions such as the mother repeatedly suffocating the child to simulate apnea or seizures or causing sepsis by putting fecal material into the child's intravenous line are examples of the horrifying nature of the syndrome.
   d. Another common presentation is when the mother simulates an illness but has not actually done anything directly to the child to cause harm. Examples include putting drops of her own blood in her child's urine or contaminating the specimen.

3. Management
   a. Medical management
      (1) Provide safety to the child and protection from further harm. Keep the child in the hospital under constant staff observation.
      (2) Review medical history in detail, and review complaints that may have been fabricated from old records, especially if presented by perpetrator.
   b. Psychiatric management
      (1) Establish an alliance with the mother or other responsible caregiver.
      (2) Use direct confrontation, indicating the inaccuracies in symptoms and possible diagnoses/laboratory findings.
      (3) Provide supportive psychotherapy for the caregiver.

22.14 Suicide

1. Definitions
   a. Suicide attempt: An act of nonfatal self-injury with intention to harm or seek attention
   b. Suicide: An intention to injure oneself resulting in death
   c. Suicidal ideation: Having the idea or wish to die, with/without a plan; but not yet initiating an attempt to harm oneself

2. Epidemiology
   a. Suicide is the second leading cause of death in persons 15 to 24 years of age.
   b. The mortality rate is 13.1 per 100,000 in this age group, accounting for 18.8% of all deaths.
   c. Suicide is uncommon in children younger than 12 years of age but does occur, with more boys than girls attempting and completing suicide.
   d. The male-to-female ratio of attempted suicide in adolescents older than 12 years of age is 1:3.

3. Methods of suicide and attempted suicide
   a. Suicide attempts: Nearly 90% of adolescent attempts are by self-poisoning with tablets, and the remaining balance by gas, poisons,

cutting, hanging, drowning, and shooting. Boys are more than twice as likely to choose active methods (firearms) than girls; girls are more likely to attempt suicide by ingestion of lethal substances.

b. Suicide: The most common method of death in adolescents is firearms, followed by hanging and suffocation, gas poisoning, and drug ingestion, and then by all other methods. Among completed suicides, 20% of boys and 30% of girls have a history of a previous attempt. The risk of death is greatest in adolescents who make attempts by active methods, but the choice of methods does not predict future attempts.

4. Clinical features: The following are considered risk factors for suicidal behavior:
   a. Male sex
   b. Increasing age or advanced pubertal development
   c. Major psychiatric disorder (depression, psychosis)
   d. Substance abuse
   e. Attempt made without likelihood of discovery
   f. Repeated attempts or attempts becoming more frequent
   g. Attempts by "active" methods (e.g., guns, hanging, cutting) with known lethality
   h. Declaration of still wanting to die
   i. Family history of suicidal behavior or affective illness
   j. History of violent or aggressive behavior
   k. Poor social support (including runaway and homeless youth)
   l. Precipitating factors such as crisis in the home and a discrepancy between family and adolescent expectations
   m. Changes in behavior or thoughts, such as "There's nothing to look forward to"; "Others will be better without me"; and "I am just a burden to you."

5. Evaluation
   a. Every child or adolescent who makes a suicide attempt, no matter how trivial, should receive a psychiatric evaluation before discharge from the emergency department (preferably by a child psychiatrist).
   b. The child should not be discharged from the emergency department until a parent or primary care provider has been interviewed. No effective treatment plan can be formulated without the parents' participation.
   c. Start the interview by asking, "What happened?" rather than "Why did you do it?" Then proceed with a review of the entire day's events, especially any arguments or disappointments and determine the following: when they first thought about killing themselves; did they tell anyone about these thoughts; how much planning was involved; who discovered the attempt and how; what does the child know about the lethality of the method; did the child write a note or give belongings away.
   d. Uncover any medical or psychiatric problems. Adolescent suicide attempters have high rates of medical illness and are more likely to have a major mental illness, especially depression, conduct disorder, and substance abuse.
   e. Assess family dysfunction (marital conflict and parent–child conflict) and family psychiatric history.

6. Management
   a. Treatment is directed first at saving life, then at finding the cause of the attempt and treating underlying psychopathology (e.g., depression).
   b. Hospitalization: A suicide attempt is almost always a reason to admit a child/adolescent to the hospital, even if only for observation.
   c. When outpatient treatment will be provided, a specific plan should be formulated before the family leaves the emergency department. Forty to 60% of patients do not keep outpatient treatment recommendations. A crisis-oriented approach has been shown to increase compliance. This includes giving a specific follow-up appointment within a few days of the attempt, with the name of the person who will see them. Also, an explanation of why follow-up is important and what problems will be addressed should be given.

22.15 Death and Dying in Children and Adolescents

1. Children's concept of death
   a. Children up to 5 years of age have virtually no concept of death. Magical thinking and egocentricity lead them to believe that they have caused the death, with consequent guilt. From 2 to 3 years, children have no understanding of death but are anxious about the separation. From 4 to 5 years, they interpret death as a long sleep or a long reversible journey. Children believe that the dead can sleep and play in heaven or underground.
   b. Children between 5 and 10 years of age begin to clarify their concept of death but are sometimes still confused ("When I die, my heart stops, I can't see, and I can't hear; but if I'm buried, how will I breathe?"). Children do not understand the universality of death.
   c. Children between 10 and 15 years of age understand the meaning of mortality. Reactions to death are mostly influenced by emotional struggles rather than intellectual capacities. They view death as a punishment for bad behavior.
2. Reactions of others to a child's death
   a. Parents usually experience an initial state of shock and denial, followed by anger ("Why my child?"), guilt ("If only I had..."), or bargaining ("If he could only live to..."). This stage is followed by normal grieving and mourning over the loss and the beginning of separation. Finally, a stage of resignation or acceptance can be reached.
   b. Perinatal or early infant deaths often produce severe distress in the parents, with difficulty in accepting that the infant is dead and recurrent thoughts about the dead child. Mourning may occur up to a year, with both parents becoming depressed and possibly experiencing marital problems.
   c. The death of a child from sudden infant death syndrome or other causes of unexpected or abrupt death produces sudden, severe grief, guilt, and bewilderment. Siblings of the dead infant/child may feel guilty and fear that they too might die.
      (1) After rapid death, parents may feel anger, which may be displaced to the physician. Mourning will include some identification with the lost person and over-idealization of the lost one.

(2) Additional reactions might include displacing attitudes toward the dead child onto the surviving children, filling the loss with another pregnancy, and emotionally withdrawing.

d. Prolonged dying: Premature mourning may occur with anticipatory grief and withdrawal of interest in the dying child. Unacceptable thoughts may arise, such as wishing the child could finally die and relieve everyone of the emotional and financial burden.

e. Siblings younger than 5 years of age feel a loss of love. They may view the death as an abandonment, punishment, or realization of unacceptable wishes. Siblings between 5 and 10 years of age are more concerned about the dying child and may also be fearful for themselves. Children may act up in response to parental withdrawal.

22.16 Indications for Hospitalization

1. The major criteria for hospitalization and commitment: danger to self; or danger to others; or unable to care for self
2. Hospitalization guidelines: The following is a compilation of guidelines from several psychiatric organizations and does not represent a set of hard-and-fast rules:
   a. Self-defeating or self-destructive behavior
   b. Inability to function in family life
   c. Highly disturbed family situation that puts the child at substantial risk
   d. A disorder of the child's cognitive, volitional, or emotional processes that grossly impairs judgment or the capacity to recognize reality or control behavior
   e. Acute disabling symptoms of mental illness, such as impaired reality testing, disordered or bizarre behavior, or psychotic organic brain symptoms, that require continuous skilled observation not possible on an outpatient basis
   f. Acute danger to property or to self or others (including suicidal or homicidal ideation, gestures, and attempts)
   g. Severely impaired social, family, educational, vocational, or developmental functioning that is unaffected by outpatient treatment or removal from home
   h. Severe physical or sexual abuse
   i. Psychosomatic or somatopsychic disorders that have become life-threatening

22.17 Pediatric Psychopharmacology

1. General principles and guidelines (Tables 22-1 to 22-9 and Box 22-1)
   a. The clinician needs to arrive at an accurate diagnosis using a multiaxial diagnostic evaluation based on DSM-IV-TR criteria before prescribing any medication. The clinician might be faced with different comorbid disorders (i.e., ADHD and mood disorders) that make careful definition and prioritization of target symptoms more complex tasks.
   b. Consultation with a child psychiatrist is often needed.
   c. The use of psychotropic medication should follow a detailed psychiatric, medical, social, cognitive, and educational evaluation of the child and the child's family.

d. Before starting treatment with a psychotropic medication, the clinician must discuss with the family and child the diagnostic findings, risks and benefits of using a particular psychotropic medication, short- and long-term adverse effects, and the availability of alternative treatments.

e. It is important for clinicians to document risks and potential benefits as well as obtain informed consent especially if they use medications not specifically addressed in the FDA guidelines (i.e., "off-label").

f. Treatment should start at the lowest possible dose and may be increased if target symptoms persist and no side effects appear. When tapering medications that can cause withdrawal reactions, it is important to discontinue medications gradually.

g. Specific current FDA treatment and follow-up recommendations for SSRIs include

(1) First 4 weeks of treatment with SSRI antidepressants: Patients should be followed weekly (in person or by telephone) to monitor severity of depression, response to treatment, and possible emergence of side effects (including suicidal ideation, self-harming behavior).

(2) Weeks 5 to 8 of treatment with SSRI antidepressants: Patients should be followed at least biweekly (preferably in person) to monitor severity of depression, response to treatment, and possible emergence of side effects.

(3) For continuing treatment (third month and beyond) with SSRI antidepressants, patients should be followed at least monthly (in person) to monitor severity of depression, response to treatment, and possible emergence of side effects.

(4) When adjusting doses (higher or lower) of SSRI antidepressants, patients should be followed weekly (in person or by telephone) to monitor severity of depression, response to treatment, and possible emergence of side effects during the first month.

REFERENCES

1. Farrington CP, Miller E, Taylor B: MMR and autism: Further evidence against a causal association. Vaccine 19:3632-3635, 2001.
2. Halsey NA, Hyman SL, Conference Writing Panel: Measles-mumps-rubella vaccine and autistic spectrum disorder: Report from the New Challenges in Childhood Immunizations Conference convened in Oak Brook, Illinois, June 12-13, 2000. Pediatrics 107:E84, 2001.
3. Taylor BMF, Farrington CP, Petropoulos M-C, et al: Autism and measles, mumps and rubella vaccine: No epidemiological evidence for a causal association. Lancet 353:2026-2029, 1999.

SUGGESTED READING

American Psychiatric Association: Diagnostic and Statistical Manual of Mental Disorders, 4th ed., text revision Washington, DC, American Psychiatric Publishing, 2000.
Brazelton TB: Crying in infancy. Pediatrics 29:579-588, 1962.
Ferber R, Kruger M: Principles and Practice of Sleep Medicine in the Child. Philadelphia, WB Saunders, 1992.
Levine MD, Carey WB, Crocker AC (eds): Developmental-Behavioral Pediatrics. Philadelphia, WB Saunders, 1983.
Lewis M (ed): Child and Adolescent Psychiatry: A Comprehensive Textbook, 3rd ed. Philadelphia, Lippincott Williams & Wilkins, 2002.
Rushton HG: Wetting and functional voiding disorders. Urol Clin North Am 22: 75-93, 1995.

22—Behavioral Disorders

Wessel MA, Cobb SC, Jackson EB, et al: Paroxysmal fussing in infancy: Sometimes called "colic." Pediatrics 14:421-434, 1954.

Wiener JM, Dulcan MK (eds): The American Psychiatric Publishing Textbook of Child and Adolescent Psychiatry, 3rd ed. Washington, DC, American Psychiatric Publishing, 2004.

WEBSITES

Autism Speaks: www.autismspeaks.org/index.php

National Institutes of Health Autism Guide: www.nimh.nih.gov

National Institute of Mental Health: www.nimh.nih.gov/publicat/schizkids.cfm

---

Box 22-1   Abbreviations Used in Psychopharmacology Tables

5-HT—serotonin (5-hydroxytryptamine)

ADHD—attention deficit hyperactivity disorder

ANC—absolute neutrophil count

MDD—major depressive disorder

bid—twice daily

BP—blood pressure

BUN—blood urea nitrogen

CBC w/diff—complete blood count with differential

Cr—creatinine

DA—dopamine

ECG—electrocardiogram

EPS—extrapyramidal symptoms

FDA—U.S. Food and Drug Administration

GABA—gamma-aminobutyric acid

GAD—generalized anxiety disorder

GI—gastrointestinal

hCG—human chorionic gonadotropin

IM—intramuscularly

IR—immediate release

IV—intravenously

LA—long acting

LFTs—liver function tests

MAOIs—monoamine oxidase inhibitors

MDD—major depressive disorder

NE—norepinephrine

NMS—neuroleptic malignant syndrome

NSAIDs—nonsteroidal anti-inflammatory drugs

OCD—obsessive-compulsive disorder

CPK—creatine phosphokinase

ODT—orally disintegrating tablets

PDD—pervasive developmental disorder

PMDD—premenstrual dysphoric disorder

PO—orally

PR—rectally

prn—as needed

PTSD—post-traumatic stress disorder

qam—every morning

qd—every day

qhs—every bedtime

qid—four times daily

qmo—every month

qwk—every week

SAD—social anxiety disorder

SR—sustained release

SSRIs—selective serotonin reuptake inhibitors

TCAs—tricyclic antidepressants

TFTs—thyroid function tests

tid—three times daily

U/A—urinalysis

VPA—valproic acid

WBC—white blood cell count

XL/XR—extended release

Drug	Brand Name/ Preparations	Dosing	Main Indications	Pharma-cokinetics	Mechanism of Action	Additional Comments/ Adverse Effects and Monitoring*
Dextro-amphetamine	**Dexedrine** 5 mg SR: 5, 10, 15 mg	**3-6 yr:** **Start:** 2.5 mg qd (0.3-1.5 mg/kg) **Increase:** 2.5 mg/ day qwk **>6 yr:** **Start:** 5 mg qd/bid **Increase:** 5 mg/ day qwk **Max:** 40 mg/day	ADHD	Onset: 30-60 min Duration: 3-6 hr	DA presynaptic release and blockade	Insomnia, decreased appetite, weight loss, depression, psychosis (rare, with very high doses) Increase in heart rate and BP (mild) Possible reduction in growth velocity with long-term use (baseline and periodic monitoring of growth recommended)
Dextro-amphetamine sulfate	**Adderall** 5, 7.5, 10, 12.5, 15, 20, 30 mg	**3-5 yr:** **Start:** 2.5 mg qam **Increase:** 2.5 mg/day qwk **>6 yr:** **Start:** 5 mg qam or bid **Increase:** 5 mg/ day qwk **Max:** 40 mg/day	ADHD	Onset: 60 min Duration: 6-8 hr	DA and norepinephrine presynaptic release and blockade	Withdrawal effects and rebound phenomena Tic disorders (rare) and psychosis (even rarer) Infrequent: headaches, dizziness, irritability, abdominal discomfort, lethargy, and fatigue

Cont'd

*The adverse effects apply to *all* stimulants.
See Box 22-1 for list of abbreviations.

Drug	Brand Name/ Preparations	Dosing	Main Indications	Pharma-cokinetics	Mechanism of Action	Additional Comments/ Adverse Effects and Monitoring*
						May lower seizure threshold Irritability that occurs 1-2 hr after dosing may indicate excessive dosing
Dextro-amphetamine saccharate	Adderall XR 5, 10, 15, 20, 25, 30 mg	>6 yr: Start: 5-10 mg qam Increase: 5-10 mg/day qwk Max: 30 mg/day	ADHD	Onset: 2-3 hr Duration: 12 hr	DA and norepinephrine presynaptic release and blockade	Capsule for Dextroamphetamine saccharate: Contents can be sprinkled on applesauce, but should be swallowed immediately without chewing
Methylphenidate	Ritalin 5, 10, 20 mg	>6 yr: Start: 0.3 mg/kg bid or 2.5-5 mg bid Increase: 0.1 mg/ kg/dose or 5-10 mg/day qwk Max: 60 mg/day	ADHD Adjunct treatment in refractory depression	Onset: 30-60 min Duration: 2-5 hr	DA and norepinephrine presynaptic release and blockade	

*The adverse effects apply to *all* stimulants. See Box 22-1 for list of abbreviations.

Methylphenidate (con't)	Ritalin SR 20 mg	>6 yr: Start: 20 mg qam Increase: 20 mg/day qwk Max: 60 mg/day	ADHD Adjunct treatment in refractory depression	Duration: 4-8 hr	As above	
	Ritalin LA 10, 20, 30, 40 mg	>6 yr: Start: 20 mg qam Increase: 10 mg/day qwk Max: 60 mg/day	ADHD Adjunct treatment in refractory depression	Duration: 8 hr	As above	
	Concerta 18, 27, 36, 54 mg	6-13 yr: Start: 18 mg qam Increase: 18 mg/day qam Max: 6-12 yr: 54 mg/day >12 yr: 72 mg/day	ADHD	Duration: 8-12 hr	As above	Concerta: Do not cut, crush, or chew— capsule is a mechanical device that pushes out medicine over time. It is not digested – patients/family will see capsule in feces.
	Daytrana patch 10, 15, 20, 30 mg	>6 yr: Start: 10 mg on for 9 hr, 15 hours between patches Increase dose each week by 10 mg Max: 30 mg on for 9 hr	ADHD	Duration: 9 hr	As above	Daytrana: Transdermal delivery. Apply to hip area 2 hr before effect is desired Remove 9 hr after application or sooner as needed

Cont'd

*The adverse effects apply to *all* stimulants.
See Box 22-1 for list of abbreviations.

22—Behavioral Disorders

Drug	Brand Name/ Preparations	Dosing	Main Indications	Pharma-cokinetics	Mechanism of Action	Additional Comments/ Adverse Effects and Monitoring
Atomoxetine HCl	**Strattera** 10, 18, 25, 40, 60 mg caps	**≤70 kg:** **Start:** 0.5 mg/kg/ day qam **Increase:** 1.2 mg/ kg/day qam **Max:** 1.4 mg/kg/ day qam **>70 kg:** **Start:** 20–40 mg qam **Increase:** 80 mg qam **Max:** 100 mg/d	ADHD	Duration: 8–12 hr	Selective NE reuptake inhibitor Not a stimulant; only non-class II FDA approved drug for ADHD	Atomoxetine HCl: Give once daily in AM or two evenly divided doses Not the same abuse potential as other stimulants Similar side effects to antidepressants (non-TCA)

*The adverse effects apply to *all* stimulants.
See Box 22-1 for list of abbreviations.

Drug	Brand Name/ Preparations	Dosing	Main Indications	Mechanism of Action	Additional Comments/ Adverse Effects and Monitoring*
Imipramine	**Tofranil** 10, 25, 50 mg	**6-12 yr:** **Range:** 1-3 mg/kg/ day ÷ tid **Start:** 1.5 mg/kg/ day ÷ tid **Increase:** 1-1.5 mg/ kg/day q3-4d **Max:** 5 mg/kg/day **>12 yr:** **Range:** 25-75 mg/ day ÷ qd-tid **Start:** 30-40 mg/day ÷ qd-tid **Increase:** 10-25 mg/ day q3-4d **Max:** 100 mg/day	Enuresis, ADHD, tic disorders, anxiety disorders, MDD	NE and DA presynaptic reuptake blockade (NE > DA)	Baseline ECG and serial ECGs throughout treatment are recommended Cardiovascular: changes in BP and ECG conduction with daily doses >3.5 mg/kg (1.0 mg/kg for nortriptyline) Anticholinergic: dry mouth, constipation, blurred vision Weight gain Withdrawal effects can occur and include severe GI symptoms, malaise Overdoses can be fatal Slightly increased risk of sudden death associated with the use of desipramine.
Desipramine†	**Norpramin** 10, 25, 50, 75, 100, 150 mg	**Range:** 100-200 mg qd **Start:** 25-75 mg qd **Increase:** 20%-30% q5d **Max:** 300 mg/day	MDD, enuresis	Anticholinergic, antihistamine, α_2 postsynaptic effects	

Cont'd

†Dosing guidelines based on adult recommendations, not defined for pediatric population.
*Comments and adverse effects apply to all tricyclic antidepressants.
See Box 22-1 for list of abbreviations.

Drug	Brand Name/ Preparations	Dosing	Main Indications	Mechanism of Action	Additional Comments/ Adverse Effects and Monitoring
Nortriptyline	Pamelor 10, 25, 50, 75 mg 10 mg/5 mL Aventyl HCl 10 mg/5 mL	Start: 6-12 yr: 1-3 mg/kg/ day ÷ tid-qid >12 yr: 30-50 mg/day ÷ qd-qid Max: 150 mg/day ÷ tid-bid Dose adjusted according to serum levels; therapeutic window 50-150 ng/m	ADHD, tic disorders, anxiety disorders	NE/5-HT reuptake blockade	Baseline ECG and serial ECGs throughout treatment are recommended Cardiovascular: changes in BP and ECG conduction with daily doses >3.5 mg/kg (1.0 mg/kg for nortriptyline) Anticholinergic: dry mouth, constipation, blurred vision Weight gain Withdrawal effects can occur and include severe GI symptoms, malaise Overdoses can be fatal Slightly increased risk of sudden death associated with the use of desipramine.
Clomipramine	Anafranil 25, 50, 75 mg	>10 yr: Range: 100-200 mg qhs (or ÷ bid) Start: 25 mg qd Increase: 25 mg/ day q4-7d Max: 3 mg/kg/day up to 100 mg/day in first 2 wk, up to 200 mg/day maintenance	OCD, trichotillomania	Same as other TCAs, 5-HT presynaptic reuptake blockade	

Drug	Brand Name/ Preparations	Dosing	Main Indications	Pharmacokinetics	Adverse Effects*	Additional Comments*
Fluoxetine	**Prozac** 10, 20, 40 mg 20 mg/5 mL	**Start:** 5-10 mg qd ×7 days **Increase:** 5-10 mg qd **Max:** 80 mg qd **Range:** 20-60 mg qd (higher range for OCD) (lower weight: slower titration, max 20-30 mg/ day)	OCD, MDD, bulimia nervosa, PMDD, panic disorder	Half-life (fluoxetine + active metabolite): 4-16 days	Worsening depression/ suicidality Activation/ agitation Anxiety Akathisia Hypomania/ mania Apathy Insomnia/ drowsiness	*Response to SSRIs in depressed patients: Onset: ≥2 wk (often ≥3 wk) at minimum effective dose Peak (MDD): Minimum 4-6 wk*
Sertraline	**Zoloft** 25, 50, 100 mg 20 mg/mL	**Start:** 25 mg qd **Increase:** 25-50 mg/day qwk **Max:** 200 mg/day	OCD, MDD, panic disorder, PTSD, PMDD, SAD	Half-life: 26 hr	GI symptoms Changes in weight/ appetite Headaches	Patients should try taking medication in the morning in case it prevents them from sleeping.

*Comments and adverse effects apply to all antidepressants.

Drug	Brand Name/ Preparations	Dosing	Main Indications	Pharmacokinetics	Adverse Effects*	Additional Comments*
Paroxetine	**Paxil** 10, 20, 30, 40 mg 10 mg/5 mL	**Start:** 10 mg qd **Increase:** 10 mg/ day q1-2wk **Max:** 60 mg/day	OCD, MDD, panic disorder, SAD, GAD, PTSD	Half-life: 24 hr	Discontinuation syndrome (dizziness, paresthesias, nausea, headache)—gradual titration, especially for Paxil	If the patient feels more tired during the day, try nighttime dose. Caution with switch to/from MAOIs (serotonin syndrome).

Fluvoxamine	**Luvox** 25, 50, 100 mg	**Start:** 25 mg qhs **Increase:** 25 mg q4-7d **Max:** <11 yr: 200 mg ÷ qd-bid >11 yr: 300 mg ÷ qd-bid	OCD	Half-life: 17-22 hr	Mechanism of Action for all SSRIs: Selectively inhibits serotonin presynaptic reuptake
Citalopram†	**Celexa** 10, 20, 40 mg 10 mg/5 mL	**Start:** 10 mg qd **Increase:** 10 mg/day qwk **Max:** 60 mg/day	MDD	Half-life: 35 hours	
Escitalopram†	**Lexapro** 5, 10, 20 mg 5 mg/5 mL	**Start:** 10 mg qd **Increase:** 10 mg/day after 1 wk **Max:** 20 mg/day	MDD, GAD	Half-life: 22-32 hr	

*Comments and adverse effects apply to all antidepressants.
†Dosing guidelines based on adult recommendations, not defined for pediatric population.
See Box 22-1 for list of abbreviations.

Drug	Brand Name/ Preparations	Dosing	Main Indications	Pharmaco-kinetics	Mechanism of Action	Adverse Effects
Bupropion	**Wellbutrin** 75, 100 mg	**Range:** 150 mg bid-tid **Start:** 75 mg qam **Increase:** 75 mg after 3 days **Max:** 150 mg tid	MDD, ADHD (second-line option for ADHD)		NE/DA presynaptic reuptake blockade	Irritability Insomnia Drug-induced seizures (in doses >6 mg/kg or 450 mg/day) Contraindications: history of bulimia, head trauma, seizures May exacerbate tic disorders *Note:* do not give second dose after 2 PM because of insomnia
	Wellbutrin SR 100, 150, 200 mg	**Range:** 150 mg bid **Start:** 150 mg qam **Increase:** 150 mg after 3 days **Max:** 200 mg bid	As above		As above	
	Wellbutrin XL 150, 300 mg	**Range:** 300 mg qam **Start:** 150 mg qam **Increase:** to 300 mg after 4 days **Max:** 450 mg qam	As above		As above	

| Trazodone | **Desyrel** 50, 100, 150, 300 mg | **Range:** 25-75 mg qhs **Start:** 12.5-25 mg **Max:** 12-18 yr: 150 mg 6-12 yr: 6 mg/kg qhs | MDD, ADHD (second-line option for ADHD) | Peak: 1-2 hr Duration: 4-9 hr | 5-HT presynaptic reuptake blockade/ 5-HT2A postsynaptic antagonism | Orthostatic hypotension Dizziness Priapism (rare) Sedation Nausea Constipation |
| Mirtazapine | **Remeron** 15, 30, 45 mg | **Range:** 15-45 mg qhs **Start:** 7.5 mg qhs | MDD Insomnia | Peak: 2 hr | 5-HT presynaptic reuptake blockade/ 5-HT2A postsynaptic antagonism | Drowsiness Weight gain |

Cont'd

Table 22-4 Antidepressants: Other—cont'd

Drug	Brand Name/ Preparations	Dosing	Main Indications	Pharmaco- kinetics	Mechanism of Action	Adverse Effects
Venlafaxine	**Effexor** 25, 37.5, 50, 75, 100 mg **Effexor XR** 37.5, 75, 150 mg (SR)	**IR:** **Range:** 150 mg bid **Start:** 37.5 mg qam **Increase:** 37.5 mg q4d **Max:** 375 mg/day **XR:** **Range:** 150 mg qd **Start:** 37.5 mg qd **Increase:** 37.5 mg/ day q4-7d **Max:** 225 mg/day	MDD		5-HT/NE presynaptic blockade	Elevated BP at higher doses Nausea Drowsiness Activation Headache Dizziness

See Box 22-1 for list of abbreviations.

Table 22-5   Alpha Agonists*

Drug	Brand Name/Preparations	Dosing	Main Indications	Pharma-cokinetics	Mechanism of Action	Adverse Effects	Additional Comments
Clonidine	**Catapres tab:** 0.025, 0.1, 0.2, 0.3 mg **Patch:** 0.1, 0.2, 0.3 mg	**Range:** 0.05-0.4 mg/day ÷ tid-qid **Start:** 0.05 mg qd **Increase:** 0.05 mg/day q3-5d **Max:** 0.4-0.5 mg/day Transdermal: dose qd	Tourette's syndrome, ADHD, PTSD, aggression/self-abuse, severe agitation, withdrawal syndromes	Onset: 30-60 min Half-life: 6-20 hr Peak: 3-5 hr	Nonspecific alpha₂ presynaptic agonist	Sedation (very common) Hypotension Bradycardia Dry mouth Confusion (with high dose) Depression Rebound hypertension with abrupt withdrawal Localized irritation with transdermal preparation	Coadministration of clonidine and beta blockers should be avoided Transdermal absorption can be erratic Use with caution in combination with methylphenidate (sudden death has been reported in a few cases using this combination) Transdermal: may need to increase dose; cutting patch size useful in adjusting dose Monitor BP

Cont'd

*No current FDA-established indications for initiating and maintaining treatment in child psychiatric disorders. These medications should be started and titrated under the supervision of a psychiatrist or neurologist. Dosing guidelines based on adult recommendations.
See Box 22-1 for list of abbreviations.

Table 22-5 Alpha Agonists—cont'd

Drug	Brand Name/ Preparations	Dosing	Main Indications	Pharma-cokinetics	Mechanism of Action	Adverse Effects	Additional Comments
Guanfacine	Tenex 1, 2 mg	**Range:** 0.5-4 mg/day ÷ bid-qid (0.09 mg/kg/day) **Start:** 0.5 mg/day **Increase:** 0.5 mg/day q3d **Max:** 4 mg/day	Tourette's syndrome, ADHD, PTSD	Onset: 2 hr Half-life: 13-14 hr Peak: 1-4 hr	Selective alpha$_2$ agonist	Sedation (less than clonidine) Hypotension (rare) Bradycardia (rare) Dry mouth Confusion Depression Rebound hypertension with abrupt withdrawal (can occur up to 4 days after d/c)	Longer duration of action than clonidine Monitor BP

| Propranolol | **Inderal** 10, 20, 40, 60, 80, 120 mg **Inderal LA** 60, 80, 120, 160 mg | **Range:** 0.5–1.0 mg/kg/day q6-8hr **Max:** 120 mg/day | Akathisia, PTSD, aggression/ self-abuse in MR/PDD, severe agitation, stage/ presentation anxiety | Postsynaptic beta blocker | High risk for bradycardia and hypotension (dose dependent) and rebound hypertension Bronchospasm (contrain-dicated in asthmatics) Nausea, vomiting Depression Allergic reactions | Monitor BP and ECG at baseline and q1-3mo |

Table 22-6 Mood Stabilizers

Drug	Brand Name/ Preparations	Dosing	Main Indications	Mechanism of Action/ Pharmacokinetics	Adverse Effects	Additional Comments/ Monitoring
Lithium	**IR:** **Lithium** 150, 300, 600 mg, 300 mg/5 mL **Eskalith** 300 mg **CR:** **Eskalith CR** 450 mg **SR:** **Lithobid SR** 300 mg	**2-11 yr:** **Start (IR + SR):** 15-60 mg/ kg/day ÷ bid-tid (or 150 mg bid-tid) **Max:** 2.4 g/day or 900 mg SR bid **>12 yr:** **Range:** 600-1200 mg/day ÷ bid-tid **Start:** IR: 300 mg qhs SR: 15-60 mg/ kg/day ÷ bid-tid **Max:** IR: 1800 mg/day SR: 900 mg bid	Bipolar disorder Mania Prophylaxis of bipolar disorder Adjunct treatment in refractory MDD Aggressive behavior Conduct disorder	Inhibition of phosphatidyl inositol and protein kinase C signaling pathways Enhancement of serotonergic transmission Half-life: 18-30 hr	Polyuria/nocturia, polydipsia, tremors, nausea, diarrhea, weight gain, drowsiness, skin abnormalities, hair loss Possible effects on thyroid (hypothyroidism) and renal functioning with long-term administration Toxicity (level >2 mEq/L) can be life-threatening and presents with nausea, vomiting, ataxia, slurred speech, blurry vision	**Laboratory studies:** CBC, BUN, Cr, U/A, TFTs, ECG Frequency: Baseline and q3-6 months **Therapeutic plasma levels:** 0.6-1.2 mEq/L Steady state takes 5-7 days to reach each time dose is changed Draw blood 12 hr after last dose **Monitoring plasma level:** First draw: 5 days after starting therapy, or increasing dose **Do not cut, crush or chew CR or SR**

| | | | | | Dehydration may cause acute lithium toxicity in children Drug interactions are very common: avoid NSAIDs | Ther: once desired blood level reached qwk X two weeks q1-2 months x 2-3 draws Thereafter: q6 months NOTE: Over time, growth and renal function may influence blood levels; make dosage changes based on clinical presentation. |
| Valproic acid | **IR:** Depakote 125, 250, 500 mg Depakene 250 mg, 250 mg/5 mL **Depakote Sprinkles** 125 mg **SR:** **Depakote ER** 250, 500 mg | **Range:** **<12 yr:** 1000-1200 mg/day ÷ bid-tid **>12 yr:** 1000-2500 mg/day ÷ bid-tid **Start:** 10-15 mg/kg/day ÷ bid-tid (qd for SR/ER) **Increase:** 5-10 mg/kg/day q4-7d | Absence seizures Bipolar disorder Aggressive behavior Conduct disorder | Inhibition of catabolic enzymes of GABA and of protein kinase C signaling Half-life: 8-16 hr | Sedation, nausea, alopecia, weight gain Liver toxicity: risk of hepatic involvement increased with age <2 yr and use of other antiseizure meds Bone marrow suppression Pancreatitis | **Laboratory studies:** CBC, LFTs, coagulation Frequency: baseline, qmo x2, then q4-6mo **Therapeutic plasma levels:** 50-125 µg/mL Steady state takes 5 days to reach after each change in dose |

Cont'd

Table 22-6 Mood Stabilizers—cont'd

Drug	Brand Name/ Preparations	Dosing	Main Indications	Mechanism of Action/ Pharmacokinetics	Adverse Effects	Additional Comments/ Monitoring
		Max: 60 mg/kg/ day *Note:* take w/ food; may open capsule but do not chew beads			Polycystic ovaries may be associated with long-term use Associated with neural tube defects in pregnancy Toxicity presents with drowsiness, weakness, lack of coordination, confusion	Draw blood 8-12 hr after last dose (any time for SR/ER) **Monitoring plasma level:** First draw: 5 days after starting therapy, or increasing dose Titration: increase dose q4-7d and check blood level each week until desired clinical and blood level reached Then: q4-6mo once desired blood level reached
Carbamazepine*	**IR:** **Tegretol** 100 (chewable), 200 mg, 100 mg/5 mL	**<6 yr:** **Range:** 10-20 mg/kg/day (200-600 mg/ day) ÷ bid-qid	Complex partial seizures Bipolar disorder	Inhibition of glial cell steroidogenesis Inhibition of alpha$_2$ receptors Blocks Na channels	Bone marrow suppression Dizziness, drowsiness, rashes, nausea	**Laboratory studies:** CBC w/diff/ platelets, LFTs, BUN/Cr, hCG (girls), TFTs, U/A

SR:
Tegretol XR
100, 200,
400 mg
Carbatrol
100, 200,
300 mg

Blocks glial
cell Ca
influx
Half-life:
13-17 hr

Max: 35 mg/
kg/day
6-11 yrs:
Range: 400-800
mg/day ÷
bid-qid
Max: 1000 mg/
day
>12 yr:
Range: 800-
1200 mg/day
÷ bid-qid
Max 1200 mg/
day
Note: Take with
food
Suspension:
divide dose qid
Dosing based on
seizure
prophylaxis

Liver toxicity
(especially <10 yr)
Skin disorders;
**Stevens-
Johnson
syndrome**
Neural tube defects
in pregnancy
Toxicity associated
with drowsiness,
nausea,
vomiting, ataxia,
nystagmus,
confusion and
seizures

Frequency: qmo ×3,
than q3-6mo
**Therapeutic plasma
levels:** 4-12 µg/mL
**Monitoring plasma
level:**
First draw 4 days after
starting therapy
Then: each week until
stable, then q3-6mo
Patient/family should
monitor for easy
bruisability, fever
Autoinduction occurs
during first 3-5 wk
(Tegretol induces
its own metabolism,
so levels can be
lower during initial
treatment. Dose
and plasma level
must be monitored
during this time.)
Must be aware of
interactions with
many other
medications
**Oral contraceptives
may lose
effectiveness**

Cont'd

Table 22-6 Mood Stabilizers—cont'd

Drug	Brand Name/ Preparations	Dosing	Main Indications	Mechanism of Action/ Pharmacokinetics	Adverse Effects	Additional Comments/ Monitoring
Oxcarbazepine*	**Trileptal** 150, 300, 600 mg 300 mg/5 mL	**Range:** 300-900 mg bid	Partial seizures Bipolar disorder	Blocks voltage-sensitive Na channels Stabilizes neural membranes and inhibits repetitive firing Decreases synaptic impulse propagation Half-life: Parent compound: 1-2.5 hr Metabolites: 8-11 hr	**Stevens-Johnson syndrome and toxic epidermal necrolysis** Hyponatremia Hyperthermia Leukopenia Thrombocytopenia Dizziness, somnolence, diplopia, fatigue, nausea, vomiting	Caution if hypersensitivity to carbamazepine Oral contraceptives may lose effectiveness Monitor thyroid function

| Lamotrigine* | Lamictal* 25, 100, 150, 200 mg | Range: 75-200 mg qd Max: 200 mg/day | Bipolar disorder Lennox-Gastaut seizures Partial seizures | Weak 5-HT3 inhibition Release of aspartate and glutamate (possibly) Half-life: 32 hr | Stevens-Johnson syndrome Pancytopenia Dizziness, ataxia, somnolence, headache, blurred vision, nausea, vomiting | **Rash:** Very gradual titration reduces risk of rash Increased risk of rash with concurrent use of VPA Lamictal dose must be adjusted Higher risk of rash in younger children **Monitor:** Laboratory studies at baseline: CBC, LFTs Advantage of Lamictal is no therapeutic plasma level monitoring |
| Topiramate* | Topamax 25, 50, 100, 200 mg 15, 25 mg (sprinkles) | Range: 50-200 mg bid Max: 200 mg bid | Bipolar disorder Partial seizures Lennox-Gastaut seizures Generalized seizures | Glutamate release antagonist GABA reuptake inhibitor Half-life: 18-24 hr | Cognitive difficulties Dizziness Sedation Weight loss | Weight loss may be beneficial side effect **Decreases oral contraceptive levels** |

*For these medications, there are no current FDA-established indications for initiating and maintaining treatment as a mood stabilizer in child psychiatric disorders. These medications should be started and titrated under the supervision of a psychiatrist or neurologist.
See Box 22-1 for list of abbreviations

Table 22-7 Antianxiety Drugs: Benzodiazepines

Drug (Duration of Action)	Brand Name/ Preparations	Dosing	Main Indications	Pharmacokinetics	Mechanism of Action	Adverse Effects^a
Alprazolam*† (Shortest-acting)	**Xanax** 0.25, 0.5, 1, 2 mg 1 mg/mL **SR: Xanax XR** 0.5, 1, 2, 3 mg	**Range: 0.25-0.5 mg** qd-tid **Max: 3.5 mg/day** Do not cut/crush/chew SR form	Anxiety disorders Adjunct treatment in refractory psychosis and in mania Severe agitation Severe insomnia Tourette's syndrome MDD	**Onset:** 1-1.5 hr **IR:** Half-life: 9-20 hr Peak: 1-2 hr **XR:** Half life: 11-16 hr Peak: 5-11 hr	Enhancement of GABA transmission by binding to unique benzodiazepine site within the GABAa receptor	Drowsiness Disinhibition Paradoxical agitation Confusion Depression Highest risk for rebound and withdrawal reactions Potential risk for abuse and dependence
Clonazepam*† (long-acting)	**Klonopin Tab:** 0.5, 1, 2 mg **Wafers:** 0.125, 0.25, 0.5, 1, 2 mg	**<10 yr or <30 kg: Start:** 0.01-0.03 mg/kg/day ÷ bid-tid **Increase:** 0.25-0.5 mg q3d **Max:** 0.1-0.2 mg/kg/day	Anxiety disorders Adjunct treatment in refractory psychosis and in mania Severe agitation Severe insomnia	**Onset:** 20-60 minutes Half-life: 22-33 hr Peak: 1-3 hr		Clonazepine: Less risk for rebound and withdrawal because of longer half-life

Drug		Indications	Dosing	Pharmacokinetics / Notes
		Tourette's disorder MDD Akathisia	>10 yr or >30 kg: Start: 0.5 mg qd-bid Increase: 0.5-1 mg q3d Max: 3 mg/day	Lorazepam: High risk for rebound and withdrawal reactions Good choice for hepatic insufficiency (no active metabolites)
Lorazepam†,‡ (short-acting)	Ativan 0.5, 1, 2 mg 2 mg/mL	Anxiety disorders Adjunct treatment in refractory psychosis and in mania Severe agitation Severe insomnia Tourette's syndrome MDD Temporary use in severe adjustment disorder with anxious mood	Range: 0.05 mg/kg PO/IV q4-8h Max: 2 mg/dose	Onset: 50 min Half-life: 10-20 hr Peak: 1-3 hr (PO)

*Adverse effects apply to all antianxiety drugs.
†The benzodiazepines have no current FDA-established indications for initiating and maintaining treatment in child psychiatric disorders. These medications should be started and titrated under the supervision of a psychiatrist or neurologist. Dosing guidelines based on adult recommendations.
‡Benzodiazepines should be tapered slowly to avoid withdrawal. Taper dose by 25% q5d (may need to go slower if patient on benzodiazepine for extended period, i.e., several months).
See Box 22-1 for list of abbreviations.

Table 22-8 Antipsychotics: Typical

Drug* (Potency)	Brand Name/ Preparations	Dosing	Indications	Adverse Effects‡	Additional Comments‡
Chlorpro-mazine† (Low)	**Thorazine (PO/IM/PR)** **Tab:** 10, 25, 50, 100, 200 mg **Soln:** 5, 10, 20, 30, 40, 100 mg/mL **IM:** 25 mg/ mL **Suppository:** 25, 100 mg	**6 mo-12 yr:** Range: 0.5 mg/kg PO/IM q4-6h prn agitation/psychosis **Max:** 6 mo-5 yr: 40 mg/ day IM 5-12 yr: 75 mg/day IM **PR:** 1 mg/kg q6-8h prn agitation/ psychosis **>12 yr:** **Agitation:** 25-50 mg PO/IM prn **Psychosis:** **Start:** 10-25 mg bid-qid or 25-50 mg IM q4-6h **Increase:** 20-50 mg/day q3-4d **Max:** 200 mg qd	Conduct disorder Agitation Psychosis	**For all typical antipsychotics:** Anticholinergic: dry mouth, constipation blurred vision Hypotension Sedation Weight gain (lower risk with molindone) EPS reactions: dystonia, rigidity, tremor, akathisia Lowering of seizure threshold Sexual dysfunction Drowsiness Tardive dyskinesia (increased risk with long-term administration) Withdrawal dyskinesia	**Thorazine:** Before IM dosing, check vital signs and ECG **General for all typical antipsychotics:** Mechanism of action: DA2 receptor blockade Monitoring: baseline laboratory studies include CBC w/diff, LFTs, TFTs, fasting lipid profile, ECG Older antipsychotics are not as effective as newer/atypical drugs at treating negative symptoms of psychosis

Drug (Potency)	Brand (Form)	Dosing	Indications	Adverse Effects	Comments
Fluphenazine (*Medium/high*)	**Prolixin** (PO/IM) 1, 2.5, 5, 10 mg; 2.5 mg/5 mL; 5 mg/mL	**Range:** <12 yr: 1.5-5 mg qd; >12 yr: 2.5-10 mg qd	PDD; Tic disorders	NMS: muscle rigidity, delirium, autonomic instability, increased creatine phosphokinase levels; Cardiac arrhythmias (QTc prolongation)	Low-potency agents more likely to have anticholinergic side effects; High-potency agents are more likely to cause EPS
Haloperidol (*High*)	**Haldol** (PO/IM) 0.5, 1, 2, 5, 10, 20 mg; 5 mg/mL	**3-12 yr:** **Range:** 0.01-0.03 mg/kg/day PO/IM ÷ bid-tid; **Max:** 0.15 mg/kg/day; **>12 yr:** **Range:** 0.5-10 mg PO/IM ÷ bid-tid; **Max:** 10 mg/d; **Agitation:** 1-5 mg q1-4hr	PDD; Conduct disorders; Psychotic disorders; Tic disorders		
Molindone (*Medium*)	**Moban** 5, 10, 25, 50, 100 mg; 20 mg/mL	**Range:** 5-50 mg tid/qid; **Max:** 225 mg/day	Conduct disorder		
Perphenazine (*High*)	**Trilafon** 2, 4, 8, 16 mg	**Range:** <12 yr: 6-12 mg/day; >12 yr: 12-22 mg/day	Psychotic disorders		

Cont'd

*No current FDA-established indications for initiating and maintaining treatment in child psychiatric disorders. These medications should be started and titrated under the supervision of a psychiatrist or neurologist. Dosing guidelines based on adult recommendations.

¹A warning from the FDA was introduced in 2000, advising against Thorazine's use as a first-line drug because of concerns over QTc interval.

²Adverse effects and comments apply to all antipsychotics in this table.

Table 22-8   Antipsychotics: Typical—cont'd

Drug (Potency)	Brand Name/ Preparations	Dosing	Indications	Adverse Effects[‡]	Additional Comments[‡]
Pimozide[§] (High)	Orap 1, 2 mg	Range: 1-5 mg/day Max: 10 mg/day	Tourette's syndrome (second line)	See previous page	
Thioridazine (Low)	Mellaril 10, 15, 25, 50, 100, 150, 200 mg	Range: 25-400 mg/ day ÷ qd-tid Max: 800 mg/day	Conduct disorder Psychotic disorders		
Thiothixene* (Medium)	Navane 1, 2, 5, 10, 20 mg 5 mg/mL	Range: 2-5 mg/day ÷ bid-tid Max: 60 mg/day	Psychotic disorders		

*No current FDA-established indications for initiating and maintaining treatment in child psychiatric disorders. These medications should be started and titrated under the supervision of a psychiatrist or neurologist. Dosing guidelines based on adult recommendations.
[†]A warning from the FDA was introduced in 2000, advising against Thorazine's use as a first-line drug because of concerns over QTc interval.
[‡]Adverse effects and comments apply to all antipsychotics in this table.
[§]Manufacturer of pimozide reported sudden unexplained deaths at >10 mg/day.
See Box 22-1 for list of abbreviations.

Drug*	Brand Name/ Preparations	Daily Dose†	Main Indications	Mechanism of Action	Adverse Effects	Monitoring
Aripiprazole	**Abilify** 5, 10, 15, 20, 30 mg 1 mg/mL	**Range:** 2.5-20 mg qd **Max:** 30 mg/ day	Psychosis (positive and negative symptoms) Bipolar disorder Tourette's syndrome Augmentation in OCD Aggression and agitation (especially in Autism/PDD)	Partial agonist at DA2 and 5-HT1A receptors Antagonism at 5-HT2A receptors	Orthostatic hypotension Weight gain Hyperglycemia Hyperlipidemia Diabetes mellitus Headache, nausea, vomiting Tachycardia Insomnia, somnolence Seizure EPS NMS Lowering of seizure threshold Hyperprolactinemia Tardive dyskinesia QTc prolongation and dysrhythmias	CBC w/diff, LFTs, ECG, prolactin, fasting lipid profile, Chem-7, weight

Cont'd

*In general, and specifically for Clozaril, do not prescribe without the guidance and supervision of a psychiatrist.
†No current FDA-established indications for initiating and maintaining treatment in child psychiatric disorders. These medications should be started and titrated under the supervision of a psychiatrist or neurologist. Dosing guidelines based on adult recommendations.
See Box 22-1 for list of abbreviations.

Drug	Brand Name/ Preparations	Daily Dose	Main Indications	Mechanism of Action	Adverse Effects	Monitoring
Clozapine	**Clozaril** 12.5, 25, 50, 100, 200 mg	**Prescribe *only* under the supervision of a psychiatrist** Range: 300-450 mg bid **Max:** 900 mg/ day	Refractory psychosis	DA and 5-HT receptor blockade 5-HT2:DA2 affinity ratio 30:1	Same as Aripiprazole **Life-threatening agranulocytosis** Significant weight gain Seizures (high risk, dose related, may require prophylaxis) Low incidence of EPS Low risk for tardive dyskinesia	**Mandatory monitoring for agranulocytosis:** see package insert for WBC and ANC monitoring frequency LFTs, ECG, prolactin, fasting lipid profile, Chem 7, weight
Olanzapine	**Zyprexa** (PO, IM, ODT*) 2.5, 5, 7.5, 10, 15, 20 mg	Range: 2.5-15 mg qd **Max:** 20 mg/ day **Agitation, acute:** Range: 2.5-10 mg PO/IM ×1 **Max:** 20 mg/24 hr	Psychosis (positive and negative symptoms) Bipolar disorder Tourette's syndrome Augmentation in OCD Autism/PDDs Aggression/ agitation	DA and 5-HT receptor blockade 5-HT2:DA2 affinity ratio 50:1	Orthostatic hypotension (particularly IM) Significant: Hyperglycemia Hyperlipidemia Diabetes mellitus Weight gain	Weight, CBC w/diff, LFTs, ECG, prolactin, fasting lipid profile, Chem 7

Quetiapine	Seroquel 25, 100, 200, 300 mg	Range: 400-800 mg/day ÷ bid-tid Max: 800 mg/day	Same as olanzapine	DA and 5-HT receptor blockade 5-HT2:D2 affinity ratio 1:1	Same as Aripiprazole Somnolence Hypercholesterolemia (significant) Possible risk of cataract formation Low incidence of EPS	Thyroid function Eye examination baseline and then q6mo Weight, CBC w/diff, LFTs, ECG, prolactin, fasting lipid profile, Chem 7
Risperidone	Risperdal (PO, IM, ODT) 0.25, 0.5, 1, 2, 3, 4 mg 1 mg/mL	Range: 0.25-6 mg/day ÷ qd-bid Max: 6 mg/day (increased risk of EPS >6 mg/day)	Same as olanzapine	DA and 5-HT receptor blockade 5-HT2:D2 affinity ratio 8:1	Same as Aripiprazole Significant risk of: EPS Weight gain Hyperprolactinemia	Prolactin (higher risk associated with Risperdal), CBC w/diff, LFTs, ECG, fasting lipid profile, Chem 7, weight
Ziprasidone	Geodon 20, 40, 60, 80 mg 20 mg/mL	Range: 40-160 mg/day ÷ bid Max: 80 mg bid Must take with food (without food, absorption can be decreased by 50%)	Same as olanzapine	DA and 5-HT receptor blockade	Same as Aripiprazole Greater risk of QTc prolongation Tends to be most weight neutral	ECG at baseline and with each increase in dose K and Mg levels at baseline CBC w/diff, LFTs, prolactin, fasting lipid profile, Chem 7, weight

Surgical Conditions in Infants and Children

23

Hannah M. Huddleston, Thomas F. Tracy, Jr., and Steven T. Cobery

23.1 Appendicitis

1. Etiology and pathophysiology
   a. The most common abdominal surgical problem in childhood
   b. Appendicitis is caused by inflammation of the appendix, usually secondary to appendiceal outlet obstruction with a fecalith and resultant overgrowth of colonic flora within the lumen of the appendix.
   c. In the child younger than 2 years of age, the appendix is usually perforated by the time the infant is brought to the emergency department. Fortunately, appendicitis in this age group is infrequent (approximately 2% of all cases).
2. Clinical features
   a. Abdominal pain: Appendiceal distention leads to abdominal pain in the periumbilical area. Peritoneal irritation from increasing inflammation corresponds with localization of the pain. This is usually the right lower quadrant (McBurney's point); however, localization of the pain will reflect where the appendix actually resides (e.g., retrocecal or pelvic appendix).
   b. Other symptoms: Nausea and vomiting (usually after abdominal pain); anorexia (fever tends to be minimal in early appendicitis)
   c. Examination: Consistent, localized, point tenderness is the cardinal, reliable sign of appendicitis. Multiple repeated examinations may be required to make the diagnosis.
      (1) Other physical signs include
         (a) Rovsing's sign: Pain in right lower quadrant with palpation of left lower quadrant
         (b) Psoas sign: Pain with right leg and hip extension while lying on left side
         (c) Obturator sign: Pain with abduction and adduction of flexed right leg
         (d) Alario's sign: Have the patient jump up and down, if possible. Pain will localize to the right lower quadrant. Inability to jump or limp with abdominal pain should raise suspicion of appendicitis.

    (2) Rectal examination: Should be done in *all* cases of abdominal pain! Purpose is to elicit pain or findings associated with a retrocecal appendix or to feel a pelvic mass, phlegmon, or abscess.

3. Laboratory/radiologic findings
   a. Complete blood count (CBC): Leukocytosis tends to be minimal in early appendicitis.
   b. Radiologic findings
      (1) Abdominal plain radiography: A calcified fecalith may be present.
      (2) Ultrasonography: A noncompressible tubular appendix greater than 6 mm on abdominal ultrasonography
      (3) Computed tomography (CT): An enlarged appendix and stranding of adjacent fat

4. Management
   a. Antibiotics
      (1) Bacterial coverage: Anaerobes, *Bacteroides*, *Clostridia*, and *Peptostreptococcus* species, as well as gram-negative aerobes, *Escherichia coli*, *Pseudomonas aeruginosa*, *Enterobacter*, and *Klebsiella* species.
      (2) Nonperforated: A single agent, such as, cefoxitin, or cefotetan, is adequate.
      (3) Perforated: If suspected, "triple antibiotics" (ampicillin, gentamicin, and clindamycin or metronidazole)
      (4) Postoperative: Antibiotics should be continued postoperatively only in cases of perforated appendicitis.
   b. Operative management: Open or laparoscopic appendectomy for early (nonperforated) appendicitis
      (1) Discharge: Patients are discharged when tolerating a regular diet, which may be as early as postoperative day 1 in cases of early appendicitis.

5. Complications/special considerations: Advanced (perforated) appendicitis with abscess formation: CT-guided abscess drainage and intravenous (IV) antibiotics with interval appendectomy in 6 to 8 weeks is an alternative to immediate appendectomy.

23.2 Pyloric Stenosis

1. Etiology and pathophysiology: hypertrophy of the pyloric muscle of the stomach, resulting in gastric outlet obstruction

2. Clinical features
   a. The classic presentation is projectile, nonbilious emesis, palpable enlargement of the pylorus (olive), and visible gastric waves on the abdomen. It usually occurs in the first 3 to 8 weeks of life and is extremely rare in the first week.
   b. Examination findings
      (1) Palpation of a hypertrophied pyloric muscle is pathognomonic. Stand on the infant's left side, elevating the feet with your left hand to relax the belly, and then gently palpate with the extended middle finger of the right hand. The pyloric mass can be displaced superiorly or inferiorly and usually lies in the midline or just to the right of the midline.

(2) If a mass is not palpable:
  (a) Give the infant a pacifier to suck or a small amount of Pedialyte. The mass is impossible to feel if the patient is crying.
  (b) Empty the stomach with a nasogastric (NG) tube.
3. Laboratory and radiologic findings
  a. If a mass is still not palpable:
    (1) Ultrasonography will demonstrate a pyloric muscle thickness of 4 mm or more and a pyloric channel length of 16 mm or more. If pyloric stenosis is not the cause of vomiting, gastroesophageal reflux may also be diagnosed by ultrasonography.
    (2) Barium upper gastrointestinal (GI) series will demonstrate an elongated and narrow pyloric channel, the "string sign."
  b. Hypokalemic, hypochloremic metabolic alkalosis can result from persistent vomiting. This should be corrected with appropriate potassium- and chloride-containing IV fluids before elective pyloromyotomy.
4. Management
  a. Treatment is a pyloromyotomy, which splits the fibers of the hypertrophied pylorus muscle, allowing relaxation of the muscle.
  b. Postoperative pyloric regimen, advancing as tolerated (modify for weight of given infant)
    (1) Nothing orally for 4 hours, then
    (2) Pedialyte, 15 mL every 2 hours for 2 feeds, then
    (3) Pedialyte or half-strength formula, 30 mL every 2 hours for 2 feeds, then
    (4) Full-strength formula, 30 mL every 2 hours for 2 feeds, then
    (5) Full-strength formula, 60 mL every 3 hours for 2 feeds, then
    (6) Formula ad libitum every 4 hours
    (7) Breast milk may be substituted for formula, but it must be measured and fed by bottle for the first 24 hours.
5. Complications/special considerations: If the duodenum is inadvertently entered during the pyloromyotomy, the infant should remain on both NG suction and IV antibiotics for a minimum of 24 hours after surgery.

23.3 Incarcerated Inguinal Hernia

1. Etiology and pathophysiology: A hernia that does not spontaneously reduce. It is the most common complication of inguinal hernia. It occurs most often during the first year of life.
2. Clinical features: Usually presents as a palpable mass. Peritoneal signs (abdominal tenderness, rebound, guarding), as well as nausea, vomiting, or diarrhea may also be presenting signs and symptoms.
  a. Examination findings: It is imperative to differentiate an incarcerated hernia from a hydrocele of the cord.
    (1) A hydrocele of the cord is often tense and the end of the hydrocele can be distinguished from the testis itself.
    (2) A rectal examination can also be helpful to distinguish the two.
    (3) If the vas and the ring are easily palpable when examining the inside of the abdominal wall at the level of the internal ring, an incarceration cannot be present.

(4) If unsure, compare palpation on the other side. Infants with hydrocele can be sent home and scheduled for elective surgery.

3. Laboratory and radiologic findings: No laboratory or imaging studies are diagnostic of an incarcerated hernia. However, a chemistry panel and a CBC are helpful to assess the patient's hydration status or possible infection.

4. Management
   a. Most, if not all, can be reduced manually, which obviates the need for emergency surgery.
   b. Reduction technique
      (1) Sedate the patient and provide adequate analgesia (parenteral).
      (2) Place the infant in Trendelenburg position. This may reduce the hernia because of the pull of the mesentery.
      (3) Have an assistant hold the infant above the knees in a frog-leg position to relax the abdominal wall.
      (4) The fingers of one hand should attempt to fix the hernia while the other hand gradually presses the incarcerated mass to reduce edema of the cord and achieve eventual reduction.
      (5) After successful reduction, the patient is almost always admitted for elective repair within 24 to 48 hours, after resolution of inguinal and scrotal edema. The infant should be monitored for reincarceration.

5. Complications/special considerations
   a. Emergency surgical intervention is required if the hernia cannot be reduced or if there is postreduction evidence of persistent intestinal obstruction or nonviable bowel.
   b. An unfortunate complication of an incarcerated hernia is potential hemorrhagic infarction of the testicle. Reduction usually reinstitutes blood flow to the testis.
   c. Incarcerated inguinal hernias in girls invariably are sliding hernias containing ovary and tube. Generally, these hernias can be repaired on a semielective basis. The blood supply to the ovary is usually not impaired.
   d. Unincarcerated hernias in premature infants
      (1) An inpatient premature infant with multiple problems may have a hernia repaired just before discharge home.
      (2) Infants with a postconceptional age (PCA) of less than 54 weeks and a history of prematurity (gestational age <38 weeks at birth) should be admitted overnight after hernia repair for apnea monitoring.
      (3) All term infants with a PCA of less than 44 weeks should also be admitted for overnight monitoring.

23.4 Foreign Bodies

1. Etiology and pathophysiology: An object ingested and lodged in the respiratory or GI tract

2. Respiratory tract
   a. Clinical features: Usually occurs in children younger than 5 years of age. Presents with a choking or coughing episode. Ten percent

of aspirated foreign bodies are in the trachea, with most located in the bronchi, most commonly on the right side.

b. Examination findings: Chest auscultation may reveal wheezing, rhonchi, or diminished breath sounds.

c. Laboratory and radiologic findings: Chest radiograph may demonstrate hyperinflation (air trapping), atelectasis, or pneumonia.

d. Management: Direct laryngoscopy and rigid bronchoscopy allow identification and removal of foreign bodies.

e. Complications/special considerations: Can rapidly lead to complete airway compromise, respiratory arrest, and death

3. Esophageal/GI foreign bodies

a. Clinical features: Objects lodge below the cricopharyngeus muscle (63% to 84%), at the aortic crossover mid-esophagus (10% to 17%), or at the lower esophageal sphincter (5% to 20%).

b. Laboratory and radiologic findings

(1) Anteroposterior and lateral chest radiographs and plain abdominal films will locate the object if it is radiopaque.

(2) A barium swallow is occasionally required, but it must be done by a skilled pediatric radiologist to avoid aspiration.

c. Management: In general, esophageal foreign bodies should be removed endoscopically, under general anesthesia. However, expert radiologists can often remove coins using balloon extraction. Miniature batteries impacted in the esophagus warrant immediate removal because they cause rapid tissue necrosis.

d. Complications/special considerations

(1) Once in the stomach, most ingested foreign bodies, with the exception of sharp objects and batteries, will safely traverse the GI tract within 4 to 5 days. The problem sites are usually the pylorus, the ligament of Treitz, and the ileocecal valve.

(2) No extraction is attempted unless the object is sharp or toxic (i.e., batteries), becomes lodged, or has not passed after 4 to 6 weeks.

(3) If, after 4 to 6 weeks, the object is still in the stomach, it may be retrieved by gastroscopy.

23.5 Intussusception

1. Etiology and pathophysiology: Longitudinal intestinal invagination upon itself in the vicinity of the ileocecal valve, usually secondary to a lead point (e.g., polyp, Peyer's patch, meconium ileus). It occurs commonly between 3 months and 2 years of age, with the highest incidence at 6 months.

2. Clinical features: The typical triad of colicky abdominal pain (alternating with periods of lethargy), abdominal "sausage-like" mass, and currant jelly stools is well known, but all these components are not invariably present.

3. Examination findings: Bimanual rectal examination is the best method for palpation of the sausage-shaped mass in the right abdomen.

4. Laboratory and radiologic findings: Air or barium enema is diagnostic and therapeutic in most infants.

5. Management
    a. Reduction is considered successful when free reflux of air or barium into the ileum is observed. Repeat attempts can be made if the child's condition will permit.
    b. The patient is always admitted for 24 hours of observation after reduction. The patient is kept NPO for the first 12 hours, and then the diet is gradually advanced. Warn parents and staff that high temperatures can follow reduction. If symptoms recur, enema reduction should be performed again. Operation is mandatory if reduction cannot be accomplished.
6. Complications/special considerations: Nonoperative reduction should not be attempted in patients with evidence of perforation, peritonitis, or sepsis.

23.6 Necrotizing Enterocolitis

1. Etiology and pathophysiology: A highly lethal disease in newborns characterized by ischemic necrosis of the GI tract frequently leading to perforation. The most commonly involved sites are the distal ileum and colon.
2. Clinical features: It is seen primarily in low–birth-weight infants, especially those with prenatal complications.
3. Examination findings: Abdominal distention is almost universal, bilious emesis and occult/gross blood in the stool may also be present. Peritonitis then ensues.
4. Laboratory and radiologic findings: Pneumatosis (intramural gas) on abdominal plain films is pathognomonic. Portal vein gas and a fixed loop of intestine on multiple films may also be seen.
5. Management: No operative management may be undertaken in the absence of intestinal necrosis or perforation.
    a. Triple antibiotic therapy with vancomycin, ampicillin, and gentamicin must be continued for at least 10 days.
    b. Patients should be monitored with serial abdominal examinations, serial abdominal films, CBCs, and blood gases.
    c. Initiate total parenteral nutrition.
    d. Peritoneal drainage for pneumoperitoneum may be attempted in very low–birth-weight infants (<1000 g) within 2 weeks of birth.
    e. Indications for surgery
        (1) Pneumoperitoneum
        (2) Clinical deterioration
        (3) Abscess formation
6. Complications/special considerations: Operation for perforation or gangrenous bowel is usually resection with end-ileostomy (or colostomy) and mucus fistula.

23.7 Meckel's Diverticulum

1. Etiology and pathophysiology
    a. Most common congenital anomaly of the GI tract, caused by failure of the vitelline duct to regress

   b. "Rule of 2s"
      (1) 2% incidence
      (2) 2 types of heterotopic mucosa (gastric and pancreatic)
      (3) 2 feet from the ileocecal valve
      (4) Usually presents by 2 years of age
2. Clinical features: Most common presentation is painless, sometimes massive, lower GI bleeding with maroon stools. Second most common presentation is intestinal obstruction.
3. Laboratory or radiologic findings: The diagnosis can be made either with a lateral contrast radiograph, umbilical ultrasonography, or a technetium-99m pertechnetate isotope scan.
4. Management: Surgical resection of symptomatic Meckel's diverticulum is the treatment of choice.
5. Complications/special considerations: may cause intestinal perforation because of secretion of gastric acid

23.8 Intestinal Obstruction, Atresias, and Stenoses

1. Etiology and pathophysiology: Box 23-1 outlines the various causes of obstruction, based on age. Atresias and stenoses are congenital anomalies that arise from failure of recanalization of intestinal lumen or failure to develop owing to vascular occlusion with resorption of the gangrenous segment. Intestinal atresia occurs in the following order of frequency: duodenum, jejunum, ileum, multiple sites, colon, and pylorus.
2. Clinical features: Present with bilious vomiting, abdominal distention, and failure to pass meconium. *Note: Bilious emesis in an infant denotes a surgical emergency until proven otherwise.*

Box 23-1 Etiology of Intestinal Obstruction in Children		
Neonate	**Infant to 24 Months**	**Toddler and Older**
Intestinal atresia/stenosis	Pyloric stenosis	Incarcerated inguinal hernia
Malrotation with volvulus	Incarcerated inguinal hernia	Appendicitis
Hirschsprung's disease	Intussusception	Adhesions
Imperforate anus	Hirschsprung's disease	Duplications
Meconium ileus	Intestinal atresia/stenosis	Malrotation
Microcolon syndrome	Congenital bands or duplications	Trauma
	Internal hernia	Granulomatous disease
	Midgut volvulus	Neoplasm
	Trauma	

3. Laboratory and radiologic findings
   a. Prenatal ultrasonography may reveal polyhydramnios.
   b. Abdominal films show a characteristic "double-bubble" sign—stomach and duodenum with gasless abdomen.
   c. Radiographic findings
      (1) Upright or left lateral decubitus and supine views of the abdomen demonstrated many dilated loops with air–fluid levels.
      (2) The level of atresia or stenosis should be confirmed by contrast enema. On plain films, the newborn colon cannot be distinguished from the small bowel because haustral markings are not yet detectable. Only by filling the colon with contrast agent can the dilated loops be accurately identified as colon or small bowel.
4. Management: After fluid resuscitation and correction of electrolyte imbalance, laparotomy may be done with resection of the proximal dilated end. End-to-end anastomosis usually is possible.
5. Complications/special considerations
   a. Associated with Down syndrome in 30% and other major anomalies in 30% to 50%
   b. Infants with cystic fibrosis and meconium ileus may have associated small bowel atresia.

23.9 Hirschsprung's Disease (Congenital Aganglionic Megacolon)

1. Etiology and pathophysiology: The absence of ganglion cells in autonomic nervous system of the gut. It most commonly involves the sigmoid colon or rectum, but can involve any part of the GI tract.
2. Clinical features: Obstruction in infants or constipation in older children
3. Examination findings: A megacolon may be palpable. Abdominal distention is almost invariably present. Avoid a rectal examination before diagnostic studies.
4. Laboratory and radiologic findings
   a. A barium enema shows a narrow rectum with a dilated colon proximally. Furthermore, failure to pass barium within 24 hours is highly suggestive of Hirschsprung's disease.
   b. The diagnosis is confirmed by suction mucosal rectal biopsy or full-thickness rectal biopsy showing an absence of ganglion cells in the submucosal plexus.
5. Management: Initial surgical management is determined by the condition of the infant. Either a temporary colostomy above the aganglionic segment or primary endorectal pull-through procedure is performed.
6. Complications/special considerations: Toxic megacolon can be a fatal complication of Hirschsprung's disease.

23.10 Meconium Ileus

1. Etiology and pathophysiology: Accounts for less than one third of all neonatal small intestinal obstructions, and occurs in about 15% of infants with cystic fibrosis

2. Clinical features
   a. Presents as an obstruction with failure to pass meconium in the first 24 to 48 hours. A maternal history of polyhydramnios may be present.
   b. The meconium may be palpable as a doughy substance in the dilated loops of distended bowel.
3. Laboratory and radiologic findings
   a. Plain film of the abdomen demonstrates bowel loops of variable size with a soap bubble appearance of the bowel contents. Calcifications on the abdominal film usually indicate meconium peritonitis resulting from an intrauterine intestinal perforation.
   b. A barium enema demonstrates a microcolon with pellet-like meconium proximally.
4. Management
   a. For simple meconium ileus, initial treatment is nonoperative with Gastrografin enemas performed under fluoroscopic control.
   b. Before the procedure, the patient should have IV hydration because Gastrografin is hyperosmolar and large fluid shifts can occur.
   c. An NG tube should also be in place and broad-spectrum antibiotics administered.
   d. Surgical relief of the obstruction is indicated in the following situations:
      (1) Failure of Gastrografin enema to relieve the obstruction
      (2) Evidence of associated atresia or perforation
      (3) A critically ill infant
5. Complications/special considerations
   a. All infants diagnosed with meconium ileus require the iontophoresis test to confirm the diagnosis of cystic fibrosis (see Chapter 16). This test is usually not practical before operation.
   b. After surgery, all infants require vigorous pulmonary therapy. When oral feedings are begun, a pancreatic enzyme preparation is given with each feeding.

23.11 Malrotation and Volvulus

1. Etiology and pathophysiology
   a. Malrotation, or failure of normal intestinal rotation and fixation during development, predisposes the infant to intestinal obstruction and other surgical emergencies.
   b. Obstruction in the infant is caused by compression of the second portion of the duodenum by Ladd's bands.
2. Clinical features
   a. In addition to acute emergencies, the condition may also present with chronic abdominal pain and intermittent nausea and vomiting, indicating intermittent volvulus or partial obstruction.
   b. Midgut volvulus is one of the most serious emergencies seen in these neonates or infants, and a delay in diagnosis of as much as a few hours can result in loss of the entire midgut.
      (1) Presents with sudden onset of bilious emesis that may become bloody, signaling intestinal necrosis.

(2) Abdominal distention and tenderness are common.

(3) On rectal examination, stool, if present, is guaiac positive.

3. Laboratory and radiologic findings

a. Plain films may demonstrate a gasless abdomen or dilated intestine. A double bubble may be present, but the duodenum is less dilated than with duodenal atresia.

b. Upper GI series provides definitive diagnosis.

4. Management

a. With shock or a clear indication for exploration, contrast studies are deferred and the patient is taken immediately for laparotomy.

b. Surgical goals include

(1) Counterclockwise rotation of the intestine to reduce the volvulus

(2) Incision of Ladd's bands, peritoneal folds anchoring the ascending colon to the duodenum

(3) Widening of the mesentery to decrease the risk of recurrent volvulus

(4) Appendectomy is necessary given the abnormal location of the appendix in the left upper quadrant after reduction.

5. Complications/special considerations: internal hernia

a. Results from entrapment of the bowel in mesenteric defects and pouches caused by lack of fixation of the right and left colonic mesentery

b. Presents as an obstruction

c. A GI contrast series usually suggests the diagnosis.

d. Repair includes reduction of the hernia and closure of the mesenteric defect to prevent recurrence.

23.12 Imperforate Anus

1. Etiology and pathophysiology

a. Defects in development of pelvic structures can lead to a variety of malformations of the genitourinary and GI systems.

b. Infants with imperforate anus are at risk for the VACTERL (vertebral, anal, cardiac, tracheoesophageal, renal, and radial limb) association of anomalies. Appropriate screening should be done in all infants with imperforate anus

2. Clinical features

a. The aforementioned defects highlight the importance of the perineal examination of the newborn. It is essential to identify a urethra and an anus in boys and a urethra, vagina, and anus in girls.

b. Infants with imperforate anus appear to have a flat bottom.

c. A rectoperineal fistula may be evident on examination.

d. Evidence of a rectourinary fistula in boys or a rectovaginal fistula in girls should be sought if no perineal fistula is present.

e. A thin anal membrane may also be evident if no fistula is found.

3. Laboratory and radiologic findings: Spine plain films should be obtained during the work-up to screen for vertebral and limb anomalies.

4. Management

a. If a rectoperineal fistula is present, or the blind-ending rectum is close to the anal membrane, repair with anoplasty can be performed.

b. If a rectogenitourinary fistula is present, a diverting colostomy is usually indicated with obliteration of the fistula and creation of a functional rectum, anus, and genitourinary system.
5. Complications/special considerations: Systemic involvement may be mild to profound and the physical examination findings may be very subtle, which makes the diagnosis and treatment of these patients difficult.

23.13 Congenital Diaphragmatic Hernia

1. Etiology and pathophysiology
   a. Formation of the diaphragm occurs at 8 to 10 weeks in the fetus. The intestines, which return to the abdomen during this time, will enter the chest if the diaphragm is not formed (persistent pleuroperitoneal canal) and prevent normal lung development.
   b. There is a male predominance.
2. Clinical features
   a. More common on the left because the left hemidiaphragm closes after the right
   b. Types
      (1) Posterolateral (through foramen of Bochdalek) is most common
      (2) Parasternal (through foramen of Morgagni) on either right or left
   c. Size can vary from 1 to 2 cm to complete absence of hemidiaphragm.
   d. Infants are born with respiratory distress (depending on severity of pulmonary hypoplasia).
   e. Physical examination reveals a scaphoid abdomen, diminished or absent breath sounds (may have bowel sounds in the chest), and heart sounds deviated to the side opposite the hernia.
3. Laboratory and radiologic findings
   a. Most congenital diaphragmatic hernias are diagnosed by prenatal ultrasonography.
   b. Plain films suggest a bubbly bowel pattern in the chest and a lack of normal intestinal gas.
4. Management
   a. Preoperative treatment
      (1) Goal is to stabilize infant for corrective operation. This usually requires gentle correction of respiratory or metabolic acidosis—secondary to hypoxia and hypothermia—as well as facilitating reversal of pulmonary hypertension.
      (2) Initiate continuous positive airway pressure or progress to orotracheal intubation and mechanical ventilation for immediate, severe respiratory distress (preductal SaO_2 <95%).
      (3) Use warming lamps to prevent hypothermia.
      (4) Aspirate stomach with an orogastric sump tube, if possible.
      (5) Alternative ventilatory strategies may be used, including high-frequency ventilation or extracorporeal membrane oxygenation.
   b. Operation
      (1) Reduction of bowel into the abdomen
      (2) Repair of the defect primarily or using muscle or artificial graft

(3) Chest tubes are optional if no air leak or bleeding persists.
  c. After surgery, wean from ventilator with slow reduction in fraction of inspired oxygen (FiO_2) to avoid vasospasm and pulmonary hypertension.
5. Complications/special considerations
  a. The mortality rate has now been reduced to 20% in expert centers.
  b. Often complicated by pulmonary hypoplasia and malrotation of intestines

23.14 Esophageal Atresia/Tracheoesophageal Fistula

1. Etiology and pathophysiology
  a. Occurs at 3 to 6 weeks of fetal life, when the trachea and lungs are developing and separating from the foregut.
  b. Classification (Fig. 23-1)
    (1) Esophageal atresia (EA) with distal tracheoesophageal fistula (TEF; 86%)
    (2) Isolated EA (7%)
    (3) Isolated TEF (4%; H-type)
    (4) EA with proximal TEF (2%)
    (5) EA with proximal and distal TEFs (<1%)
2. Clinical features
  a. Infants with EA display drooling, return of undigested feeds, choking with feedings, and inability to pass an NG tube.
  b. Infants with a TEF aspirate frequently, may become cyanotic with feeding, and develop aspiration pneumonia.
3. Laboratory and radiologic findings
  a. EA is diagnosed by observing a coiling NG tube in the proximal pouch on radiography. A paucity of gastric and bowel gas will be noticed on the abdominal film in isolated EA.
  b. TEF with EA is identified by the presence of gastric and proximal small bowel air.
  c. H-type TEF may be identified with contrast studies or bronchoscopy.
4. Management
  a. Preoperative treatment
    (1) Prevent recurrent aspiration by elevating the head and suctioning saliva with continuous sump drainage.
    (2) Administer broad-spectrum antibiotics and vitamin K.
    (3) Vigorous chest physical therapy
  b. Operation
    (1) Place gastrostomy, if needed, to facilitate ventilation.
    (2) An extrapleural division and closure of the TEF with end-to-end anastomosis of the esophagus is performed, avoiding tension.
    (3) If EA is present, a delayed anastomosis may be considered. Gastrostomies or stenting NG tubes are not uniformly placed.
5. Complications/special considerations: Infants must be screened for VACTERL anomalies.

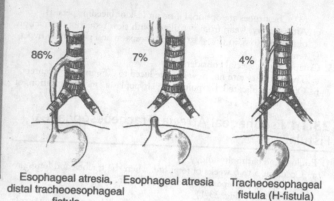

86%   7%   4%

Esophageal atresia, distal tracheoesophageal fistula   Esophageal atresia   Tracheoesophageal fistula (H-fistula)

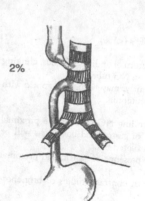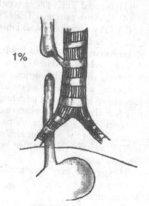

2%   1%

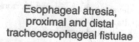

Esophageal atresia, proximal and distal tracheoesophageal fistulae   Esophageal atresia, proximal tracheoesophageal fistula

Figure 23-1 The major types and approximate incidences of tracheoesophageal malformations in neonates. (Modified from Rudolph AM [ed]: Pediatrics, 18th ed. Norwalk, Conn, Appleton & Lange, 1987.)

23.15 Abdominal Wall Defects

1. Etiology and pathophysiology: Table 23-1 summarizes the etiology and pathophysiology of the most common abdominal wall defects.
2. Clinical features: See Table 23-1 for comparison.
3. Laboratory and radiologic findings: Most often physical examination can differentiate between these three defects. However, occasionally an abdominal CT is indicated for both diagnosis and operative planning.
4. Management
   a. Umbilical hernia: Indications for surgical repair
      (1) Incarceration (very rare)
      (2) Persistent hernias beyond 5 years of age
      (3) Protruding hernias in 3- to 4-year-old children with large fascial defects
   b. Any omphalocele or gastroschisis is repaired operatively.
      (1) Preoperative management
         (a) Infants with gastroschisis are placed feet-first into a bowel bag to conserve heat and measure fluid losses.
         (b) They should be placed on their left side after examination of the mesentery to prevent torsion and volvulus.
         (c) Those with omphalocele should have the sac covered with a barrier-type dressing to prevent hypothermia.
         (d) IV hydration with balanced salt solution and colloid is essential.
         (e) GI decompression by NG tube is imperative to minimize further GI distention and prevent aspiration of gastric contents.

Table 23-1 Clinical Findings in Omphalocele and Gastroschisis

Factor	Umbilical Hernia	Omphalocele	Gastroschisis
Cause	Failure of closure of the fascial ring through which the umbilical cord passes	Failed fusion of lateral embryonic folds	Failure of umbilical coelom formation
Location	Umbilical ring	Umbilical ring	Lateral to cord
Defect size	Small	Large (2-10 cm)	Small (2-4 cm)
Sac	None	Present	Absent
Contents	Bowel	Liver, bowel	Bowel, gonads
Malrotation	No	Present	Present
Associated anomalies	Unusual	Common (30%-70%)	Unusual (10%-15%)

Modified from O'Neill JA Jr, Grosfeld JL, Fonkalsrud EW, et al: Principles of Pediatric Surgery, 2nd ed. St. Louis, Mosby, 2003.

(f) Systemic IV antibiotics (ampicillin/gentamicin) are given to protect contaminated amnion or viscera.

(g) Rule out associated anomalies, particularly in neonates with an omphalocele.

(2) Operative management: Defects should be closed primarily.

5. Complications/special considerations: Alternatively, if the abdomen is too small to accommodate the viscera, a Silastic silo may be placed to suspend the intestines outside the abdomen. The viscera are then gradually returned to the abdomen and the abdominal wall is closed.

23.16 Biliary Atresia

1. Etiology and pathophysiology
   a. Obstruction of bile flow due to absence or hypoplasia of intrahepatic or extrahepatic bile ducts
   b. Etiology is thought to be an inflammatory process in utero, although the specific cause is unknown.
   c. Important to identify biliary atresia (BA) early (before 6 weeks of age) to maximize outcome after surgical therapy

2. Clinical features
   a. Persistent jaundice with acholic stools and dark urine devoid of urobilinogen
   b. Firm hepatomegaly by 4 weeks and splenomegaly by 6 weeks
   c. Physical findings of portal hypertension with ascites after 6 months

3. Laboratory and radiologic findings
   a. Laboratory findings: A conjugated hyperbilirubinemia is the rule for BA. Other causes of conjugated and unconjugated hyperbilirubinemia are summarized in Box 23-2.
   b. Radiographic findings
      (1) Ultrasonography may demonstrate absence of a gallbladder; however, the diagnosis of BA is not excluded by the presence of a gallbladder.
      (2) DISIDA (technetium-99m diisopropyl iminodiacetic acid) scintiscan will demonstrate failure of excretion of radioisotope into the intestine.
   c. Percutaneous liver biopsy will reveal bile duct proliferation and periportal fibrosis. This is useful to differentiate BA from neonatal hepatitis.
   d. Diagnostic laparotomy
      (1) Includes operative cholangiography and a wedge biopsy of the liver
      (2) If BA is diagnosed, proceed with Kasai hepatic portoenterostomy.

4. Management: Kasai hepatic portoenterostomy
   a. Goal of operation is to connect microscopic biliary ductules that lie within the bifurcation of the portal vein to a limb of intestine, establishing biliary drainage.
   b. Outcomes are best if procedure is performed before 8 weeks of age.
   c. Kasai procedure may be definitive therapy for one third of patients presenting before 8 weeks.
   d. One third of patients who receive a Kasai procedure improve for months to years, but then require liver transplantation.

Box 23-2 Differential Diagnosis of Neonatal Jaundice

Unconjugated Hyperbilirubinemia	Conjugated Hyperbilirubinemia
Excess production	Cholestasis
Hemolytic anemia	Systemic infection
Reduced uptake	Metabolic disease
Drugs	Total parenteral nutrition
Impaired conjugation	Genetic diseases
Physiologic	Neonatal hepatitis
Genetic-metabolic disorders	Obstruction
Diffuse disease	Biliary atresia
	Choledochal cyst
	Inspissated bile plug syndrome
	Biliary compression/stenosis

5. Complications/special considerations
   a. Orthotopic liver transplantation is indicated for infants who present late or in whom the Kasai procedure fails to establish biliary drainage.
   b. Current data indicate that portoenterostomy should be performed regardless of the age at presentation.

23.17 Hydrocephalus

1. Etiology and pathophysiology
   a. Two general classifications
      (1) Obstructive/noncommunicating: The cerebrospinal fluid (CSF) flow is prevented from exiting the brain at some point along its normal pathway to the arachnoid granulations (lateral ventricle → foramen of Monro → third ventricle → sylvian aqueduct → fourth ventricle → foramen of Magendie or Luschka → basal cisterna).
      (2) Communicating: Overproduction or underabsorption of CSF causes a system wide increase in CSF-containing spaces.
   b. The etiology of hydrocephalus is quite variable and its causes are numerous.
      (1) Chiari I/II malformations
      (2) Dandy-Walker cyst
      (3) Aqueductal stenosis
      (4) Postinfectious (neonatal meningitis)
      (5) Posthemorrhagic (germinal matrix hemorrhage of prematurity)
      (6) Tumors (e.g., medulloblastoma, colloid cyst, astrocytoma, germinomas)
2. Clinical features
   a. The patient often presents with macrocephaly.
   b. In infants, irritability, spontaneous vomiting, and failure to thrive are common presentations. A bulging fontanelle is indicative of high intracranial pressure (ICP).

    c. In older children, headache, nausea, vomiting, poor head control, and lethargy are common presentations.

    d. In severe acute hydrocephalus, apnea and bradycardia can often be life-threatening.

    e. A striking sign of high ICP, which is the hallmark of hydrocephalus in children, is the "setting sun" sign, which is upgaze palsy bilaterally, light/near dissociation of the papillary reflex, and vertical nystagmus.

    f. The sixth cranial nerve is most often affected.

3. Laboratory and radiologic findings

    a. A CT of the brain, without contrast, is diagnostic of hydrocephalus.

    b. Masses, hemorrhage, and asymmetry of ventricles may allow differentiation between obstructive and communicating hydrocephalus.

4. Management

    a. Symptomatic hydrocephalus is managed with a ventriculoperitoneal shunt. A small catheter is placed occipitally into the right lateral ventricle and connected to a pressure-regulating valve. The outlet of the valve is connected to a subcutaneous catheter, which drains into the abdominal cavity.

    b. The outlet of the shunt can be placed in any sterile cavity or space if the abdomen prohibits placement there. Ventriculoatrial, ventriculopleural, and even ventriculo-gallbladder shunts have been placed.

    c. A third ventriculostomy is an "internal" shunt that bypasses the sylvian aqueduct and fourth ventricle by creating a foramen in the floor of the third ventricle, connecting the third ventricle with the basal cisterns. This is an option for obstructive hydrocephalus caused by obstruction in these areas.

5. Complications/special considerations: Shunt infection is a common complication, affecting 25% to 50% of shunted patients.

    a. Risks include reduction of intelligence quotient, seizures, and death.

    b. Treatment includes removal of shunt hardware after placement of an extraventricular drain and IV antibiotics until cultures are clear for greater than 10 days.

    c. Skin flora (coagulase-negative staphylococci) are the most common pathogens.

SUGGESTED READING

Dillon PW, Tracy TF Jr: Biliary atresia. In Oldham KT, Colombani PM, Foglia RP, Skinner MA (eds). Principles and Practice of Pediatric Surgery. Philadelphia, Lippincott Williams and Wilkins, 2005, pp 1475-1493.

Tracy TF Jr: Abdominal wall defects. In Oldham KT, Colombani PM, Foglia RP, (eds). Surgery of Infants and Children: Scientific Principles and Practice. Philadelphia, Lippincott-Raven, pp 1083-1093.

Weber TR, Tracy TF, Keller MS: Groin hernias and hydroceles. In Ashcraft KW, Holcomb GW, Murphy JP (eds). Pediatric Surgery, 4th ed. Philadelphia, Elsevier Saunders, 2005, pp 697-705.

WEBSITES

www.bms.brown.edu/pedisurg/
www.clsnyder.com/media/Main.swf
www.home.coqui.net/titolugo/handbook.htm

Toxicologic Emergencies

24

*Robert O. Wright, Gregory R. Lockhart,
and William J. Lewander*

24.1 Introduction

1. Epidemiology
   a. Approximately 6,000,000 children ingest a potentially toxic substance each year. In pediatrics, poisonings occur most frequently in the 1- to 5-year-old age group and are generally accidental. A second peak occurs from age 13 years into adulthood, frequently due to intentional suicide attempts. Poisonings occur but are rare in the 6- to 12-year-old group.
   b. The American Association of Poison Control Centers recently reported a 24-per-year annual poisoning fatality rate for children younger than 6 years of age. Children 13 to 19 years of age have an annual fatality rate of 64/year.
   c. Preschoolers are more likely to ingest nontoxic substances or nontoxic amounts of toxic substances.
   d. The most common exposures in children are cosmetics/personal care items, household cleaning substances, analgesics, plants, and cough/cold preparations.
   e. The most common lethal exposures in children are due to hydrocarbons, antidepressants, fumes/gases (e.g., carbon monoxide), insecticides, and analgesics.
2. Diagnosis and evaluation: Overview
   a. Assess and stabilize the airway, breathing, and circulation (ABCs) first, then proceed.
   b. Any patient who presents with unknown, sudden-onset multisystem disease should be suspected of poisoning until proven otherwise.
   c. Toxic ingestions may present as unexplained seizures, dysrhythmia, or coma. In any patient in whom poisoning is suspected, trauma should be suspected because altered consciousness may lead to trauma.
   d. Many areas of the country have regional poison centers that can assist in the management of unknown, complicated, or severe poisonings. Regional poison centers should also be consulted for the management of more basic issues, such as when to give ipecac or charcoal.

e. History
  (1) What was ingested, if known?
  (2) When was it ingested (i.e., time)?
  (3) How much was ingested (number of pills/liquid)?
    (a) Did the family bring in the medicine/agent?
    (b) Always assume the worst-case scenario. If the family states 10 to 15 pills, assume 15 were taken. If the bottle is missing 20 tablets, assume 20 were taken.
    (c) A swallow for a 3-year-old is approximately 5 mL; for a 10-year-old, 10 mL; and for an adolescent, 15 mL.
  (4) Symptoms (vomiting, lethargy, excitement, etc.)
  (5) Was this a suicide attempt or gesture?
  (6) Past medical history, especially any history of heart, lung, kidney, gastrointestinal (GI), or central nervous system (CNS) disease that may complicate management. Ask about previous poisonings.
f. Physical examination
  (1) Vital signs are very important and may give clues to diagnosis.
    (a) Tachycardia: Stimulants or anticholinergics
    (b) Hypoventilation: Narcotics, depressants
    (c) Fever: Anticholinergic, aspirin, stimulants, and so on
  (2) Breath: Alcohol, hydrocarbons, and cyanide have distinctive odors.
  (3) Eyes
    (a) Are the pupils large or small? Dilated pupils may indicate sympathomimetic or anticholinergic ingestion. Small pupils are associated with narcotics.
    (b) Is there nystagmus? (phenytoin or phencyclidine)
  (4) Cardiac: dysrhythmias
    (a) Bradycardia may mean a beta blocker, cholinergic, or calcium channel blocker.
    (b) Tachycardia may mean a stimulant or anticholinergic.
    (c) A widened QRS or a prolonged PR interval may indicate a tricyclic antidepressant (TCA).
  (5) Skin and mucous membranes: Dry may indicate anticholinergic; very moist may indicate a cholinergic or sympathomimetic agent.
  (6) Bowel sounds: Decreased may indicate an anticholinergic or narcotic.
  (7) Neurologic (gait, reflexes, mental status): Is the patient stimulated/sedated?
g. Toxidromes: Collections of signs and symptoms, called *toxidromes*, may point to a specific ingestant. Examples are given in Table 24-1.
h. Laboratory studies
  (1) Glucose
    (a) Low in alcohols, oral hypoglycemics, aspirin (may also cause hyperglycemia), beta blockers, insulin
    (b) May be high in iron and calcium channel blockers
  (2) Electrolytes
    (a) Toxins may alter electrolytes (lithium may cause hypokalemia).
    (b) May induce high–anion-gap metabolic acidosis. High anion gap mnemonic is MUDPPILES (methanol, uremia, diabetes, paraldehyde, phenformin, iron/isoniazid, lactic acid, ethylene glycol, salicylates).

Table 24-1 **Toxidromes**	
Toxin	**Clinical Findings**
Iron	Diarrhea, bloody stools, metabolic acidosis, hematemesis, coma, abdominal pain, leukocytosis, hyperglycemia
Opioids	Coma, respiratory depression, miosis, track marks, bradycardia, absent or decreased bowel sounds
Organophosphates	Miosis, cramps, salivation, urination, bronchorrhea, lacrimation, defecation, bradycardia
Salicylates	Hyperventilation, fever, diaphoresis, tinnitus, hypoglycemia or hyperglycemia, vomiting blood, altered mental status, metabolic acidosis, respiratory alkalosis
Phencyclidine	Muscle twitching, rigidity, agitation, bidirectional nystagmus, hypertension, tachycardia, prolonged psychosis, blank stare, myoglobinuria, increased creatine phosphokinase
Tricyclic antidepressants	Dryness of mucosa, vasodilation, hypotension, seizures, ileus, alteration of mental status, pupillary dilation, arrhythmias, widened QRS interval (findings may be similar to anticholinergic toxins)
Theophylline	Nausea, vomiting, tachycardia, tremor, convulsions, metabolic acidosis, hypokalemia, electrocardiographic abnormalities
Adrenergic storm (cocaine, amphetamines, phenylpropanolamine)	Pupillary dilation, hyperthermia, agitation, diaphoresis, seizures, tremor, anxiety, tactile hallucinations, dysrhythmias, active bowel sounds, track marks, hypertension
Sedative-hypnotics	Respiratory depression, coma, hypothermia, disconjugate eye movements
Anticholinergics	Dryness of mucous membranes and skin, tachycardia, fever, arrhythmias, urinary and fecal retention, mental status change, pupillary dilation, flushing

Adapted and modified from Goldfrank LR, Flomenbaum NE, Lewin NA, et al (eds): Goldfrank's Toxicological Emergencies, 4th ed. Norwalk, Conn, Appleton & Lange, 1990, p 66.

(3) Arterial blood gas (ABG)
  (a) Confirm respiratory depression.
  (b) Determine patient's acid-base status.
(4) Kidney, ureter, and bladder: Radiopaque pill fragments may be seen. The mnemonic is CHIPPED (calcium/chloral hydrate, heavy metals [including lead], iron, Pepto Bismol, phenothiazines, enteric-coated pills, dental amalgam).
(5) Electrocardiogram (ECG)
  (a) Prolonged QTc, PR, or widened QRS may appear with TCA.
  (b) Heart block or bradyarrhythmias may be seen with calcium channel blockers.
  (c) Tachyarrhythmias occur with sympathomimetics.
  (d) Ischemia may be seen in cocaine toxicity.
(6) Liver function tests (LFTs)
  (a) Obtain a baseline in acetaminophen ingestion.
  (b) LFT results may be elevated earlier in certain liver toxins (e.g., mushrooms, herbal teas).
(7) White blood cell (WBC) count
  (a) An elevated WBC count occurs in iron overdose.
  (b) Many unknown ingestants present similarly to infections, especially aspirin and cocaine.
(8) Toxicology screen: Urine and serum
  (a) Specify the specific toxin if one is suspected.
  (b) A toxicology screen should be obtained in all unknown cases.
  (c) A toxicology screen alone should not guide management, however. Clinical evaluation in conjunction with laboratory results should guide management. Most toxins will *not* appear on a routine toxicology screen.
(9) Bedside tests
  (a) Ferric chloride added to a urine sample can detect aspirin (purple color).
  (b) Methemoglobin can be detected by placing drops of blood on white filter paper; in a positive test the blood will appear chocolate-brown.

3. Management: General strategies
  a. Remember the ABCs. Administer oxygen, and place the patient on a cardiorespiratory monitor. Consultation with the regional poison center is recommended in all potentially toxic ingestions.
  b. Provide supportive care (mechanical ventilation in respiratory failure; glucose if hypoglycemic).
    (1) Prevent absorption or decontamination (activated charcoal, gastric lavage, whole-bowel irrigation).
    (2) Enhance elimination (dialysis, ionized diuresis).
    (3) Interrupt or alter metabolism (ethanol in methanol or ethylene glycol poisoning).
    (4) Provide specific antidotes (naloxone in opiate poisoning).
  c. Glucose treatment should be routine with depressed mental status of unknown origin. Try to draw serum level just before treatment (also consider naloxone).

d. Ipecac is generally *not* advisable in the emergency department. Most children will vomit within 20 minutes of administration. Vomiting may persist for hours and may interfere with subsequent oral treatments, such as charcoal, or a specific antidote. Impending coma, seizures, caustics, most hydrocarbons, and respiratory depressants are contraindications to using ipecac.

e. Gastric lavage may be performed if less than 1 hour has passed since ingestion. A large-bore Ewald tube improves pill fragment retrieval. Lavage is contraindicated in caustics and most hydrocarbons. If more than 1 hour has passed, proceed with other treatment such as charcoal, if indicated. If patient is unable to protect airway or there is impending airway compromise from seizure or depressed mental status, intubate before lavage/charcoal.

f. Activated charcoal: 1 g/kg up to 60 g. Charcoal can be mixed with juice or soft drinks to make it more palatable. Many toxins will adsorb to charcoal. Elemental toxins such as iron and heavy metals will not. Alcohols and hydrocarbons also bind poorly.

g. Forced diuresis consists of fluids and diuretics but is *very rarely* recommended. It may cause pulmonary edema.

h. Ion trapping: Urine alkalinization for weak acids (barbiturates, aspirins) traps the toxin in the renal tubules and is commonly recommended. Urine acidification for weak bases (phencyclidine, amphetamine) is not advised and may be detrimental.

i. Hemoperfusion/hemodialysis: Most common indications are severe poisoning with theophylline (hemoperfusion) or salicylate, lithium, methyl alcohol, or ethylene glycol (hemodialysis).

4. Specific antidotes and treatments are given in Table 24-2.

24.2 Acetaminophen

1. Pathophysiology and overview of toxicity
   a. Overdose causes centrilobular hepatic necrosis.
   b. There are three stages to toxicity.
      (1) In the first stage (1 to 12 hours), symptoms may be minimal and consist of vomiting/nausea or mild right upper quadrant pain.
      (2) In the second stage (24 to 72 hours), liver enzymes elevate.
      (3) In the final stage (after 72 hours), fulminant liver failure ensues, and patients may develop bleeding disorders, hypoglycemia, and hepatic encephalopathy.
   c. Toxicity
      (1) A toxic ingestion is 140 mg/kg in acute overdose. In multiple-dose ingestions or sustained-release form, toxic amounts are not well defined.
      (2) Toxicity is due to the formation of a reactive metabolite when usual metabolic pathways are overwhelmed by overdosage. Toxicity is mainly hepatic. Renal toxicity has also been described.

2. Management
   a. Treatment of acetaminophen overdose depends on interpretation of acetaminophen serum levels using the Rumack-Matthew

Table 24-2   Specific Antidotes and Treatments for Poisoning

Poison	Antidote	Dose	Comment
Acetaminophen	N-acetylcysteine	140 mg/kg loading then 70 mg/kg every 4 hr 17 times	Most effective within 10-16 hr of ingestion
Arsenic (heavy metals)	BAL (British Anti-Lewisite)	300-600 mg/m²/day IM every 4-8 hr	BAL contains peanut oil and dimercaprol
Atropine	Physostigmine	Initial dose 0.5-2 mg IV	Use with caution; it may produce asystole, bradycardia, or seizure
Benzodiazepines	Flumazenil	0.01 mg/kg IV	Avoid in seizure disorder, or coingestion of seizure-inducing agent
Beta blockers	Glucagon	150 μg/kg up to 10 mg IV; titrate to effect If effective, give loading dose/hr as maintenance drip	Stimulates cyclic adenosine monophosphate synthesis, increasing cardiac contractility
Calcium channel blocker	Calcium chloride (CaCl) or Glucagon/ atropine	CaCl 10% solution 0.25 mL/kg IV; repeat once in 10 min See above	Optimal dose of CaCl is unknown; repeat dose to effect Calcium extravasation may cause tissue necrosis
Carbon monoxide	Oxygen	100% by face mask or hyperbaric oxygen	Consult poison center for hyperbaric indications
Digitalis	Digoxin immune Fab (Digibind)	Based on amount ingested	Consult poison center before use
Iron	Deferoxamine	Initial dose 40-90 mg IM or slow IV, maximum dose 1 g; then 15 mg/kg/hr IV	May cause hypotension; forms excretable complex
Isoniazid	Pyridoxine	Dose matches ingested isoniazid dose; 5 g if ingested dose unknown	Only effective anticonvulsant

Lead	CaEDTA BAL	1 ampule/250 mL D_5W; 5-mL ampule over 1 hr (20% solution), 1.0–1.5 g/m^2/day IM every 4 hr or IV drip	Dilute to less than 3% solution; may chelate calcium, magnesium, and zinc as well as lead
			Contains peanut oil
Methanol/ethylene glycol	Ethanol	300–600 mg/m^2/day IM every 4-8 hr 1 mL/kg of 100% ethanol diluted in glucose solution to 10%; maintain blood level of 100 mg/dL	Prevents formation of formic acid/ oxalates; competes for alcohol dehydrogenase
Nitrates (methemoglobinemia)	Methylene blue	1-2 mg/kg of 1% solution IV over 5 min	May be ineffective in glucose-6-phosphate dehydrogenase deficiency; may cause hemolysis in neonates
Opiates	Naloxone	Adults, 2.0 mg IV; children up to 2 yr, 0.1 mg/kg IV, then 2.0 mg IV	Continuous drip may be necessary
Organophosphates	Atropine Pralidoxime	Adults, 0.5-2 mg IV; children, 0.02 mg/kg IV (minimum dose 0.15 mg IV; maximum dose 2 mg IV) Adults, 1 g IV; children, 25-50 mg/kg IV	Blocks acetylcholine; up to 5 mg IV every 15 min may be necessary in a critically ill adult patient Cleaves alkly phosphate–cholinesterase bond; up to 500 mg/hr may be necessary in a critically ill adult
Tricyclic antidepressants	Sodium bicarbonate (NaHCO$_3$)	50 mEq IV in adult; 1 mEq/kg IV in child then continous drip, approximately 50 mEq/– NaHCO$_3$ to start	Optimal dose is unknown; may repeat dose to effect maximum serum pH 7.55; mix with solution 0.2% normal saline

CaEDTA, calcium disodium ethylenediamine tetraacetic acid; IM, intramuscularly; IV, intravenously.
Adapted and modified from Haddad LM, Winchester J (eds): Clinical Management of Poisoning and Drug Overdose. Philadelphia, WB Saunders, 1990, based on the American College of Emergency Physicians poster on poisonings, Dallas, 1980.

nomogram (Fig. 24-1). *This nomogram should be used only in patients with single-dose ingestions.*

b. It is crucial that serum acetaminophen levels be obtained at least 4 hours postingestion to plot the level properly on the nomogram. Patients falling below the line on the nomogram need no treatment.

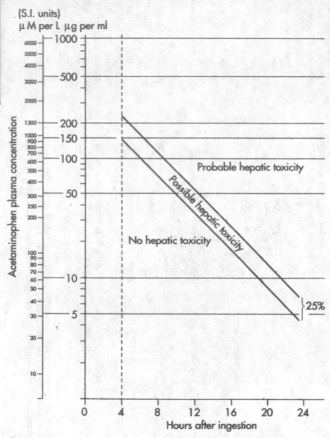

Figure 24-1 Rumack-Matthew nomogram for acetaminophen poisoning: semilogarithmic plot of plasma acetaminophen levels versus time. *Cautions for the use of this chart:* (1) Time coordinates refer to time after ingestion. (2) Serum levels drawn before 4 hours may not represent peak levels. (3) Graph should be used only in relation to a single acute ingestion. (4) The *lower solid line* 25% below the standard nomogram is included to allow for possible errors in acetaminophen plasma assays and estimated time from ingestion of an overdose. (From Rumack BH, Matthew H: Acetaminophen poisoning and toxicity. J Pediatr 55:871-876, 1975.)

Patients at or above the line should receive N-acetylcysteine (NAC; 140 mg/kg loading, then 70 mg/kg/dose orally every 4 hours for 17 doses). NAC is malodorous and unpleasant to swallow orally. Nasogastric tube placement or antiemetics are often necessary to carry out the NAC regimen. A 48 hour intravenous (IV) regimen is also available and ensures delivery, but anaphylactoid reactions to this are possible.

c. Any level above the toxic line of the nomogram should be treated for a full 18-dose course. Subsequent acetaminophen levels do *not* determine discontinuation of NAC.

d. The Rumack nomogram does not apply to chronic ingestions or to extended-release preparations; management of these patients should be made in conjunction with a regional poison center.

e. Activated charcoal can still be used with NAC; some authorities recommend increasing the dose by 40% when used in conjunction with activated charcoal.

f. LFTs should be monitored daily; baseline liver functions should be sent when a toxic ingestion is established. Blood urea nitrogen (BUN) and creatinine should also be monitored because the toxic metabolite may cause renal toxicity.

24.3 Salicylates

1. Pathophysiology and overview of toxicity
   a. Patients may confuse salicylates and acetaminophen. Whenever a history of ingesting one of these agents is given, levels of both should be checked. If a patient carries an odor of wintergreen, this is a possible clue for salicylate ingestion (e.g., Ben-Gay).
   b. Aspirin causes a central stimulation of respiratory drive, resulting in a respiratory alkalosis.
   c. Salicylates interfere with the Krebs cycle (uncouple oxidative phosphorylation) and thus will cause a metabolic acidosis with an accumulation of lactic acid. Profound electrolyte disturbances may be seen. Fever and hypoglycemia may occur.
   d. Most ingestions have a mixed picture of respiratory alkalosis and metabolic acidosis. However, children often present solely with a metabolic acidosis.
   e. Neurotoxicity may result in mental status change, seizures, tinnitus, or hearing loss. Other CNS findings include nausea, vomiting, lethargy, and coma.
   f. Cerebral and pulmonary edema are the leading causes of fatality.

2. Management
   a. Obtain salicylate levels 2 and 6 hours postingestion. If rising, monitor every 2 to 4 hours.
   b. ABGs, electrolytes, and glucose should be obtained.
   c. Mild toxicity is seen at 30 to 60 mg/dL. Moderate toxicity is generally considered likely at levels above 60 mg/dL. Severe toxicity is seen above 100 mg/dL. Levels do not correspond exactly with symptoms. Patients with chronic ingestions may have symptoms of severe toxicity at levels of 40 mg/dL.

   d. Symptomatic patients (metabolic acidosis, mental status change, tinnitus, fever) should have *immediate* treatment, consisting of activated charcoal and urine alkalinization.
   e. Multidose charcoal may enhance elimination and shorten serum half-life.
   f. Alkaline diuresis causes ion trapping and increases renal clearance of salicylic acid. A urinary pH of 7 to 8 should be obtained by hydrating with IV solutions containing bicarbonate. The maximum serum pH should be 7.55.
   g. Hypokalemia stimulates aldosterone secretion, increasing hydrogen ion secretion and acidifying urine. Treatment with supplemental potassium may be necessary to maintain alkalotic urine.
   h. As a guideline, begin with D_5W 0.2% normal saline with 50 mEq/L $NaHCO_3$ and 20 to 40 mEq/L KCl. If adding more than 50 mEq/L $NaHCO_3$, use D_5W.
   i. Hemodialysis may be used in severe toxicity (altered mental status, significant metabolic acidosis, pulmonary edema, or seizures). Levels greater than 100 mg/dL require dialysis regardless of symptoms. Patients with chronic toxicity may require dialysis at lower levels.
   j. Patients who cannot tolerate large sodium loads required for alkalinization, have renal insufficiency, or in whom alkalotic urine pH cannot be maintained should also be treated with dialysis.

24.4 Hydrocarbons

1. Pathophysiology and overview of toxicity
   a. The primary toxicologic insult is pulmonary, due to aspiration. Propensity for aspiration is indirectly proportional to viscosity—the lower the viscosity the higher the propensity for aspiration.
   b. Toxicity can be divided into straight carbon chain (aliphatic) or cyclic structures (aromatic). Aromatic compounds have more associated neurotoxicity.
   c. Halogenation increases toxicity. For example, carbon tetrachloride is toxic to the liver. Fluorinated compounds are more cardiotoxic.
   d. Respiratory involvement in severe forms may manifest as acute respiratory distress syndrome and require intubation.
   e. Direct CNS toxicity may further complicate management by depressing respiratory drive.
2. Clinical features
   a. Symptoms are usually pulmonary, but specific toxins may injure other organ symptoms.
   b. Initial symptoms include coughing, choking, grunting, retractions, and nasal flaring. Symptoms of respiratory distress may be delayed.
3. Management
   a. Give oxygen; monitor oxygenation by pulse oximetry and arterial blood gases.
   b. Chest radiographs should be obtained immediately in symptomatic patients and 4 hours postingestion in asymptomatic patients. Most patients with aspiration (88%) will have abnormalities on chest radiography by this time.

   c. GI decontamination is controversial. For aliphatic hydrocarbons, decontamination is usually contraindicated unless the overdose is large (>5 mL/kg). Compounds with high viscosity pose less aspiration risk. These include camphor, carbon tetrachloride, benzene, and pesticides containing hydrocarbons. Consultation with the regional poison center is recommended.

24.5 Iron

1. Pathophysiology and overview of toxicity
   a. Iron is rapidly absorbed, with peak levels occurring 2 to 6 hours postingestion.
   b. Serum iron is bound to numerous proteins; free unbound iron is toxic to living tissue. If the ingestion is large enough to saturate the total iron-binding capacity (TIBC), toxicity may occur.
   c. Toxicity generally is seen at doses greater than 20 to 60 mg/kg. A lethal dose is 180 mg/kg or greater.
2. Clinical features: There are four clinical stages of iron toxicity:
   (1) First stage: Occurs within 1 to 4 hours, with direct toxicity on the GI mucosa involving vomiting (which may be heme positive), diarrhea, and abdominal pain.
   (2) Second stage: Improvement in symptoms may occur, and the patient may be asymptomatic up to 36 hours.
   (3) Third stage: Free iron disrupts mitochondrial function, poisoning cells. Venous pooling and third spacing occurs. GI bleeding, hypovolemic shock, metabolic acidosis, and cardiac, renal, and hepatic failure may also be seen. Death may occur.
   (4) Fourth stage: This last stage may be delayed for weeks to months and consists of GI scarring, particularly the pylorus, from the direct toxic effects of iron, which may lead to bowel obstruction.
3. Diagnosis and laboratory findings
   a. Laboratory data should consist of complete blood count (CBC), glucose, electrolytes, TIBC, and LFTs. A blood type and cross may be needed in severe ingestions.
   b. Serum iron should be drawn 4 hours postingestion. If it is elevated, it should be monitored every 2 to 4 hours.
   c. Abdominal radiographs may reveal radiopaque pill fragments.
   d. Toxic ingestions are associated with peripheral WBC counts greater than 15,000/mm^3 and serum glucose greater than 150 mg/dL, but normal values do not rule out toxicity.
   e. A serum iron greater than 350 µg/dL is generally considered elevated. A level of 500 µg/dL requires treatment regardless of symptoms. Symptomatology should be the major consideration in the initiation of treatment. Symptomatic patients with levels below 500 µg/dL should also be treated.
   f. A serum iron greater than the TIBC is also considered toxic and is a useful guideline for treatment with deferoxamine. *However, a serum iron lower than the TIBC may still be toxic*; thus, the TIBC should not be used as the sole basis for initiating treatment.

4. Management
   a. Use IV deferoxamine, an iron-chelating agent that binds free iron to form nontoxic ferrioxamine, which is excreted by the kidneys. Ferrioxamine can be detected by "vin rosé" appearance of the urine.
   b. For unknown ingestions, a deferoxamine challenge (40 mg/kg intramuscularly) may be given and urine examined for vin rosé color. A positive deferoxamine challenge may not always be visually detectable.
   c. The deferoxamine dose is generally 15 mg/kg/hr as a continuous drip. Higher doses may be necessary for severe symptoms or very high iron levels.
   d. Rapid deferoxamine infusions may cause hypotension or an anaphylactoid reaction, but these are *not* indications for terminating treatment. Temporary cessation to treat these complications is recommended, but the infusion should be restarted when the patient is stable.
   e. Slowing the rate of infusion and adequate hydration may prevent hypotension. Diphenhydramine (Benadryl), epinephrine, and steroids will treat anaphylactoid reactions.
   f. Whole-bowel irrigation (polyethylene glycol) speeds removal of tablets in the bowel. This is given by nasogastric tube with the patient seated, at a rate of 500 mL/hr in children younger than 6 years of age, 1000 mL/hr for 7- to 12-year-olds, and 1500 mL/hr for children older than 12 years. Antiemetics or gastric-emptying medications (metoclopramide) may be needed.
   g. Free iron is not dialyzable; hemodialysis of ferrioxamine may be efficacious. Deferoxamine must be continued during dialysis for treatment to be effective.
   h. Activated charcoal will not bind iron but may be used in the setting of coingestants.

24.6 Tricyclic Antidepressants

1. Pathophysiology, overview of toxicity, and clinical features
   a. The most commonly used are imipramine, desipramine, amitriptyline, and nortriptyline.
   b. A significant overdose is a medical emergency. The cardiotoxic effects are responsible for the majority of fatalities in TCA overdose and generally occur with ingestions of 10 to 20 mg/kg.
   c. TCAs block the reuptake of norepinephrine and serotonin, thus allowing an accumulation of aminergic transmitter at CNS sites.
   d. Anticholinergic effects occur and initial symptoms may be tachycardia, dry mouth/skin, fever, mydriasis, and mental status change.
   e. TCAs inhibit fast sodium channels and slow-phase zero depolarization in ventricular myocardium. *The hallmark of TCA overdose is a prolonged QRS interval* (>100/msec is a sign of severe toxicity). PR and QT intervals can also be prolonged. Ventricular tachycardia, bradycardia, and torsades de pointes are occasionally seen.
   f. Poor myocardial contractility may lead to pulmonary edema, which large fluid volumes may exacerbate.

g. CNS effects occur early; patients present with confusion/delirium progressing to coma.

h. Seizures are common and most are brief; repetitive seizures may require intervention.

2. Management

a. All patients should receive oxygen and ECG monitoring.

b. IV access should be obtained and fluid given at no more than a maintenance rate.

c. Patients with depressed mental status or who are combative/delirious should be intubated.

d. Gastric lavage and activated charcoal (1 g/kg up to 60 g). Ipecac is contraindicated.

e. The mainstay of treatment for cardiac arrhythmias is $NaHCO_3$. Alkalinization to a blood pH of 7.5 may reduce the incidence of cardiac arrhythmias. *An IV bolus of $NaHCO_3$ (1 mEq/kg) is the treatment of choice for acute ventricular arrhythmias.*

f. As a guideline, mix two ampules (total 100 mEq $NaHCO_3$) in 1 L D_5W and run at maintenance rate. Alkalinization is maintained until the patient is stable for 24 hours.

g. Drugs for seizure control include benzodiazepines (lorazepam 0.1 mg/kg). Phenobarbital (10 to 20 mg/kg loading dose) may be useful as a second-line drug.

h. The use of flumazenil is contraindicated in mixed ingestions of TCAs and benzodiazepines. The reversal of the benzodiazepine may induce a seizure by unmasking TCA CNS toxicity.

i. The use of physostigmine for anticholinergic toxicity is contraindicated in TCA overdose.

24.7 Lead

1. Overview of toxicity: Lead poisoning results mainly from the ingestion of lead-based paint or plaster in the form of household dust. Soil, contaminated water, and paint chips may also result in significant exposure (see section on Screening in Chapter 2). Children 1 to 3 years of age are most vulnerable.

2. Pathophysiology and clinical features

a. Symptoms include lethargy, irritability, abdominal pain, constipation, and anorexia.

b. Lead inhibits erythropoiesis by interfering with heme synthesis. Concomitant iron deficiency worsens anemia. These effects are reversible with removal of lead and institution of iron therapy.

c. Neurobehavioral deficits have been described with lead levels as low as 10 µg/dL.

d. Acute encephalopathy is due to cerebral edema from diffuse vasculitis, increasing capillary permeability. Severe toxicity may lead to seizures or behavioral disturbances. Lumbar punctures are contraindicated.

e. Peripheral neuropathy is characterized by motor weakness with little or no sensory change and is rare in children. Peripheral neuropathy is more common in sickle cell anemia.

    f. Renal toxicity is manifested primarily as proximal renal tubular injury. Fanconi's syndrome may ensue as a result of lead toxicity. Acute renal insults are reversible, but late lead nephropathy may lead to interstitial nephritis, renal scarring, and kidney failure.

3. Diagnosis and laboratory findings

    a. A CBC, serum iron, TIBC, or ferritin study should be obtained to assess anemia. BUN and creatinine tests are useful to assess renal toxicity.

    b. Knee radiographs will detect lead lines (increased densities due to calcification in the distal femur, proximal tibia, and proximal fibula). These lines are present with chronic exposure.

    c. An abdominal radiograph can be used to screen for intestinal lead in acute exposures.

4. Management

    a. The most important step in the treatment of any child with lead poisoning is to *identify and remove the source*. Removing the child from the site of a home renovation or inspections of the home by the board of health are crucial treatments of lead toxicity.

    b. Commonly used chelating agents for lead toxicity include calcium disodium ethylenediamine tetraacetic acid (CaEDTA), British Anti-Lewisite (BAL), D-penicillamine, and dimercaptosuccinic acid (DMSA).

    c. Indication for inpatient chelation therapy is a venous blood lead level of 45 μg/dL or more.

    d. Inpatient chelation consists of combination BAL/CaEDTA therapy. CaEDTA may be given alone in asymptomatic patients with lead levels below 70 μg/dL.

    e. For symptomatic patients and all patients with levels of 70 μg/dL or more, CaEDTA should be given in combination with BAL. *The first dose of BAL should be given before the CaEDTA.*

    f. If the lead level is 45 to 70 μg/dL or more in an asymptomatic patient, CaEDTA may be used without BAL.

    g. Outpatient therapy with DMSA can be performed only in asymptomatic patients and only if the home environment is known to be lead-free.

    h. Outpatient chelation (Table 24-3) can be used for a venous blood lead level of 25 to 44 μg/dL or more. At present, indications for treatment are controversial and should be made in conjunction with the regional poison center or state health department.

24.8 Caustics

1. Pathophysiology and overview of toxicity

    a. Toxicity is related to pH. The degree of the burn is multifactorial and depends on the concentration, molarity, quantity ingested, form of the agent, and the presence of food in the stomach.

    b. Alkalis cause a liquefactive necrosis of fat and protein that may penetrate deep into tissue.

    c. Acids cause a superficial corrosion and coagulation necrosis that limits penetration into the deeper tissues. However, severe tissue destruction may still be seen.

Chelator	Dose	Treatment Length	Complications/Precautions
CaEDTA	1.0–1.5 g/m²/day; continuous IV infusion	5 days	Potential renal toxicity; maintain good hydration; monitor blood urea nitrogen/creatinine/calcium/urinalysis
BAL (British Anti-Lewisite)	300–600 mg/m²/day IM every 4–8 hr	3–5 days	Contraindicated in peanut allergy; may cause fever, granulocytopenia, paresthesias, salivation, conjunctivitis, headache, nausea, abdominal pain; avoid in glucose-6-phosphate dehydrogenase deficiency
D-Penicillamine	20–40 mg/kg/day orally 3 times per day	Weeks	Contraindicated in penicillin allergy; avoid giving with dairy products or iron; may cause rash, nausea, vomiting, leukopenia, or thrombocytopenia
DMSA (dimercaptosuccinic acid)	30 mg/kg/day orally three times per day, then 20 mg/kg/day orally two times per day	First 5 days, next 14 days; multiple courses may be necessary	Neutropenia; may cause liver toxicity; monitor liver function tests

CaEDTA, calcium disodium ethylenediamine tetraacetic acid; IM, intramuscularly; IV, intravenously.

    d. Some agents may have other toxicologic properties, such as neuro-toxicity.

2. Management

    a. Given the vast array of caustic cleaning agents, consultation with the regional poison center is recommended.

    b. Avoid induced vomiting. Use of milk or water is controversial because it may lead to emesis.

    c. Neutralization with the opposing base or acid is contraindicated.

    d. Patients with evidence of esophageal burns (drooling, vomiting, oropharyngeal burns) require a referral to a specialist trained in endoscopy because perforation and stricture formation may occur.

24.9 Ophthalmologic Exposures

1. Clinical features and management:

    a. Alkalotic agents generally cause more severe injury, although acidic burns can cause significant damage.

    b. Irrigation for 30 minutes with copious amounts of sterile saline is the initial management. Consider the use of a Morgan lens with a topical ophthalmic anesthetic such as tetracaine to facilitate adequate irrigation.

    c. The pH of tears should be checked and irrigation continued until the pH is 7.0. Visual acuity should be documented.

    d. Referral to an ophthalmologist is suggested for all significant exposures.

24.10 Carbon Monoxide

1. Pathophysiology and overview of toxicity

    a. Carbon monoxide (CO) is colorless and odorless. Poisoning is seen in patients exposed to fires, exhaust from internal combustion engines, or cigarette smoke.

    b. CO combines with cytochrome oxidase (producing cellular asphyxia and anaerobic metabolism), with myoglobin, and with hemoglobin in competition with oxygen. Metabolic acidosis and tissue hypoxemia ensue.

2. Clinical features and diagnosis

    a. Patients typically have mild flulike symptoms with headache and dizziness. In more severe cases patients present with mental status changes, seizures, or frank coma. Levels of 20% to 30% carboxyhemoglobin will generally induce mild to moderate symptoms. Some patients may become comatose at levels as low as 35%, whereas others may be relatively normal with levels as high as 55%.

    b. Pulse oximetry will read carboxyhemoglobin as oxygenated hemoglobin and is thus inaccurate in CO poisoning.

    c. Diagnosis is confirmed by co-oximetry of venous or arterial blood.

    d. ABG analysis may calculate oxygen saturation and give a *falsely normal* value.

3. Management

    a. Asymptomatic patients with levels below 25% can be treated with 100% oxygen. The half-life of carboxyhemoglobin is roughly 4 hours at room air temperature. On 100% oxygen it is 1.5 hours, and it is 30 minutes with 100% oxygen at three atmospheres (hyperbaric oxygen).

b. Hyperbaric oxygen should be considered in symptomatic patients and in all patients with a 40% or greater carboxyhemoglobin, regardless of symptomatology.

c. The management of asymptomatic patients with carboxyhemoglobin between 25% and 40% is controversial; some experts recommend hyperbaric oxygen. Others prefer 100% high-flow oxygen. Consultation with the regional poison center is recommended.

24.11 Cyanide

1. Pathophysiology and overview of toxicity
   a. Cyanide is a contributor in many smoke inhalation injuries and occasionally the main intoxicant. Hydrogen cyanide gas is produced by the pyrolysis of polyurethane, polyacrylonitrile, silk, and wool cyanide salts. Nitrile solvents, superglue, and nitroprusside are other sources of cyanide.
   b. Cyanide inhibits cytochrome oxidase, the terminal respiratory mitochondrial enzyme. Other effects, such as inhibition of glycolysis, contribute to toxicity.
2. Clinical features: Onset of symptoms may be extremely rapid and include flushing, dizziness, headache, tachypnea, and tachycardia. Ultimately seizure, coma, metabolic acidosis, and death ensue.
3. Management
   a. Treatment consists of sequestering cyanide as cyanomethemoglobin, then converting it to the less toxic compound thiocyanate. Nitrites are used to produce methemoglobin levels of about 30%.
   b. The cyanide antidote kit consists of amyl nitrite, sodium nitrite, and sodium thiosulfate.
   c. Amyl nitrite is inhaled for 15 to 30 seconds every 60 seconds until sodium nitrite is given (0.15 to 0.33 mL/kg [maximum 10 mL] of 3% solution IV over 2 to 4 minutes, followed immediately by sodium thiosulfate 1.1 to 2 mL/kg of a 25% solution).
   d. Sodium nitrite should not exceed the recommended dose because fatal methemoglobinemia may ensue.

SUGGESTED READING

Abbruzzi G, Stork CM: Pediatric toxicologic concerns. Emerg Med Clin North Am 20:223-247, 2002.

Goldfrank LR, Flomenbaum NE, Lewin NA, et al (eds): Goldfrank's Toxicologic Emergencies, 7th ed. New York, McGraw-Hill, 2002.

Tenenbein M: Recent advancements in pediatric toxicology. Pediatr Clin North Am 46:1179-1188, vii, 1999.

WEBSITE

Rocky Mountain Poison and Drug Center (RMPDC): www.rmpdc.org

General Approach to Trauma

Aris C. Garro and Thomas H. Chun

1. History
   a. Resuscitative efforts are often undertaken without the benefit of a history (e.g., unwitnessed event, patient too injured or too young, parents unavailable). Information should be obtained from witnesses or medical transport personnel regarding the circumstances of the incident.
   b. The mnemonic AMPLE is recommended to obtain information quickly:

      Allergies
      Medications
      Past medical history
      Last meal
      Events leading up to the injury

2. Physical examination of the trauma victim: a systematic approach
   a. *Primary survey:* ABCDEs. The following steps should be followed in the order presented. Any abnormality should prompt an intervention to correct it and then a return to the beginning of the primary survey to repeat ABCDEs for any changes.
      (1) Airway (and cervical spine protection)
         (a) Patency: Normal speech indicates a patent airway. If airway is not patent, check for signs of obstruction (noisy respiration, inadequate air exchange). Also ascertain whether patient will continue to be able to maintain the airway (e.g., smoke inhalation or decreasing level of consciousness).
         (b) Cervical spine: It is at this step that cervical spine (C-spine) protection using a hard collar should be performed in victims of significant trauma. Patients brought to the hospital without spinal immobilization cannot be presumed to be free of significant spinal injury.
      (2) Breathing: Note respiratory rate and oxygen saturation; observe chest for uneven movement; auscultate chest.
      (3) Circulation: Note heart rate, blood pressure, adequacy of pulses and capillary refill.
      (4) Disability
         (a) Level of consciousness: Use the AVPU scale:
            (i) Alert
            (ii) Verbal stimuli response: Patient not alert but responds when spoken to

          (iii) Painful stimuli response: patient not alert but responds to painful stimuli (e.g., sternal rub, nail squeeze, intravenous line placement).

          (iv) Unresponsive

       (b) Neurologic deficit

          (i) Pupil size and reactivity

          (ii) Four-extremity gross motor function

          (iii) Sensory deficit

   (5) Exposure/environment: Completely undress the patient but keep ambient temperature adequate to prevent hypothermia.

  b. *Secondary survey* (Table 25-1): Presented here in a "head-to-toe" fashion; memorize and call out positive and negative findings. Frequently reassessing the ABCs and vital signs is also recommended. If any abnormality occurs, the primary survey should be repeated from the beginning.

3. Radiographic evaluation of the patient with blunt trauma

  a. Common radiographs

   (1) C-spine: The following criteria should be applied to pediatric patients with C-spine injury older than 9 years of age. In the younger patient, use these criteria only in the context of other clinical factors (e.g., mechanism of injury, cooperativeness of patient). There should be a low threshold for radiographic evaluation of the C-spine in very young children.

       (a) Criteria for clinical clearance of the C-spine

         .(i) Patient is alert and cooperative

          (ii) Patient is not intoxicated

          (iii) Patient is without midline neck tenderness

          (iv) Patient has a negative neurologic examination

          (v) Patient is without significant (distracting) injuries

       (b) If patients meet the preceding criteria, the neck should be flexed, extended, and rotated in both directions. If there is then no pain on neck movements, radiographs are not necessary (C-spine is cleared clinically).

       (c) All patients not meeting the preceding criteria or who have pain with movements should have their C-spine evaluated radiographically.

       (d) If there are no fractures on the C-spine radiographs, the C-spine should again be evaluated, starting from the beginning of the assessment. If the C-spine again cannot be cleared clinically, the cervical collar should remain in place.

   (2) Chest radiograph: Provides information regarding potentially significant injuries (e.g., pneumothorax, great vessel injuries, rib fractures, pulmonary contusions)

   (3) Pelvic radiograph: Any mechanism of injury consistent with pelvic injury should be evaluated with a pelvic radiograph.

   (4) Extremity radiographs: Based on suspected injuries

  b. Computed tomography (CT)

   (1) Head CT

       (a) Indications: History of loss of consciousness or altered level of consciousness. In a younger child, include the caregiver

Body Area	Inspect For	Palpate For	Auscultate For	Test For
Head	Raccoon eyes* Battle's sign* Laceration Hematoma Deformity	Hematoma Laceration Skull fracture		
Face	Laceration Deformity Asymmetry	Bony tenderness/step-off Orbital deformity/step-off		Midface instability
Eyes	Exophthalmos Enophthalmos Hyphema Globe laceration Lens dislocation			Visual acuity Pupil reactivity Extraocular movements
Ears	Laceration Pinna hematoma Hemotympanum* CSF otorrhea*			
Nose	Laceration Nosebleed Septal hematoma CSF rhinorrhea*	Bone/cartilage tenderness		

Mouth	Soft tissue laceration Loose/missing teeth Presence of foreign body	Loose teeth (tapping on a fractured tooth will produce pain) Jaw tenderness/deformity	
Neck	Laceration Hematoma Tracheal deviation Venous distention	Carotid pulsation Cervical spine tenderness/ deformity Tracheal deviation Subcutaneous emphysema	Bruit Stridor
Chest	Symmetry Flail segments Laceration	Rib and clavicle deformity/ tenderness Subcutaneous emphysema	Bilateral breath sounds Heart sounds
Abdomen	Laceration Ecchymosis Previous scars	Tenderness Distention	Bowel sounds
Pelvis	Symmetry Deformity	Femoral pulse Tenderness Stability to anteroposterior and lateral compression	
Rectal		Tone Bony fragments Prostate position	Occult blood
Genitourinary	Meatal blood Hematoma Laceration	Tenderness (penile and testicular)	Hematuria (urine dipstick or urinalysis)

*Indicator of possible basilar skull fracture.
CSF, cerebrospinal fluid.

Continued

Body Area	Inspect For	Palpate For	Auscultate For	Test For
Extremities	Color Deformity Laceration Hematoma Effusion	Temperature Pulses Bony tenderness		Capillary refill
Back	Ecchymosis Laceration	Bony tenderness (spine and posterior ribs) Costovertebral angle tenderness		Ankle-brachial index
Neurologic				Level of consciousness Pupil reactivity Motor function Sensation Reflexes Babinski's sign

report of any change from baseline mental status (e.g., fussiness, inconsolability, decreased feeding).
(b) Interpretation: A negative head CT in a patient with normal results on neurologic examination is reassuring that serious morbidity or mortality resulting from the head injury is unlikely (although not absolute proof).
(c) Discharge: Patients who have not had a loss of consciousness and are alert with no other significant injuries can be discharged home with a reliable guardian. Give written instructions regarding indicators to watch for and when to return for immediate reevaluation.
(2) Neck CT: Indication—considered in patients who are unlikely to meet criteria for C-spine clearance or if radiographic views are technically difficult to obtain
(3) Abdomen CT
(a) Indication: Considered in patients who are clinically stable but have a potential (by mechanism of injury, history, or examination) intra-abdominal injury
(b) Contraindication: Patients who are unstable, those with peritonitis, or those with clear indications for surgical exploration (e.g., gunshot wound to the abdomen)

SUGGESTED READING

American College of Surgeons Committee on Trauma: Advanced Trauma Life Support Course. Chicago, American College of Surgeons, 1997.
Cantor RM, Leaming JM: Evaluation and management of pediatric major trauma. Emerg Med Clin North Am 16:229-256, 1998.
Tepas JJ: Pediatric trauma. In Feliciano DV, Moore EE, Mattox KL (eds): Trauma. Stamford, Conn, Appleton & Lange, 1996.

Child Maltreatment 26

Shelly D. Martin and
Christine Barron

26.1 Introduction

Child maltreatment encompasses all forms of child abuse and neglect. This chapter focuses on two common forms: child physical and child sexual abuse.

1. Child physical abuse is defined as the infliction of physical injury on a child that is not an accident. This includes burning, hitting, pinching, shaking, kicking, beating, or otherwise harming a child.
2. Child sexual abuse is defined as an act of a sexual nature on or with a child for the sexual gratification of the perpetrator or a third party. Included is any form of anal, genital, or oral contact to or by the child, exhibitionism, voyeurism, or using the child for the production of pornography.

26.2 Epidemiology and Risk Factors

1. Of the approximately 1 million substantiated cases of abuse and neglect reported in 2003, approximately 19% were physical abuse and 10% were sexual abuse.[3]
   a. Physical abuse: The age group of birth to 3 years accounts for the highest rate of abuse, with abusive head trauma as the leading cause of mortality and morbidity.
   b. Sexual abuse
      (1) Seventy-five percent of reported victims are female.[3]
      (2) Male perpetrators are more common, and nearly 76% of all perpetrators of sexual abuse were relatives, friends, or neighbors.[3]
      (3) An increasing trend of children sexually abusing other children has been noted. Forty percent of offenders who sexually molested a child younger than 6 years of age were juveniles.[1,2]

---

*The opinions and assertions contained herein are the private views of the authors and are not to be construed as those of the Departments of Defense, Army, Air Force, or Navy; the Armed Forces Center for Child Protection; the National Naval Medical Center; or Walter Reed Army Medical Center.

2. Risk factors
   a. Physical abuse: Risk factors for child physical abuse include
      (1) Poor parenting skills
      (2) Lack of understanding of normal developmental abilities of children
      (3) Family stress: Poverty, social isolation, domestic violence, and substance abuse
      (4) Crying: A parent may get frustrated and resort to abuse as a means to quiet the child.
   b. Sexual abuse: Children at higher risk include
      (1) Those who have a diminished capacity to resist or disclose. This includes children who are preverbal, developmentally delayed, or physically handicapped.
      (2) Those with exposure to known perpetrators

26.3 Diagnosis

1. Presentation
   a. Physical abuse: A wide variety of presenting signs and symptoms should be considered in the differential diagnosis, especially when medical care is not sought in an appropriate and timely fashion, the history is incongruent with the child's injuries or the child's developmental abilities, or injuries are patterned and in different stages of healing or in areas uncommonly seen in accidental injuries.
   b. Acute sexual assault: Children who present within 72 hours of a sexual assault should be referred to an emergency department or child protection program for the collection of forensic specimens.
   c. Chronic sexual abuse or delayed disclosure: Often children do not immediately disclose when they have been sexually abused and can present with a medical or behavioral complaint that is concerning for sexual abuse.
   d. Behavioral indicators are nonspecific and similar to symptoms due to other stressors. However, some behaviors to consider include
      (1) Fears and phobias, especially of circumstances related to abuse
      (2) Nightmares or other sleep disturbances
      (3) Appetite changes or eating disorders
      (4) Enuresis or encopresis, problems with toileting
      (5) Decline in school performance
      (6) Depression, social isolation or withdrawal, suicidality
      (7) Excessive anger, aggression
      (8) Running away from home
      (9) Promiscuous behavior or substance abuse
      (10) Post-traumatic stress disorder
2. History: As is true for all of medicine, making the diagnosis of child abuse relies on the history. Information should be collected in a non-judgmental manner to include history of presenting complaint, physical and behavioral review of systems, past medical history, developmental history, family history, and social history.
3. Interviewing: Interview everyone separately when possible, including each caretaker, the patient, and other potential witnesses.

a. Interviewing the parent/caregiver
   (1) When obtaining detail about the injury, be sure to identify all caregivers present at the time of the injury.
   (2) When obtaining social history, ask about potential risk factors for abuse.
   (3) Pay particular attention to changing histories or shifting blame.
   (4) Also note injury being blamed on the injured child or siblings.
b. Interviewing the child
   (1) *Interview the child at his or her developmental level.* Use his or her terms for body parts. Sit at eye level and take time to establish rapport with neutral topics (i.e., ask about where they live, pets, school, favorite activities, etc.).
   (2) *Use nonleading, open-ended questions,* such as what, who, where, and when. Do not ask direct or leading questions. Maintain a "Then what happened" approach. Avoid any demonstration of emotion. Document the child's statements verbatim in the medical record.
   (3) *Reassure the child* that he or she did the right thing by telling you, and whatever happened was not his or her fault.
c. Recantations: Children will often recant in an effort to minimize the disruption to the family, feeling guilty because their disclosure causes stress, sadness, or outrage for others involved.

4. Physical examination: Complete a full physical examination, including a thorough skin examination, in a child-friendly examination room. All injuries should be documented to include description, size, and location. Photographs are ideal, but if equipment is not available, drawings of any concerning injury should be completed.
a. Physical abuse (Table 26-1)
   (1) Carefully inspect for recognizable patterns of injury (bruises or burns), bilateral injuries, circumferential injuries, and injuries in different stages of healing.
   (2) Concerning injuries include bruising or injury to the scalp, face, pinna, or genitals, frenula tears, extremity tenderness or deformity, and abdominal pain/tenderness.
b. Sexual abuse: Note that most sexually abused children have no physical findings. The absence of physical findings *does not* rule out sexual abuse.
   (1) Know useful examination positions (supine frog-leg, prone knee-chest, lithotomy) and techniques (labial separation, labial traction).
   (2) Use a good light source with magnification. A colposcope is ideal, but other light sources can be helpful, such as an otoscope head, handheld or headpiece lens, or magnifying fluorescent light.
   (3) Know genital anatomy and normal developmental variations.
       (a) All girls are born with a hymen that usually fits into one of five categories: Crescentic, circumferential, fimbriated, sleevelike, or septate.
       (b) Newborn hymens are fleshy and redundant secondary to maternal estrogen effect.
       (c) Prepubertal hymens are very sensitive to touch and have thinner tissue because of low estrogen concentrations.

Injury	Differential Diagnosis	Clinical Points
Bruising	Accidental injury in mobile children Coagulation disorders (hemophilia, idiopathic thrombocytopenic purpura, von Willebrand's disease, ingested anticoagulants, vitamin K deficiency) Dye or ink Birth marks (Mongolian spots, café au lait spots) Phytophotodermatitis Connective tissue disorders (Ehlers-Danlos syndrome) Folk medicine (coining) Contact dermatitis	Document size and location of each lesion. Measure with a ruler for accuracy. Document the color of the lesion. Keep in mind color cannot be used to determine the age of a bruise. If edema and erythema are present, you can assert that an injury is acute. If there are bruises that are acute and fading, you can likely state that the lesions occurred on at least two different occasions, but you cannot say more than that.
Burns	Accidental Infection (impetigo, epidermolysis bullosa, staphylococcal scalded skin syndrome) Folk medicine (cupping, moxibustion) Fixed drug reactions Phytophotodermatitis	Burns concerning for abuse have the following characteristics: Symmetric injury (i.e., stocking-and-glove) Patterned (dip burns, objects) Well-demarcated Mechanism of burn is unexplained based on developmental level of the child

Continued

Injury	Differential Diagnosis	Clinical Points
Fractures	Birth trauma Accidental trauma Congenital or acquired disorders (osteogenesis imperfecta, leukemia) Infection (osteomyelitis, septic arthritis) Vitamin or mineral deficiency (rickets, scurvy, Menkes' syndrome)	Fractures highly suggestive for abuse include metaphyseal, rib, sternum, scapular, vertebral body and spinous process, and medial and lateral clavicular. Additional fractures suggestive of abuse include multiple, bilateral, and symmetric, fractures of different ages; fractures of hand and feet; and complex skull fractures (depressed, comminuted) without appropriate history. The radiographic appearance of a fracture provides information as to the mechanism of injury and therefore the plausibility, or implausibility, of the history.
Intracranial bleeding	Motor vehicle crash Aneurysm Tumor or vascular malformations Glutaric aciduria type I Coagulopathy	The triad of intracranial hemorrhage, retinal hemorrhage, and diffuse axonal injury implies abusive head trauma as a mechanism of injury in the absence of a medical etiology to explain. Often, there are no external signs of injury. Contact epidural and subdural hemorrhages are seen in accidental injury with or without skull fracture. Short falls are not likely to cause massive head injury.

(d) Pubertal hymens are thickened and usually fimbriated and folded owing to the renewal of the estrogen effect.

(e) There is no such thing as a "virgin test." A negative hymenal examination is often seen despite a history of sexual abuse or consensual sexual activity. Hymenal tears and notches may indicate penetrating trauma, but their absence does not rule it out.

(f) Completing genital examinations as part of all general well-child visits will improve practitioner comfort level and increase the ability to identify normal variations.

(4) Know abnormal findings that can mimic sexual abuse (Table 26-2).

    (a) *All lesions are not sexual abuse.* Although some lesions may be concerning for sexual abuse (human papillomavirus, herpes), they are not diagnostic. Other lesions may be present that are not caused by abuse: viral exanthems, bacterial infections (streptococcal vaginitis), molluscum contagiosum, Behçet's syndrome, lichen sclerosis.

    (b) *Erythema and irritation are nonspecific.*

(5) Potential indicators of sexual abuse

    (a) Genital or rectal pain, bleeding, trauma, or infection

    (b) Sexually transmitted diseases in prepubertal or non–sexually active children can be diagnostic of sexual abuse (see also Chapter 19). Note that bacterial vaginosis, *Gardnerella* infection, and candidiasis are unlikely to be due to abuse. Diseases suspect for sexual abuse include

        (i) Gonorrhea and syphilis (unless acquired perinatally)

        (ii) Condyloma acuminatum (unless acquired perinatally)

        (iii) *Chlamydia trachomatis* and *Trichomonas vaginalis* infection

        (iv) Herpes simplex 1 or 2 (indicates possible abuse, but may be transmitted by nonsexual means)

    (c) Sexual behavior in young children (such as engaging in or acting out intercourse or other sex acts or sexual coercion) that is developmentally inappropriate

5. Diagnostic imaging: Radiographic imaging may be necessary for suspected physical injury.

  a. Occult skeletal injury

    (1) Children younger than 2 years of age with concerns for physical abuse require a complete skeletal survey to identify occult trauma.

    (2) A selective approach to imaging is indicated in children older than 2 years of age because of the dramatic decrease in *occult* skeletal injuries in older children.

    (3) Children younger than 2 years of age who had a skeletal survey completed for acute abusive injuries should have a repeat skeletal survey performed 2 weeks later to identify acute trauma that may have been missed on the initial study.

  b. Central nervous system (CNS) imaging for suspected head trauma

    (1) A computed tomography (CT) scan is helpful to identify acute CNS injuries, particularly hemorrhage.

Table 26-2 Genital Examination Findings

| | | Findings | | | |
| | | | | Sexual Abuse | |
	Anatomic Variations	Nontraumatic	Traumatic, Not Sexual Abuse	Acute	Chronic
Vaginal	Periurethral and perihymenal bands, small hymenal mounds adjacent to vaginal ridges, perineal midline raphe, hymenal tags or flaps, imperforate hymen, labial adhesions, notches or clefts in anterior half of hymen	Lichen sclerosis, genital hemangiomas, urethral prolapse, vaginitis, infection (bacterial or viral), foreign bodies	Straddle injury, accidental penetrating injury, female circumcision	Lacerations, abrasions, ecchymoses or edema of hymen or surrounding structures, hymenal transactions, petechiae	Complete, healed transaction of hymen, notches of hymen >50% of hymenal diameter, scarring of hymen or other genital structures, absent or attenuated hymen
Penile	Pink pearly penile papules	Urethritis, contact dermatitis, acrodermatitis enteropathica, infection (bacterial and viral)	Accidental injury (i.e., zipper)	Edema, petechiae, abrasions	Scarring
Anal	Diastasis ani (smooth areas at 6 and 12 o'clock), skin tags, visible pectinate line, anal dilation, failure of midline fusion	Erythema, midline skin tags, increased pigmentation, venous congestion, anal dilation with stool in the rectum, rectal prolapse	Superficial fissures secondary to constipation, fissures secondary to Crohn's disease or ulcerative colitis or other medical conditions	Lacerations, edema, abrasions, ecchymoses, fissures that extend past the anal verge, post-traumatic hemorrhoid-like tags	Scars, dilation ≥20 mm without rectal stool, loss of symmetric rugal pattern, loss of subcutaneous fat

(2) Magnetic resonance imaging (MRI) can be used to identify chronic injury or deep structure injury. MRI can also be useful in determining the age of intracranial injuries, and should be performed 3 to 5 days after suspected injury.

c. Imaging for intra-abdominal injuries due to suspected abdominal trauma: Abdominal CT scan, upper gastrointestinal series, and ultrasonography are useful modalities to determine the presence and extent of abdominal injury. Occult abdominal injury may be present despite a lack of external signs of injury.

6. Laboratory studies
   a. Physical abuse
      (1) Prothrombin time, partial thromboplastin time, and complete blood count are useful, particularly when bruising is present.
      (2) Liver function tests have proven useful as a screening tool for occult abdominal injury, prompting further investigation with imaging studies. Amylase, lipase, and urinalysis may be useful when pancreatic or kidney injury is suspected.
      (3) Other laboratory studies may be indicated to rule out medical causes of injury (e.g., calcium, phosphorus, vitamin D, factor levels, organic or amino acids).
   b. Sexual abuse
      (1) When indicated by history or physical findings, culture for *Neisseria gonorrhoeae* (throat, anus, vagina/urethra as indicated), and *Chlamydia* (vagina and anus as indicated). Testing can also be done with urine DNA tests.
      (2) Serologic tests for syphilis, hepatitis, and human immunodeficiency virus (HIV), and a pregnancy test should be performed if the history warrants.
      (3) *Symptomatic children* should be investigated for other genital infections, such as *Trichomonas*, herpes virus, condyloma acuminatum, *G. vaginalis*, and *Candida*.

26.4 Management

1. Immediate management: Emergent issues require prompt medical intervention. Initially provide medical treatment for life-threatening injuries (head trauma, abdominal trauma, and large area burns).
2. Ensure the safety of the patient and other children in the same environment.
3. Short-term management: With acute sexual assault, prophylaxis for sexually transmitted diseases (including HIV) and emergency contraception should be considered.
4. Long-term management: Some abusive injuries (i.e., abusive head trauma) have long-term neurologic sequelae, and early intervention services are needed.
5. Make the appropriate referrals for (short- and long-term) counseling.

26.5 Mandatory Reporting

Report suspect injuries to the appropriate child protective service agency.
All states have mandatory reporting laws for primary care physicians and
other professionals who *suspect* abusive injuries. The goal is the child's
safety; you *do not need* to confirm the diagnosis of child maltreatment before
reporting.

REFERENCES

1. Hunter JA, Figueredo AJ, Malamuth NM, Becker JV: Juvenile sex offenders:
   Toward the development of a typology. Sex Abuse 15(1):27-48, 2003.
2. Rogers C, Tremain T: Clinical interventions with boy victims of sexual abuse. In
   Stuart I, Greer J (eds): Victims of Sexual Aggression. New York, Van Nostrand
   Reinhold, 1984.
3. U.S. Department of Health and Human Services, Children's Bureau: Child Mal-
   treatment 2003: Reports from the States to the National Child Abuse and Neglect
   Data System. Washington, DC, U.S. Government Printing Office, 2005.

SUGGESTED READING

Adams JA, Harper K, Knudson S, Revilla J: Examination findings in legally confirmed
child sexual abuse: It's normal to be normal. Pediatrics 94:310-317, 1994.

American Academy of Pediatrics: Visual Diagnosis of Child Abuse on CD-ROM,
2nd ed. Elk Grove Village, Ill, American Academy of Pediatrics, 2003.

Berenson AB: Normal anogenital anatomy. Child Abuse Negl 22:589-596, 1998.

Botash ASL: Evaluating Child Sexual Abuse: Education Manual for Medical Professionals. Baltimore, Johns Hopkins University Press, 2000.

Heger A, Emans SJ, Muram, D (eds): Evaluation of the Sexually Abused Child.
New York, Oxford University Press, 2000.

Hobbs C, Wynne JM: Physical Signs of Child Abuse: A Color Atlas, 2nd ed. Philadelphia, WB Saunders, 2001.

Jenny C, Hymel K, Ritzen A, et al: Analysis of missed cases of abusive head trauma.
JAMA 281:621-626, 1999.

Kleinman PK: Diagnostic Imaging of Child Abuse, 2nd ed. St. Louis, Mosby, 1998.

Labbe J: Determining whether a skin injury could be physical abuse. Contemp Pediatr
20(5):27-49, 2003.

Reece RM, Ludwig S (eds): Child Abuse: Medical Diagnosis and Management. Philadelphia, Lippincott Williams & Wilkins, 2001.

Sugar NF, Taylor JA, Feldmen KW: Bruises in infants and toddlers: Those who don't
cruise rarely bruise. Arch Pediatr Adolesc Med 153:399-403, 1999.

Appendices

Appendix I: Vital Signs

Appendix I·A: Temperature Conversion Formulas

To convert degrees Celsius to degrees Fahrenheit:
  $(9/5 \times temperature) + 32$
To convert degrees Fahrenheit to degrees Celsius:
  $(temperature - 32) \times 5/9$

Appendix I-B: Heart Rates and ECG Parameters in Children

Age	Heart Rate (bpm)*	QRS Axis*	PR Interval (sec)*	QRS Duration (sec)†	Lead V₁ R-Wave Amplitude (mm)†	Lead V₁ S-Wave Amplitude (mm)†	Lead V₁ R/S Ratio	Lead V₆ R-Wave Amplitude (mm)†	Lead V₆ S-Wave Amplitude (mm)†	Lead V₆ R/S Ratio
0-7 days	95-160 (125)	+30 to 180 (110)	0.08-0.12 (0.10)	0.05 (0.07)	13.3 (25.5)	7.7 (18.8)	2.5	4.8 (11.8)	3.2 (9.6)	2.2
1-3 wk	105-180 (145)	+30 to 180 (110)	0.08-0.12 (0.10)	0.05 (0.07)	100.6 (20.8)	4.2 (10.8)	2.9	7.6 (16.4)	3.4 (9.8)	3.3
1-6 mo	110-180 (145)	+10 to +125 (+70)	0.08-0.13 (0.11)	0.05 (0.07)	9.7 (19)	5.4 (15)	2.3	12.4 (22)	2.8 (8.3)	5.6
6-12 mo	110-170 (135)	+10 to +125 (+60)	0.10-0.14 (0.12)	0.05 (0.07)	9.4 (20.3)	6.4 (18.1)	1.6	12.6 (22.7)	2.1 (7.2)	7.6
1-3 yr	90-150 (120)	+10 to +125 (+60)	0.10-0.14 (0.12)	0.06 (0.07)	8.5 (18)	9 (21)	1.2	14 (23.3)	1.7 (6)	10

*Normal range and (mean).
†Mean and (98th percentile).
Data from Park MK: Pediatric Cardiology for Practitioners, 3rd ed. St. Louis, Mosby, 1996; and Davignon A, Rautaharju P, Boisselle E, et al: Normal ECG standards for infants and children. Pediatr Cardiol 1:123-152, 1979.

Continued

Appendix I

Appendix I-B:　Heart Rates and ECG Parameters in Children—cont'd

Age	Heart Rate (bpm)*	QRS Axis*	PR Interval (sec)*	QRS Duration (sec)†	Lead V₁ R-Wave Amplitude (mm)†	Lead V₁ S-Wave Amplitude (mm)†	Lead V₁ R/S Ratio	Lead V₆ R-Wave Amplitude (mm)†	Lead V₆ S-Wave Amplitude (mm)†	Lead V₆ R/S Ratio
4-5 yr	65-135 (110)	0 to +110 (+60)	0.11-0.15 (0.13)	0.07 (0.08)	7.6 (16)	11 (22.5)	0.8	15.6 (25)	1.4 (4.7)	11.2
6-8 yr	60-130 (100)	-15 to +110 (+60)	0.12-0.16 (0.14)	0.07 (0.08)	6 (13)	12 (24.5)	0.6	16.3 (26)	1.1 (3.9)	13
9-11 yr	60-110 (85)	-15 to +110 (+60)	0.12-0.17 (0.14)	0.07 (0.09)	5.4 (12.1)	11.9 (25.4)	0.5	16.3 (25.4)	1.0 (3.9)	14.3
12-16 yr	60-110 (85)	-15 to +110 (+60)	0.12-0.17 (0.15)	0.07 (0.10)	4.1 (9.9)	10.8 (21.2)	0.5	14.3 (23)	0.8 (3.7)	14.7
>16 yr	60-100 (80)	-15 to +110 (+60)	0.12-0.20 (0.15)	0.08 (0.10)	3 (9)	10 (20)	0.3	10 (20)	0.8 (3.7)	12

Appendix I-C: **Respiratory Rates**

Age (yr)	Respiratory Rate (breaths/min)
0-1*	24-38
1-3	22-30
4-6	20-24
7-9	18-24
10-14	16-22
14-18	14-20

*Slightly higher respiratory rates in the neonatal period (i.e., 40-50 breaths/min) may be normal in the absence of other signs and symptoms.
Data from Bardella IJ: Pediatric advanced life support: A review of the AHA recommendations. Am Fam Physician 60:1743-1750, 1999.

Appendix I-D: **Blood Pressure**

Blood pressure levels for the 95th percentile of blood pressure for boys aged 1 to 17 years by percentile of height.

Age (yr)	Systolic Blood Pressure (mm Hg) by Percentile of Height			Diastolic Blood Pressure (mm Hg) by Percentile of Height		
	5th	50th	95th	5th	50th	95th
1	98	103	106	54	56	58
2	101	106	110	59	61	63
3	104	109	113	63	65	67
4	106	111	115	66	69	71
5	108	112	116	69	72	74
6	109	114	117	72	74	76
7	110	115	119	74	76	78
8	111	116	120	75	78	80
9	113	118	121	76	79	81
10	115	119	123	77	80	82
11	117	121	125	78	80	82
12	119	123	127	78	81	83
13	121	126	130	79	81	83
14	124	128	132	80	82	84
15	126	131	135	81	83	85
16	129	134	137	82	84	87
17	131	136	140	84	87	89

The 95th percentile is 1.645 SD over the mean.
Data from National Institutes of Health, National Heart, Lung, and Blood Institute: Fourth Report on the Diagnosis, Evaluation, and Treatment of High Blood Pressure in Children and Adolescents. NIH publication no. 05-5267. Bethesda, Md, National Institutes of Health, 2005.

Continued

Appendix I-D: Blood Pressure—cont'd

Blood pressure levels of the 95th percentile of blood pressure for girls aged 1 to 17 years by percentile of height.

Age (yr)	Systolic Blood Pressure (mm Hg) by Percentile of Height			Diastolic Blood Pressure (mm Hg) by Percentile of Height		
	5th	50th	95th	5th	50th	95th
1	100	104	107	56	58	60
2	102	105	109	61	63	65
3	104	107	110	65	67	69
4	105	108	112	68	70	72
5	107	109	113	70	72	74
6	108	111	115	72	74	76
7	110	113	116	73	75	77
8	112	115	118	75	76	78
9	114	117	120	76	77	79
10	116	119	122	77	78	80
11	118	121	124	78	79	81
12	119	123	126	79	80	82
13	121	124	128	80	81	83
14	123	126	129	81	82	84
15	124	127	131	82	83	85
16	125	128	132	82	84	86
17	125	129	132	82	84	86

The 95th percentile is 1.645 SD over the mean.
Data from National Institutes of Health, National Heart, Lung, and Blood Institute: Fourth Report on the Diagnosis, Evaluation, and Treatment of High Blood Pressure in Children and Adolescents. NIH publication no. 05-5267. Bethesda, Md, National Institutes of Health, 2005.

Appendix II: Growth Charts

Appendix II-A: Length and Weight Conversion Formulas

1 lb = 454 g; 1 kg = 2.2 lb. To convert pounds to grams, multiply by 454. To convert kilograms to pounds, multiply by 2.2. To convert inches to centimeters, multiply by 2.54.

Appendix II-B: Stature and Weight for Boys, Birth to 36 Months

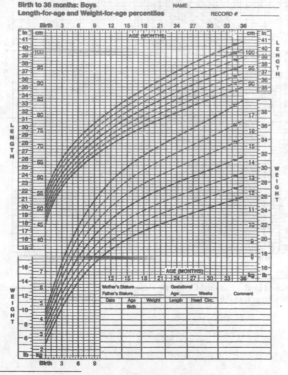

Birth to 36 months: Boys
Length-for-age and Weight-for-age percentiles

Developed by the National Center for Health Statistics in collaboration with the National Center for Chronic Disease Prevention and Health Promotion, 2000.

Appendix II-C: Stature and Weight for Girls, Birth to 36 Months

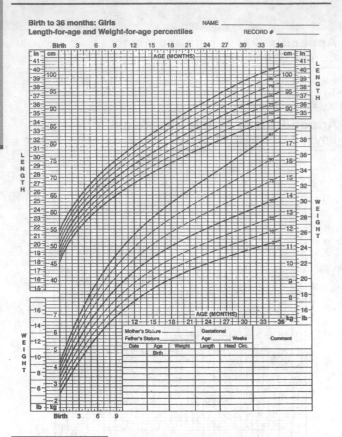

Developed by the National Center for Health Statistics in collaboration with the National Center for Chronic Disease Prevention and Health Promotion, 2000.

Appendix II-D: Stature and Weight for Boys, 2 to 20 Years

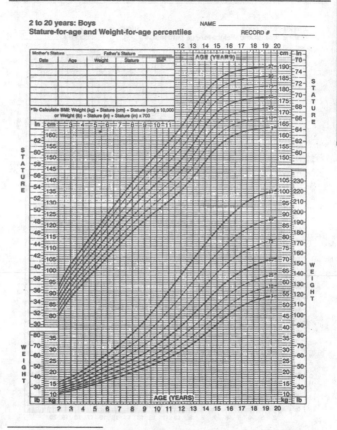

2 to 20 years: Boys
Stature-for-age and Weight-for-age percentiles

Developed by the National Center for Health Statistics in collaboration with the National Center for Chronic Disease Prevention and Health Promotion, 2000.

Appendix II-E: Stature and Weight for Girls, 2 to 20 Years

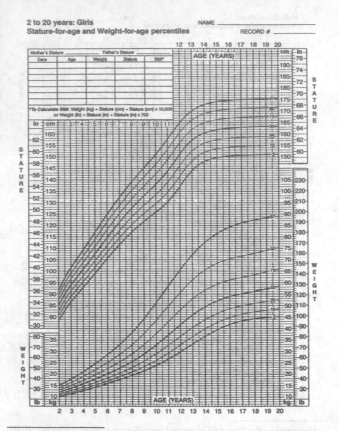

Developed by the National Center for Health Statistics in collaboration with the National Center for Chronic Disease Prevention and Health Promotion, 2000.

Appendix II-F: Body Mass Index

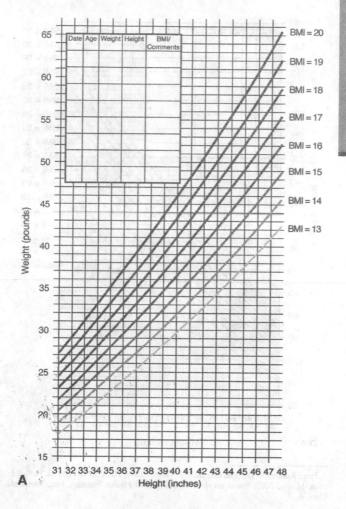

Date	Age	Weight	Height	BMI/Comments

Appendix II-F: Body Mass Index—cont'd

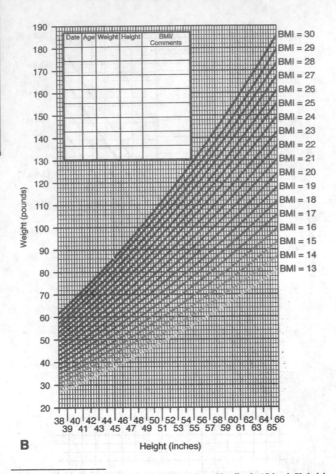

From Robertson J, Shilkofski N: The Harriet Lane Handbook, 17th ed. Philadelphia, Mosby, 2005; based on data from Portland Health Institute, Inc., Portland, Oregon.

Appendix II-G: Head Circumference, 2 to 18 Years

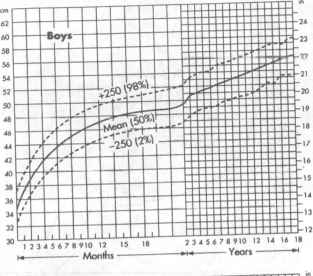

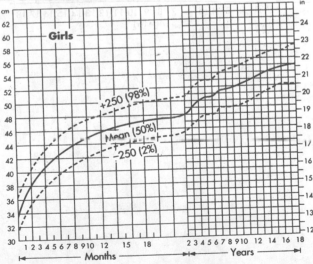

Appendix II-H: Height Velocity Curves

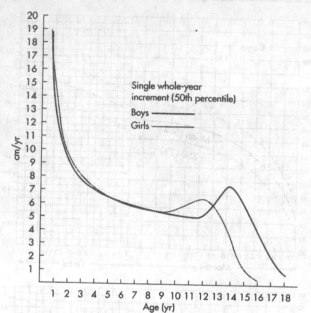

Appendix III: Body Surface Area Nomogram

Approximate relation of surface area and weight in individuals of average bodily proportions.

Weight			Weight		
kg	lb	Area (m²)	kg	lb	Area (m²)
2	4.4	0.12	25	55	0.93
3	6.6	0.20	30	66	1.07
4	8.8	0.23	35	77	1.20
5	11	0.25	40	88	1.32
6	13	0.29	45	99	1.43
7	15	0.33	50	110	1.53
8	18	0.36	55	121	1.62
9	20	0.40	60	132	1.70
10	22	0.44	65	143	1.78
15	33	0.62	70	154	1.84
20	44	0.79			

Appendix IV: Timing of Tooth Eruption

	Deciduous Teeth: Eruption		Deciduous Teeth: Shedding		Permanent Teeth: Eruption	
	Maxillary	Mandibular	Maxillary	Mandibular	Maxillary	Mandibular
Central incisors	6-8 mo	5-7 mo	7-8 yr	6-7 yr	7-8 yr	6-7 yr
Lateral incisors	8-11 mo	7-10 mo	8-9 yr	7-8 yr	8-9 yr	7-8 yr
Cuspids	16-20 mo	16-20 mo	11-12 yr	9-11 yr	11-12 yr	9-11 yr
1st premolar	—	—	—	—	10-11 yr	10-12 yr
2nd premolar	—	—	—	—	10-12 yr	11-13 yr
1st molars	10-16 mo	10-16 mo	10-11 yr	10-12 yr	6-7 yr	6-7 yr
2nd molars	20-30 mo	20-30 mo	10-12 yr	11-13 yr	12-13 yr	12-13 yr
3rd molars	—	—	—	—	17-22 yr	17-22 yr

The sexes are combined, although girls tend to be slightly more advanced (at least with respect to tooth eruption) than boys. Averages are approximate values derived from various studies.

Data from Behrman RE, Vaughan VC, Nelson WE (eds): Nelson's Textbook of Pediatrics, 13th ed. Philadelphia, WB Saunders, 1987.

Appendix V:
Sexual Maturation and Tanner Staging

Appendix V-A: Boys

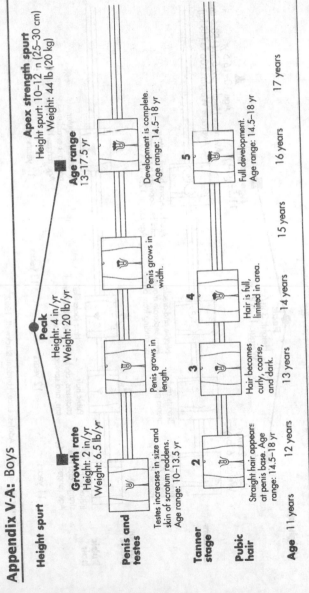

Height spurt

Apex strength spurt: Height spurt: 10–12 n (25–30 cm)
Weight: 44 lb (20 kg)

Age range 13–17.5 yr

Peak
Height: 4 in/yr
Weight: 20 lb/yr

Growth rate
Height: 2 in/yr
Weight: 6.5 lb/yr

Penis and testes

Testes increases in size and skin of scrotum reddens. Age range: 10–13.5 yr

Penis grows in length.

Penis grows in width.

Development is complete. Age range: 14.5–18 yr

Tanner stage   2   3   4   5

Pubic hair

Straight hair appears at penis base. Age range: 14.5–18 yr

Hair becomes curly, coarse, and dark.

Hair is full, limited in area.

Full development. Age range: 14.5–18 yr

Age 11 years 12 years 13 years 14 years 15 years 16 years 17 years

Redrawn from Tanner JM: Growth at Acolescence. London, Blackwell, 1962.

Appendix V-B: Girls

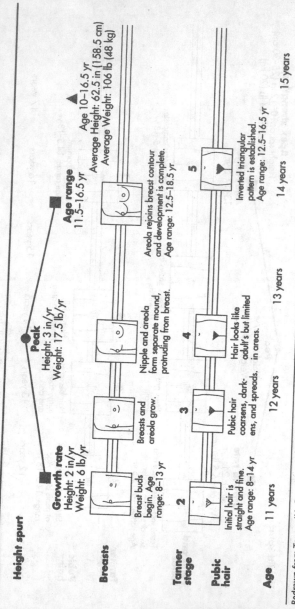

Height spurt

Growth rate
Height: 2 in/yr
Weight: 6 lb/yr

Peak
Height: 3 in/yr
Weight: 17.5 lb/yr

Age range
11.5–16.5 yr

Age 10–16.5 yr
Average Height: 62.5 in (158.5 cm)
Average Weight: 106 lb (48 kg)

Breasts

2 — Breast buds begin. Age range: 8–13 yr

3 — Breasts and areola grow.

Peak — Nipple and areola form separate mound, protruding from breast.

Areola rejoins breast contour and development is complete. Age range: 12.5–18.5 yr

Tanner stage 2 3 4 5

Pubic hair

2 — Initial hair is straight and fine. Age range: 8–14 yr

3 — Pubic hair coarsens, darkens, and spreads.

4 — Hair looks like adult's but limited in areas.

5 — Inverted triangular pattern is established. Age range: 12.5–16.5 yr

Age 11 years   12 years   13 years   14 years   15 years

Redrawn from Tanner JM: Growth at Adolescence. London, Blackwell, 1962.

Appendix VI:
Nutritional
Reference Material

Component (per dL)	Recommended Daily Dietary Allowances (0-6 mo)	Human Milk Values (Variable)	"Humanized" Formulas Enfamil (Mead-Johnson) with Iron	Similac (Ross) with Iron	Whole Milk (3.5% Fat)
Calories (kcal)	117 kcal/kg	67-75	67	68	66
Protein (g)	2.2 g/kg	1.1	1.5	1.6	3.5
Fat, total (g)	Not listed	4.5	3.7	3.6	3.5-3.7
Saturated		2.2	1.2	1.4	2.2
Unsaturated		2.3	2.5	2.2	1.3
Cholesterol (mg)	Not listed	7-47			10-35
Carbohydrate (g) (Lactose)	Not listed	6.8	7	7.1	4.9
Calcium (mg)	300	34	55	58	118
Phosphorus (mg)	240	14	46	43	92
Sodium (mg)	Not listed	16	28	25	50
Potassium (mg)	Not listed	51	69	75	137
Magnesium (mg)	60	4	4	4	12
Iron (mg)	10	0.05	1.2	1.2	0.05
Copper (µg)	Not listed	40	60	40	30
Zinc (mg)	3	0.3-0.5	0.4	0.5	0.3-0.5
Iodine (µg)	35	3	7	10	5
Vitamin A (IU)	1400	200	170	250	140
Thiamine (mg)	0.3	0.016	0.05	0.07	0.17
Riboflavin (mg)	0.4	0.036	0.06	0.1	0.17
Niacin (mg)	5	0.1	0.8	0.7	0.1

Pyridoxine (mg)	0.3	0.01	0.04	0.04	0.06
Folacin (mg)	0.05	0.005	0.01	0.005	0.005
Vitamin B_{12} (µg)	0.3	0.03	0.2	0.2	0.4
Vitamin C (mg)	35	4	5	6	1
Vitamin D (IU)	400	2	42	40	Fortified 42
Vitamin E (IU)	4	0.2	1.3	1.5	0.04
Vitamin K (µg)	Not listed	1.5	6	9	6

Modified from Hoekelman RA, Friedman SB, Nelson NM, Seidel HM: Primary Pediatric Care, 2nd ed. St. Louis, Mosby, 1992.

HUMAN MILK AND FORTIFIERS (PER LITER)

Formula	kcal/oz (kcal/mL)	Protein Source	Fat Source	Carbohydrate Source	Suggested Uses
Enfamil Human Milk Fortifier (per pkt) (Mead Johnson)	3.5 kcal/mL	Whey protein isolate Na caseinate	From caseinate	Corn syrup solids	Fortifier for preterm human milk
Preterm Human Milk + Similac Human Milk Fortifier (1 pkt/ 25 mL) (Ross)	24 (0.8)	Human milk protein Nonfat milk Whey protein concentrate	Human milk fat MCT oil	Lactose Corn syrup solids	Preterm infants

MCT, medium-chain triglyceride.

PRETERM INFANT FORMULAS (PER LITER)

Formula	kcal/oz (kcal/mL)	Protein Source	Fat Source (%)	Carbohydrate Source (%)	Suggested Uses
Enfamil Premature LIPIL (with iron) (Mead Johnson)	24 (0.8)	Nonfat milk Whey protein concentrate	MCT oil (40) Soy oil (30) HO vegetable oil (27) DHA and ARA (3)	Corn syrup solids (60) Lactose (40)	Preterm infants
Similac Special Care Advance (with iron) (Ross)	24 (0.8)	Nonfat milk Whey protein concentrate	MCT oil (50) Soy oil (30) Coconut oil (18) DHA (0.25) ARA (0.4)	Corn syrup solids (50) Lactose (50)	Preterm infants

Continued

ARA, arachidonic acid; DHA, docosahexaenoic acid; HO, high-oleic; MCT, medium-chain triglyceride.

COW'S MILK-BASED FORMULAS (PER LITER)

Formula	kcal/oz (kcal/mL)	Protein Source	Fat Source (%)	Carbohydrate Source (%)	Suggested Uses
America's Store Brand Infant Formula (Wyeth Nutritionals)	20 (0.67)	Nonfat milk Whey protein concentrate	Palm or palm olein oil Coconut oil HO safflower oil or HO sunflower oil	Lactose	Infants with normal GI tract
Enfamil with iron (Mead Johnson)	20 (0.67)	Nonfat milk Whey protein concentrate	Soy oil Palm olein oil (44) Soy oil (19.5) Coconut oil (19.5) HO sunflower oil (14.5)	Lactose	Infants with normal GI tract
Enfamil LIPIL (with iron) (Mead Johnson)	20 (0.67)	Nonfat milk Whey protein concentrate	Palm olein oil (44) Soy oil (19.5) Coconut oil (19.5) HO sunflower oil (14.5) DHA and ARA (2.5)	Lactose	Infants with normal GI tract
Enfamil LactoFree LIPIL (Mead Johnson)	20 (0.67)	Milk protein isolate	Palm olein oil (44) Soy oil (19.5) Coconut oil (19.5) HO sunflower oil (14.5) DHA and ARA (2.5)	Lactose Rich starch Maltodextrin	Infants with lactose malabsorption

Good Start Supreme (Nestle)	20 (0.67)	Enzymatically hydrolyzed reduced minerals Whey	Palm olein oil (47) Soy oil (26) Coconut oil (21) HO safflower oil or HO sunflower oil (6)	Lactose (70) Maltodextrin (30)	Infants with normal GI tract
Similac Advance (Ross)	20 (0.67)	Nonfat milk Whey protein concentrate	HO safflower oil (41) Soy oil (30) Coconut oil (28) DHA (0.15) ARA (0.4)	Lactose	Infants with normal GI tract
Similac Lactose Free (Ross)	20 (0.67)	Milk protein isolate	HO safflower oil (41) Soy oil (30) Coconut oil (28) DHA (0.15) ARA (0.4)	Maltodextrin (55) Sucrose (45)	Infants with lactose malabsorption

Continued

ARA, arachidonic acid; DHA, docosahexaenoic acid; GI, gastrointestinal; HO, high-oleic.

SOY-BASED INFANT FORMULAS (PER LITER)

Formula	kcal/oz (kcal/mL)	Protein Source	Fat Source (%)	Carbohydrate Source (%)	Suggested Uses
America's Store Brand Soy Infant Formula (Wyeth Nutritionals)	20 (0.67)	Soy protein isolate L-Methionine	Palm or Palm olein oil Coconut oil HO sunflower oil or HO safflower oil	Corn syrup solids Sucrose	Infants with cow's milk allergy, galactosemia, or lactose malabsorption
Isomil Advance (Ross)	20 (0.67)	Soy protein isolate L-Methionine	Soy oil HO safflower oil (41) Soy oil (30) Coconut oil (28) DHA (0.15) ARA (0.4)	Corn syrup (80) Sucrose (20)	Infants with cow's milk allergy, galactosemia, or lactose malabsorption

ARA, arachidonic acid; DHA, docosahexaenoic acid; HO, high-oleic.
Data from Barness LA: Nutrition update. Pediatr Rev 15:321-326, 1994; also adapted from Robertson J, Shilkofski N: The Harriet Lane Handbook, 17th ed. Philadelphia, Mosby, 2005.

Appendix VI-B: Examples of Various Formulas and Their Uses—cont'd

CASEIN HYDROLYSATE INFANT FORMULAS (PER LITER)

Formula	kcal/oz (kcal/mL)	Protein Source	Fat Source (%)	Carbohydrate Source (%)	Suggested Uses
Alimentum Advance (Ross)	20 (0.67)	Casein hydrolysate L-Cystine L-Tyrosine L-Tryptophan	Safflower oil (38) MCT oil (33) Soy oil (28) DHA (0.15) ARA (0.4)	Sucrose (70) Modified tapioca starch (30)	Infants with food allergies, protein or fat malabsorption
Nutramigen made from powder (Mead Johnson)*	20 (0.67)	Casein hydrolysate L-Cystine L-Tyrosine L-Tryptophan	Palm olein oil (44) Soy oil (19.5) Coconut oil (19.5) HO sunflower oil (14.5) DHA and ARA (2.5)	Corn syrup solids (86) Modified corn starch (14)	Infants with food allergies or protein malabsorption
Pregestimil liquid (Mead Johnson)†	24 (0.8)	Casein hydrolysate L-Cystine L-Tyrosine L-Tryptophan	MCT oil (55) Soy oil (35) HO safflower (10)	Corn syrup solids (75) Modified corn starch (25)	Infants with food allergies, protein or fat malabsorption requiring additional calories

*Pediatric Products Handbook, 1990 (Evansville, Ind, Mead Johnson).
†Mead Johnson letter, January 1989 (Mead Johnson Nutritionals). Powder form only; to make normal dilution (20 kcal/oz), add 9 7 g of powder to each 60 mL of water.
ARA, arachidonic acid; DHA, docosahexaenoic acid; HO, high-oleic; MCT, medium-chain triglyceride.
Data from Barness LA: Nutrition update. Pediatr Rev 15:321-326, 1994; also adapted from Robertson J, Shilkofski N: The Harriet Lane Handbook, 17th ed. Philadelphia, Mosby, 2005.

Appendix VI-C: Other High-Calorie Formulas and Caloric Boosters

1. Special formulas to increase calorie intake
   a. PediaSure—30 cal/oz
      (1) Casein/whey protein: 30 g of protein/L
      (2) Hydrolyzed corn starch, sucrose: 325 mOsm/kg
   b. Ensure—32 cal/oz
      (1) Casein/soy protein
      (2) 14% cal as protein, 32% cal as fat, 54% CHO
      (3) Corn syrup, sucrose: 470 mOsm/kg
   c. Sustacal—30 cal/oz
      (1) Casein/soy protein
      (2) 24% cal as protein, 21% cal as fat, 55% CHO
      (3) Sucrose, corn syrup: 620 mOsm/kg
2. Calorie boosters for infants
   a. Polycose (glucose polymers)
      (1) 1 tablespoon = 6 g (23 cal/tablespoon)
      (2) 2 tablespoons Polycose + 8 oz of whole milk/formula
      (3) 30 cal/oz, 1.0 g of protein/oz
      (4) Must be titrated, can cause diarrhea
   b. Medium-chain triglycerides (MCT oil)
      (1) 215 cal/oz
      (2) Must be titrated, can cause diarrhea
   c. Supermilk
      (1) 1 cup nonfat milk (protein) + 1 quart whole milk
      (2) 28 cal/oz, 1.8 g of protein/oz
      (3) High renal solute load
   d. Carnation Instant Breakfast (CIB)
      (1) 8 oz of whole milk + 1 package of CIB
      (2) 32 cal/oz, 1.8 g protein/oz
   e. Super fruit
      (1) 1 jar pureed fruit + 2 tablespoons powdered formula + 1 tablespoon corn oil
      (2) 300 cal/serving

Appendix VII:
Developmental
Reference Material

Appendix VII-A: Age-Based Developmental Milestones

Age	Gross Motor	Fine and Visual Motor	Language	Social/Adaptive
1 mo	Raises head slightly from prone, makes crawling movements, lifts chin up	Has tight grasp, follow to midline	Alerts to sound (e.g., by blinking, moving, startling)	Regards face
2 mo	Holds head in midline, lifts chest off table	No longer clenches fist tightly, follows object past midline	Smiles after being stroked or talked to	Recognizes parents
3 mo	Supports on forearms in prone, holds head up steadily	Holds hands open at rest, follows in circular fashion	Coos (produces long vowel sounds in musical fashion)	Reaches for familiar people for objects, anticipates feeding
4-5 mo	Rolls front to back, back to front, sits well when propped, supports on wrists and shifts weight	Moves arms in unison to grasp, touches cube placed on table	Orients to voice 5 mo: orients to bell (localizes laterally), says "ah-goo," razzes	Enjoys looking around environment
6 mo	Sits well unsupported, puts feet in mouth in supine position	Reaches with either hand, transfers, uses raking grasp	Babbles 7 mo: orients to bell (localizes indirectly)	Recognizes strangers
9 mo	Creeps, crawls, cruises, pulls to stand, pivots when sitting	Uses pincer grasp, probes with forefinger, holds bottle, finger feeds	Understands "no," waves bye-bye 8 mo: "dada/mama" indiscriminately 10 mo: "dada/mama" discriminately; orients to bell (directly) 11 mo: one word other than "dada/mama"	Starts to explore environment, plays pat-a-cake

Age	Gross Motor	Fine Motor	Language	Personal/Social
12 mo	Walks alone	Throws objects, lets go of toys, hand release, uses mature pincer grasp	Follows one-step command with gesture, uses two words other than "dada/mama" *14 mo:* uses three words	Imitates actions; comes when called, cooperates with dressing *15-18 mo:* uses spoon and cup
15 mo	Creeps upstairs, walks backward	Builds tower of two blocks in imitation of examiner, scribbles in imitation		
18 mo	Runs, throws toy from standing without falling	Turns two to three pages at a time, fills spoon and feeds self	Follows one-step command without gesture, uses four to six words and immature jargoning (runs several unintelligible words together) Knows 7-20 words, knows one body part, uses mature jargoning (includes intelligible words in jargoning)	Copies parent in tasks (e.g., sweeping, dusting), plays in company of other children
21 mo	Squats in play, goes up steps	Builds tower of five blocks, drinks well from cup	Points to three body parts, uses 2-word combinations, has 20-word vocabulary	Asks to have food and to go to toilet
24 mo	Walks up and down steps without help	Turns pages one at a time, removes shoes, pants, etc., imitates swim stroke	Uses 50 words, 2-word sentences, uses pronouns (I, you, me) inappropriately, points to five body parts, understands two-step command	Parallel play
30 mo	Jumps with both feet off floor, throws ball overhand	Unbuttons, holds pencil in adult fashion, differentiates horizontal and vertical line	Uses pronouns (I, you, me) appropriately, understands concept of "one," repeats two digits forward	Tells first and last names when asked, gets self drink without help

Continued

Appendix VII

Appendix VII-A: Age-Based Developmental Milestones—cont'd

Age	Gross Motor	Fine and Visual Motor	Language	Social/Adaptive
3 yr	Pedals tricycle, can alternate feet when going up steps	Dresses and undresses partially, dries hands if reminded, draws a circle	Uses three-word sentences; uses plurals, past tense, knows all pronouns, minimum 250 words, understands concept of "two"	Group play, shares toys, takes turns, plays well with others, knows full name, age, sex
4 yr	Hops, skips, alternates feet going downstairs	Buttons clothing fully, catches ball	Knows colors, says song or poem from memory, asks questions	Tells "tall tales," plays cooperatively with a group of children
5 yr	Skips, alternating feet, jumps over low obstacles	Ties shoes, spreads with knife	Prints first name, asks what a word means	Plays competitive games, abides by rules, likes to help in household tasks

Data from Capute A, Biehl RF: Functional developmental evaluation: Prerequisite to habilitation. Pediatr Clin North Am 20:3-26, 1973; Capute AJ, Accardo PJ: Linguistic and auditory milestones during the first two years of life: A language inventory for the practitioner. Clin Pediatr (Phila) 17:847-853, 1978; Capute AJ, Shapiro BK, Wachtel RC, et al: The Clinical Linguistic and Auditory Milestone Scale (CLAMS): Identification of cognitive defects in motor-delayed children. Am J Dis Child 140:694-698, 1986; Capute AJ, Palmer FB, Shapiro BK, et al: Clinical Linguistic and Auditory Milestone Scale: Prediction of cognition in infancy. Dev Med Child Neurol 28:762-771, 1986.
Adapted from Barone MA (ed): The Harriet Lane Handbook, 14th ed. St. Louis, Mosby, 1996.

Appendix VII-B: Ontogeny of Neonatal Reflexes

Reflex	Clinical Description	Age (mo) Presents	Age (mo) Disappears
Primitive			
Palmar group	Stimulus to palm of hand→flexion of fingers and closure of hand	Birth	4
Plantar grasp	Stimulus to hallucal area of foot→flexion of toes	Birth	9
Automatic stepping	Involuntary "walking"	Birth	2
Crossed extension	Supine: stimulus to sole of foot→flexion, abduction, and extension of contralateral limb	Birth	2
Galant	Linear noxious stimulus usually applied paravertebrally in caudal direction→withdrawal response of trunk with "curving away" of trunk	Birth	3-6
Moro	Neck extension→flexion of arms followed by extension	Birth	4
Asymmetric tonic neck	Turn head to one side→extension of the arm and leg on the face side and flexion of the arm and leg on the occiput side ("fencing position")	Birth	4
Symmetric tonic neck	Neck extension→extension of upper extremities and flexion of lower extremities; neck flexion→flexion of upper extremities and extension of lower extremities	5	8
Lower extremity placing	Anterior aspect of tibia and dorsum of foot moved along a table edge→ flexion→extension and then placing the foot on the table surface	1 day	
Upper extremity placing	Anterior aspect of radius and dorsum of hand moved along a table edge→ flexion→extension and then placing the hand on the table surface	3	

Continued

Appendix VII-B: Ontogeny of Neonatal Reflexes—cont'd

Reflex	Clinical Description	Age (mo) Presents	Age (mo) Disappears
Postural responses			
Landau	Prone→head extension then trunk, hip, and leg extension	3	12-24
Head righting	Head held midline and upright	4-6	
Derotational righting	Head or legs are rotated to one side→segmental rolling of rest of body	4	
Anterior propping	Sitting position→arms extend forward with hands placed on floor	6	
Lateral propping	Sitting→moved off center of gravity toward side→extension of arm with hand placed to prevent falling over	8	
Posterior propping	Sitting→moved off center of gravity backward→arms extend backwards to prevent fall	10	
Parachute	Held prone→moved quickly toward floor→extension of arms to "break fall"	8-9	

Appendix VII-C: Denver Developmental Assessment (Denver II)*

Since the Denver Developmental Screening Test (DDST) first appeared in 1967, it has undergone major revisions and restandardizations. A version titled Revised-Prescreening Developmental Questionnaire II (R-PDQ II) can be used by parents as a prescreening tool. It is designed to identify between 15% and 30% of the children screened as suspect for a developmental delay. In the appropriate setting, it can be used by parents as they wait to be seen by the provider (see figure). A modification of the original DDST, the Denver II, can be used as a primary or secondary stage screening instrument (e.g., after parental report on the R-PDQ II). The 125-item Denver II is divided into four major domains: gross motor, language, fine motor, and personal-social. The age was determined at which 25%, 50%, 75%, and 90% of children could perform the item in each domain. The test form has an age scale corresponding to the American Academy of Pediatrics (AAP) recommended health maintenance visits.

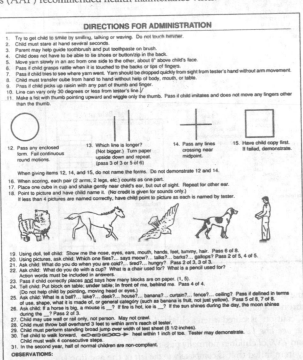

DIRECTIONS FOR ADMINISTRATION

1. Try to get child to smile by smiling, talking or waving. Do not touch him/her.
2. Child must stare at hand several seconds.
3. Parent may help guide toothbrush and put toothpaste on brush.
4. Child does not have to be able to tie shoes or button/zip in the back.
5. Move yarn slowly in an arc from one side to the other, about 8" above child's face.
6. Pass if child grasps rattle when it is touched to the backs or tips of fingers.
7. Pass if child tries to see where yarn went. Yarn should be dropped quickly from sight from tester's hand without arm movement.
8. Child must transfer cube from hand to hand without help of body, mouth, or table.
9. Pass if child picks up raisin with any part of thumb and finger.
10. Line can vary only 30 degrees or less from tester's line.
11. Make a fist with thumb pointing upward and wiggle only the thumb. Pass if child imitates and does not move any fingers other than the thumb.

12. Pass any enclosed form. Fail continuous round motions.
13. Which line is longer? (Not bigger.) Turn paper upside down and repeat. (pass 3 of 3 or 5 of 6)
14. Pass any lines crossing near midpoint.
15. Have child copy first. If failed, demonstrate.

When giving items 12, 14, and 15, do not name the forms. Do not demonstrate 12 and 14.

16. When scoring, each pair (2 arms, 2 legs, etc.) counts as one part.
17. Place one cube in cup and shake gently near child's ear, but out of sight. Repeat for other ear.
18. Point to picture and have child name it. (No credit is given for sounds only.)
    If less than 4 pictures are named correctly, have child point to picture as each is named by tester.

19. Using doll, tell child: Show me the nose, eyes, ears, mouth, hands, feet, tummy, hair. Pass 6 of 8.
20. Using pictures, ask child: Which one flies?... says meow?... talks?... barks?... gallops? Pass 2 of 5, 4 of 5.
21. Ask child: What do you do when you are cold?... tired?... hungry? Pass 2 of 3, 3 of 3.
22. Ask child: What do you do with a cup? What is a chair used for? What is a pencil used for?
    Action words must be included in answers.
23. Pass if child correctly places and says how many blocks are on paper. (1, 5).
24. Tell child: Put block on table; under table; in front of me, behind me. Pass 4 of 4.
    (Do not help child by pointing, moving head or eyes.)
25. Ask child: What is a ball?... lake?... desk?... house?... banana?... curtain?... fence?... ceiling? Pass if defined in terms of use, shape, what it is made of, or general category (such as banana is fruit, not just yellow). Pass 5 of 8, 7 of 8.
26. Ask child: If a horse is big, a mouse is __? If fire is hot, ice is __? If the sun shines during the day, the moon shines during the __? Pass 2 of 3.
27. Child may use wall or rail only, not person. May not crawl.
28. Child must throw ball overhand 3 feet to within arm's reach of tester.
29. Child must perform standing broad jump over width of test sheet (8 1/2-inches).
30. Tell child to walk forward, ⟵○⟶○⟶○⟶ heel within 1 inch of toe. Tester may demonstrate.
    Child must walk 4 consecutive steps.
31. In the second year, half of normal children are non-compliant.

OBSERVATIONS:

*From Frankenberg WE, Dodds JB: The Denver II: A major revision and standardization of the Denver Developmental Screening Test. Pediatrics 89:1, 1992.

SCORING THE DENVER II

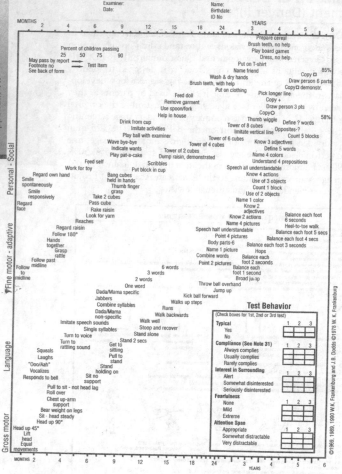

Appendix VII

1. A vertical line is drawn connecting the top and bottom age markers at the child's chronologic age.

2. "Caution": A "caution" is scored when a child fails (or refuses to do) an item on which the *age line falls on or between* the 75th and 90th percentile (i.e., more than 75% of children normally pass that item at a younger age).

3. "Delay": Any item failed that is *completely to the left* of the age line (i.e., the child failed an item that 90% of the children normally pass at a younger age) is considered a delay.

4. Suggested guidelines in interpreting the test
   a. Normal
      (1) No delays and a maximum of one Caution
      (2) Conduct routine rescreening at next well-child visit.
   b. Suspect
      (1) Two or more Cautions and/or one or more Delays
      (2) Because communities' and programs' priorities differ in types or severity of problems they seek to identify in screening, it will be necessary to adjust Suspect criteria to achieve their goals most efficiently. Tables of percentages of Cautions and Delays that may be expected for different demographic groups are proved in the *Denver II Technical Manual*.
      (3) Rescreen in 1 to 2 weeks to rule out temporary factors such as fatigue, fear, or illness.
   c. Untestable
      (1) Refusal scores on one or more items completely to the left of the age line or on more than one item intersected by the age line in the 75% to 90% area
      (2) Rescreen in 1 to 2 weeks.
5. Referral considerations: If, upon rescreening, the test result is again Suspect or Untestable, whether or not to refer should be determined by the clinical judgment of the supervising professional based on:
   a. Profile of test results (which items are Cautions and Delays);
   b. Number of Cautions and Delays;
   c. Rate of past development;
   d. Other clinical considerations (clinical history, examination, etc.); and
   e. Availability of referral resources.

Monitoring the screening program is discussed in the *Denver II Technical Manual*. The use of such monitoring is strongly recommended to assist the supervising professional in establishing and adjusting referral criteria. Detailed instructions to administer and score the test are provided in the *Denver II Training Manual*. The manual should be used to ensure accuracy and reliability in administration of the test. These materials are available from DDM, Inc., P.O. Box 6919, Denver, CO 80206-0919; (303) 355-4729 or (800) 419-4729.

Appendix VII-D: A Screening Tool for Language (CLAMS: 10 to 36 mo Language Screen)

The CLAMS (Clinical Linguistic and Auditory Milestone Scale) was created to assess language skills from 1 to 36 months of age. For practical purposes, illustrated here is the test for 10 to 36 months, the most useful age range. Scoring is done by calculating the basal age as the highest age group in which a child accomplishes all of the test tasks correctly. The age equivalent is then determined by adding the decimal number (recorded in parenthesis) next to each correctly scored item passed at age groups beyond the basal age to the basal age itself. Each of these age equivalents is then divided by the child's chronologic age and multiplied by 100 to determine a developmental quotient (DQ). A DQ less than 70 constitutes delay and warrants referral.

Age (mo)	CLAMS Item	Yes	No
10	Understands "no" (.03)	—	—
	Uses "dada" appropriately (0.3)	—	—
	Uses "mama" appropriately (0.3)	—	—
11	One word (other than "mama" and "dada" (1.0)	—	—
12	One-step command with gesture (0.5)	—	—
	Two-word vocabulary (0.5)	—	—
14	Three-word vocabulary (1.0)	—	—
	Immature jargoning (1.0)	—	—
16	Four- to six-word vocabulary (1.0)	—	—
	One-step command without gesture (1.0)	—	—
18	Mature jargoning (0.5)	—	—
	7- to 10-word vocabulary (0.5)	—	—
	Points to one picture (0.5)*	—	—
	Knows body parts (0.5)	—	—
21	20-word vocabulary (1.0)	—	—
	Two-word phrases (1.0)	—	—
	Points to two pictures (1.0)*	—	—
24	50-word vocabulary (1.0)	—	—
	Two-step command (1.0)	—	—
	Two-word sentences (1.0)	—	—
30	Uses pronouns appropriately (1.5)	—	—
	Concept of one (1.5)*	—	—
	Points to seven pictures (1.5)*	—	—
	Two digits forward (1.5)*	—	—
36	250-word vocabulary (1.5)	—	—
	Three-word sentence (1.5)	—	—
	Three digits forward (1.5)*	—	—
	Follows two prepositional commands (1.5)*	—	—

*Indicates CLAMS item that must be demonstrated by the child to receive credit.

Appendix VII-E: Relationships of Psychodevelopmental Theories to Normal Development and Behavioral Problems						
	Theories of Development			Developmental Area		
Age	Freud	Eriksor	Piaget	Language	Motor	Behavioral Problems
Birth–18 mo	Oral	Basic trust vs. mistrust	Sensorimotor	Body actions, crying, naming, pointing (preverbal)	Reflex sitting reaching, grasping, walking	Autism, depression, colic, disorders of attachment, feeding or sleeping problems
18 mo–3 yr	Anal	Autonomy vs. shame, doubt	Symbolic (preoperational)	Sentences; telegraph jargon (output restrictions)	Climbing, running	Separation issues, negativism, fearfulness, constipation, shyness, withdrawal
3–6 yr	Oedipal	Initiative vs. guilt	Intuition (preoperational)	Connective words, can be readily understood (differentiation)	Increased coordination; tricycle, jumping	Enuresis, encopresis, anxiety, aggressive acting out, phobias, nightmares
6–11 yr	Latency	Industry vs. inferiority	Concrete operational	Subordinate sentences, reading and writing, language reasoning	Increased skills; sports, recreational cooperative games	School phobias, obsessive reactions, conversion reactions, depressive equivalents
12–17 yr	Adolescence (genital)	Identity vs. role confusion	Formal operational (abstract)	Abstract reasoning, using language, abstract manipulation	Refinement of skills	Delinquency, promiscuity, schizophrenia, anorexia nervosa, suicide

Appendix VIII: Preventive Pediatric Health Care

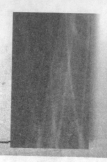

Appendix VIII-A: Recommendations for Preventive Pediatric Health Care

Each child and family is unique; therefore, these recommendations are designed for the care of children who are receiving competent parenting, have no manifestations of any important health problems, and are growing and developing in satisfactory fashion. Additional visits may become necessary if circumstances suggest variations from normal.

These guidelines represent a consensus by the Committee on Practice and Ambulatory Medicine in consultation with national committees and sections of the American Academy of Pediatrics. The Committee emphasizes the great importance of continuity of care in comprehensive health supervision and the need to avoid fragmentation of care.

AGE[1]	Prenatal[1]	Newborn[2]	2-4 d[3]	By 1 mo	2 mo	4 mo	6 mo	9 mo	12 mo	15 mo	18 mo	24 mo	3 yr	4 yr	5 yr	6 yr	8 yr	10 yr	11 yr	12 yr	13 yr	14 yr	15 yr	16 yr	17 yr	18 yr	19 yr	20 yr	21 yr
Infancy[4]													**Early Childhood[4]**			**Middle Childhood[4]**			**Adolescence[4]**										
HISTORY																													
Initial/interval	•	•	•	•	•	•	•	•	•	•	•	•	•	•	•	•	•	•	•	•	•	•	•	•	•	•	•	•	•
MEASUREMENTS																													
Height and weight		•	•	•	•	•	•	•	•	•	•	•	•	•	•	•	•	•	•	•	•	•	•	•	•	•	•	•	•
Head circumference		•	•	•	•	•	•	•	•	•	•	•																	
Blood pressure													•	•	•	•	•	•	•	•	•	•	•	•	•	•	•	•	•
SENSORY SCREENING																													
Vision	S	S		S	S	S	S	S	S	S	S	S	O[6]	O	O	O	O	O	S	O	S	S	O	S	S	O	S	S	S
Hearing	O[7]	S		S	S	S	S	S	S	S	S	S	O	O	O	O	•	•	•	•	•	•	•	•	•	•	•	•	•
DEVELOPMENTAL/ BEHAVIORAL ASSESSMENT[8]																			•	•	•	•	•	•	•	•	•	•	•
PHYSICAL EXAMINATION[9]	•	•	•	•	•	•	•	•	•	•	•	•	•	•	•	•	•	•	•	•	•	•	•	•	•	•	•	•	•
PROCEDURES—GENERAL[10]																													
Hereditary/metabolic screening[11]		←→																											
Immunization[12]		•	•	•	•	•	•	•	•	•	•	•	•	•	•	•	•	•	←————14————→										→
Hematocrit or hemoglobin[13]							→								•	•	•	•	←—————15—————→										
Urinalysis															•	•	•	•											
PROCEDURES—PATIENTS AT RISK																													
Lead screening[16]							→																						
Tuberculin test[17]											•		•	•	•	•	•	•	•	•	•	•	•	•	•	•	•	•	•
Cholesterol screening[18]															•	•	•	•	•	•	•	•	•	•	•	•	•	•	•
STD screening[19]																			•	•	•	•	•	•	•	•	•	•	•
Pelvic examination[20]																									←——20——→				
ANTICIPATORY GUIDANCE[21]	•	•	•	•	•	•	•	•	•	•	•	•	•	•	•	•	•	•	•	•	•	•	•	•	•	•	•	•	•
Injury prevention[22]	•	•	•	•	•	•	•	•	•	•	•	•	•	•	•	•	•	•	•	•	•	•	•	•	•	•	•	•	•
Violence prevention[23]	•	•	•	•	•	•	•	•	•	•	•	•	•	•	•	•	•	•	•	•	•	•	•	•	•	•	•	•	•
Sleep positioning counseling[24]	•	•	•	•	•	•	•																						
Nutrition counseling[25]		•	•	•	•	•	•	•	•	•	•	•	•	•	•	•	•	•	•	•	•	•	•	•	•	•	•	•	•
DENTAL REFERRAL[26]									←—————————																				

Appendix VIII

Key: ● = to be performed; * = to be performed for patients at risk; S = subjective, by history; O = objective, by a standard testing method; ←●→ = the range during which a service may be provided, with the dot indicating the preferred age.

NB: Special chemical, immunologic, and endocrine testing is usually carried out on specific indications. Testing other than newborn (e.g., inborn errors of metabolism, sickle disease) is discretionary with the physician.

The recommendations in this statement do not indicate an exclusive course of treatment or standard of medical care. Variations, taking into account individual circumstances, may be appropriate. Copyright ©1999 by the American Academy of Pediatrics, Committee on Practice and Ambulatory Medicine.

From American Academy of Pediatrics, Committee on Practice and Ambulatory Medicine: Recommendations for preventive pediatric health care. Pediatrics 105:645-646, 2000.

1. A prenatal visit is recommended for parents who are at high risk, for first-time parents, and for those who request a conference. The prenatal visit should include anticipatory guidance, pertinent medical history, and a discussion of benefits of breast-feeding and planned method of feeding per AAP statement "The Prenatal Visit" (1996).

2. Every infant should have a newborn evaluation after birth. Breast-feeding should be encouraged and instruction and support offered. Every breast-feeding infant should have an evaluation 48 to 72 hours after discharge from the hospital to include weight, formal breast-feeding evaluation, encouragement, and instruction as recommended in the AAP statement "Breastfeeding and the Use of Human Milk" (1997).

3. For newborns discharged in less than 48 hours after delivery per AAP statement "Hospital Stay for Healthy Term Newborns" (1995).

4. Developmental, psychosocial, and chronic disease issues for children and adolescents may require frequent counseling and treatment visits separate from preventive care visits.

5. If a child comes under care for the first time at any point on the schedule, or if any items are not accomplished at the suggested age, the schedule should be brought up to date at the earliest possible time.

6. If the patient is uncooperative, rescreen within 6 months.

7. All newborns should be screened per the AAP Task Force on Newborn and Infant Hearing statement "Newborn and Infant Hearing Loss: Detection and Intervention" (1999).

8. By history and appropriate physical examination: if suspicious, by specific objective developmental testing. Parenting skills should be fostered at every visit.

9. At each visit, a complete physical examination is essential, with infant/early unclothed, older child undressed and suitably draped.

10. These may be modified, depending upon entry point into schedule and individual need.

11. Metabolic screening (e.g., thyroid, hemoglobinopathies, phenylketonuria, galactosemia) should be done according to state law.

12. Schedule(s) per the Committee on Infectious Diseases, published annually in the January edition of Pediatrics. Every visit should be an opportunity to update and complete a child's immunizations.

13. See AAP Pediatric Nutrition Handbook (1998) for a discussion of universal and selective screening options. Consider earlier screening for high-risk infants (e.g., premature infants and low birth weight infants). See also "Recommendation to Prevent and Control Iron Deficiency in the United States," MMWR 1998;47(RR-3):1-29.

14. All menstruating adolescents should be screened annually.

15. Conduct dipstick urinalysis for leukocytes annually for sexually active male and female adolescents.

16. For children at risk of lead exposure, consult the AAP statement "Screening for Elevated Blood Levels" (1998). In addition, screening should be done in accordance with state law where applicable.

17. Tuberculosis testing per recommendations of the Committee on Infectious Diseases, published in the current edition of

Red Book: Report of the Committee on Infectious Diseases. Testing should be done upon recognition of high-risk factors.

18. Cholesterol screening for high-risk patients per AAP statement "Cholesterol in Childhood" (1998). If family history cannot be ascertained and other risk factors are present, screening should be at the discretion of the physician.

19. All sexually active patients should be screened for sexually transmitted diseases (STDs).

20. All sexually active female patients should have a pelvic examination. A pelvic examination and routine Pap smear should be offered as part of preventive health maintenance between the ages of 18 and 21 years.

21. Age-appropriate discussion and counseling should be an integral part of each visit for care per the AAP *Guidelines for Health Supervision III* (1998).

22. From birth to age 12, refer to the AAP injury prevention program (TIPP) as described in *A Guide to Safety Counseling in Office Practice* (1994).

23. Violence prevention and management for all patients per AAP statement "The Role of the Pediatrician in Youth Violence Prevention in Clinical Practice and at the Community Level" (1999).

24. Parents and caregivers should be advised to place healthy infants on their backs when putting them to sleep. Side positioning is a reasonable alternative but carries a slightly higher risk of SIDS. Consult the AAP statement "Positioning and Sudden Infant Death Syndrome (SIDS): Update" (1996).

25. Age-appropriate nutrition counseling should be an integral part of each visit per the AAP *Handbook of Nutrition* (1998).

26. Earlier initial dental examinations may be appropriate for some children. Subsequent examinations as prescribed by dentist.

Appendix VIII-B: Recommended Childhood and Adolescent Immunization Schedule, United States

Vaccine	Birth	1 mo	2 mo	4 mo	6 mo	12 mo	15 mo	18 mo	24 mo	4-6 yr	11-12 yr	13-14 yr	15 yr	16-18 yr
Hepatitis B [1]	HepB	HepB		HepB[1]			HepB				HepB series			
Diphtheria, tetanus; pertussis [2]			DTaP	DTaP	DTaP		DTaP	DTaP		DTaP	Tdap	Tdap		Tdap
Haemophilus influenzae type b [3]			Hib	Hib	Hib[3]	Hib								
Inactivated poliovirus [4]			IPV	IPV	IPV		IPV			IPV				
Measles, mumps, rubella [4]						MMR				MMR	MMR			
Varicella [5]							Varicella				Varicella			
Meningococcal [6]									MPSV4		MCV4		MCV4	
Pneumococcal [7]			PCV	PCV	PCV	PCV			PCV		PPV			
Influenza [8]						Influenza (yearly)				Influenza (yearly)				
Hepatitis A [9]											HepA series			
Human papillomavirus [10]														

Range of recommended ages

■ Catch-up immunization

■ 11 to 12-year-old assessment

- - - Vaccines within broken line are for selected populations

Any dose not administered at the recommended age should be administered at any subsequent visit, when indicated and feasible. ■ Indicates age groups that warrant special effort to administer those vaccines not previously administered. Additional vaccines might be licensed and recommended during the year. Licensed combination vaccines may be used whenever any components of the combination are indicated and other components of the vaccine are not contraindicated and if approved by the Food and Drug Administration for that dose of the series. Providers should consult the respective Advisory Committee on Immunization Practices (ACIP) statement for detailed recommendations. Clinically significant adverse events that follow immunization should be reported through the Vaccine Adverse Event Reporting System (VAERS). Guidance about how to obtain and complete a VAERS form is available at http://www.vaers.hhs.gov or by telephone, 800-822-7967.

1. **Hepatitis B vaccine (HepB). AT BIRTH:** All newborns should receive monovalent HepB soon after birth and before hospital discharge. **Infants born to mothers who are hepatitis B surface antigen (HBsAg)-positive** should receive HepB and 0.5 mL of hepatitis B immune globulin (HBIG) within 12 hours of birth. **Infants born to mothers whose HBsAg status is unknown** should receive HepB within 12 hours of birth. The mother should have blood drawn as soon as possible to determine her HBsAg status; if HBsAg-positive, the infant should receive HBIG as soon as possible (no later than age 1 week). **For infants born to HBsAg-negative mothers,** the birth dose can be delayed in rare circumstances, but only if a physician's order to withhold the vaccine and a copy of the infant's original HBsAg-negative laboratory report are documented in the infant's medical record. **FOLLOWING THE BIRTH DOSE:** The HepB series should be completed with either monovalent HepB or a combination vaccine containing HepB. The second dose should be administered at age 1–2 months. The final dose should be administered at age ≥24 weeks. It is permissible to administer four doses of HepB (e.g., when combination vaccines are given after the birth dose); however, if monovalent HepB is used, a dose at age 4 months is not needed. **Infants born to HBsAg-positive mothers** should be tested for HbsAg and antibody to HbsAg after completion of the HepB series, at age 9–18 months (generally at the next well-child visit after completion of the vaccine series).

2. **Diphtheria and tetanus toxoids and acellular pertussis vaccine (DTaP).** The fourth dose of DTaP may be administered as early as age 12 months, provided 6 months have elapsed since the third dose and the child is unlikely to return at age 15–18 months. The final dose in the series should be administered at age ≥4 years. **Tetanus toxoid, reduced diphtheria toxoid, and acellular pertussis vaccine (Tdap adolescent preparation)** is recommended at age 11–12 years for those who have completed the recommended childhood DTP/DTaP vaccination series and have not received a Td booster dose. Adolescents aged 13–18 years who missed the age 11–12-year Td/Tdap booster dose should also receive a single dose of Tdap if they have completed the recommended childhood DTP/DTaP vaccination series. **Subsequent Td** boosters are recommended every 10 years.

3. **Haemophilus influenzae type b conjugate vaccine (Hib).** Three Hib conjugate vaccines are licensed for infant use. If PRP-OMP (PedvaxHIB or ComVax [Merk]) is administered at ages 2 and 4 months, a dose at age 6 months is not required. DTaP/Hib combination products should not be used for primary immunization in infants at ages 2, 4, or 6 months but may be used as boosters after any Hib vaccine. The final dose in the series should be administered at age ≥12 months.

4. **Measles, mumps, and rubella vaccine (MMR).** The second dose of MMR is recommended routinely at age 4–6 years but may be administered during any visit, provided at least 4 weeks have elapsed since the first dose and both doses are administered at or after age 12 months. Those who have not previously received the second dose should complete the schedule by age 11–12 years.

5. **Varicella vaccine.** Varicella vaccine is recommended at any visit at or after age 12 months for susceptible children (i.e., those who lack a reliable history of chickenpox). Susceptible persons aged ≥13 years should receive two doses administered at least 4 weeks apart.

6. **Meningococcal vaccine (MCV4).** Meningococcal conjugate vaccine (MCV4) should be administered to all children at the 11–12-year-old visit as well as to unvaccinated adolescents at high school entry (15 years of age). Other adolescents who wish to decrease their risk for meningococcal disease may also be vaccinated. All college freshmen living in dormitories should also be vaccinated, preferably with MCV4, although **meningococcal polysaccharide vaccine (MPSV4)** is an acceptable alternative. Vaccination against invasive meningococcal disease is recommended for children and adolescents aged ≥2 years with terminal complement deficiencies or anatomic or functional asplenia and for certain other high risk groups (see *MMWR* 2005;54[RR-7]); use MPSV4 for children aged 2–10 years and MCV4 for older children, although MPSV4 is an acceptable alternative.

Continued

7. **Pneumococcal vaccine.** The heptavalent **pneumococcal conjugate vaccine (PCV)** is recommended for all children aged 2-23 months and for certain children aged 24-59 months. The final dose in the series should be administered at age ≥12 months. **Pneumococcal polysaccharide vaccine (PPV)** is recommended in addition to PCV for certain high-risk groups (see *MMWR* 2000;49[RR-9];1-35).

8. **Influenza vaccine.** Influenza vaccine is recommended annually for children aged ≥6 months with certain risk factors (including, but not limited to, asthma, cardiac disease, sickle cell disease, human immunodeficiency virus infection, diabetes, and conditions that can compromise respiratory function or handling of respiratory secretions or that can increase the risk for aspiration), health care workers, and other persons (including household members) in close contact with persons in groups at high risk (see *MMWR* 2005;54[RR-8];1-55). In addition, healthy children aged 6-23 months and close contacts of healthy children aged 0-5 months are recommended to receive influenza vaccine because children in this age group are at substantially increased risk for influenza-related hospitalizations. For healthy persons aged 5-49 years, the intranasally administered, live, attenuated influenza vaccine (LAIV) is an acceptable alternative to the intramuscular trivalent inactivated influenza vaccine (TIV) (see *MMWR* 2005;54[RR-8];1-55). Children receiving TIV should be administered a dosage appropriate for their age (0.25 mL if aged 6-35 months or 0.5 mL if aged ≥3 years). Children aged ≤8 years who are receiving influenza vaccine for the first time should receive two doses (separated by at least 4 weeks for TIV and at least 6 weeks for LAIV).

9. **Hepatitis A vaccine (HepA).** HepA is recommended for all children at age 1 year (i.e., 12-23 months). The two doses in the series should be administered at least 6 months apart. States, countries, and communities with existing HepA vaccination programs for children aged 2-18 years are encouraged to maintain these programs. In these areas, new efforts focused on routine vaccination of 1-year-old children should enhance, not replace, ongoing programs directed at a broader population of children. HepA is also recommended for certain high-risk groups (see *MMWR* 1999;48[RR-12];1-37).

10. Quadrivalent human papillomavirus (types 6, 11, 16, 18) recombinant vaccine (Gardasil) should be given to all girls at age 11-12 and to all females aged 13-26 who have not been previously vaccinated. The vaccine is indicated for the prevention of cervical cancer and genital warts caused by the human papilloma virus (HPV) types 6, 11, 16, or 18. Gardasil is an intramuscular injection for administration to the thigh or upper arm. The schedule consists of three 0.5-mL doses, with the second dose given 2 months after the first, and the final dose administered 6 months after the initial dose.

Modified from Centers for Disease Control and Prevention: Recommended childhood and adolescent immunizaton schedule—United States, 2006. MMWR Morb Mortal Wkly Rep 54(52):Q1-Q4, 2006.

Appendix VIII-C: Catch-up Childhood and Adolescence Immunization Schedules; United States

CATCH-UP SCHEDULE FOR CHILDREN AGED 4 MONTHS TO 6 YEARS

Vaccine	Minimum age for dose 1	Minimum Interval between Doses			
		Dose 1 to Dose 2	Dose 2 to Dose 3	Dose 3 to Dose 4	Dose 4 to Dose 5
Diphtheria, tetanus, pertussis	6 wk	4 wk	4 wk	6 mo	6 mo[1]
Inactivated poliovirus	6 wk	4 wk	4 wk	4 wk[2]	
Hepatitis B[3]	Birth	4 wk	8 wk (and 1E wk after first dose)		
Measles, mumps, rubella	12 mo	4 wk			
Varicella	12 mo				
Haemophilus influenza type b[5]	6 wk	4 wk: if first dose administered at age <12 mo 8 wk (as final dose): if first dose administered at age 12–14 mo No further doses needed if first dose administered at age ≥15 mo	4 wk6: if current age <12 mo 8 wk (as final dose)6: if current age ≥12 mo and second dose administered at age <-5 mo No further doses needed if previous dose administered at age ≥15 mo	8 wk (as final dose): This dose necessary only for child en aged 12 mo–5 yr who received 3 doses before age 12 mo	

Continued

Appendix VIII-C: Catch-up Childhood and Adolescence Immunization Schedules; United States—cont'd

Vaccine	Minimum age for dose 1	Minimum Interval between Doses			
		Dose 1 to Dose 2	Dose 2 to Dose 3	Dose 3 to Dose 4	Dose 4 to Dose 5
Pneumococcal[7]	6 wk	4 wk: if first dose administered at age 12 mo and current age <24 mo 8 wk (as final dose); if first dose administered at age ≥12 mo or current age 24–59 mo No further doses needed for healthy children if first dose administered at age ≥24 mo	4 wk: if current age <12 mo; if 8 wk (as final dose); if current age ≥12 mo No further doses needed for healthy children if previous dose administered at age ≥24 mo	8 wk (as final dose): This dose necessary only for children aged 12 mo–5 yr who received 3 doses before age 12 mo	

1. **DTaP.** The fifth dose is not necessary if the fourth dose was administered after the fourth birthday.
2. **IPV.** For children who received an all-IPV or all-oral poliovirus (OPV) series, a fourth dose is not necessary if the third dose was administered at age ≥4 years. If both OPV and IPV were administered as part of a series, a total of 4 doses should be administered, regardless of the child's current age.
3. **HepB.** Administer the 3-dose series to all persons aged <19 years if they were not previously vaccinated.
4. **MMR.** The second dose of MMR is recommended routinely at age 4-6 years but may be administered earlier if desired.
5. **Hib.** Vaccine not generally recommended for children ages ≥5 years.
6. **Hib.** If current age is >12 months and the first 2 doses were **PRP-OMP** (PedvaxHIB or ComVax [Merck]), the third (and final) dose should be administered at age 12-15 months and at least 8 weeks after the second dose.
7. **PCV.** Vaccine is not generally recommended for children aged ≥5 years.

CATCH-UP SCHEDULE FOR CHILDREN AGED 7 TO 18 YEARS

Vaccine	Minimum Interval between Doses		
	Dose 1 to Dose 2	Dose 2 to Dose 3	Dose 3 to Booster Dose
Tetanus, diphtheria[1]	4 wk	6 mo	6 mo: if first dose administered at age <12 mo and current age <11 yr, otherwise 5 yr
Inactivated poliovirus[3]	4 wk	4 wk	IPV[2,3]
Hepatitis B	4 wk	8 wk (and 16 wk after first dose)	
Measles, mumps, rubella	4 wk		
Varicella[4]	4 wk		

1. **Td.** Tdap adolescent preparation may be substituted for any dose in a primary catch-up series or as a booster if age appropriate for Tdap. A 5-year interval from the last Td dose is encouraged when Tdap is used as a booster dose.
2. **IPV.** For children who received an all-IPV or all-oral poliovirus (OPV) series, a fourth dose is not necessary if the third dose was administered at age ≥4 years. If both OPV and IPV were administered as part of a series, a total of 4 doses should be administered, regardless of the child's current age.
3. **IPV.** Vaccine is not generally recommended for persons aged ≥18 years.
4. **Varicella.** Administer the 2-dose series to all susceptible adolescents aged ≥13 years.

Modified from Centers for Disease Control and Prevention: Recommended childhood and adolescent immunization schedule—United States, 2006. MMWR Morb Mortal Wkly Rep 54(52):Q1–Q4, 2006.

Appendix IX: Guidelines for Pediatric Resuscitation

Appendix IX-A: Overview, Quick Calculations

1. Rapid weight calculation (kg): 50th percentile for patients ≤10 years of age: 9 + (2 × age)
2. Lower limit systolic blood pressure: 70 + (2 × age)
3. Endotracheal tube (ETT)
   Size: 4 + (age/4) = internal diameter of tube = size of ETT (mm)
   Distance to insert ETT (mm) = 3× internal diameter
   Uncuffed tube until age 8 years (cricoid cartilage narrowest part of airway)
   Cuffed tube after age 8 years (vocal cords narrowest part of airway)
   Recommended laryngoscope selection
   Premature infants: Miller 0
   Infants: Miller 1
   Older children: Miller 2
   After 8 years of age: Straight (Miller) or curved (Macintosh) blade, size 2 or 3
4. Broselow tape (if available): Placed head-to-toe along a patient, Broselow tape is color-coded, with each color bar indicating approximate weight, equipment sizes, and medication doses as well as infusion rates for a child of that size.

Appendix IX-B: Basic Cardiopulmonary Resuscitation (CPR)

1. CPR is an attempt to provide blood flow to the vital organs while efforts to restore spontaneous circulation are underway.
2. CPR is believed to work through direct chest compression of the heart between the vertebral column and the anterior chest wall, or through changes in intrathoracic pressure associated with compression and relaxation of the chest wall.
3. Proper chest compressions require exerting enough force to push child's chest to one third to one half of the depth of the chest. Properly performed CPR probably provides about one third of the normal cardiac output.

INFANT CPR (<1 YEAR OF AGE)

1. Ensure or establish a patent airway.
2. Ventilate by bag-valve-mask or endotracheal tube.

832

3. Check for pulses at the brachial artery (mid, medial humerus) or femoral artery (inguinal fold). If absent, begin chest compressions.
4. Infant chest compressions:

   Infant should be on a hard surface.

   Chest compressions are performed with two thumbs over the lower half of the sternum approximately one fingerbreadth below the nipple line and with hands encircling the chest. This is preferred over compression with two fingers (ring and middle) over the sternum.

   Depth of compression is one third to one half of the depth of child's chest (corresponds to 0.5 to 1 inch).

   Compression rate is at least 100 per minute (count: 1, 2, 3...).

   Five compressions for one ventilation.

CHILD CPR (1 TO 8 YEARS OF AGE)

1. Ensure or establish a patent airway.
2. Ventilate by bag-valve-mask or endotracheal tube.
3. Check for pulse at the carotid artery lateral to the thyroid cartilage on either side of the neck. If absent, begin chest compression.
4. Child chest compressions:

   Child should be placed on a firm surface.

   In the child 1 to 8 years of age, compressions are applied midway between the xiphoid notch and the nipple line, with care to avoid the xiphoid process.

   Depth of compression is one third to one half of the depth of child's chest (corresponds to 1 to 1.5 inch).

   One hand is used to compress the lower half of the sternum.

Drug	Dose (IV) (mg/kg)	Comments
Adjuncts (First)		
Atropine (vagolytic)	0.01-0.02 Min: 0.1 mg Max: 1 mg	Prevents bradycardia and reduces oral secretions, may increase HR
Lidocaine (optional anesthetic)	1-2	Blunts ICP spike, cough reflex, and CV effects of intubation; controls ventricular dysrhythmias
Sedative/Hypnotic (Second)		
Thiopental	1-7	May cause hypotension; myocardial depression (barbiturate); decreases ICP and cerebral blood flow; use low dose in hypovolemia (1-2 mg/kg); may increase oral secretions, cause bronchospasm and laryngospasm; contraindicated in status asthmaticus
or		
Ketamine	1-4	May increase ICP, BP, HR, and oral secretions; (general anesthetic); causes bronchodilation, emergence delirium; give with atropine; contraindicated in eye injuries
or		
Midazolam (benzodiazepine)	0.05-0.1	May cause decreased BP and HR and respiratory depression; amnestic properties; benzodiazepines reversible with flumazenil (seizure warning applies)
or		
Fentanyl (opiate)	2-5 μg/kg	Fewest hemodynamic effects of all opiates; chest wall rigidity with high dose or rapid administration; opiates reversible with naloxone (seizure warning applies); do not use with MAO inhibitors

Paralytics (third)*

Rocuronium	0.6-1.2	Onset 30-60 sec, duration 30-60 min; coadministration with sedative; may reverse in 30 min with atropine and neostigmine; minimal effect on HR or BP; precipitates when in contact with other drugs, so flush line before and after use
or Pancuronium	0.1-0.2	Onset 70-120 sec, duration 45-90 min; contraindicated in renal failure, tricyclic antidepressant use; may reverse in 45 min with atropine and neostigmine
or Vecuronium	0.1-0.2	Onset 70-120 sec, duration 30-90 min; minimal effect on BP or HR; may reverse in 30-45 min with atropine and edrophonium
or Succinylcholine	1-2	Onset 30-60 sec, duration 3-10 min; increases ICP, irreversible; contraindicated in burns, massive trauma, neuromuscular disease, eye injuries, malignant hyperthermia, and pseudocholinesterase deficiency *Risk:* lethal hyperkalemia in undiagnosed muscular dystrophy

*Nondepolarizing neuromuscular blockers, except succinylcholine, which is depolarizing.
BP, blood pressure; CV, cardiovascular; HR, heart rate; ICP, intracranial pressure; MAO, monoamine oxidase.

Appendix IX-D: Medication/Treatment Protocols in Emergencies

Asthma/croup

Epinephrine: (1:1000) 0.01 mL/kg SQ q20min ×3 (max. 0.3 mL/dose)
Terbutaline: 0.01 mg/kg SQ (max. 0.5 mg); Drips: 10 µg/kg over 10 min load; increase as necessary by 0.2 µg/kg/min up to 3-6 µg/kg/min

Metaproterenol (Alupent) 5%:
0.01-0.02 mL/kg to max. 1 mL ⎫
Albuterol (Ventolin) 0.5%: ⎬ Nebulized in NS to 3 mL q20-30min, ×3, monitor HR
0.01-0.03 mL/kg to max. 1 mL ⎭

Aminophylline: Load 5-7 mg/kg over 20 min IV

Drip: <1 year [(age in wk × 0.2) + 5] mg/kg/24 hr

>1 year 0.9-1.1 mg/kg/hr

>9 year 0.6-0.7 mg/kg/hr

Methylprednisolone (Solumedrol): 1-2 mg/kg/dose q6h
Racemic epinephrine: 0.25-0.50 mL in 2.5-4.0 mL NS aerosol

Analgesia

Ketamine: 1-2 mg/kg IV over 60 sec or 4-5 mg/kg IM
Meperidine (Demerol): 1 mg/kg/dose IV IM q3-4h
Midazolam (Versed): 0.05 mg/kg IV; 0.2-0.5 mg/kg intranasally
Morphine: 0.1 mg/kg/dose IM, IV, SQ q2-4h

Seizures/increased intracranial pressure

Phenobarbital: 10-20 mg/kg IV load, max. load 30-40 mg/kg
Phenytoin (Dilantin): 10-20 mg/kg IV load (in NS), rate of infusion <0.1 mL/kg/min
Paraldehyde: 0.3 mL/kg/dose PR mixed 1:1 with mineral oil via glass syringe; 150 mg (0.15 mL)/kg IV; max. dose of 1-2 g/kg during 2-6 hr
Mannitol: 0.25 g/kg IV; may repeat ×1 to max. dose of 7 mL
Dexamethasone (Decadron): 0.5-1.0 mg/kg IV load, follow with 0.25 mg/kg IV q6h
Diazepam (Valium): 0.1-0.3 mg/kg IV, PR q10-15min, up to 1.0 mg/kg
Lorazepam (Ativan): 0.05-0.1 mg/kg IV, IM; max. dose 4 mg; may repeat after 15-20 min

Hypoglycemia (after drawing 3 mL in purple top, on ice for insulin, glucagon, cortisol, and growth hormone)

Dextrose: (D_{10}) 2-5 mL/kg IV, IO or (D_{25}) 2 mL/kg IV, IO
Glucagon: 0.03-0.1 mg/kg IV, IM, SQ (max. 1.0 mg)

Diabetes (diabetic ketoacidosis)

Insulin (regular): 0.05-0.1 U/kg initially; then 0.05-0.3 U/kg/hr IV drip

Hypertensive emergency (check blood pressure yourself ×2 with proper cuff)

Diazoxide: 1-3 mg/kg rapid IV push q5-15min, max. 5 mg/kg
Hydralazine: 0.2-0.6 mg/kg IV, IM q4-6h
Nifedipine: 0.25-0.5 mg/kg/dose PO, SL q10-15min, max. 10 mg ×3
Nitroprusside: start at 1.0 µg/kg/min, then titrate.

Intravenous fluids

Load: NS or LR 20 mL/kg, or albumin 5% or Plasmanate 10 mL/kg

Maintenance: 1st 10 kg 100 mL/kg/24 hr
                 2nd 10 kg 50 mL/kg/24 hr; >20 kg 20 mL/kg/24 hr

Parkland burn formula: 4 mL/kg/% burn: $\frac{1}{2}$ 1st 8 hr, $\frac{1}{2}$ next 16 hr
                        If less than maintenance, add to maintenance fluids

Sepsis/meningitis/septic shock

Ampicillin: 100 mg/kg IV load then 100-400 mg/kg/24 hr ÷ q4-6h

Gentamicin: 2.5 mg/kg/dose IV (q12h <7 days, q8h >7 days)

Cefotaxime: 50 mg/kg IV, then 75-150 mg/kg/day ÷ q6h

Ceftriaxone: 75 mg/kg IV load then 100 mg/kg/24 hr ÷ q12h

Dexamethasone: 0.15 mg/kg before antibiotics then q6h × 4 days
(bacterial meningitis)

Blood products

10 mL/kg RBCs will raise hematocrit 5%

0.1 U/kg platelets will raise platelet count 25,000/mm^3

1 U/kg of factor VIII concentrate will raise level 2%

Hyperkalemia (K^+ >7 or ECG changes)

Kayexalate: 1-2 g/kg/day PO, PR ÷ q6h (use alone in mild cases with no
ECG changes) $NaHCO_3$: 1 mEq/kg IV (add in moderate cases,
i.e., peaked T waves)

Calcium gluconate 10%: 0.5 mL/kg IV over 3 min (max. 10 mL)
(for severe cases, i.e., absent P waves, wide QRS, arrhythmias)

16 mL $D_{25}W$ + 1 unit regular insulin to be given at 1 mL/kg

Hyponatremia

3% NaCl: 6-12 mL/kg will raise serum Na^+ 5-10 mEq/L

Na^+ deficit = (Na^+ desired − Na^+ observed) × 0.6 × wt (kg)

Volume of 3% NaCl to correct = 2 × Na^+ deficit

Give $\frac{1}{3}$ over 1st hr if symptomatic

Miscellaneous/ingestions

Diphenhydramine (Benadryl): For anaphylaxis or phenothiazine OD
1-2 mg/kg IV (max. 300 mg/day)

Ipecac: 9 mo-1 yr: 10 mL; 1-12 yr: 15 mL; >12 yr: 30 mL with 4-6 oz clear
fluid, repeat ×1 after 30 min

Charcoal: 1 g/kg with cathartic (Mg citrate 2-4 mL/kg or Mg sulfate
250 mg/kg) mixed in a slurry

Heparin: 100 U/kg IV bolus followed by 10-25 U/kg/hr as infusion or
100 U/kg/dose IV q4h

Drug/Intervention	First or Loading Dose	Route	Comments
Adenosine	0.1 mg/kg	IV/IO	Repeat dose: 37.5-50 µg/kg q1-2min up to 3× (max 12 mg); or 0.2 mg/kg rapid flush to central circulation; SVT
Amiodarone	5 mg/kg	IV/IO	Maximum single dose 0.5 mg in child and 1 mg in adolescents; may repeat once; SVT; unstable VT and VF
Atropine	0.02 mg/kg	IV/IC/ETT	Minimum 0.1 mg/dose (max 0.4 mg/kg or 2 mg); bradycardia
Bretylium	5 mg/kg	IV (slowly)	May increase to 10 mg/kg if defibrillation unsuccessful
Lidocaine	1 mg/kg	IV/IO/ETT	Drip: 20-50 µg/kg/min; wide-complex tachycardia
Procainamide (100 and 500 mg/mL)	15 mg/kg	IV/IO	Load over 30-60 min; drip: 20-80 g/kg/min; SVT, VT
Cardioversion	0.5 J/kg		Double energy for subsequent attempts, up to 4 J/kg; SVT or VT (with pulses) accompanied by poor perfusion, hypotension, or heart failure
Defibrillation	2 J/kg		4 J/kg for subsequent attempts
Automatic external defibrillator	150-200 J		For children >8 yr of age; VF/pulseless VT

ETT, endotracheal tube; IC, intracardiac; IO, intraosseous; IV, intravenous; SVT, supraventricular tachycardia; VF, ventricular fibrillation; VT, ventricular tachycardia.

Drug	First or Loading Dose	Route	Comments
Epinephrine	0.01 mg/kg IV 0.1 mg/kg ETT	IV/IO/ETT	Repeat the same dose every 3 to 5 min during cardiopulmonary resuscitation; drip: 0.1-1 μg/kg/min; asystole, bradycardia
Calcium chloride 10% (= 100 mg/mL or 27.2 mg/mL elemental Ca)	20 mg/kg (0.2 mL/kg of 10% solution)	IV	Give slowly
Glucose	0.5-1 g/kg	IV/IO	1-2 mL/kg 50%; 2-4 mL/kg 25%; 5-10 mL/kg 10%
Magnesium sulfate (500 mg/mL)	20-50 mg/kg	IV/IO	Max. 2 g/dose; rapid infusion for torsades de pointes VT or hypomagnesemia; asthma treatment, 10- to 20-min infusion
Sodium bicarbonate	1 mEq/kg/dose	IV/IO	Infuse slowly and only if ventilation is adequate
Digoxin (digitalize)	20-40 μg/kg	IV	IM load (½ initially, ¼ every 8 hr ×2) then ¼ of loading dose daily + twice daily Oral dose: 2 mg/kg
Furosemide (Lasix)	1 mg/kg	IV/IM	
Naloxone	≤5 yr or ≤20 kg: 0.1 mg/kg ≥5 yr or ≥20 kg: 2.0 mg	IV/IO	For opiate overdose; use small repeated doses (0.01-0.03 mg/kg) titrated to desired effect; for total reversal of narcotic effect Max. 1 mg for infant, 10 mg for children
Propranolol	0.1 mg/kg	IV	To maintain PDA in infants with critical aortic stenosis
Prostaglandin E₁	0.05-0.1 μg/kg/min	IV	Drip: 0.01-0.05 μg/kg/min; maintains PDA in infants with cyanotic congenital heart disease; causes apnea and hypotension
Verapamil	0.1-0.3 mg/kg/dose	IV	Over 2 min, may repeat every 30 min (avoid if age <3 yr or concurrent use of beta blockers)

ETT, endotracheal tube; IM, intramuscular; IO, intraosseous; IV, intravenous; PDA, patent ductus arteriosus.

Appendix IX-G: Medications to Maintain Cardiac Output: Drips

Rules of Drips:
1. (15 mg × pt wt in kg) in 250 mL distillate; 1 mL/hr = 1 µg/kg/min
2. (1.5 mg × pt wt in kg) in 250 mL distillate; 1 mL/hr = 0.1 µg/kg/min
3. (0.15 mg × pt wt in kg) in 250 mL distillate; 1 mL/hr = 0.01 µg/kg/min

Drug	First or Loading Dose	Route	Comments
Dobutamine hydrochloride	2-20 µg/kg/min	IV	α-Adrenergic action predominates at higher infusion rates
Dopamine hydrochloride	2-20 µg/kg/min	IV	
Milrinone	50-75 µg/kg	IV	Drip: 0.5-0.75 µg/kg/min; monitor for hypotension during loading dose; consider infusion without loading dose
Norepinephrine	0.1-2 µg/kg/min	IV/IO	
Sodium nitroprusside	1-8 µg/kg/min	IV/IO	Do not mix with normal saline; monitor blood pressure closely

IO, intraosseous; IV, intravenous.

Appendix IX-H: Overview of Resuscitation in the Delivery Room

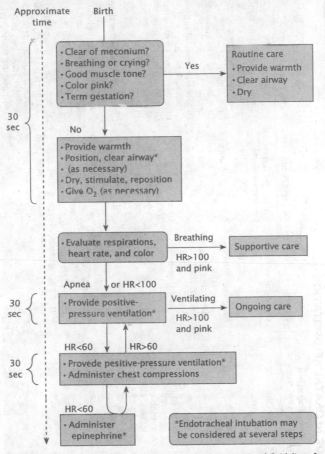

From Niermeyer S, Kattwinkel J, Van Reempts P, et al: International Guidelines for Neonatal Resuscitation: An excerpt from the Guidelines 2000 for Cardiopulmonary Resuscitation and Emergency Cardiovascular Care: International Consensus on Science. Pediatrics 2000;106(3):E29.

MEDICATIONS FOR NEONATAL RESUSCITATION

Medication	Concentration to Administer	Route	Dosage/Prep	Rate/Precautions
Epinephrine *Caution:* Two routes Two dosages	1:10,000	Umbilical vein	0.1-0.3 mL/kg IV Draw up in 1-mL syringe	Give rapidly Follow with a 0.5- to 1-mL flush of normal saline to ensure the drug reaches the blood
	1:10,000	Endotracheal route acceptable while IV access is being established	0.3-1 mL/kg via ETT Draw up in 3-mL or 5-mL syringe	Give rapidly Give directly into endotracheal tube Follow with several positive-pressure breaths
Volume expanders	Normal saline (recommended) Acceptable: Ringer's lactate, O Rh-negative packed RBCs	Umbilical vein	10 mL/kg Draw estimated volume needed into large syringe(s)	Give over 5 to 10 minutes Give by syringe or infusion pump
Sodium bicarbonate	0.5 mEq/mL (4.2% solution)	Large vein with good blood return; usually the umbilical vein	2 mEq/kg/dose Prepare 20-mL prefilled syringe or two 10-mL prefilled syringes	Give slowly, no faster than 1 mEq/kg/min Give only if newborn lungs are being adequately ventilated
Naloxone hydrochloride (Narcan)	1.0 mg/mL	IV route preferred IM route acceptable, but delayed onset of action	0.1 mg/kg Prepare 1 mL of 1.0 mg/mL solution in a 1-mL syringe	Never give by ETT Give rapidly Do not give to newborn of mother suspected of being addicted to narcotics or on methadone maintenance; this may result in the newborn having seizures

ETT, endotracheal tube; IM, intramuscular; IV, intravenous.

Appendix IX-I: After Airway, Breathing, Circulation: Asystole and Pulseless Arrest Decision Tree

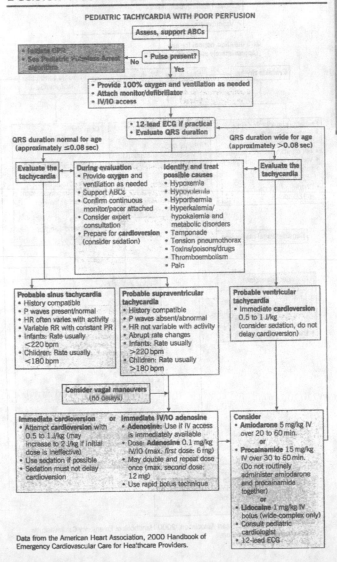

PEDIATRIC TACHYCARDIA WITH POOR PERFUSION

Assess, support ABCs

- **Initiate CPR**
- **See Pediatric Pulseless Arrest algorithm**

← No — **Pulse present?**

Yes ↓

- Provide 100% oxygen and ventilation as needed
- Attach monitor/defibrillator
- IV/IO access

↓

- 12-lead ECG if practical
- Evaluate QRS duration

QRS duration normal for age (approximately ≤0.08 sec) ←→ **QRS duration wide for age (approximately >0.08 sec)**

Evaluate the tachycardia

During evaluation
- Provide oxygen and ventilation as needed
- Support ABCs
- Confirm continuous monitor/pacer attached
- Consider expert consultation
- Prepare for **cardioversion** (consider sedation)

Identify and treat possible causes
- Hypoxemia
- Hypovolemia
- Hypothermia
- Hyperkalemia/hypokalemia and metabolic disorders
- Tamponade
- Tension pneumothorax
- Toxins/poisons/drugs
- Thromboembolism
- Pain

Evaluate the tachycardia

Probable sinus tachycardia
- History compatible
- P waves present/normal
- HR often varies with activity
- Variable RR with constant PR
- Infants: Rate usually <220 bpm
- Children: Rate usually <180 bpm

Probable supraventricular tachycardia
- History compatible
- P waves absent/abnormal
- HR not variable with activity
- Abrupt rate changes
- Infants: Rate usually >220 bpm
- Children: Rate usually >180 bpm

Probable ventricular tachycardia
- Immediate **cardioversion** 0.5 to 1 J/kg (consider sedation, do not delay cardioversion)

Consider vagal maneuvers (no delays)

Immediate cardioversion *or* **Immediate IV/IO adenosine**

Immediate cardioversion
- Attempt **cardioversion** with 0.5 to 1 J/kg (may increase to 2 J/kg if initial dose is ineffective)
- Use sedation if possible
- Sedation must not delay cardioversion

Immediate IV/IO adenosine
- **Adenosine:** Use if IV access is immediately available
- Dose: **Adenosine** 0.1 mg/kg IV/IO (max. *first dose:* 6 mg)
- May double and repeat dose once (max. *second dose:* 12 mg)
- Use rapid bolus technique

Consider
- **Amiodarone** 5 mg/kg IV over 20 to 60 min. *or*
- **Procainamide** 15 mg/kg IV over 30 to 60 min. (Do not routinely administer amiodarone and procainamide together) *or*
- **Lidocaine** 1 mg/kg IV bolus (wide-complex only)
- Consult pediatric cardiologist
- 12-lead ECG

Data from the American Heart Association, 2000 Handbook of Emergency Cardiovascular Care for Healthcare Providers.

PEDIATRIC TACHYCARDIA WITH ADEQUATE PERFUSION

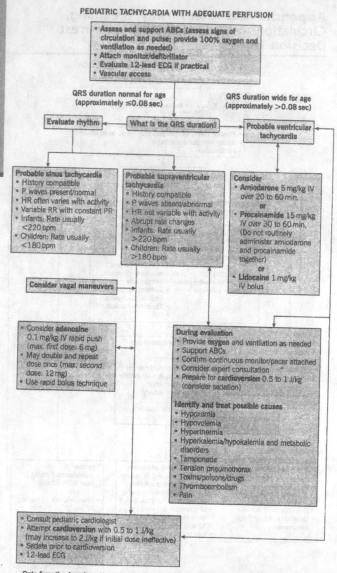

- Assess and support ABCs (assess signs of circulation and pulse; provide 100% oxygen and ventilation as needed)
- Attach monitor/defibrillator
- Evaluate 12-lead ECG if practical
- Vascular access

QRS duration normal for age (approximately ≤0.08 sec)

QRS duration wide for age (approximately >0.08 sec)

Evaluate rhythm ← What is the QRS duration? → Probable ventricular tachycardia

Probable sinus tachycardia
- History compatible
- P waves present/normal
- HR often varies with activity
- Variable RR with constant PR
- Infants: Rate usually <220 bpm
- Children: Rate usually <180 bpm

Probable supraventricular tachycardia
- History compatible
- P waves absent/abnormal
- HR not variable with activity
- Abrupt rate changes
- Infants: Rate usually >220 bpm
- Children: Rate usually >180 bpm

Consider
- Amiodarone 5 mg/kg IV over 20 to 60 min.
  or
- Procainamide 15 mg/kg IV over 30 to 60 min. (Do not routinely administer amiodarone and procainamide together)
  or
- Lidocaine 1 mg/kg IV bolus

Consider vagal maneuvers

- Consider adenosine 0.1 mg/kg IV rapid push (max. first dose: 6 mg)
- May double and repeat dose once (max. second dose: 12 mg)
- Use rapid bolus technique

During evaluation
- Provide oxygen and ventilation as needed
- Support ABCs
- Confirm continuous monitor/pacer attached
- Consider expert consultation
- Prepare for cardioversion 0.5 to 1 J/kg (consider sedation)

Identify and treat possible causes
- Hypoxemia
- Hypovolemia
- Hyperthermia
- Hyperkalemia/hypokalemia and metabolic disorders
- Tamponade
- Tension pneumothorax
- Toxins/poisons/drugs
- Thromboembolism
- Pain

- Consult pediatric cardiologist
- Attempt cardioversion with 0.5 to 1 J/kg (may increase to 2 J/kg if initial dose ineffective)
- Sedate prior to cardioversion
- 12-lead ECG

Data from the American Heart Association, 2000 Handbook of Emergency Cardiovascular Care for Healthcare Providers.

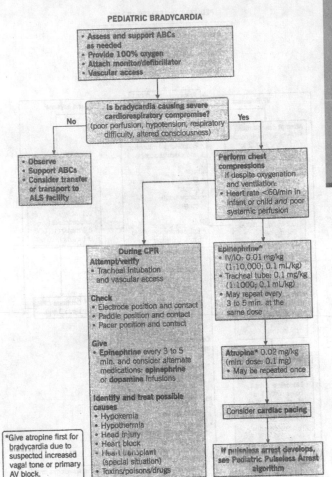

PEDIATRIC BRADYCARDIA

- Assess and support ABCs as needed
- Provide 100% oxygen
- Attach monitor/defibrillator
- Vascular access

Is bradycardia causing severe cardiorespiratory compromise? (poor perfusion, hypotension, respiratory difficulty, altered consciousness)

No

- Observe
- Support ABCs
- Consider transfer or transport to ALS facility

Yes

Perform chest compressions
If despite oxygenation and ventilation:
- Heart rate <60/min in infant or child *and* poor systemic perfusion

During CPR

Attempt/verify
- Tracheal intubation and vascular access

Check
- Electrode position and contact
- Paddle position and contact
- Pacer position and contact

Give
- Epinephrine every 3 to 5 min. and consider alternate medications: epinephrine or dopamine infusions

Identify and treat possible causes
- Hypoxemia
- Hypothermia
- Head injury
- Heart block
- Heart transplant (special situation)
- Toxins/poisons/drugs

Epinephrine**
- IV/IO: 0.01 mg/kg (1:10,000; 0.1 mL/kg)
- Tracheal tube: 0.1 mg/kg (1:1000; 0.1 mL/kg)
- May repeat every 3 to 5 min. at the same dose

Atropine* 0.02 mg/kg (min. dose: 0.1 mg)
- May be repeated once

Consider cardiac pacing

If pulseless arrest develops, see Pediatric Pulseless Arrest algorithm

*Give atropine first for bradycardia due to suspected increased vagal tone or primary AV block.

Data from the American Heart Association, 2000 Handbook of Emergency Cardiovascular Care for Healthcare Providers.

Appendix IX

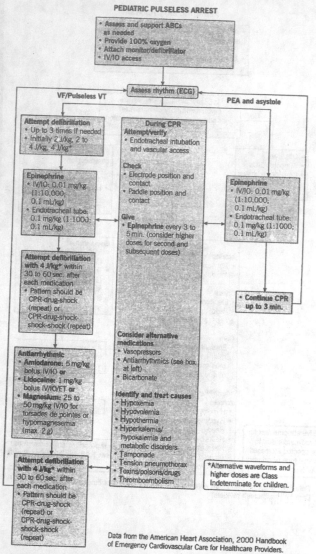

PEDIATRIC PULSELESS ARREST

- Assess and support ABCs as needed
- Provide 100% oxygen
- Attach monitor/defibrillator
- IV/IO access

↓

Assess rhythm (ECG)

VF/Pulseless VT

Attempt defibrillation
- Up to 3 times if needed
- Initially 2 J/kg, 2 to 4 J/kg, 4 J/kg*

Epinephrine
- IV/IO: 0.01 mg/kg (1:10,000; 0.1 mL/kg)
- Endotracheal tube: 0.1 mg/kg (1:1000; 0.1 mL/kg)

Attempt defibrillation with 4 J/kg* within 30 to 60 sec. after each medication
- Pattern should be CPR-drug-shock (repeat) or CPR-drug-shock-shock-shock (repeat)

Antiarrhythmic:
- **Amiodarone:** 5 mg/kg bolus IV/IO
- **Lidocaine:** 1 mg/kg bolus IV/IO/ET or
- **Magnesium:** 25 to 50 mg/kg IV/IO for torsades de pointes or hypomagnesemia (max. 2 g)

Attempt defibrillation with 4 J/kg* within 30 to 60 sec. after each medication
- Pattern should be CPR-drug-shock (repeat) or CPR-drug-shock-shock-shock (repeat)

During CPR
Attempt/verify
- Endotracheal intubation and vascular access

Check
- Electrode position and contact
- Paddle position and contact

Give
- Epinephrine every 3 to 5 min. (consider higher doses for second and subsequent doses)

Consider alternative medications
- Vasopressors
- Antiarrhythmics (see box at left)
- Bicarbonate

Identify and treat causes
- Hypoxemia
- Hypovolemia
- Hypothermia
- Hyperkalemia/hypokalemia and metabolic disorders
- Tamponade
- Tension pneumothorax
- Toxins/poisons/drugs
- Thromboembolism

PEA and asystole

Epinephrine
- IV/IO: 0.01 mg/kg (1:10,000; 0.1 mL/kg)
- Endotracheal tube: 0.1 mg/kg (1:1000; 0.1 mL/kg)

- Continue CPR up to 3 min.

*Alternative waveforms and higher doses are Class Indeterminate for children.

Data from the American Heart Association, 2000 Handbook of Emergency Cardiovascular Care for Healthcare Providers.

SUGGESTED READING

American Heart Association: 2005 Guidelines for Cardiopulmonary Resuscitation and Emergency Cardiovascular Care. Part 12: Pediatric advanced life support. Circulation. 112:IV167-IV187, 2005.

Hazinski MF, Zaritsky AL, Nadkarni VM, et al (eds): PALS Provider Manual. Dallas, American Heart Association, 2002.

Lee PC, Chen SA, Chiang CE, et al: Clinical and electrophysiological characteristics in children with atrioventricular nodal reentrant tachycardia. Pediatr Cardiol 24:6-9, 2003.

Richman PB, Nashed AH: The etiology of cardiac arrest in children and young adults: Special considerations for ED management. Am J Emerg Med 17:264-270, 1999.

Rockney RM, Alario AJ, Lewander WJ: Pediatric advanced life support. Part I: Airway, circulation, and intravascular access. Am Fam Physician 43:1223-1230, 1991.

Rockney RM, Alario AJ, Lewander WJ: Pediatric advanced life support. Part II: Fluid therapy medications and dysrhythmias. Am Fam Physician 43:1712-1720, 1991.

Strange GR, William RA, Lelyveld S, Schafermeyer RW: Pediatric Emergency Medicine: A Comprehensive Study Guide. New York, McGraw-Hill, 2002.

Strasburger JF: Cardiac arrhythmias in childhood. Drugs 42:974-983, 1991.

Index

Note: Page numbers followed by the letter b refer to boxes, those followed by the letter f refer to figures, and those followed by the letter t refer to tables.

Index

Index

Index

Index

Index

Index

Key Telephone Numbers

This is a listing of the phone numbers of departments and individuals in the hospital who might be needed for immediate consultation.

Department

Admitting

Anesthesia

CCU

ECG

EEG

ER

ICU

Information

IV Team

Laboratory

   Chemistry

   Hematology

   Microbiology

   Other

Medical Records

Nuclear Medicine

Paging

Pathology

Pharmacy

Physical Therapy

Pulmonary Function

Radiology

Recovery Room

Respiratory Therapy

Security

Social Service

Sonography

Other

Nursing Stations

_____
_____
_____
_____
_____
_____
_____
_____

House Staff

_____
_____
_____
_____
_____
_____
_____
_____

Attending Staff

_____
_____
_____
_____
_____
_____
_____
_____
_____
_____
_____
_____